Biomechanics of Diarthrodial Joints
Volume I

Van C. Mow Anthony Ratcliffe
Savio L-Y. Woo
Editors

Biomechanics of Diarthrodial Joints

Volume I

In Two Volumes
With 366 Figures

Springer-Verlag
New York Berlin Heidelberg
London Paris Tokyo Hong Kong

Van C. Mow
Orthopaedic Research Laboratory
Departments of Mechanical Engineering
and Orthopaedic Surgery
Columbia University
New York, NY 10032, USA

Anthony Ratcliffe
Orthopaedic Research Laboratory
Department of Orthopaedic Surgery
Columbia College of Physicians
& Surgeons
New York, NY 10032, USA

Savio L-Y. Woo
Division of Orthopaedics
University of California, San Diego
La Jolla, CA 92093, USA

Printed on acid-free paper.

Softcover reprint of the hardcover 1st edition 1990

Camera-ready copy prepared by the authors using LaTex.

9 8 7 6 5 4 3 2 1

ISBN-13:978-1-4612-8015-6 e-ISBN-13:978-1-4612-3448-7
DOI:10.1007/978-1-4612-3448-7

Preface

Historical folklore indicates that Asklepios (circa 900 BC), the first western doctor of ancient Greece, treated many patients with rheumatic diseases of joints[1,2]. Later, Hippocrates (circa 400 BC), who claimed to have learned from Asklepios, used the term arthritis in reference to joint diseases: "When the disease of arthritis strikes, acute inflammation and pain attacks the joints of the body...". Indeed, arthritic joint disease dates much farther back into antiquity than Asklepios. Many modern anthropologists have noted degenerative joint disease in the fossils of Neanderthal man (archanthropus europeus petraloniensis) and even in those of dinosaurs.

More recent scientific studies on joints date back to the work of the great English anatomist Hunter who wrote "The Structure and Diseases of Articular Cartilage" in the Philosophical Transactions of London in 1743. The notion that osteoarthritis results from the wearing away of cartilage was copiously documented by the histological observations of the German physician Ecker in 1843. This idea was further supported by Pommer (1927) who felt that mechanical stresses played important roles in the initiation and propagation of cartilage lesions leading to osteoarthritis. This same conclusion was reached by the assembled distinguished experts at a National Institutes of Health Workshop held in 1986[3].

Biomechanical studies of joint materials such as articular cartilage, ligaments, meniscus and bone began in earnest during the 20th century. Hirsch is largely credited to be the most influential individual in promoting orthopaedic biomechanics research as we know it today. Since then, more recent investigators have led the way to modern biomechanics research in diarthrodial joints. We are indeed pleased that some of these eminent researchers have contributed to these volumes.

In 1969, Leon Sokoloff wrote:

> "The morphological characteristics of the lesions [on the joint surface] allow no serious question that mechanical factors are instrumental in causing the abrasion and reshaping of joint characteristics of osteoarthritis. From the mechanical view, this requires an analysis of the stress acting on the joints, the material properties, and lubrication."[4]

In the past twenty years, a vast amount of research has appeared dealing with these topics. Striking advances have occurred through specialized and interdisciplinary studies on connective tissues from the macroscopic to the molecular level. In these two volumes on diarthrodial joints, we feel we have selected a good representation of topics currently considered to be important areas of research. While the coverage of these volumes is not encyclopaedic, they do include numerous topics on joint function, joint evaluation and joint materials such as articular cartilage, tendon, ligaments, meniscus, bone. However, some topics are not included due to limited space in these volumes and time availability at the First World Congress on Biomechanics.

The First World Congress provided an excellent and timely opportunity to discuss the biomechanics of diarthrodial joints in a comprehensive manner. In 1990, the theories used to model these joint materials are sophisticated and the experimental methods used to determine their properties are complex. These chapters provide a snap-shot of the latest thinking on these topics. The invited contributors are leaders in their fields of specialization and some young investigators have been chosen for the promise of their ideas. We believe these volumes do present many new ideas and theories as we know them today. There are some materials which appear to be contradictory or inconsistent; such is the nature of science. The readers of these volumes will be treated to a wide array of fascinating topics to gain new and refreshing insights into an old subject. These are the objectives of our two volumes on the Biomechanics of Diarthrodial Joints.

Acknowledgements

We wish to thank all the authors for their outstanding contributions to these volumes. We especially wish to thank Dr. Robert J. Foster of the Orthopaedic Research Laboratory of Columbia University for his hard work in the production of these two volumes. We also wish to thank Dr. Zvi Ruder, editor of the engineering series of Springer Verlag, New York, for his encouragement and cooperation in producing these books.

Van C. Mow, Ph.D.
Anthony Ratcliffe, Ph.D.
Columbia University
New York, New York

Savio L-Y. Woo, Ph.D.
University of California, San Diego
La Jolla, California

1. Lyons, AS and Petrucelli, RJ, II: Medicine, An Illustrated History, Harry N. Abrams, Inc, Publishers, New York, 1978.
2. Rigatos, G, Kappou, I, Thouas, RV: The History of Greek Rheumatology, The Hellenic Society of Rheumatology, Publishers, Athens, 1987.
3. Brandt, KD and Mankin, HJ, J Rheum, 13:1127-1160, 1987.
4. Sokoloff, L: The Biology of Degenerative Joint Disease, University of Chicago Press, Chicago and London, 1969.

Contents

Volume I

Part II Cartilage Biomechanics

Volume II

Part III Bone Biomechanics

Contributors

K-N. An Mayo Medical School, Rochester, Minnesota 55905, U.S.A.

S.P. Arnoczky Laboratory for Comparative Orthopaedic Research, The Hospital for Special Surgery, New York, New York 10021, U.S.A.

E. Askari Department of Theoretical and Applied Mechanics, Kimball Hall, Cornell University, Ithaca, New York 14853, U.S.A.

G.A. Ateshian Orthopaedic Research Laboratory, Department of Orthopaedic Surgery, Columbia University, New York, New York 10032, U.S.A.

L. Blankevoort Biomechanics Section, Institute of Orthopaedics, Univeristy of Nijmegen, P.O. Box 9101, 6500 HB, Nijmegen, The Netherlands

R.D. Boyd Bone and Joint Center, Henry Ford Hospital, Detroit, Michigan 48202, U.S.A.

T.D. Brown Department of Orthopaedic Surgery, University of Iowa, Iowa City, Iowa 52242, U.S.A.

D.B. Burr Indiana University, School of Medicine, Department of Anatomy, Medical Science Building, Indianapolis, Indiana 46202-5120, U.S.A.

D.L. Butler University of Cincinnati, Noyes-Giannestras Biomechanics Laboratories, Cincinnati, Ohio 45221-0048, U.S.A.

D.R. Carter Mechanical Engineering Department, Stanford University, Stanford, California 94305-4021, U.S.A.

K.Y. Chern Orthopaedic Research Laboratory, Department of Orthopaedic Surgery, Columbia University, New York, New York 10032, U.S.A.

W.D. Comper Department of Biochemistry, Monash University, Clayton, Vic. 3168, Australia

S.C. COWIN Department of Mechanical Engineering, City College of the City University of New York, New York, New York 10031, U.S.A.

J.D. CURREY Department of Biology, University of York, York, YO1 5DD, England

D. DOWSON Department of Mechanical Engineering, The University of Leeds, Leeds LS2 9JT, West Yorkshire, England

A.E. ENGIN Department of Biomechanics and Mechanics, Department of Engineering Mechanics, The Ohio State University, Columbus, Ohio 43210, U.S.A.

G.A.M. FINERMAN Biomechanics Research Section, Division of Orthopaedic Surgery, University of California at Los Angeles, Los Angeles, California 90024, U.S.A.

D.C. FITHIAN Orthopaedic Research Laboratory, Department of Orthopaedic Surgery, Columbia University, New York, New York 10032, U.S.A.

C.B. FRANK Department of Surgery, Faculty of Medicine, University of Calgary HSC, Calgary, Alberta, Canada T2N 4N1

E.H. FRANK Continuum Electromechanics Group, Department of Electrical Engineering and Computer Science, Massachusetts Institute of Technology, Cambridge, Massachusetts 02139, U.S.A.

D. FYHRIE Bone and Joint Center, Henry Ford Hospital, Detroit, Michigan 48202, U.S.A.

S.A. GOLDSTEIN Biomechanics, Trauma and Sports Medicine Laboratory, Orthopaedic Surgery, The University of Michigan, AnnArbor, Michigan, 48109-0486, U.S.A.

J.F. GOREK Biomechanics Research Section, Division of Orthopaedic Surgery, University of California at Los Angeles, Los Angeles, California 90024, U.S.A.

P.E. GRIMSHAW Continuum Electromechanics Group, Department of Electrical Engineering and Computer Science, Massachusetts Institute of Technology, Cambridge, Massachusetts 02139, U.S.A.

A.J. GRODZINSKY Continuum Electromechanics Group, Department of Electrical Engineering and Computer Science, Massachusetts Institute of Technology, Cambridge, Massachusetts 02139, U.S.A.

Y. GUAN University of Cincinnati, Noyes-Giannestras Biomechanics Laboratories, Cincinnati, Ohio 45221-0048, U.S.A.

D.A. HART Department of Microbiology and Infectious Diseases, Faculty of Medicine, University of Calgary HSC, Calgary, Alberta, Canada T2N 4N1

W.C. HAYES Orthopaedic Biomechanics Laboratory, Department of Orthopaedic Surgery, Charles A. Dana Research Institute, Beth Israel Hospital and Harvard Medical School, Boston, Massachusetts 02215, U.S.A.

S.J. HOLLISTER Biomechanics, Trauma and Sports Medicine Laboratory, Orthopaedic Surgery, The University of Michigan, AnnArbor, Michigan, 48109-0486, U.S.A.

M.H. HOLMES Department of Mathematical Sciences, Rensselaer Polytechnic Institute, Troy, NY 12180-3590, U.S.A.

J.S. HOU Orthopaedic Research Laboratory, Department of Orthopaedic Surgery, Columbia University, New York, New York 10032, U.S.A.

R. HUISKES Biomechanics Section, Institute of Orthopaedics, Univeristy of Nijmegen, P.O. Box 9101, 6500 HB, Nijmegen, The Netherlands

J.T. JENKINS Department of Theoretical and Applied Mechanics, Kimball Hall, Cornell University, Ithaca, New York 14853, U.S.A.

J.M. KABO Biomechanics Research Section, Division of Orthopaedic Surgery, University of California at Los Angeles, Los Angeles, California 90024, U.S.A.

M.A. KELLY Orthopaedic Research Laboratory, Department of Orthopaedic Surgery, Columbia University, New York, New York 10032, U.S.A.

N. KIKUCHI The Department of Mechanical Engineering and Applied Mechanics, The University of Michigan, AnnArbor, Michigan, 48109-0486, U.S.A.

J.L. KUHN Biomechanics, Trauma and Sports Medicine Laboratory, Orthopaedic Surgery, The University of Michigan, AnnArbor, Michigan, 48109-0486, U.S.A.

M.K. KWAN Division of Orthopaedics and Rehabilitation, University of California, San Diego, and Veterans Administration Medical Center, La Jolla, California, 92093, U.S.A.

W.M. Lai Orthopaedic Research Laboratory, Departments of Orthopaedic Surgery and Mechanical Engineering, Columbia University, New York, New York 10032, U.S.A.

D.A. MacKenna Division of Orthopaedics, Univerisity of California, San Diego, San Diego VA Medical Center and M & D Coutts Institute for Joint Reconstruction, La Jolla, California 92093, U.S.A.

A.F.T. Mak Rehabilitation Engineering Centre, Hong Kong Polytechnic, Hung Hom, Kowloon, Hong Kong

K.L. Markolf Biomechanics Research Section, Division of Orthopaedic Surgery, University of California at Los Angeles, Los Angeles, California 90024, U.S.A.

T.A. Maxian Department of Mechanical Engineering, Aeronautical Engineering, and Mechanics, Rensselaer Ploytechnic Institute, Troy, New York 12180-3590, U.S.A.

K.J. McLeod Musculo-Skeletal Research Laboratory, Department of Orthopaedics, Health Sciences Center, State University of New York at Stony Brook, Stony Brook, New York 11794-8181, U.S.A.

B.F. Morrey Mayo Medical School, Rochester, Minnesota 55905, U.S.A.

L. Mosekilde Department of Connective Tissue Biology, Institute of Anatomy, University of Aarhus, DK-8000 Aarhus C, Denmark

V.C. Mow Orthopaedic Research Laboratory, Departments of Orthopaedic Surgery and Mechanical Engineering, Columbia University, New York, New York 10032, U.S.A.

J.J. O'connor Department of Engineering Science, University of Oxford, Oxford OX1 3PJ, England

J.M. Owens Orthopaedic Research Laboratory, Department of Orthopaedic Surgery, Columbia University, New York, New York 10032, U.S.A.

S.L. Phillips Continuum Electromechanics Group, Department of Electrical Engineering and Computer Science, Massachusetts Institute of Technology, Cambridge, Massachusetts 02139, U.S.A.

E.L. Radin Bone and Joint Center, Henry Ford Hospital, Detroit, Michigan 48202, U.S.A.

A. Ratcliffe Orthopaedic Research Laboratory, Department of Orthopaedic Surgery, Columbia University, New York, New York 10032, U.S.A.

V.O. Ribitsch Department of Physical Chemistry, University Graz, A - 8010 Graz, Austria

C.T. Rubin Musculo-Skeletal Research Laboratory, Department of Orthopaedics, Health Sciences Center, State University of New York at Stony Brook, Stony Brook, New York 11794-8181, U.S.A.

M.S. Shapiro Biomechanics Research Section, Division of Orthopaedic Surgery, University of California at Los Angeles, Los Angeles, California 90024, U.S.A.

B.D. Snyder Orthopaedic Biomechanics Laboratory, Department of Orthopaedic Surgery, Charles A. Dana Research Institute, Beth Israel Hospital and Harvard Medical School, Boston, Massachusetts 02215, U.S.A.

L.J. Soslowsky Orthopaedic Research Laboratory, Department of Orthopaedic Surgery, Columbia University, New York, New York 10032, U.S.A.

R.L. Spilker Department of Mechanical Engineering, Aeronautical Engineering, and Mechanics, Rensselaer Ploytechnic Institute, Troy, New York 12180-3590, U.S.A.

J-K. Suh Department of Mechanical Engineering, Aeronautical Engineering, and Mechanics, Rensselaer Ploytechnic Institute, Troy, New York 12180-3590, U.S.A.

P.A. Torzilli Department of Biomechanics, Hospital for Special Surgery, New York, New York 10021, U.S.A.

M.E. Vermilyea Department of Mechanical Engineering, Aeronautical Engineering, and Mechanics, Rensselaer Ploytechnic Institute, Troy, New York 12180-3590, U.S.A.

A. Viidik Department of Connective Tissue Biology, Institute of Anatomy, University of Aarhus, DK-8000 Aarhus C, Denmark

J.A. Weiss Division of Orthopaedics, Univerisity of California, San Diego, San Diego VA Medical Center and M & D Coutts Institute for Joint Reconstruction, La Jolla, California 92093, U.S.A.

M. Wong Rehabilitation R&D Center, Palo Alto, Veterans Affairs Medical Center, Palo Alto, California 94304, U.S.A.

S.L-Y. Woo Division of Orthopaedics, Univerisity of California, San Diego, San Diego VA Medical Center and M & D Coutts Institute for Joint Reconstruction, La Jolla, California 92093, U.S.A.

A. Zavatsky Hertford College, University of Oxford, Department of Engineering Science, Oxford OX1 3PJ, England

W.B. Zhu Orthopaedic Research Laboratory, Department of Orthopaedic Surgery, Columbia University, New York, New York 10032, U.S.A.

ACKNOWLEDGEMENTS FOR PERMISSIONS

Springer-Verlag wishes to thank the publishers and authors listed below for their copyright permission and endorsement to use their previously published figures in this book. Their invaluable help in this matter has made the publication of these volumes possible. The figures and/or pictures listed below are reprinted with permission from the following:

Chapter 2:

Figure 8 reprinted with permission from Raven Press - Journal of Orthopaedic Research; Reproduced with Permission (Matyas; 1990) - Figure 7 from "The Developmental Morphology of a 'Periosteal' Ligament Insertion: Growth and Maturation of the Tibial Insertion of the Rabbit Medial Collateral Ligament" (J.R. Matyas, D. Bodie, M. Anderson, C.B. Frank).

Chapter 3:

Figures 13 and 14 reprinted with permission from Raven Press; from "Knee Ligaments: Structure, Function, Injury and Repair", edited by D. Daniel et al. (1990); Figure 13 from Figure 18-6, in "The Response of Ligaments to Injury: Healing of the Collateral Ligaments" (Woo, et al.; 1990); Figure 14 from Figure 18-8, in "The Response of Ligaments to Injury: Healing of the Collateral Ligaments" (Woo, et al.).

Figures 10, 15 and 16 reprinted with permission from The Journal of Bone and Joint Surgery; Figure 10 from Figure 11, in "The biomechanical and morphological changes in the medial collateral ligament of the rabbit after immobilization and remobilization" (Woo et al.), 69-A, pp. 1200-1211, 1987. Figure 15 from Figure 1, and Figure 16 from Figure 8, in "The quadriceps-anterior cruciate ligament interaction: an In-Vitro kinematic study of the quadriceps stabilized knee" (Shoemaker et al.) - in review for Journal Bone and Joint Surgery.

Chapter 4:

Figure 14 reprinted with permission from J.B. Lippincott Company; from "Veterinary Surgery", Vol. 12, #3, p.117; 1983.

Figure 5 reprinted with permission from Franklin Institute Press; from "Exercise Sports Sciences Reviews".

Figure 1 reprinted with permission from Journal of Bone and Joint Surgery; Vol. 62-A, p. 262, Figure 2 (Butler/Noyes/Grood).

Figure 3 reprinted with permission from Journal of Bone and Joint Surgery; Vol. 64-A, p. 263, Figure 6 (Fukubayashi/Torzilli, et al.).

Figures 4a and 4b reprinted with permission from Journal of Bone and Joint Surgery; Vol. 63-A, p. 1261 (Grood/Noyes/Butler/Suntay).

Figure 7 reprinted with permission from Journal of Bone and Joint Surgery; vol. 63-A, p. 1259, Figure 2 (Grood/Noyes/Butler/Suntay).

Figure 8a reprinted with permission from Journal of Bone and Joint Surgery; Vol. 58-A, p. 1079, Figures 2-A & 2-B (Noyes/Grood).

Figure 8b reprinted with permission from Journal of Bone and Joint Surgery; Vol. 58-A, p. 1079, Figures 2-B, 2-C, 3. (Noyes/Grood).

Figure 16 reprinted with permision from Journal of Orthopaedic Research; Vol. 7, p. 76.; 1989.

Figure 9 reprinted with permission from J.B. Lippincott Company; from "Clinical Orthopaedics and Related Research", Vol. 123, p. 164; 1977.

Figures 6, 12, and 13 reprinted with permission from Journal of Biomechanics; from Figures 6,12 and 13 from "The Journal of Biomechanics", Volume 20, 1987, P.561; Volume 19, 1986, P.427; and Volume 19, 1986, P.429. Pergamon Press, PLC.

Figure 2 reprinted with permission from The Journal of Biomechanical Engineering, Volume 102, P.279.

Chapter 5:

Figures 1,7,8,9,10 reprinted with permission from The Journal of Bone and Joint Surgery, Boston, MA; from Vol. 72A, #4, April 1990 - pp. 557-567 by Markolf/Gork/Cabo/Shapiro - Figures 1,3,2,4,5 respectively.

Chapter 7:

Figure 4 reprinted by permission of the Council of the Institution of Mechanical Engineers from proceedings of the IMECHE; IMECHE 1989, "Exponential Law Representation of Tensile Properties of Human Meniscus", p. 90 Fig. 5. On behalf of the Institution of Mechanical Engineers,

Chapter 8:

Figures 1,3 reprinted with permission from Lea & Febiger, Philadelphia, PA; 1989. From "Basic Biomechanics" ,Figure 2-5, p. 34 and Figure 2-1, p. 32.

Figures 2,6,7 reprinted with permission from Eular Publishers and Pfizer Corp.; Eular Bulletin, Vol. XVII, No.1, pp. 9,11,12 - Figures 1,3,4 ("Molecular Structure"); 1988.

Figure 8 reprinted with permission from Biorheology, Vol. 17, p. 115 Fig. 3, "Drag Induced Compression of Articular Cartilage During Permeature Exp"(Lai/Mow; 1980); Pergamon Press PLC.

Figure 4 reprinted with permission from Raven Press New York - Figure 1.3 from "Fundamentals of Articular Cartilage and Meniscus Biomechanics" (Mow/Fithian/Kelly) from Articular Cartilage and Knee Joint Function: Basic Science and Arthroscopy; 1990.

Figure 1 from Figure 2-5, pg. 34 from Hultkrantz, W.: Ueber die Spaltrichtungen der Gelenkknorpel. Verh. Anat. Ges., 12:248, 1898. In Basic Biomechanics of the Musculoskeletal System, 2nd edition. Edited by M. Nordin and V.J. Frankel. Philadelphia; reprinted with permission from Lea & Febiger, 1989.

Figure 3 from Figure 2-1, pg. 32 from Hultkrantz, W.: Ueber die Spaltrichtungen der Gelenkknorpel. Verh. Anat. Ges., 12:248, 1898. In "Basic Biomechanics of the Musculoskeletal System", 2nd edition. Edited by M. Nordin and V.J. Frankel. Philadelphia; reprinted with permission from Lea & Febiger, 1989.

Chapter 9:

Figure 8 adapted with permission from Journal of Biomechanics from Figures 8 & 9 in Volume 20, #6, pp. 615-627, "Cartilage Electromechanics, Electrokinetic Transduction and The Effects of Electrolyte pH and Ionic Strength" (E.H. Frank, A.J. Grodzinsky; 1987); Pergamon Press PLC.

Figure 6 adapted with permission from Raven Press, Ltd.; from Figures 8b and 9b in "Swelling of Articular Cartilage and Other Connective Tissues: Electromechanochemical Forces" (S.R. Eisenberg, A.J. Grodzinsky) in "Journal of Orthopaedic Research", Volume 3, pages 148-159; 1985.

Chapter 12:

Figures 4, 5, and 6 reprinted with permission from Elsevier Science Publishers; figures 5 and 6 from MS RFS 000142 "Osmotic Flow Caused by Polyelectrolytes" (Williams/Comper); Figure 4 from Figure 2 MS RFS 000141 "Osmotic Flow Caused by Chondroitin Sulfate Proteoglycan Across Well-Defined Nuclepore Membranes" (Comper/Williams).

Part I
Ligaments, Tendons, and Menisci

Chapter 1

Structure and Function of Normal and Healing Tendons and Ligaments

A. Viidik

The structure and function of tendons and ligaments are intimately interrelated. The structural arrangement of these parallel-fibered collagenous tissues is similar to rope-building; from the α chains in the collagen molecule itself up to the level of fibrils the principle is thus helicality that changes handedness on consecutive levels of organization. This arrangement, which is comparable to rope-tightening, renders stability and strength to the tissue - collagen is the strongest protein in the mammalian organism. On higher levels of organization there is "only" planar waviness, which contributes to the properties during the initial part of the stress-strain curve.

A considerable part of the viscoelasticity in these tissues is due to the ground substance with its hydrophilic proteoglycans. Also other structural features contribute to these properties. Interfibrillar sliding and shear between the fibers and/or fibrils and the ground substance takes place during the initial part of the stress-strain curve. At higher strain levels also the polypeptide chains (alpha-helices) show viscoelastic behavior.

One important question regarding the physiological functioning of tendons and ligaments is whether there is a reasonable safety margin between the highest stresses these structures are subjected to normally *in vivo* and their ultimate tensile strengths; here the whole functional units, *i.e.* bone-tendon-muscle-tendon-bone and bone-ligament-bone, must be taken into consideration. The knowledge we have is reached by interpolation from various measurements, which are not from derived the same experimental setup. The safety margin seems, however, to be large.

Another key question is to what extent these structures respond to physical stimuli (training) and lack of such stimuli (immobilization) as well as to hormonal disturbances and the aging process. From what we know it must be concluded that both tendons and ligaments are quite dynamic tissues, which respond metabolically and undergo remodelling.

The mechanical properties of these tissues are highly dependent on their structural integrity, *i.e.* the parallel-fiberedness (with its in this context minor helicality and waviness) and continuity. The healing of a lesion in a ligament or a tendon is, therefore, in relative terms rather slow. The developing scar tissue, with its initial random pattern of fibers, is by necessity much less ideally organized. Although this pattern becomes with time more oriented in the direction of the applied physiological stresses during the maturation and remodelling phases of healing, it is doubtful whether the strength of intact tissues is ever reached. The healing process in soft connective tissues is quite different from callus formation during fracture healing in bone.

It is thus clear that the structure and function of normal and healing ligaments are so intimately interrelated with each other that any biomechanical study in this field should take these relations into account.

Structural organization

Tendons and ligaments are unique in the respect that most of their substance is pure type I collagen. They are, therefore, the tissues of choice for the study of the mechanical properties of this collagen. This study is simplified by the parallel arrangement of fibers in a number of the tendons and ligaments in the mammalian body, while some of them exhibit geometrical "aberrations". This provides us with opportunities to study the interaction between structure and function type I collagen. None of the other collagens nor any of the other connective tissue components is available for study in "pure" form.

This section does not contain an extensive set of references to original research reports, only a few key references and references relevant to the mechanical functioning of the tissues are given. The reader is referred to reviews on this topic, *e.g.* by Bailey & Etherington 1980, Frank *et al.* 1987, Gelbermann *et al.* 1987, Labat-Robert & Robert 1988, Nimni & Harkness 1988, Ruggeri & Benazzo 1984, Viidik 1973, 1978, 1979a, 1980b, Viidik *et al.* 1982.

Tissue components

Connective tissues consist of cells and an extracellular matrix, where fibrillar structures are embedded into a ground substance. While the cells perform the important functions in most other tissues, in tendons and ligaments, which have mechanical functioning as their main task, this role is vested in the fibrillar structures of the extracellular matrix. The cells do the "house-keeping" in these tissues.

Type I collagen molecule is the predominant building unit in tendons and ligaments. There are, however, a number of other tissue components present, They contribute to those properties, which are important for the physiological *in vivo* functioning, while their importance for the strength of these tissues is minimal.

The collagens

While collagen up to the middle of the 1970s was considered to be one molecule, it has developed to become a whole family of molecules. There are now two major groups, the fiber-forming collagens and the "other" collagens, which do not form regular fibers.

The fiber-forming collagens are type I (in tendons, ligaments, muscle, skin, blood vessel walls, trabeculae in visceral organs, scar and granulation tissues, and bone), type II (in cartilage), and type III (in the sheaths of tendons and ligaments, muscle, skin, blood vessel walls, scar and granulation tissues and probably in visceral organ trabeculae).

The first subgroup of the "other" collagens is the basement membrane collagens (types IV and V). Type IV collagen is present in fiber bundle sheaths in tendons and ligaments.

The second subgroup is the "minor" collagens, presently consists of 6-7 different types. All of them are not yet fully characterized. They seem to have interactions between cellular and extracellular elements as main role; residing on the borderlines between cells, fibrous structures and ground substance. The one associated with these tissue is type XII, which has been found in the cDNA library of the tendon fibroblast. This collagen, which appears to be homologous to type IX in cartilage, might provide a coupling between cells and extracellular fibrillar structures. No obvious mechanical functions on tissue level have been reported for any of these "minor" collagens.

Collagen is quantified by the colorimetric measurement of an amino acid, hydroxyproline, which is with minor exceptions unique for collagen. These molecules do not introduce an error in measurements on tendons and ligaments. Although the amount of hydroxyproline varies between collagen types, this method is precise for these tissues, where type I collagen most of the collagen mass.

The quantitative assessments of amounts of different types of collagen are less precise, involving cyanobromide digestion followed by electrophoretic or chromatographic separation. Staining tissue sections with specific antibodies against different collagen types gives a visual impression of the distributions within a tissue, although some cross-reacting might occur.

Other tissue components

The only non-collagenous fibrillar structure of importance in connective tissues is elastin. This protein is present in very small amounts if at all in most tendons and ligaments (it is, of course, present in the walls of their blood vessels). It is present in *e.g.* rat tail tendons in amounts of less than 0.07 mg/g wet weight, if at all. In a few ligaments, most notably *ligamentum nuchae* and *ligamenta flava*, elastin is a dominant tissue component. This is reflected in the mechanical properties of these ligaments, which are quite different from those of other ligaments. While a regular tendon or ligament has a strength of about 60 MPa and a strain value of 0.10-0.20 at the point of maximum strength, the corresponding values for *ligamentum nuchae* are 2.4 MPa and 1.25 respectively. The elastic stiffness of these two tissues are 700 and 7.5 N/mm^2 respectively.

There is a number of methods to quantify elastin. Most of them depend on the fact that elastin is much more resistant to chemical degradation than collagen and other connective tissue components; the non-soluble residue is taken to be elastin. The only reliable method for quantification is to measure desmosines by amnio acid analysis. The desmosines are unique for elastin and are formed as intramolecular cross-links by aldol condensation.

Fibronectin and laminin are large glycoproteins, which seem to function on the borderlines between cells, fibrous structures and ground substance. They are thought to facilitate interactions between cells and their surrounding extracellular matrix. Fibronectin inhibits collagen fibrillogenesis and play a role in the regulation of fiber formation. The amount of fibronectin seems to be relatively plentiful in developing tissues; it might also have regulatory functions during early wound healing. Laminin binds to type IV collagen and cell membranes They are analyzed with immunohistochemical techniques; there are no quantitative assays available.

Proteoglycans form the "core" of the ground substance. Its structure is polyanionic; the polysaccharide chains thus repel one another. Small amounts in a solution can therefore fill rather large domains. Because of their pronounced hydrophilic properties they regulate the amount of water in the tissue. Most of our knowledge of the proteoglycans is derived from studies on cartilage, where they are present in dominating amounts. Due to the fact that very small amounts of proteoglycans are present in tendons and ligaments (about 3 mg/g dry weight), our knowledge of the properties of those present in these tissues is meagre. The proteoclygans associated with type I collagen are small monomers contains almost exclusively dermatan sulphate. The usual method to quantify proteoglycans is to measure the amount of uronic acid in the tissue.

The type I collagen molecule

The type I collagen molecule consists of three linear (*i.e.* non-branching) chains of about 1000 amino acid residues each. Two of the chains are identical α1(I) chains, while the third one, α2(I) is slightly different with respect to its amino acid sequence. This molecule, which can thus be designated $[\alpha1(I)]_2\alpha2(I)$, is the only fiber-forming collagen not having three identical α chains. Type II and III are thus $[\alpha1(II)]_3$ and $[\alpha1(III)]_3$ respectively.

The major part of each α chain is wound into a *left-handed* helix with a pitch of 0.89 nm. The helical parts of the α chains are then wound together into the $[\alpha1(I)]_2\alpha2(I)$ collagen molecule, a *right-handed* super-helix with a pitch of 8.7 nm. The steric condition making the very tight packing possible is that every third amino acid residue is the small glycine; they connect by hydrogen bonds to amides of peptide bonds in adjacent chains. The short end parts of the chains are not helical; they remain in "random" order and form the telopeptides of the molecules.

The sequence for the helical part of the molecule can be written thus as a repeat of Gly-X-Y, where X and Y are other amino acid residues, quite frequently one of the imino acids, proline (in either position) and hydroxyproline (almost always in the Y position). This repeating sequence is important for the stability of the molecule. Experiments with synthetic peptides has shown that the stability of the peptide falls gradually from being highest for Gly-Pro-Hyp via Gly-Pro-Pro, Gly-Pro-Y and Gly-X-Pro to Gly-X-Y, which least stable. By blocking the hydroxylation of proline to hydroxyproline the resulting collagen molecule is instable already at physiological temperatures.

The importance of the imino acids for the stability of collagen under physiological conditions is shown by the analysis of the amount of them versus the thermal stability of tissues. The number of imino acid residues per 1000 is for calf skin 232; its denaturing temperature (for collagen in solution) is 39 ∘C and its shrinkage temperature is 65 ∘C. The correspon-ding figures are for shark skin 191, 29 and 35, while they are only 155, 16 and 40 for cod skin. It is not clear yet how these figures relate to changes in mechanical properties. It has, however, been shown instances that mechanical strength and shrinkage temperature correlate in other instances, although differences in cross-linking patterns might be a confounding factor.

Microfibrils and fibrils

The supramolecular arrangement of type I collagen is not entirely established. A number of models have been proposed (see Brodsky *et al.*, Woodhead-Galloway 1984). The two current ones are the distorted microfibril and the quasihexagonal models. Calculations have shown that x-ray diffraction data do not yet have resolution enough to resolve the question. Morphologic studies using a variety of techniques at the electron microscopic level have, on the other hand, have described diagonal clefts inside fibrils, which suggests a helical organization of microfibrils. The microfibril model will, therefore, be used in this discussion.

Microfibrils are primarily aggregated as five strands of molecules, with clusters of residues with hydrophobic side chains playing a major role for the assembly. By elevating the temperature of a solution of collagen from 4 to 37 °C, the electrostatic forces of the hydrophobic interactions increase and microfibrils are formed. The aggregation occurs in "quarter-stagger" fashion, *i.e.* with a displacement of the molecules by 67 nm (= 1 D) from one strand to the next (viewing the microfibril as a planar sheet).

The whole helical part of a molecule is 4.34 D long, which corresponds to 4 x 234 + 75 residues. This leaves gaps of 0.66 D (~44 nm) between two consecutive molecules in a strand. The telopeptides are in these spaces, probably being dislocated laterally. This results in 0.6 D gap and 0.4 D overlap regions. This agrees well with theoretical calculations, which have demonstrated that the hydrophobic interactions are at maximum, when the stagger is 234 residues.

The five strands of molecules in the microfibril, viewed above as a planar sheet, are *in vivo* wound together into a *left-handed* super-super-helix. The diameter of the microfibril is about 4 nm; its length is unknown. This microfibril, held together mainly by hydrophobic interactions, has very low mechanical strength. The strength and stability during maturation of the microfibrils are achieved by the development of intermolecular cross-links.

The prerequisite for the formation of a cross-link is the oxidative deamination of [hydroxy]lysine residues in the telopeptides to [hydroxy]allysines ([B-hydroxy] α-aminoadipic acid-δ-semialdehydes), mediated by lysyl oxidase and requiring collagen in fibrillar form. The primary cross-link, an aldimine, is formed between a [hydroxy]allysine (on a telopeptide) and a [hydroxy]lysine in the helical part of a molecule. The resulting aldimine cross-link is further stabilized by an Amadori re-arrangement to a ketoimine, provided the participating deaminated residue is a hydroxyallysine. The amounts of the different types depends on the degree of telopeptide lysine hydroxylation and does not reflect differences in collagen genotypes. The ketoimine is more stable against physico-chemical influences; differences in mechanical behavior have not been investigated.

Cross-link formation can be blocked pharmacologically by *e.g.* β-aminopropionitrile and D-penicillamine. Already formed aldimine cross-links can be split by D-penicillamine. Chronic feeding of animals with β-aminopropionitrile (present in sweet beans and other members of the *Lathyrus* family) renders them lathyritic; their tendons and ligaments show only a fraction of the normal tensile strength. Treatment with D-penicillamine renders tissues containing aldimine cross-links weaker.

Fibrils have a diameter of 30-150 nm and show on electron micrographs the cross-striation with a periodicity of 67 nm (1 D) characteristic for the fiber-forming collagens (Fig. 1). The packing of fibrils follows, at least in the surface layers of the fibril, a helical pattern: The microfibrils are wound together into a *right-handed* super-super-super-helix, the pitch of which is about 1090 nm. There is no evidence for any intermediate level of packing. Even if the basic pattern is parallel-fibrilled, there is a certain amount of undulation (Fig. 1).

The full extent of the mechanisms holding fibrils together is not established; the distances between microfibrils allows cross-links between adjacent microfibrils, but there are probably also other contributing factors, *e.g.* weaker bonds and interactions, proteoglycans, and probably glycoproteins. The proteoglycans are seen as regularly spaced (with the same distance as the D period) thin filaments; they appear to surround the neighboring collagen fibrils. The material surrounding the fibril has considerable mechanical properties; when single fibrils are extended to failure, the sheath still holds (Barenberg *et al.* 1978).

Fibers, fiber bundles and tendons/ligaments

The fibrils are packed into fibers, the structural unit on the next level of the organizational hierarchy. With a diameter of 1-10 μm it is the smallest unit seen in the light microscopy. The fibers are in turn assembled into primary and secondary bundles or fascicles, at times tertiary bundles or secondary fascicles, and ultimately into the tendon or ligament itself.

Most authors consider that there is on these hierarchical levels a gentle, planar and in the relaxed specimen almost sinusoidal waviness but

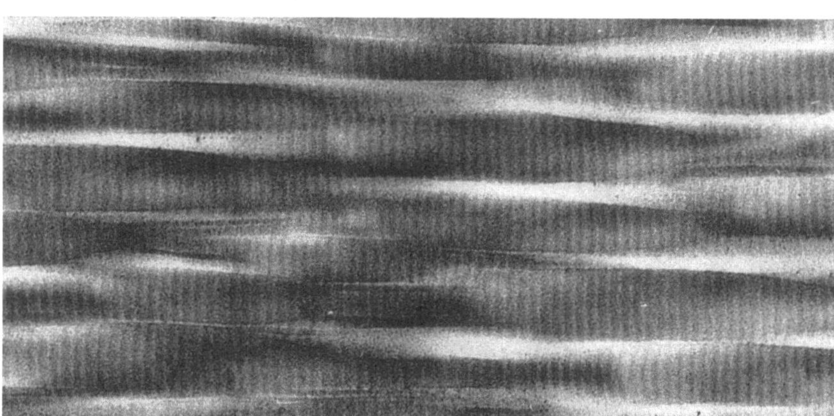

Fig. 1. Electron micrograph of rat tail tendon showing slight undulation of the fibrils along the longitudinal axis (24,000 x).

no helicality (Fig. 2). Recently, however, Yahia & Drowin (1989) presented evidence that there could be a combined helical and planar waviness in the fascicles of the anterior cruciate ligament and the patellar tendon. Although they discuss "fibrils" it is evident from their SEM micrographs that the helical pattern is in *fibers*. It is well-known that the bundles of fascicles in some ligaments (most typically the cruciate ligaments in the knee joint) are wound in a more or less spiral manner is not the rule, it is rather an exception.

There is some controversy regarding the nature of the planar waviness. Diamant *et al.* (1972) suggested that this waveform is a zig-zag rather than sinusoidal, *i.e.* a rather regular bending, which in some tissues would occur every 100 μm. This avenue of research has been pursued especially by the Bristol group (see *e.g.* Gathercole *et al.* 1974, Gathercole & Keller 1978). These reports have inspired to some modelling of tendon mechanical function, using bars, hinges and springs as elements. It is difficult to see a biochemical basis (or a basis on fibrillar level) for such a structural arrangement. The Bristol group reported themselves that the crimp length decreased, when smaller fiber bundles were teased out of the same tendon. The present author has been able to reproduce this zig-zag pattern by varying the histotechnical procedure, at times with zig-zag and sinusoidal waves in the same section (Fig. 3). On the other hand, smooth waviness was always present when sectioning the same tissues on a freezing microtome and viewing them without further processing (with crossed polars and the Nomarski interference contrast technique (Viidik 1978, 1980b).

The distances between the fibrils excludes the possibility that the fibers are held together by cross-links. The interfibrillar matrix, especially the proteoglycans in it, probably plays the major role. It has been shown that fibrils can be dispersed in a dilute acid solution, when parts of the interfibrillar matrix has been removed by chelating agents. Further, it can

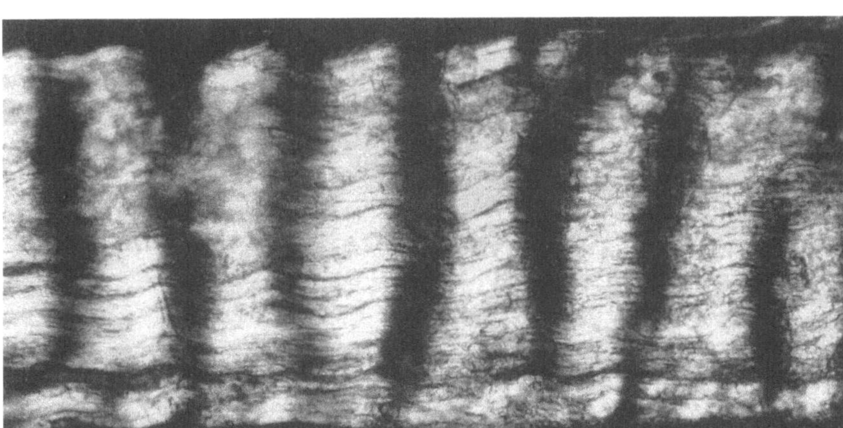

Fig. 2. Micrograph in polarized light of a relaxed tendon fiber bundle (250 x).

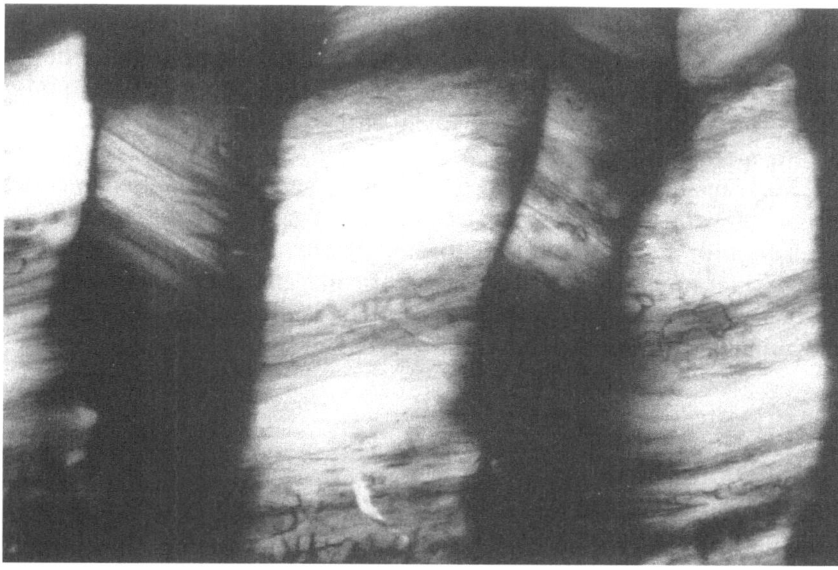

Fig. 3. Micrograph in polarized light of a relaxed tendon fiber bundle exhibiting smooth sinusoidal waviness concomitantly with sharp zig-zag patterns (550 x).

be seen in scanning electron microscopy that the fibers tend to open up into fibrils, when the "loose" proteoglycans are removed by crude bacterial α-amylase or hyaluronidase.

There are on higher hierarchical levels sheaths, the structure of which resembles "woven fabric", containing collagen, elastin and proteoglycans. The collagen is of types I, III and IV. The fiber arrangement could be described as criss-cross, with fiber dimensions increasing with hierarchical level. Filament-like particles of proteoglycans cross-connect and surround collagen fibrils here. Their nature is not known. While type I collagen is associated with dermatan sulphate in small amounts, type III is associated with larger amounts of mainly heparan sulphate. It could, therefore, seem reasonable to assume that the sheaths contain larger amounts of proteoglycans and with more variety in composition than that of tendons.

There is no universally accepted terminology for these hierarchical levels. According to Gelberman *et al.* (1987) the levels can be divided into (i) visceral paratenon enveloping a fascicle, (ii) parietal paratenon with one or more fascicles inside, (iii) endotenon with fascicle(s?), blood vessels and nerves, and (iv) epitenon (with the whole tendon inside). This might be an oversimplification. Clark & Sidles (1990) found that the sheaths of larger fascicles were covered by "more layers of membrane" but that "this distinction often broke down". They also found that the sheaths were not always complete but extended into the ligament tissue "almost randomly as septa". This observation might explain why it has been difficult to attain a common terminology.

The important feature in this somewhat confusing organization of the subunits in tendons and ligaments is that there is no lateral coupling between fascicles; they can slide freely past each other, which is optimal from a mechanical point of view.

It can thus be concluded that the substance of tendons and ligaments, with the exception of the elastic ligaments, consists of type I collagen with small amounts of proteoglycans and glycoproteins in the interfibrillar ground substance. The other collagens and elastin are present in the sheaths, blood vessels and other surrounding and at times intermingling tissues.

Mechanical properties

When discussing the mechanical properties of tendons and ligaments in detail, it is important to start with considering the experimental foundation for acquiring data from biomechanical testing. The inherent problems have been discussed in detail previously (see Viidik 1973, 1979b, 1987a, 1987b). Only key points will, therefore, be highlighted in relation to stress-strain behavior and the viscoelastic and plastic properties of these tissues.

Stress-strain behavior

Original length and strain measurements

One key point for the analysis of load-deformation data acquired from *in vitro* testing of tendons or ligaments is the definition of original length of the tissue specimen. This length is crucial for the transformation of deformation data to strain values. The commonly used method is to compute this length as the sum of the distance between the clamps at zero deformation and the length the moving clamp travels until a well-defined point on the load-deformation curve is reached. This point is usually taken as where the load has reached a small predefined value, most often the minimum load (typically one grid unit on the chart paper) the recording equipment can discern from zero load. Errors are caused by variations in specimen size and amplification levels (Viidik 1979b).

Less amplification-sensitive methods use intersects between calculated curves or lines and the deformation axis of the raw load-deformation curve (Viidik 1990). These include the approximated tangent and the superimposed derivate (a straight line) for the initial part of the load-deformation curve. Further precision can hardly be attained by using an intermediarily calculated stress-deformation curve, except when there are large variations in the cross-sectional areas of the specimens.

The "ideal" initial length would, from a physiological point of view, be the length the tissue has *in vivo*. The difficulty is, however, to determine unambiguously the physiological "prestress" present. Such a tension in tendons most probably varies with muscle tone and the degree of flexion or extension in the adjacent joints. Schatzker & Brånemark (1969) demonstrated by intravital techniques that in the anesthetized rabbit the smooth surface of a tendon became wavy only after transection. This suggests that the *in vivo* resting prestress stretches the tendon to a point somewhere on the toe part of the stress-strain curve (see below). The magnitude of this prestress is unknown; *in vivo* studies do not help, since there are no precise and noninvasive measuring techniques. The prestress in ligaments should depend on joint position and varies from joint to joint. There seems to be no prestress in knee joint ligaments (Kennedy *et al.* 1977, Lewis 1982), while spinal ligaments, especially *ligaments flava*, are under constant stress (Åkerblom 1948).

There is thus no possibility to establish the extent of prestress present in these tissues. The best possible avenue is to develop a reproducible empirical method along the lines discussed above, taking care to avoid introducing bias when comparing groups with disparate properties.

Another key point is how deformation is measured. The conventional method is to record the distance the moving clamp travels. Some materials testing machines have an output from the cross-head for this purpose; a slack in the mechanics may introduce significant errors with respect to the initial movement (in relation to the force recorded simultaneously). Other techniques use LVDTs coupled to the stationary and moving cross-bars, which eliminates this error. Both methods have, however, other sources of error. In case some slippage of the specimen occurs in the clamps, this is included into the deformation measurement. Further, the deformation of the transducer is included in the measurement; it can be significant when most of the range of the transducer is utilized. This source of error is eliminated by mounting the LVDT on the clamps; this might, however, interfere with the force measurement.

A non-contact video technique seems to solve these problems, at least for measuring surface strains. The specimen, with markings on key points, is continuously videorecorded and analyzed in a video dimension analyzer, which translates the distance between two markers into an output voltage (Woo *et al.* 1976, 1983). With repeated runs of the videotape different parts of the specimen can be analyzed separately and inhomogeneities in strain development be detected. The possible source of error is then the synchronization with the force recording.

Cross-sectional area and stress measurements

Also the methods to measure cross-sectional areas of specimens may introduce errors and biases (for review see Viidik 1979b, 1987a, 1987b). One inherent problem is that the cross-sectional areas of tendons and ligaments are seldom uniform and they may also vary considerably along the specimen length. Planimetric methods are destructive and can be used only on the end surfaces of specimens. Calliper measurements assume a reasonably regular cross-sectional area (round, ellipsoid or rectangular) or require approximations. Also a double calliper technique, by which the specimen is gently squeezed into a rectangle, is possible. Another difficulty, pronounced especially with the last mentioned technique, is that these tissues are somewhat compressible; careful standardization is necessary.

These problems can be overcome to a certain extent by using indirect methods of measurement and calculate an average area for the tested length. The volume can be calculated by the principle of Archimedes. Another method is to measure wet weight and *either* calculate the area using a known or assumed density (expressing stress in *e.g.* N/mm^2) *or* use weight per unit length as area parameter ("stress" in *e.g.* N/(mg/mm)). To eliminate the influence of non-collagenous tissue elements (*e.g.* variations in amount of water) from the calculations "stress" can be expressed in newton per unit collagen per unit length. The last mentioned methods render inter-laboratory comparisons difficult, if not impossible, but may be useful for comparisons between groups (see Viidik 1980a, 1982). The best future method might be to measure the cross-section of the specimen repeatedly with laser-based technique while rotating the specimen (Woo SL-Y, *personal communication*).

The stress-strain curve related to structural changes

The stress-strain curve for parallel-fibred collagenous tissue starts insidiously with a shallow toe segment, convex towards the strain axis. The very first part of it is seldom included, because the method to define the starting point of the curve cuts it off (see above). The completely relaxed tendon shows a rather regular waviness, which becomes shallower already before any force can be recorded (Viidik & Ekholm 1968, Viidik 1972, 1973, 1980a). The common cutoff is indicated on Fig. 4 as the small rectangle at the origo of the stress-strain curve.

The transition from the toe segment to the linear segment is gradual, but the waviness is straightened out before the latter segment is entered (Fig. 5). The transition is most often determined by visual approximation. A more precise method to use is to determine the "tangent" modulus, $\delta\sigma/\delta\epsilon$, which should increase gradually during the toe segment and then remain constant during the linear segment of the curve.

A number of methods have been used to characterize and/or quantify the toe segment of the curve. Wertheim (1947) was the first to suggest an exponential function to describe the stress-strain curve:

$$\epsilon^2 = c_1\sigma^2 + c_2\sigma \qquad (1)$$

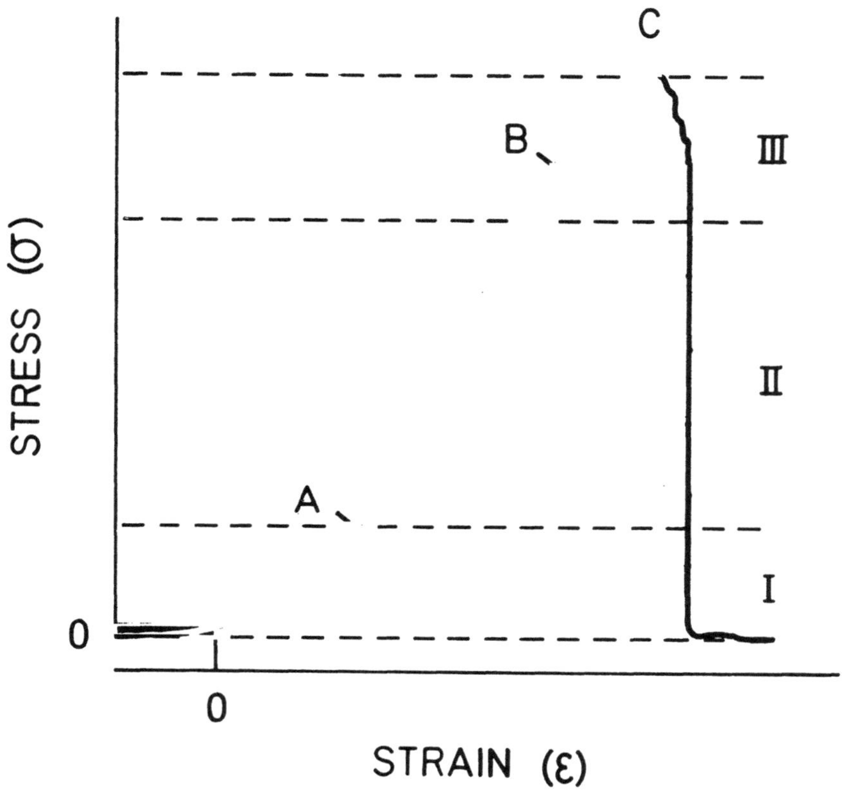

Fig. 4. Stress-strain curve for a tendon a finite speed. 0 is the starting point of the curve. A and B are the start and end of the linear segment. C is the point of ultimate stress. I, II, and III are the three for structural changes.

where ϵ is strain, σ stress and c_i are constants in my notation. Other expressions have been suggested later, *e.g.* by Morgan (1960)

$$\epsilon = c_3\sigma^{0.812} \tag{2}$$

and Elden (1968)*

$$\sigma = c_4\epsilon^2 \tag{3}$$

Later Fung (1967, 1968, 1972, 1981) developed his "quasi-linear" viscoelasticity law for soft biological tissues. Since he had observed that there is a linear relationship between stress and corresponding "tangent moduli", he could formulate a basic equation by reducing the dynamic stress-strain curve to the one for infinitely slow strain rate:

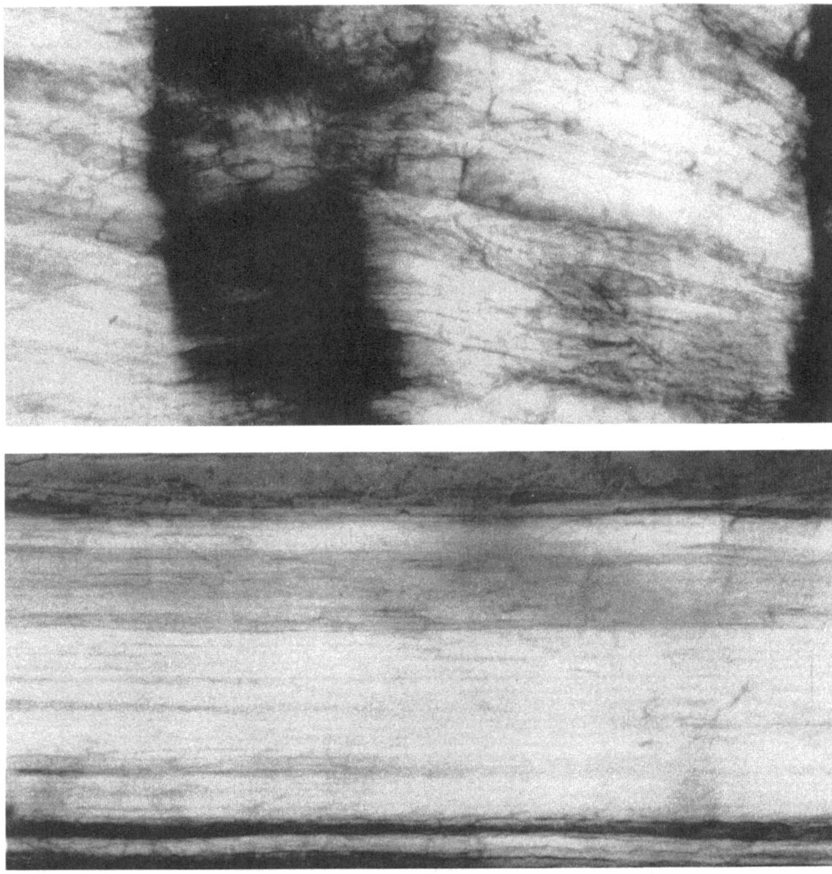

Fig. 5. Micrographs in polarized light of tendons (top) completely relaxed and (bottom) elongated into the linear segment of the σ/ϵ curve (750 x). The tendons were processed according to Viidik & Ekholm.

$$d\sigma_L/d\lambda = c_5\sigma_L(1+c_6) \tag{4a}$$

where σ_L is Lagrangian stress and λ extension ratio, {length of specimen under strain}/{original or relaxed length}. Strain is then calculated

$$\epsilon = (\lambda^2 - 1)/2 \tag{4b}$$

Fung performed the basic experiments on rabbit mesentery. No one has yet used this approach extensively to analyze the toe segment of stress-strain curves for tendons and ligaments. Haut & Little (1969), Stromberg & Wiederhielm (1969), Viidik *et al.* (1982) have used the "tangent modulus" for analyzing the stress-strain behavior of canine ligaments, mice tail tendons and collagen membranes, respectively. Fung's "quasi-linear" viscoelasticity law has also been applied in modified form successfully for analysis of dynamic experiments on tendons (Haut & Little 1972). It is, therefore, worthwhile to discuss the possible modifications Fung has suggested. Eq(4a) is after deleting the insignificant intercept c_5c_6 in Eq(4a) and integration written

$$\sigma_L = \sigma_{L\delta}\, e\, \exp\{c_5(\lambda-\lambda_\delta)\} \quad (1 \leq \lambda \leq \lambda_1)) \tag{4c}$$

where subscript δ indicates a specific extension ratio and its corresponding stress value. It might, however, be necessary in some cases to describe the stress response by two linear segments, *e.g.* by

$$d\sigma_L/d\lambda = c_7(\sigma + c_8) \quad (1 \leq \lambda \leq \lambda_2)$$

$$d\sigma_L/d\lambda = c_9(\sigma + c_{10}) \quad (\lambda_2 \leq \lambda \leq \lambda_3) \tag{4d}$$

but that could indicate that the tissue in question should be characterized by some other method, the two linear segments being two approximations for a continuous nonlinear phenomenon. Such quantification of the toe segment would yield more detailed data for the elucidation of the effects of *e.g.* pharmacological intervention or age-related physiological changes.

The linear segment, *i.e.* the A-B segment in Fig. 4, should be considered as an approximation of a very small gradual increase followed by a similar decrease. That this is the case is more obvious from data for other tissues, *e.g.* skin, where the points A and B have clearly "merged" into an inflection point. The parameter commonly derived from the linear segment is the elastic or linear stiffness. These terms signify that this stiffness is not the modulus of elasticity, which by definition belongs to an elastic material, while tendons and ligaments exhibit pronounced viscous and some plastic components (see below).

A few authors have reported for stress-strain curves from rat tail tendons a second linear segment, which is less steep than the first one. The present author has never been able to reproduce such curves under normal conditions, only after irregularities in the protocol for preserving the tendons in the time period between sacrifice and testing (Viidik, unpublished data).

There are no further light microscopical changes during the linear segment, except for a few minor strands regaining waviness toward the end of this segment (early ruptures of a few bundles). Stretching occurs now on lower hierarchical levels, the fibrillar and molecular ones. Viidik & Ekholm (1968) measured fibril period lengths from electron micrographs of rabbit hind limb tendons. They were processed relaxed and while under tension (strain level relaxed and 0.0-0.10). The periodicity of the fibrils is extended from 67 nm up to 72.5 nm. This agrees with Cowan *et al.* (1955) who reported from a low-angle x-ray diffraction pattern study that the reflection pattern increased proportionally with specimen length. Nemetschek and co-workers (Nemetschek *et al.* 1978, Riedl *et al.* 1980) later performed similar measurements on rat tail tendons from x-ray diffraction patterns recorded while gradually stretching the specimens. A synchrotron was used as the powerful x-ray source. They found the increase to occur throughout the stress-strain curve (strain range 0-0.11), although the initial part of the strain versus period length curve was somewhat shallow.

These results indicate that the fibrils is elongated, when the specimen is stretched, but they do not determine on which hierarchical level the elongation occurs. Cowan *et al.* (1955) also studied the wide-angle pattern, which reflects the winding of the triple helix. The axial periodicity of 0.286 nm of the dried fiber increased to about 0.31, when the fiber was stretched. Here the increase starts at a strain of about 0.03. When the low-angle pattern has increased about 10 percent, the wide-angle pattern has gained only 4.3 percent.They also noted that the resting length wide-angle pattern was restored immediately after relaxation. The collagen structure is thus affected by tensile straining on all hierarchical levels.

The part of the curve from the end of the linear segment to the point of ultimate stress (B-C in Fig. 4) is characterized by a bending off toward the strain axis. Here waviness is gradually seen in an increasing number of the fiber bundles, which suggests a gradual rupturing of the specimens. There seems to be a recoil phenomenon, since Viidik & Ekholm (1968) noted that there were in the highest strain group fibrils with very short period lengths, down to 61 nm. This phenomenon begins near the end point of the linear segment of the curve.

To summarize: There are three regions of structural changes, which relate to tensile testing of parallel-fibred tissues (*cf.* Fig. 4).I: Straightening out of the light microscopical fiber bundle waviness, II: Elongating the helical structure on fibrillar and macromolecular levels, and III: Failure of fibrils and fibers in gradually increasing numbers resulting in recoil on all hierarchical levels. The transitions between these regions is gradual.

Viscoelasticity and plasticity

Stress-strain experiments designed for investigating the mechanical properties of tendons and ligaments up to the point of failure are normally performed on from a mechanical point of view fresh tissues, *i.e.* without previous *in vitro* strain history. A protocol, which includes non-destructive loading prior to loading until failure, would introduce a significant error, since such loading wound distort the lower part of the stress-strain curve. This becomes obvious when analyzing the viscoelasticity and plasticity, which are rather pronounced in tendons and ligaments.

It is well established that tendons and ligaments are non-linear viscoelastic solids, with some plastic or strain-hardening phenomena in the initial (preconditioning phase) (see *e.g.* Fung 1981, Viidik 1980a).

Initial phase and preconditioning

Protocols employing repeated non-destructive testing up to a predesigned level of stress or strain (below region III in Fig. 4) include procedures for preconditioning in order to ensure reproducibility. This can be achieved by (i) loading the specimen to that level and unloading a number of times, (ii) exhausting the creep phenomenon at that level (once if the point is defined in stress, a number of times if in strain), or (iii) perform stress relaxation at that level a number of times.

When performing cyclic loading-unloading a number of times the hysteresis becomes smaller, the loading curve steeper, and the stress-strain curves move gradually to the right (Freestone A, B, Viidik A, 1973, 1980a). The creep phenomenon and the stress relaxation become gradually less pronounced. The changes are largest between the first few cycles. After 6-10 cycles a steady state is achieved. Then this steady state level is stable until the tissue starts to decay. The loading-unloading cycles before and after stress relaxation or creep phenomenon experiments are reproducible, even after such a cycle has lasted for more than 24 hours (Viidik, unpublished data).

This preconditioning is lasting under *in vitro* conditions. Whether there is any recovery under *in vivo* conditions is not known. It can be hypothesized that the lack of circulation and thereby restoration of full hydration (water being squeezed out from the specimen during tensile testing) plays a role. It is otherwise difficult to find an explanation for why the corresponding changes occurring during limbering-up and subsequent sports activities are reversible.

The stationary, reproducible phase

Repeated loading-unloading stress-strain curves are reproducible during this phase. This is shown in Fig. 6 as the loading (solid) curve up to σ_R,ϵ_R, followed by the unloading (dashed) curve, with a hysteresis between them, caused by viscous elements and energy dissipation.

The two theoretical extremes for testing such a non-linear visco-elastic solid are at strain rates $\epsilon \rightarrow \infty$ and $\epsilon \rightarrow 0$. The viscous elements are "locked" in the first instance, rendering the curve steep. They are continuously exhausted in the second instance, which results in a shallower curve. This is shown schematically in Fig. 7a. When the point (σ_0,ϵ_0) is reached and the "machine" stopped instantaneously, stress relaxation occurs, if ϵ_0 is kept constant (Fig. 7b), while creep occurs, if σ_0 is kept constant (which requires continuous adjustment of ϵ) (Fig. 7c).

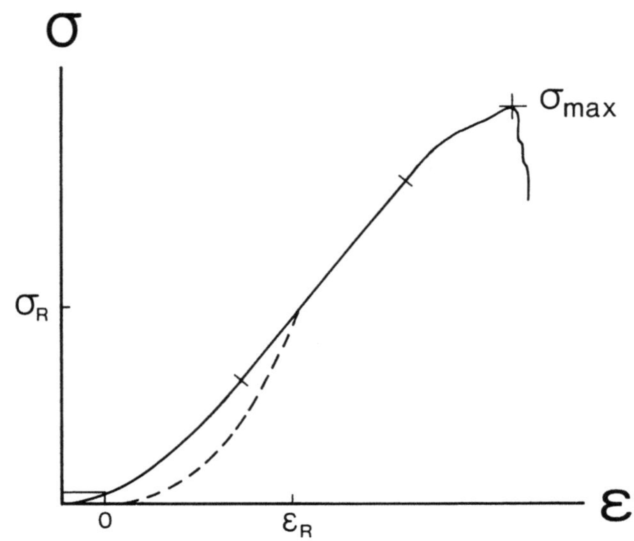

Fig. 6. Schematic stress-strain curve for parallel-fibred collagenous tissue. It has been preconditioned to (σ_R/σ_R), from which the stress relaxation and creep experiments in Fig. 7 begin.

Models

Mathematical models and Fung's law

A number of models has been developed to analyze the interrelationship between the elastic and viscous components in tissue behavior. A number of descriptive mathematical models have been proposed to satisfy specific experimental conditions.It has been difficult to find meaningful structural or functional correlations to the parameter values derived from these mathematical exercises. Further, they have had no value in interlaboratory comparisons.

Fung introduced a broader approach to the mathematical characterization of the properties of soft tissues (Fung 1967, 1968, 1972, 1981, for review see also Viidik 1980a, 1987a) by formulating his "quasi-linear" viscoelasticity law. This equation, which has been proved valid for a number of different tissue, can be written as

$$\sigma(t) = f\{\epsilon(t)\} + f'\{\epsilon(t-\tau);t,\tau\} \qquad (5)$$

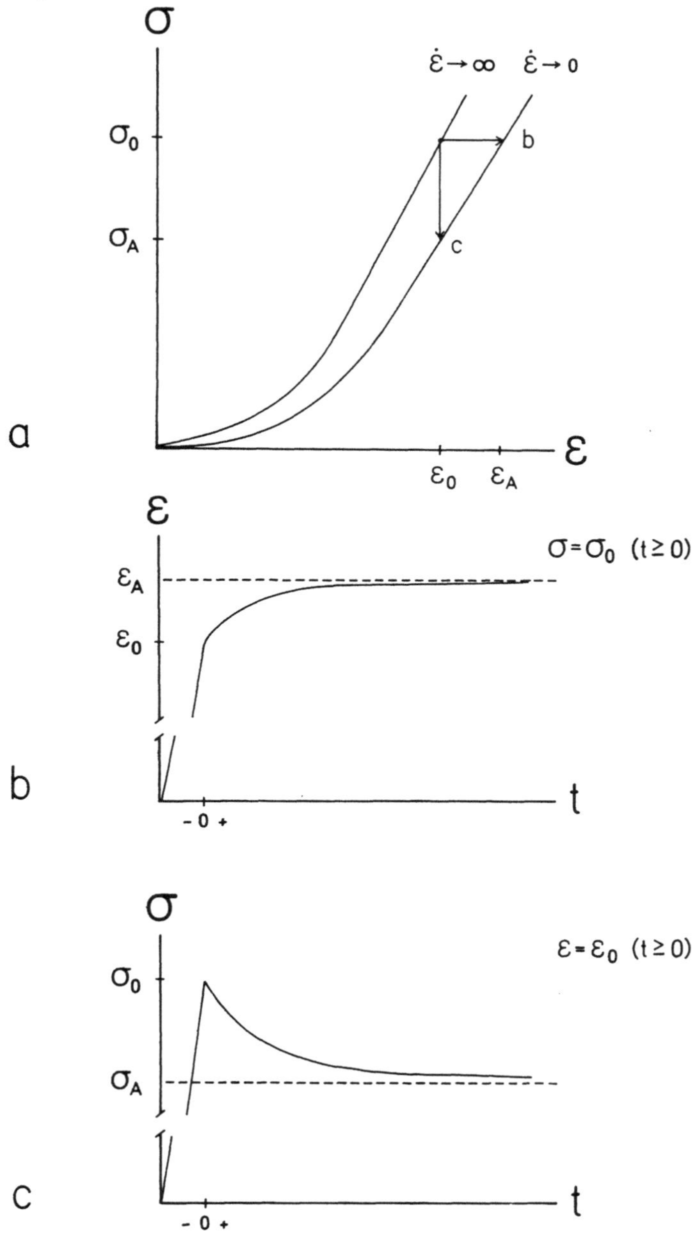

Fig. 7. (a) Theoretical tensile loading curves at infinitely high and low strain rates, (b) stress relaxation, and (c) creep. (From Viidik 1980c).

where σ(t) and ϵ(t) are the stress and strain at time t, $f\{\epsilon(t)\}$ is a function of ϵ and t, and $f'\{\epsilon(t-\tau);t,\tau\}$ is a function of the whole time history, $\epsilon(t-\tau)$. A "reduced relaxation function" was incorporated into this mathematical representation to take the strain-history-dependent part of the stress-strain relationship into account. A considerable number of tissues and experimental protocols have been analyzed with this method. The hysteresis in cyclic loading-unloading did not, however, have the strain rate dependence of linear viscoelastic materials. Fung overcame this discrepancy by introducing a continuous spectrum of relaxation times. While Fung mostly used soft tissues, such as rabbit mesentery, Haut & Little (1972) later used Fung's law with minor modifications to analyze the behavior of rat tail tendons.

Discrete models

Discrete models using ideal elements of elasticity, viscosity and plasticity has had an appeal for biologists, more than engineers in need to visualize tissue properties and the couplings between them. Alfrey & Gurnee (1957) used such discrete models to discuss the mechanical behavior of macromolecules, while Alexander (1962) found that a Kelvin element in series with a linear spring could describe the properties of the sea anemone body wall qualitatively. Viidik (1968a) proposed a model, which accounted qualitatively for both the initial and stationary phase behavior (with respect to elastic, viscous and plastic elements). Later, Freestone *et al.* (1969a, 1969b) developed this model further and verified it experimentally and semiquantitatively. In brief, the stationary phase consists of a Kelvin element in series with a nonlinear array of springs (to account for the toe segment of the stress-strain curve) and a friction element (for the loading to unloading reversion). The equation for it can be written as

$$d\sigma/dt + \sigma(\phi + C_K)/\eta = (d\epsilon/dt)\phi + \epsilon C_K\phi/\eta_K - C_K\psi/\eta_K \tag{6}$$

where C_K and η_K are the constants for Kelvin element spring and dashpot, ϕ is the step-function "constant" for the nonlinear spring array and ψ is another step function (for elaboration of the constants, see Freestone *et al.* 1969a, Viidik 1980a).

The present discussion will be confined to two special cases, those for stress relaxation and creep within the linear part of the curve (*cf.* Fig. 7). Eq(6) can then be written, with subscripts 0 and A for the starting and asymptotic values respectively, for stress relaxation as

$$\ln(\sigma-\sigma_A) = \ln(\sigma_0-\sigma_A) - (C_E+C_K)t/\eta_K \tag{6a}$$

where C_K is ϕ for the linear part, and for creep as

$$\ln(\epsilon_A-\epsilon) = \ln(\epsilon_A-\epsilon_0) - C_K t/\eta_K \tag{6b}$$

Eq(6a) can be rewritten as

$$\sigma = (\sigma_0-\sigma_A)^{-\beta t} + \sigma_A \tag{7}$$

where β is $-(C_K+C_E)/\eta_K$, the shape parameter and in a lin-ln plot the tangent of the stress relaxation curve, which becomes a straight line. Correspondingly Eq(6b) can be rewritten as

$$\epsilon = \epsilon_A - (\epsilon_A-\epsilon_0)^{-\delta t} \tag{8}$$

where δ is $-C_K/\eta_K$, corresponding to β in Eq(7).

It is quite popular to evaluate stress relaxation and creep phenomena from rather short experiments, typically 10 minutes or less. To undertake long-term experiments requires a tissue, the properties of which do not deteriorate during the experiment. Anterior cruciate ligaments from mature rabbits is such a tissue. The stress-strain curves are, after proper preconditioning, identical before and after 20 hours of stress relaxation or creep at a level of 100 newton (about one third of ultimate strength), provided a 10 minute relaxation period is allowed before the second cyclic loading-unloading (Viidik *unpublished data*). The results of two stress relaxation experiments, lasting 12 and 1,200 minutes respectively, on the same ligament are shown in Fig. 8 (left panels). It is obvious that the shape parameters (*cf.* Eq(7)) are quite different; the asymptote was nine percent lower. Two similar creep experiments (*cf.* Eq(8) on another ligament are also given in Fig 8 (right panels). Also here the difference between the two asymptote levels was nine percent.

It seems, therefore, not safe to develop a model based on such data on short-term experiments only. Further analysis of these data suggest that there might be more than one viscous component, at least one rather rapid component and another slower one. The behavior is even more complex for skin, where there seems to be an array of components, especially at lower stress values (Viidik & Quirinia *unpublished data*). This agrees with the concept that a proteoglycans have a pronounced influence on the viscous properties (see below the discussion on the T-jump technique), since the relative amount of proteoglycans is sizably larger in skin than tendons and ligaments.

T-jump analysis

Early attempts to elucidate temperature dependence in the analysis of viscoelastic properties of tendons failed to show any changes in these properties in the wide range of 0-37 °C. Here separate experimental stress relaxation or creep runs on the same or different specimens were used.

It became later, with the development of the T-jump method, evident that the existing changes had been confounded by inter-experiment and/or inter-specimen variations. McCrum and coworkers (Cohen *et al.* 1974, 1975) developed this method and analyzed it in detail (Cohen *et al.* 1976, Hooley 1977); Cohen & Hooley (1979) then integrated these results in an broader model for the viscoelasticity in tendons.

They avoided the scatter, which is inherent in the earlier used methodologies, by imposing small, abrupt temperature changes on a specimen during creep experiments. Temperature changes do not alter the geometry of a specimen during a single run. They were further able to use this method for studies of the toe segment of the stress-strain curve.

The activation energy (ΔH) was calculated, when the two temperatures were T_1 and T_2 and the corresponding strain rates were measured to be $d\epsilon_1/dt$ and $d\epsilon_2/dt$, from

$$(d\epsilon_1/dt)/(d\epsilon_2/dt) = \exp\{(\Delta H/R)(-1/T_1-1/T_2)\} \qquad (9a)$$

where R is the gas constant. With ΔT as $(T_1\text{-}T_2)$ the equation can be written as

$$\ln\{(d\epsilon_1/dt)/(d\epsilon_2/dt)\} = \{\Delta H/(RT_1T_2)\}\Delta H \qquad (9b)$$

which is a straight line with the slope being ΔH (kJ/mol).

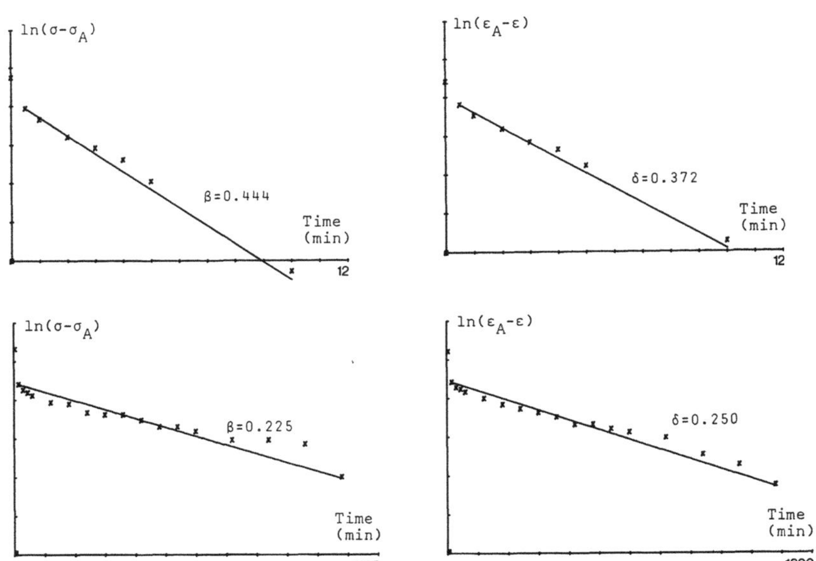

Fig. 8. *Left panel* Stress relaxation and *right panel* creep data. The in ln-lin plots are in each panel are for the same ligament, after 12 (upper) and 1,200 (lower) minute experiments.

They found in creep experiments at stress levels corresponding to the toe segment of the stress-strain curve the activation energy to be about 50 kJ/mol, while this figure for linear segment stress levels were about 135 kJ/mol. This difference suggests that there could be at least two components in the creep phenomenon in tendons. These figures should be compared with the activation energies found for a water-hyaluronic acid gel (an approximation for the ground substance) and for a tape of pure collagen, which were 20-40 and about 140 kJ/mol respective. They suggested that the mechanisms were (i) interfibrillary sliding and shear with the interfibrillar gel and (ii) fibrillar creep, which is compatible with data from light and electron microscopic and x-ray diffraction studies of stretched tendons (Cowan *et al.* 1955, Viidik & Ekholm 1968, Viidik 1972, Nemetschek *et al.* 1978, Riedl *et al.* 1980).

This technique merits wider use, because it could provide further insight into viscoelastic behavior of parallel-fibred collagenous tissues. It could thus be employed for studies of *in vitro* manipulated tissues, *e.g.*. after enzymatic removal or modification of the interfibrillar matrix and changes in the cross-linking pattern. Such studies would enable further development of tissue behavior models.

Mechanical functioning in vivo

Most *in vitro* investigations of the stress-strain properties of tendons and ligaments deal with the whole stress-strain curve; some have even confined their scope to the point of ultimate tensile strength. The main reason for studying the properties of an isolated tendon or ligament in the whole stress-strain range is to describe the tissue as such. These tissues, however, function *in vivo* as parts of a functional unit, bone-tendon-muscle-tendon-bone or bone-ligament-bone. The healthy tendon or ligament is seldom the weakest link in such a unit, provided the tensile stress is applied along the line of main fiber direction. Tendons from small rodents might be an exception, the explanation to which should rather be sought from morphological arrangements (*i.e.* the structure of the insertion into the bone and the architecture of the adjacent bone) than from differences in tendon structure and biochemical properties. The calcaneal tendon, when the whole functional unit is tested *in vitro*, has been found prone to rupture in rats (Barfred 1971a) but not in other animals (*e.g.* Davidsson 1955, Viidik 1969).

The tissue separation in bone-ligament-bone specimens has in most instances been reported to occur in one of the insertions of the anterior cruciate ligament in rabbits (*e.g* Viidik *et al.* 1965, Viidik 1968b) and the posterior cruciate ligament in rats (Rundgren, 1974). This ligament in primates ruptures in mid substance, however (Noyes *et al.* 1974). The studies by Alm *et al.* on dog anterior cruciate ligaments demonstrate that the axis of loading is important. They could by varying the degree of flexion change the tensile strength dramatically; the strength decreases, when the fiber bundles are loaded more and more unevenly. Also skeletal maturity may play a role. Woo *et al.* (1986) found that the medial collateral ligament failed as insertion fractures before epiphysis closure but most often in mid substance after closure. This also illustrates ligament to ligament differences, since the rabbits of Viidik (1968b) had closed epiphyses.

The accidental tendon and ligament ruptures seen in man are probably mainly due to uneven distribution of forces on the fiber bundles, since the violent external force in most cases is applied as a combination or bending and torque on the joint and the ligament (or tendon). The other factors discussed above should also be considered, especially when the trauma has occurred without any such force. Whether the "spontaneous" achilles tendon rupture, seen mostly in sedentary middle-aged men, occurs in a healthy or previously diseased tendon is not yet firmly established.

Knowledge of the normal and maximal *in vivo* capabilities and safety margins is important for traumatological assessment. There is no solid information available regarding ligaments. The following discussion will, therefore, be limited to tendons.

Laboratory investigations

Correlating in vivo and in vitro data

Elliott & Crawford (1955) found that there was a strong correlation between the maximum force a muscle could produce during isometric tetanic stimulation and the size of the tendon. They also found that tendons of fusiform muscles had smaller cross-sectional areas relative to muscle strength than those of penniform muscles (*cf.* the difference between extensor and flexor muscles regarding the effects of physical training discussed below). Harkness (1968) estimated from these data that the tensile strength of a tendon is about four times the maximum force of its muscle. Hirsch (1974) came to the same conclusion after measuring the maximum force of the muscle *in vivo* and testing its tendon *in vitro*.

The safety margin during normal functioning is thus considerable and that the normal functioning occurs during the toe segment of the stress-strain curve and reaches occasionally into the linear segment.

Invasive techniques

The information regarding *in vivo* stress-strain behavior is meagre. Barnes & Pinder (1974) measured, after implanting a buckle-shaped transducer around the forelimb common digital extensor muscle tendon of a horse, tension peaks. They found that the one occurring just after impact in the support phase to have a high load rate. Simon (1978) calculated in to be during walking up to 800 N/sec and it more than doubled during trotting. Strain in tendons was measured by Kear & Smith (1975) with an implanted flexible bridge transducer. They recorded from the forelimb lateral extensor muscle tendon in sheep and found a maximum strain of 0.026 and a corresponding strain rate of 0.44/sec.

These findings agree with the results of the previously discussed combined *in vivo* and *in vitro* studies, *i.e.* the functional working range of a tendon is largely confined to the toe segment of the stress-strain curve, even if a "physiological pretension" is present.

Indirect calculations

Human data have been acquired by indirect calculations, based on kinesiological (joint angle, angular accelerations) and anatomical (weights, distances, centers of gravity) data. Barfred (1971b) based his calculations on a cinematographic recording of a person, who ruptured an achilles tendon partially when during running suddenly altering running direction. The ordinary running push-offs were calculated to be about 2,000 N, while the injury occurred at 4,340 N. This value relates well to the ultimate tensile strength of this tendon, which Stucke (1950) by *in vitro* testing found to be about 4,000N.

Some other such calculations are less credible at our present stage of knowledge of tendon properties. Grafe (1969) thus claimed that the maximum load on the two achilles tendons was 10,500 N during the take-off to the second half of a double somersault. This would mean that one of the tendons would be subjected to more than 5,250 N in case of unintentional asymmetry and that achilles tendon injuries would be a rather common athletics injury. This figure should be compared with the maximum *in vitro* tensile strength of about 4,000 N reported by Stucke (1950). One possible difference might be that the viscous elements participate more during dynamic *in vivo* loading than during static *in vitro* loading. It is doubtful whether the capacity to absorb energy increases that much during dynamic loading. The evaluation of these conflicting results is difficult, since data on energy absorption are lacking in both studies.

Conclusions derived from such indirect calculations should, therefore, be interpreted with caution and await confirmation from actual force and strain data from a suitable animal model is available.

Influence of physical stimuli on normal tissues

Physical training

Physical exercise has besides the well-known local effects (for review see Viidik 1986) also systemic effects on connective tissues, both biochemical and biomechanical. The *systemic* influence of training in man can be recorded in *e.g.* the skin of the medial side of the upper arm as increased elastic stiffness and effectiveness (Suominen *et al.* 1978). Hydroxyproline concentration increases at the same time. Such an increased concentration has also been reported in trained mice (Kiiskinen & Heikkinen 1976).

There is no consistent pattern in the reports regarding the *local* influence of physical training. Increased strength of have been reported for rabbit (Viidik 1967) and dog (Tipton *et al.* 1970) ligaments and those in male rats (Tipton *et al.* 1974), while no such effect was found for female rats (Booth & Tipton 1969). Likewise, while there are effects on tendons in rabbits (Viidik 1967, 1969), no changes were found in mice (Kiiskinen 1977). A plausible explanation is differences between species and between tendon and ligament types.

Woo *et al.* (1980, 1982) demonstrated that the initial flexor stiffness of flexor tendons did not increase in trained pigs compared to sedentary ones, while there was a pronounced effect on extensor tendons. By comparing these two types of tendons they found that the extensor tendons were initially less stiff than the flexor tendons. The stiffness of extensor tendons increased after training to the same level as that of both trained and control flexor tendons. These result are in agreement with Elliott & Crawford (1965), who noted that the maximum tetanic contraction force in flexor muscles is higher than in extensors. The normal functional demand seems to be higher on flexor than extensor muscles, since they have a higher collagen content per unit tendon length.

It might be concluded that some tendons have reached their "trainability" limit during habitual living, while others are less heavily used and therefore have the potential to respond to physical training.

Our knowledge of the effects of training on the viscoelastic properties of tendons is nonexisting and that of ligaments limited. Viidik (1968b) found the stress relaxation in rabbit anterior cruciate ligaments more pronounced after exercise. This implies that the viscous component is larger, which could result in a larger safety margin in dynamic loading. Confirmative dynamic testings should be performed.

Immobilization

It becomes evident from reviewing the literature on the effects of immobilization on tendons and ligaments that physical stimuli are required to maintain the balance of the continuous biochemical turnover processes. The responses of a joint and its periarticular tissues seem to be quite different: While the periarticular tissues stiffen, the ligaments weaken.

The periarticular tissues of an immobilized joint stiffen, which results in joint contracture, with concomitant loss of water and proteoglycans (measured as hexosamines) and an increase of reducible cross-links in an unchanged collagen mass (Akeson *et al.* 1974, 1977).

The ligaments and their insertions into bone weaken considerably (*e.g.* Tipton *et al.* 1970, Laos *et al.* 1971, Noyes *et al.* 1974, Noyes 1977, Woo *et al.* 1975, 1982, Larsen *et al.* 1987). No comprehensive data are available on the corresponding biochemical events.

One major problem with interpreting these results is the differentiation between the effects of immobilization: the osteoporosis at the insertion site and the changes in the ligament. Noyes *et al.* (1974) studied primate anterior cruciate ligaments and found that the incidence of femoral avulsions increased after immobilization, while the percentage of ruptures in the ligament substance decreased. Noyes (1977) subsequently analyzed the insertion sites histologically and found no evidence for changes; no quantitative assessment was made. He found, on the other hand, pronounced bone resorption in the tibial insertion of the medial collateral ligament. Larsen *et al.* (1987) also noted an increase of avulsion type failures in their study of cruciate ligaments in rats.

Woo *et al.* (1982) showed conclusively that the ligament substance as such was drastically weakened by testing the lateral collateral ligament without its bone insertions and the medial one as a bone-ligament-bone complex. In the last mentioned study both the isolated ligament and the complex showed a considerably shallower toe segment, lower elastic stiffness, ultimate load and failure energy. Most of these parameters decreased by about two thirds compared to controls for the medial ligament and less for the lateral one. The changes seem to occur in the ligament substance, since the cross-sectional area was not decreased.

These changes are, however not irreversible. Both Noyes *et al.* (1974) and Larsen *et al.* (1987) demonstrated that retraining is possible. The primates of Noyes *et al.* (1974) had recovered after 5 months of normal life in cages (the only length of time tested) from eight weeks of immobilization. The rats of Larsen *et al.* (1987) recovered after six weeks of training following four weeks of immobilization. The data do not allow for conclusions whether there are species differences or whether the prognosis for recovery depends on immobilization time or whether to what extent an active training program accelerates recovery.

These data show that immobilization effects are twofold, one on the ligament substance and an additional one on the insertions, and that recovery from the effects is possible.

Wound healing

The purpose of wound healing is to restore continuity of the tissue between the wound edges after a trauma. This occurs in most tissues by a connective tissue scar, which bridges the defect. This healing results in mechanically weak tissues in a scar that is stronger than the original tissue. The restoration of the strong, dense parallel-fibered collagenous structure of tendons and ligaments is on the other hand difficult, if not impossible to attain (for review see *Viidik & Gottrup* 1986).

Normal healing

Granulation tissue is cellular and vascular. It contains collagen fibers laid down in a random pattern and shows, especially in the early phases of organization, some "unscheduled" waviness (Frank *et al.* 1983a, Hutton & Ferris 1984). Hirsch (1974) studied the tendon of the short peroneal muscle in rabbits and found that the increase of breaking load of tendons increased very slowly and had attained 2, 7, 13, 38 and 67 percent of the intact value after 7, 14, 28, 56 and 168 days respectively. Using the medial collateral ligament in rabbits Frank *et al.* (1983a) found similar values, 60 and 70 percent of the intact value after 98 and 280 days of healing. The latter study also reported on the fiber structure (studied light microscopically). The fiber pattern tended with time become more regular, but even after 280 days could some irregularities be seen. Similar irregularities persist in ligaments beyond 98 days of healing (Frank *et al.* 1983b). How the new fibrils attach to the "old" tissue is not clear.

The failure to heal rapidly is caused by the inability of the reparative process to make a parallel-fibered "scar". Also for intact tissues there is a pronounced interrelationship between fiber orientation and mechanical properties. Fig. 9 illustrates such a drastic difference between a parallel-fibred tendon and skin, a three-dimensional meshwork. "Stress" is in both instances calculated as load per unit collagen per unit specimen length so that the difference of collagen concentration is eliminated. Also minor changes in the fiber pattern are important. Fig. 10 shows the differences in mechanical properties of skin when tested along (TR) and at a right angle (LO) to the main fiber direction in the meshwork.

Influence of physical stimuli on healing

Mechanical exercising as well as the lack of it influences profoundly the mature intact tendon or ligament. Such stimuli seem to be even more important for the healing tissue. Woo *et al.* (1981) showed in a study on healing flexor tendons in the dog that the strength after immobilization was 21 percent of that of the intact tendon, while passive motion resulted in an increase to 33 percent. Gelberman *et al.* subsequently showed that the rate of healing is enhanced already one week of healing.

Similar results have been reported for ligaments. Vailas *et al.* (1981) found that the separation force for healing medial collateral ligaments after two weeks of casting followed by six weeks of exercise was 111 percent of the intact value. The corresponding value after eight weeks in cast was only 54 percent. These figures should, however be recalculated

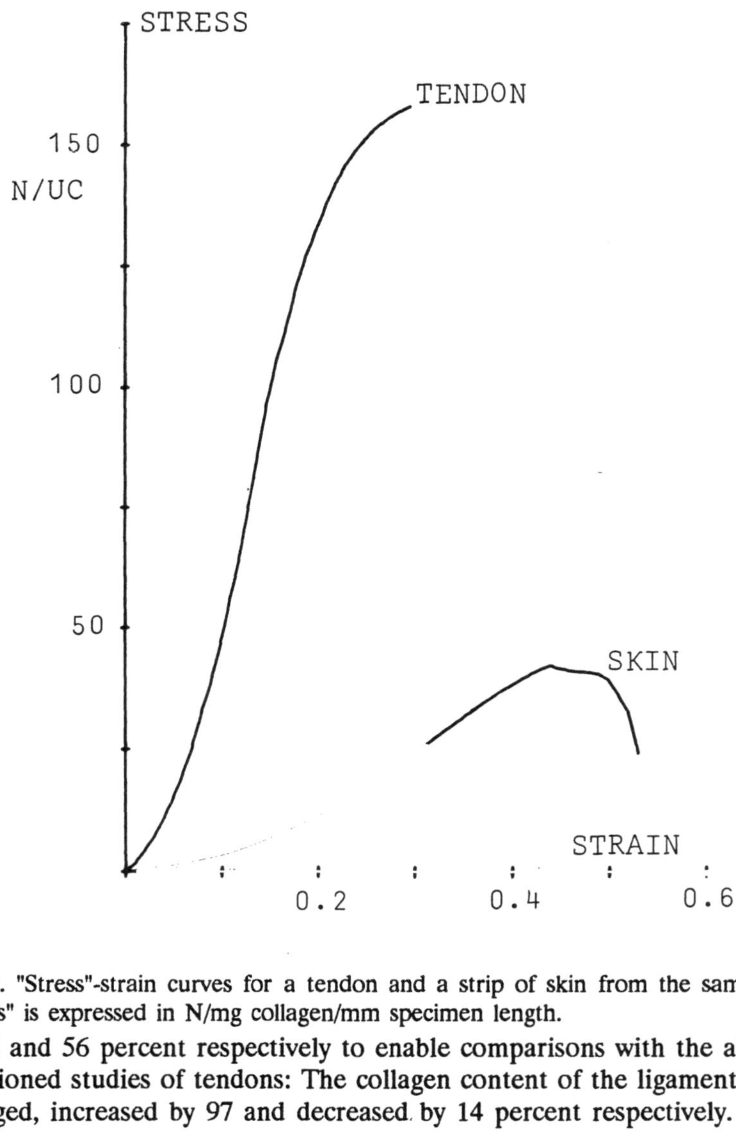

Fig. 9. "Stress"-strain curves for a tendon and a strip of skin from the same rat. "Stress" is expressed in N/mg collagen/mm specimen length.

to 64 and 56 percent respectively to enable comparisons with the above-mentioned studies of tendons: The collagen content of the ligaments had changed, increased by 97 and decreased by 14 percent respectively.

Other influences on healing

A large number of other factors influence the formation of granulation tissue and the healing process. Most of them are negative and include hypoxia, corticosteroids and other pharmacological agents (*e.g.* non-steroid antiinflammatory drugs [NSAIDs] and D-penicillamine), diabetes mellitus, and aging. Little is known about the effects on the mechanical properties of healing tendons and ligaments.

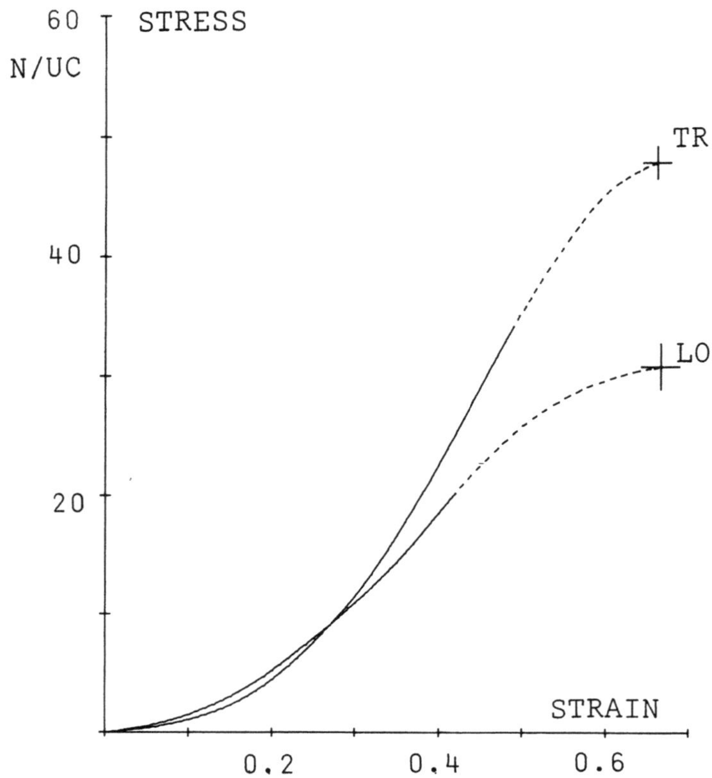

Fig. 10. "Stress"-strain curves for strips of skin from the same rat, tested along (TR) and at a right angle to the main fiber direction. "Stress" is expressed in n/mg collagen/mm specimen length.

Hypoxia is well-known to impair healing and occurs as an effect of *e.g.* traumatologic or diabetic lesions to blood vessels. The normal increase of scar strength can be severely impaired and threaten the survival of the healing tissue. Quirinia & Viidik (1989, 1990) developed an ischemic skin flap model, in which the tensile strength of the wound is "normally" decreased by about 40 percent, as are the other mechanical parameters. Hyperbaric oxygen in the early phase of healing improved the mechanical properties significantly. It remains to develop a corresponding model for tendons or ligaments, tissues which normally are by far less vascular than skin.

Carlstedt (1987) found that indomethacin, a NSAID, increased the tensile strength of healing plantaris longus tendon in the rabbit. Larsen & Viidik (1988) came to the same conclusion regarding healing of skin wounds. It should be noted that this effect is quite contrary to that on callus formation after fracture.

There are numerous reports in the literature on attempts to improve normal wounds in a variety of tissues. Most of them have failed. One exception is electromagnetic stimulation, which Frank *et al.* (1983c) found to stimulate healing medial collateral ligaments in rabbits somewhat.

Concluding remark

We need our connective tissue and in good shape whatever we do. This discussion has focused on the mechanical properties of tendons and ligaments and the underlying structural basis for these properties. It would be worthwhile to remember that there are also other connective tissue structures in the organism, which we need as much as we need our tendons and ligaments. To quote Arcadi (1952):

"If by some magic solution one could dissolve all the connective tissue of the body, all that would remain would be a mass of slimy epithelium, quivering muscle and frustrated nerve cells."

There would not even be any bone or cartilage.

References

Åkerblom B: Standing and Sitting Posture. Stockholm, Nordiska Bokhandeln, 1948.

Akeson WH, Woo SL-Y Maiel D, Matthews JV: Biomechanical and biochemical changes in the periarticular connective tissue during contracture development in the immobilized rabbit knee. Conn Tiss Res 1974;2:315-323.

Akeson WH, Amiel D, Mechanic GL, Woo SL-Y, Harwood FL & Hamer ML: Collagen cross-linking alterations in joint contractures: Changes in the reducible cross-links in periarticular connective tissue collagen after nine weeks of immobilization. Conn Tiss Res 1977;5:15-20.

Alexander RM: Visco-elastic properties of the body-wall of sea anemones. J exp Biol 1962;39:373-386.

Alfrey T, Gurnee EF: Molecular structure and mechanical behaviour of macromolecules, in Remington JW (ed): Tissue Elasticity. Washington, Amer Phys Soc, 1957;12-32.

Arcadi: Quoted from Hansen TM: Cyclophosphamide and Collagen. Copenhagen, Lægeforeningens Forlag, 1979.

Bailey AJ, Etherington DJ: Metabolism of collagen and elastin, in Florkin M, Neuberger A (eds): Comprehensive Biochemistry, Vol 19B, Part I, Protein Metabolism. Amsterdam, Elsevier, 1980, pp 299-408.

Barenberg SA, Filisko FE Geil PH: Ultrastructural deformation of collagen. Conn Tiss Res 1878;6:25-35.

Barfred T: Experimental rupture of the achilles tendon. Acta Orthop Scand 1971a;42:528-543.

Barfred T: Kinesiological comments on subcutaneous ruptures of the achilles tendon. Acta Orthop Scand 1971b;42:397-405.

Barnes GRG,Pinder DN: In vivo tendon tension and bone strain measurement and correlation. J Biomechanics 1974;7:35-42.

Booth FW, Tipton CM: Effects of training and 17-B estradiol upon heart rates, organ weights, and ligamentous strength of female rats. Intern Zschr angew Physiol 1969;27:187-197.

Brodsky B, Tamaka S, Eikenberry EF: X-ray diffraction as a tool for studying collagen structure, in Nimni ME (ed): Collagen Vol I Biochemistry. Boca Raton, CRC Press, 1988, pp 95-112.

Carlstedt CA: Mechanical and chemical factors in tendon healing. Effects of indomethacin and surgery in the rabbit. Acta Orthop Scand 1987;58:Suppl 224.

Clark JM, Sidles JA: The interrelation of fiber bundles in the anterior cruciate ligament. J Orthop Res 1990;8:180-188.

Cohen RE, Hooley CJ, McCrum NG: The mechanism of the viscoelastic deformation of collagenous tissue. Nature 1974,247:59-61.

Cohen RE, Hooley CJ, McCrum NG: Mechanism of the viscoelastic deformation of collagenous tissue, in Atkins EDT, Keller A (eds): Structure of Fibrous Biopolymers. London, Butterworths, 1975, pp 251-254.

Cohen RE, Hooley CJ, McCrum NG: Viscoelastic creep of collagenous tissue. J Biomechanics 1976:9:175-184.

Cohen RE, Hooley CJ: A model for creep behaviour of tendon. Int J Biol Macromol 1979;1:123-132.

Cowan PM, North ACT, Randall JT: X-ray diffraction studies of collagen fibres. Symp Soc Exp H Biol 1955;9:115-126.

Davidsson L: Über die subkutanen Sehnen-Rupturen und die Regeneration der Sehne. Ann Chir Gynaec Fenniae 1956; Suppl 6.

Diamant J, Keller A, Baer E, Litt M, Arridge RGC: Collagen: ultrastructure and its relation to mechanical properties as a function of ageing. Proc Roy Soc Lond B 1972;180:293-315.

Elden HR: Physical properties of collagen fibers, in Hall DA (ed): International Review of Connective Tissue Research, Vol 4. New York, Academic Press, 1968, pp 283-348.

Elliott DH, Crawford GNC: The thickness and collagen content of tendon relative to the strength and cross-sectional area of muscle. Proc Roy Soc Lond B 1965;162:137-146.

Frank C, Woo SL-Y, Amiel D, Harwood F, Gomez M, Akeson W: Medial collateral ligament healing. A multidisciplinary assessment in rabbits. Am J Sports Med 1983a;11:379-389.

Frank C, Amiel D, Akeson WH: Healing of the medial collateral ligament of the knee. A morphological and biochemical assessment in rabbits. Acta Orthop Scand 1983b;54:917-923.

Frank C, Schachar N, Dittrich D, Shrive N, DeHaas W, Edwards G: Electromagnetic stimulation of ligament healing in rabbits. Clin Orthop Rel Res 1983c;175:263-272.

Frank C, Woo SL-Y, Andriacchi T, Brand R, Oakes B, Dahners L, DeHaven K, Lewis J, Sabiston P: Normal ligament: structure, function, and composition, in Woo SL-Y, Buckwalter JA (eds): Injury and Repair of the Musculoskeletal Soft Tissues. Park Ridge, American Academy of Orthopaedic Surgeons, 1987, pp 45-101.

Frisén M, Mägi M, Sonnerup L, Viidik A: Rheological analysis of soft collagenous tissues. Part I: Theoretical considerations. J Biomechanics 1969;2:13-20.

Frisén M. Mägi M, Sonnerup L, Viidik a: Rheological analysis of soft collagenous tissues. Part II: Experimental evaluations and verifications. J Biomechanics 1969;2:21-28.

Fung YCB: Elasticity of soft tissues in simple elongation. Amer J Physiol 1967;213: 1552-1544.

Fung YCB: Biomechanics, its scope, history and some problems of continuum mechanics in physiology. App Mech Rev 1968;21-1-20.

Fung YCB: Stress-strain history relations of soft tissues in simple elongation, in Fung YCB, Perrone N, Anliker M (eds): Biomechanics: its foundations and objectives. Englewood Cliffs, Prentice-Hall, 1972, pp 181-208.

Fung YC: Biomechanics - Mechanical properties of living tissues. New York, Springer-Verlag, 1981.

Gathercole LJ, Keller A: X-ray diffraction effects related to superstructure in rat tail tendon collagen. Biochim Biophys Acta 1978;535:253-271.

Gathercole LJ, Keller A, Shah JS: The periodic pattern in native tendon collagen; correlation of polarizing with scanning electron microscopy. J Microscopy 1974;102:95-106.

Gelbermann R, Goldberg V, An K-N, Banes A: Tendon, in Woo SL-Y, Buckwalter JA (eds): Injury and Repair of the Musculoskeletal Soft Tissues. Park Ridge, American Academy of Orthopaedic Surgeons, 1987, pp 5-40.

Gelberman RH, Woo SL-Y, Lothringer K, Akeson WH, Amiel D: Effects of early intermittent passive mobilization on healing canine flexor tendons. J Hand Surg 1982;7:170-175.

Grafe H: Aspekte zur Ätiologie der subkutanen Achillessehnenruptur. Zbl Chir 1969;94:1073-1082.

Haut RC, Little RW: A constitutive equation for collagen fibers. J Biomechanics 1972;5:423-430.

Harkness RD: Mechanical properties of collagenous tissues. in Gold BS (ed): Treatise on Collagen, Vol 2 Biology of Collagen Part A. London, Academic Press, 1968, pp 247-310.

Hirsch G: Tensile properties during tendon healing. Acta Orthop Scand 1974;Suppl 153.

Hooley CJ: The Viscoelastic Behaviour of Tendon, *thesis,* Oxford University, 1977.

Hutton P, Ferris B: in Bucknail TE, Ellis H (eds): Wound Healing for Surgeons. London, Ballière Tindall, 1984, pp 286-296.

Kennedy JC, Hawkins RJ, Willis RB: Strain gauge analysis of knee ligaments. Clin Orthop Rel Res 1977;129:225-229.

Kiiskinen A: Physical training and connective tissues in young mice. Physical properties of Achilles tendons and long bones. Growth 1977;44:123-137.

Kiiskinen A, Heikkinen E:Physical training and connective tissues in young mice. Brit J Derm 1976;95:525-529.

Labat-Robert J, Robert L: Interactions between structural glycoproteins and collagen, in Nimni ME (ed): Collagen, Vol I Biochemistry, Boca Raton, CRC Press, 1988,173-186.

Laos GS, Tipton CM, Cooper RR: Influence of physical activity on ligament insertions in the knees of dogs. J Bone Joint Surg 1971;53A:275-286.

Larsen AQ, Viidik A: The influence of diclofenac sodium and indomethacin on healing incisional wounds in skin. Eur Surg Res 1988;20:Suppl 1:58-59.

Larsen NP, Forwood MR, Parker AW: Immobilization and retraining of cruciate ligaments in the rat. Acta Orthop Scand 1987;58:260-264.

Lewis JL: A note on the application and evaluation of the buckle transducer for knee ligament force. J Biomech Engng 1982;104:125-128.

Morgan FR: The mechanical properties of collagen fibres: stress-strain curves. J Soc Leather Trades' Chem 1960;44:170-182.
Nemetschek T, Jonak R, Nemetschek-Gansler H, Riedl H: Über die Bestimmung von Langperioden-Änderungen am Kollagen. Z Naturforsch 1978;33C:928-936.
Nimni ME, Harkness RD: Molecular structures and functions of collagen, in Nimni ME (ed): Collagen, Vol I Biochemistry. Boca Raton, CRC Press, 1988, pp 1-77.
Noyes FR: Functional properties of knee ligaments and alterations induced by immobilization. Clin Orthop Rel Res 1977;123:240-242.
Noyes FR, Torvik PJ, Hyde WB, De Lucas JL: Biomechanics of ligament failure. II: An analysis of immobilization, exercise and reconditioning effects in primates. J Bone Joint Surg 1974;56A:1406-1418.
Qurinia A, Viidik A: Hyperbaric oxygen improves the healing of ischaemic flaps but not incisional wounds in skin. Eur Surg Res 1989;21:Suppl 2:81-82.
Qurinia A, Viidik A: Design of an ischaemic double flap model, an investigation of blood flow and biomechanical properties, in Hvid I (ed): Proceedings of the 7th Meeting of the European Society of Biomechanics. Aarhus, Aarhus University, *in press*.
Riedl H, Nemetschek T, Jonak R: A mathematical model for the changes of the long-period structure in collagen, in Viidik A, Vuust J (eds): Biology of Collagen, London Academic Press, 1980, pp 289-296.
Ruggeri A, Benazzo F: Collagen-proteoglycan interaction, in Ruggeri a, Motta PM (eds): Ultrastructure of the Connective Tissue Matrix. Boston, Martinus Nijhoff, 1984, pp 113-125.
Rundgren Å: Physical properties of connective tissue as influenced by single and repeated pregnancies in the rat. Acta Physiol Scand 1974;Suppl 417.
Simon PJ: The Mechanics of Tendon Function in Health and Disease, *thesis*, Massey University, Palmerston North, New Zealand, 1978.
Suominen H, Heikkinen E, Moisio H, Viljama K: Physical and chemical properties of skin in habitually trained and sedentary 31- to 70-year-old men. Brit J Derm 1978;99:147-154.
Stucke K: Über das elastische Verhalten der Achillessehne im Belastungsversuch. Langenbecks Arch klin Chir 1950;265:579-599.
Tipton CM, James SL, Mergner W, Tchang TK: Influence of exercise on strength of medial collateral knee ligaments of dogs. Am J Physiol 1970;218:894-901.
Tipton CM, Matthes RD, Sandage DS: In situ measurement of junction strength and ligament elongation in rats. J Appl Physiol 1974;37:758-761.
Viidik A: The effect of training on the tensile strength of isolated rabbit tendons. Scand J Plast Reconstr Surg 1967;1:141-147.
Viidik A: A rheological model for uncalcified parallel-fibred collagenous tissue. J Biomechanics 1968a;1:3-11.
Viidik A: Elasticity and tensile strength of the anterior cruciate ligament in rabbits as influenced by training. Acta Physiol Scand 1968b;74:372-380.
Viidik A: Tensile properties of achilles tendon systems in trained and untrained rabbits. Acta Orthop Scand 1969;40:261-272.
Viidik A: Simultaneous mechanical and light microscopic studies of collagen fibers. Z Anat Entwickl-Ges 1972;136:204-212.
Viidik A: Functional properties of collagenous tissues, in Hall DA, Jackson DS (eds): International Review of Connective Tissue Research. New York, Academic

Press, 1973;6:127-215.
Viidik A: On the correlation between structure and mechanical function of soft connective tissues. Verh Anat Ges 1978;72:75-89.
Viidik A: Connective tissues - possible implications of the temporal changes for the aging process. Mech Age Dev 1979a;9:267-285.
Viidik A: Biomechanical behavior of soft connective tissues, in Akkaş N (ed): Progress in Biomechanics. Alphen aan den Rijn, Sijthoff & Nordhoff, 1979b, pp 75-113.
Viidik A: Mechanical properties of parallel-fibred collagenous tissues, in Viidik A, Vuust J (eds): Biology of Collagen. London, Academic Press, 1980a, pp 237-255.
Viidik A: Interdependence between structure and function in collagenous tissues, in Viidik A, Vuust J (eds): Biology of Collagen. London, Academic Press, 1980b, pp 257-280.
Viidik A: Age-related changes in connective tissues, in Viidik A (ed): Lectures on Gerontology, Vol 1, Part A, On the Biology of Ageing. London, Academic Press, 1982, pp 173-211.
Viidik A. Adaptability of connective tissues, in Saltin B (ed): Biochemistry of Exercise - Metabolic Regulation and its Practical Significance. Camagne, Human Kinetics Publishers, 1986, pp 545-562.
Viidik A: Properties of tendons and ligaments, in Skalak R, Chien S (eds): Handbook of Bioengineering. New York, McGraw-Hill, 1987a, pp 6.1-6.19.
Viidik A: Biomechanics of tendons and other soft tissues - testing methods and structure-function interdependence, in Bergmann G, Kölbel R, Rohlmann A (eds): Biomechanics: Basic and applied Research. Dordrecht, Martinus Nijhoff, 1987b, pp 59-72.
Viidik A: Connections between muscle and bone, in Payne PA (ed): Concise Encyclopaedia on Biomedical and Biological Measurement Systems. Oxford, Pergamon Press, *in press*.
Viidik A, Danielsen CC, Oxlund H: On fundamental and phenomenological models, structure and mechanical properties of collagen, elastin and glycosaminoglycans. Biorheology 1982;19:437-451.
Viidik A, Ekholm R: Light and electron microscopic studies of collagen fibers under strain. Z Anat Entwickl-Ges 1968;127:154-164.
Viidik A, Gottrup F: Mechanics of healing soft tissue wounds, in Schmid-Schönbein GR, Woo SL-Y, Zweifach BW (eds): Frontiers in Biomechanics. New York, Springer-Verlag, 1986, pp 262-279.
Viidik A, Sandqvist L, Mägi M: Influence of postmortal storage on the tensile strength characteristics and histology of rabbit ligaments. Acta Orthop Scand 1965;Suppl 79.
Wertheim MG: Mémoire sur l'élasticité et la cohésion des principaux tissus du corps humain. Chim Phys 1947;21:385-414.
Woo SL-Y, Akeson WH, Amiel D, Convey FR, Matthews JV: The connective tissue response to immobility: A correlative study of the biomechanical and biochemical measurements of the normal and immobilized rabbit knee. Arth and Rheum 1975;18:257-264.
Woo SL-Y, Akeson WH, Jemmott GF: Measurements of nonhomogeneous directional mechanical properties of articular cartilage in tension using a video-dimensional analyzer. J Biomech 1976;9:785-791.

Woo SL-Y, Ritter MA, Maiel D, Sanders TM, Gomez MA, Kuei SC, Garfin SR, Akesson WH: The biomechanical and biochemical properties of swine tendons - long term effects of exercise on the digital extensors. Conn Tiss Res 1980;7:177-183.

Woo SL-Y, Gomez MA, Woo Y-K, Akeson WH: Mechanical properties of tendons and ligaments. II. The relationship between immobilization and exercise on tissue remodeling. Biorheology 1982;19:397-408.

Woo SL-Y, Gomez MA, Seguchi Y, Endo CM, Akeson WH: Measurement of mechanical properties of ligament substance from a bone-ligament-bone preparation. J Orthop Res 1983;1:22-29.

Woo SL-Y, Orlande CA, Gomez MS, Frank CB, Akeson WH: Tensile properties of medial collateral ligament as a dunction of age. J Orthop Res 1986;4:333-341.

Woodhead-Galloway J: Two theories of the structure of the collagen fibril, in Hukins DWL (ed): Connective Tissue Matrix. Deerfield Beach, Weinheim, 1984 133-160.

Yahia L-H, Dorwin G: Microscopical investigation of canine anterior cruciate ligament ant patellar tendon: collagen fascicle morphology and architecture. J Orthop Res 1989;7:243-251.

Chapter 2

The Biology of Tendons and Ligaments

C.B. Frank, and D.A. Hart

Introduction

As noted in the previous chapter and as reviewed extensively elsewhere (Frank 1985, 1988; Akeson 1984), both tendons and ligaments are highly complex structures with a number of unique functional characteristics. While similar in many ways, tendons and ligaments have some important differences in both structure and function which should be appreciated. Further, it is important to recognize that despite their relatively simple appearances, tendons and ligaments are not homogeneous, static structures that simply serve to connect different elements of the musculoskeletal system. Instead, they are both structurally and biologically heterogeneous and surprisingly dynamic in their responses to the environment.

In this chapter, we present an overview of normal tendon and ligament cell biology, pointing out some of their surprising heterogeneities before providing examples of the normal dynamic responses of these tissues to a variety of stimuli (eg. during growth and maturation, loading and inflammation). We will also provide some insights into new approaches which will undoubtedly reveal much more about the biology of these tissues -- an area which has lagged behind the understanding of their functions.

Tendon and Ligament Heterogeneity

Gross Appearances

Tendons and ligaments belong to a family of skeletal structures known as "dense connective tissues" (Akeson 1984). This classification is based partly on the gross appearances of these tissues and partly on their microscopic nature.

Grossly, both tendons and ligaments are similar in appearing to be firm white bands or cords of connective tissue stretching between their respective points of attachment (Figure 1). In the case of tendons, these attachments are to muscle at one end and bone at the other, with the tendon usually being named by the name of its muscle (eg. extensor digitorum longus tendon). Ligaments, on the other hand, are distinguished by being attached to bone at both ends, usually spanning a diarthrodial joint, and being named by those points of boney attachment (eg. calcaneofibular ligament). As noted elsewhere (Frank 1985, 1988), many ligaments have been named based on a variety of factors other than these attachments, such as: shapes (eg. deltoid), relationships to joints (eg. collateral), and relationships to each other (eg. cruciate). At this point in time there is no reasonable biological classification system of tendons or ligaments.

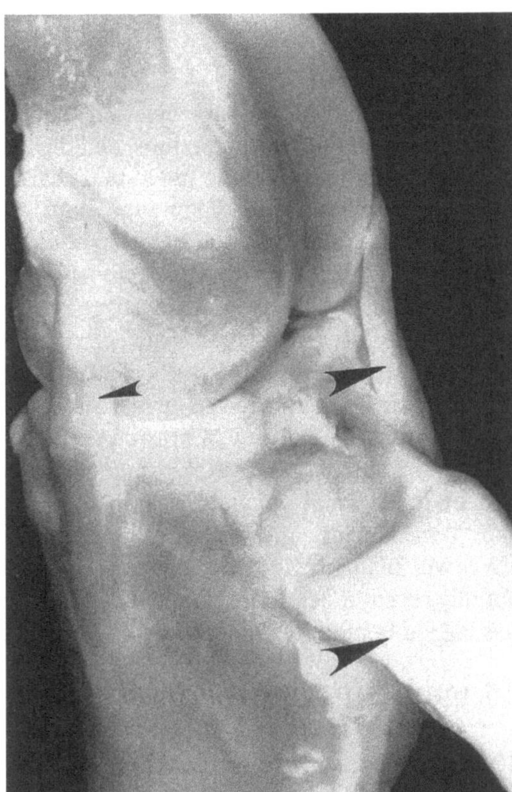

Figure 1: Photograph of a rabbit knee joint, showing apparently similar dense white ligamentous (small arrow) and tendonous (large arrows) structures.

On closer inspection, tendons and ligaments have other similarities in that both appear to be composed of nearly parallel fibers of connective tissue elements which, in many structures, appear to be organized into definite "bundles" or even larger "bands" (Jackson 1984). In other situations, however, both tendons and ligaments do not appear to have these subdivisions (eg. capsular ligaments are very difficult to separate). In those cases, this homogeneous gross appearance may be somewhat misleading and may be a function of the gross masking of internal tendon or ligament architecture by surface layers of tissue known as epitenon (Gelberman 1988) in the case of tendons, and epiligament (Berger 1984) in the case of ligaments. In some situations, such as in the cruciate ligaments of the knee joint, this surface structure is further obscured by the presence of surrounding synovium but subdivisions may become apparent when the structure is seen in cross-section (Yahia 1989; Kennedy 1974).

With surface layers still intact, one of the most striking features of both tendons and ligaments are their white glistening appearances. As compared with surrounding tissues, they are therefore easily perceived to be much less vascular (ie. less red) than most other tissues, having only occasional vessels on their surfaces. Similarly, tendons and ligaments probably have very subtle innervation, which is easily disrupted and thus easily missed at the time of gross dissection. Despite these impressions, with careful histological inspection, both fine vascularity and fine innervation of ligaments can be revealed (Frank 1988; Bray R 1990, 1990a).

Microscopic Appearances

Midsubstance Similarities

As noted in the previous chapter, both tendons and ligaments are similar histologically in their substance and are characterized by having relatively sparsely distributed cells, separated by nearly parallel arrangements of largely collagenous matrix. It is this relative paucity of cells (as compared with other connective tissues) and organization of matrix that led to the grouping of tendons and ligaments into one family of tissues. In this chapter we will not concentrate on the characteristics of that dense matrix but, rather, we will discuss some characteristics of the cells that are found within that matrix in both tendons and ligaments.

The midsubstance of both tendons and ligaments contain cells which have been variably called fibroblasts by some and fibrocytes by others (Amiel 1983). These generic descriptions differ only in their implied proliferative and metabolic potential with "blastic" cells presumably having the more dynamic connotation. Unfortunately, there do not seem to be any definite criteria for this separation in these tissues -- a deficiency with important implications in terms of growth and healing potential. Unpublished data in our laboratory suggests that there are only a very small number of midsubstance cells in an adolescent rabbit medial collateral ligament (MCL) with *in situ* proliferative capability, as estimated by *in vivo* pulsed H^3-thymidine uptake (Figure 2A). With *in vitro* incubation in H^3-proline, a collagen precursor, it would appear that a much higher percentage of these same midsubstance cells are metabolically active (Frank 1988a). It is of course unknown whether these represent activities of unique cell types, or whether there is a single cell population in different phases of proliferation and metabolic activity. Based on this evidence, however, we speculate that there is more than one major type of fibrous cell present in adolescent ligament midsubstance. The most common cells can be considered "blastic" metabolically, but are not rapidly proliferative. The second cell type may be less blastic and may or may not be from the same population.

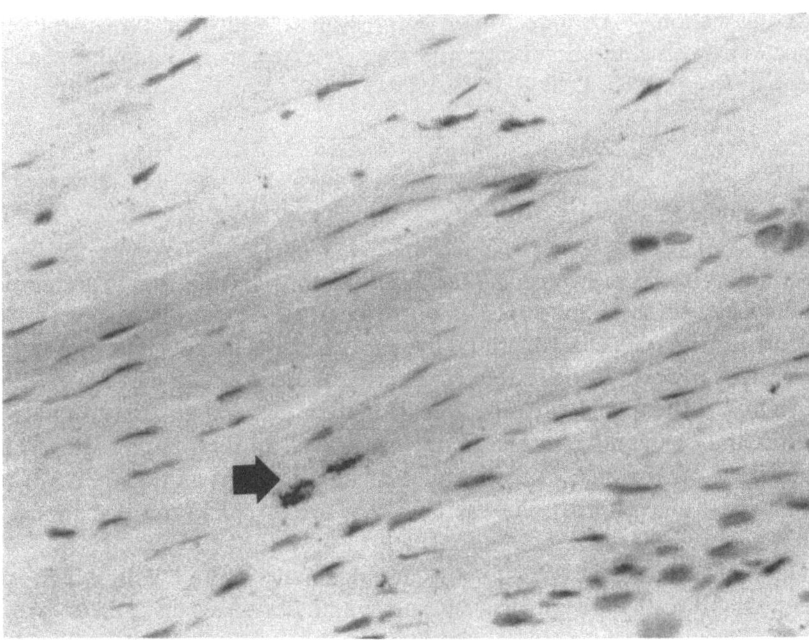

Figure 2A: Autoradiograph of adolescent rabbit MCL midsubstance from an animal pulsed with H^3-thymidine 48 hours prior to sacrifice. Only rarely are midsubstance cells (black arrow) seen to pick up this label (presumably since they are not replicating very actively).

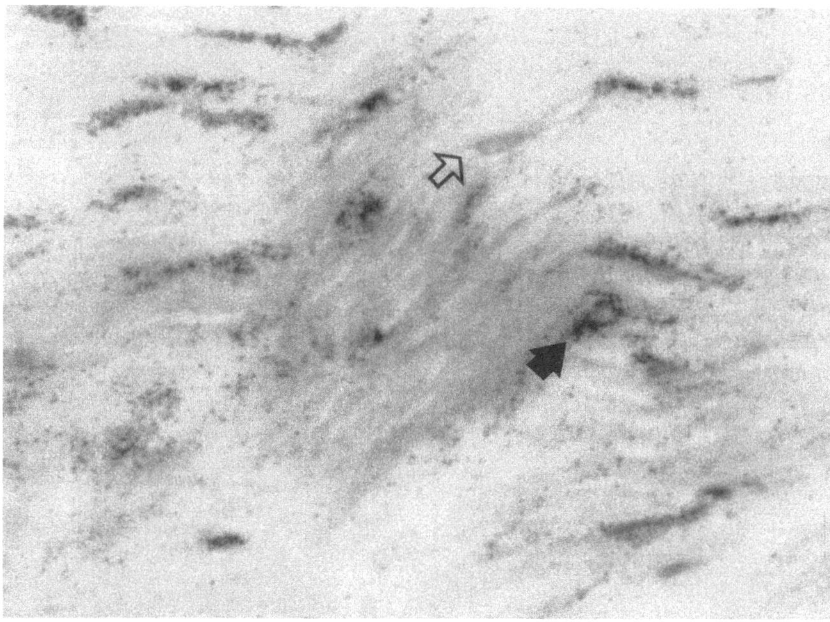

Figure 2B: Autoradiograph of rabbit MCL midsubstance after 12 hour in vitro incubation in H^3-proline. Note that about 90% of cells appear to have incorporated label in this sample (eg. dark arrow), suggesting that they were metabolically active during this interval. Some cells did not incorporate label (open arrow), possibly an artefact or possibly an indication that not all cells were active in the tissue over this interval.

Midsubstance Heterogeneity

Careful inspection of any single midsubstance tendon or ligament sample shows an interesting spectrum of subtle differences in cell sizes and shapes (Figure 3). Many of these differences are only apparent, of course, and can be attributed to cutting artefacts in which cells are sectioned at slightly different locations in their thickness, or at slightly different orientations. Some of these differences, however, may be "real" and may account for some of the subtle differences in the cell populations that are noted above metabolically. As with metabolic experiments, therefore, even simple histology suggests that there may be some sort of ligament or tendon cell "subtypes" which remain to be defined.

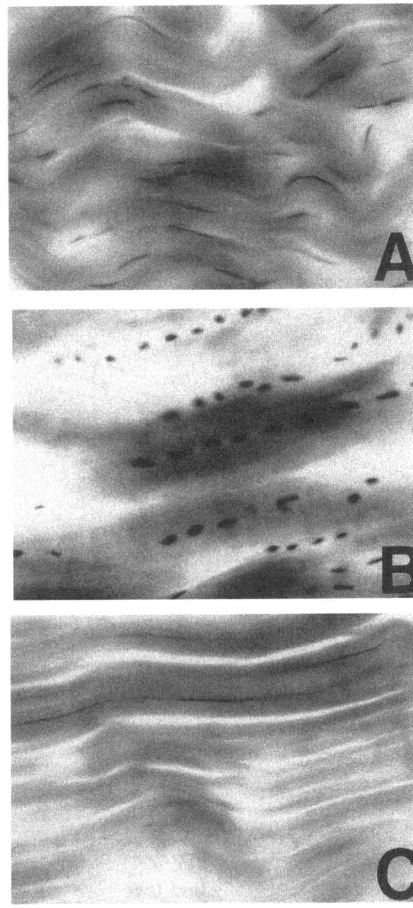

Figure 3: Histologic appearances of the midsubstance of (A) MCL, (B) ACL, and (C) patellar tendon, in the 1 year old rabbit. Note the differences in nuclear shapes between tissues as noted elsewhere by Amiel and co-workers (1983).

Structure-Specific Cell Shapes

Comparing midsubstance samples of several different rabbit ligaments and tendons reveals some not-so-subtle differences in cellular sizes, shapes and relationships (Amiel 1983). In some tissues, cells appear to be more independent than in others with most cells appearing to be isolated in a "sea of matrix". In other tissues, cells are more clearly organized in "chains", much like a series of cars in a train and much more clearly being associated within the matrix interfibrillar space.

While many of these tissues have not been sectioned serially in a thorough enough manner to make any definitive statement in this regard, evidence in the rabbit MCL (Bray D 1990) suggests that most cells, even in midsubstance, are interconnected in some way (Figure 4A). So-called "gap junctions" have also been seen at these MCL intercellular interfaces (Figure 4B), suggesting that at least some populations of cells within the MCL share communicative links. The histologic impression that ligament cells are independent may therefore be erroneous.

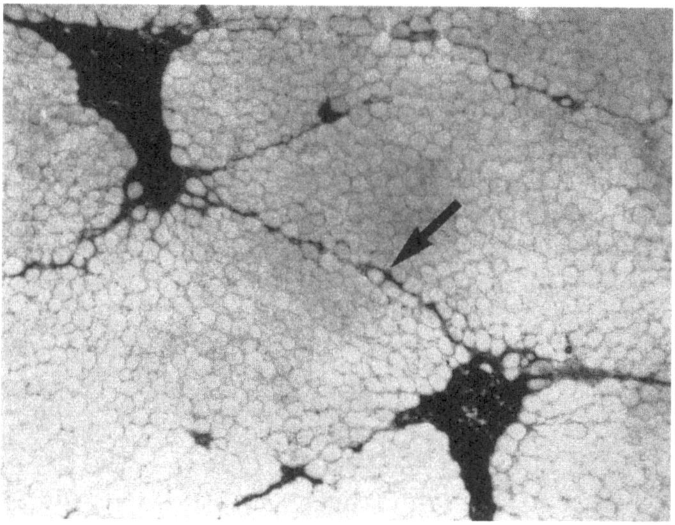

Figure 4A: Transmission E.M. photograph of ruthenium red stained MCL cross section showing apparent connections of cell processes (magnification X 16,000). Photo courtesy D. Bray.

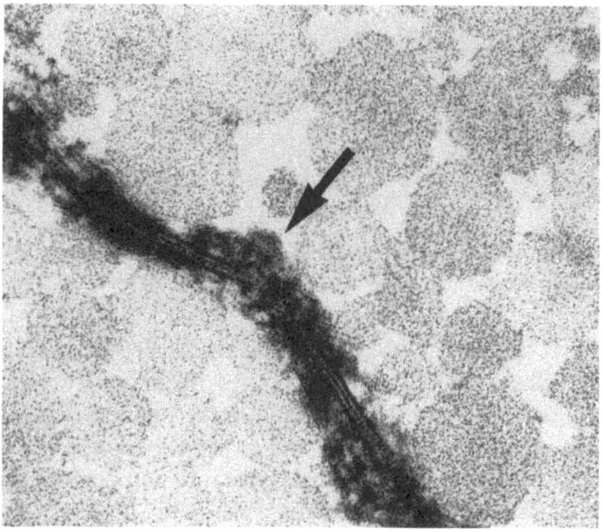

Figure 4B: High power transmission E.M. photograph of ruthenium red stained MCL section showing a junction of cell processes between two cells (magnification X 160,000). Photo courtesy D. Bray.

Tissue Surfaces

Whereas all of the observations noted above refer to tissue midsubstance in a three dimensional sense, it must be pointed out that tendons and ligaments are probably not homogeneous either radially or longitudinally. In the radial direction, both types of tissues are bounded by a unique layer of cells and matrix known as the epitenon (Gelberman 1988) for certain tendons, and epiligament (Matyas 1990) in the case of the rabbit MCL (Figure 5). Other tendons and ligaments may instead (or in addition) have an additional surface layer of synovium on them -- depending on their locations and, no doubt, on their functions.

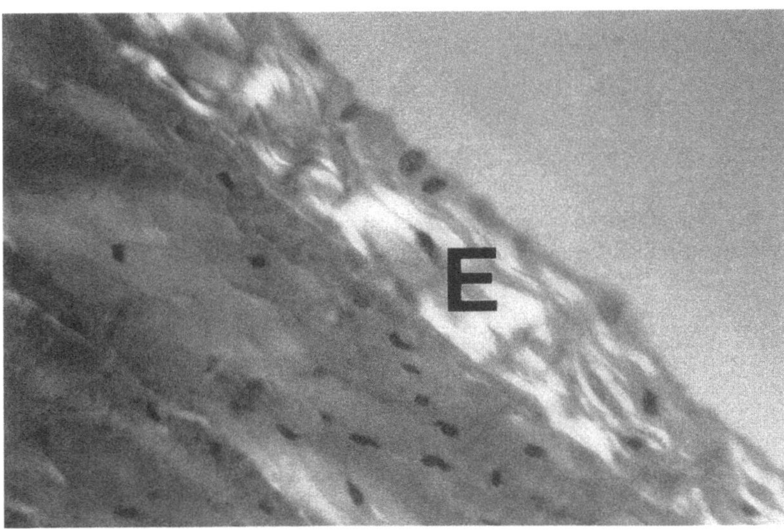

Figure 5: Photograph of MCL epiligament with polarizing light, showing unique organization of this surface layer (cross-sectional view -- magnification X 250).

In the case of the rabbit MCL, this surface layer has been shown to be quite vascular (Bray 1990a), and, like other ligaments (Schultz 1984) has been shown to contain certain specialized nerve endings (Bray 1990) which may function in both pain perception and in proprioception (Brand 1986). It is distinct from the underlying ligament substance in being hypercellular and containing much more blastic appearing cells. This impression is supported by the previously noted H^3-thymidine and H^3-proline experiments, which confirm that this layer is indeed more metabolically active and appears to have greater proliferative ability than the midsubstance itself. Based on these biological differences, it would be argued that this layer is not truly a part of the ligament substance but, instead, is a unique structure onto itself. On the other hand, based on its structural approximation and on evidence that it appears to be intermittently anchored to the classically defined MCL substance, the view can be defended that this layer *is* ligamentous (Matyas 1990, 1990a). We would further submit that, based on its complex biology, that the epiligament is almost certainly a very important component of these dense connective tissue complexes -- possibly even being analogous to, or continuous with, periosteum of bone.

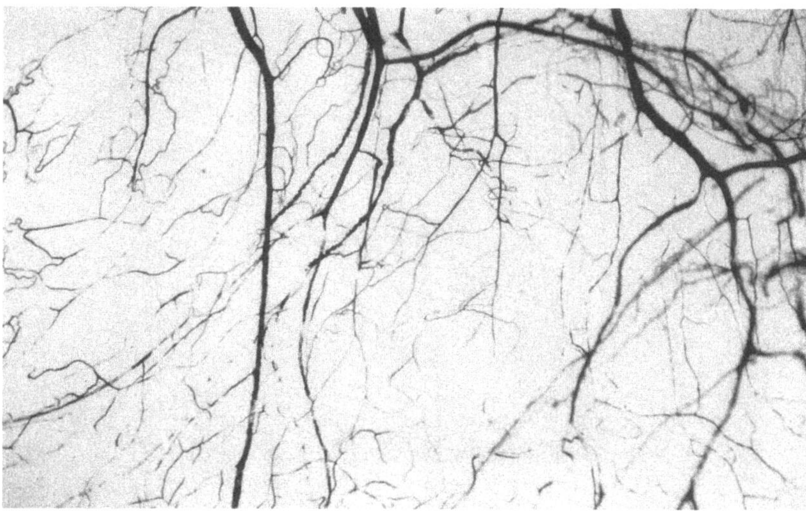

Figure 6: Vascular injection of rabbit MCL epiligament showing relatively rich blood supply. Photo courtesy R. Bray.

Insertions into Bone

As tendons or ligaments approach bones, their structural and material properties are known to change (Woo 1988) as do their appearances. Grossly, these tissues appear to simply "merge" into bones. On closer inspection, however, it is appreciated that the mechanisms by which this all-important attachment takes place is unique and dynamic. As an area of potential stress concentration, this uniqueness and dynamism is not surprising.

As noted in the classical works of Cooper (1970) and others (Matyas 1990), it is clear that the cell biology of so-called "fibrocartilagenous insertions" of tendons and ligaments is complex and probably involves more than one cell phenotype. Four cellular zones of these insertions have been described from ligament substance through a zone of fibrocartilage to a zone of calcified fibrocartilage into bone (Figure 7). The sizes and distributions of these zones is probably insertion-specific and may well depend on a variety of environmental factors (such as loading, etc.).

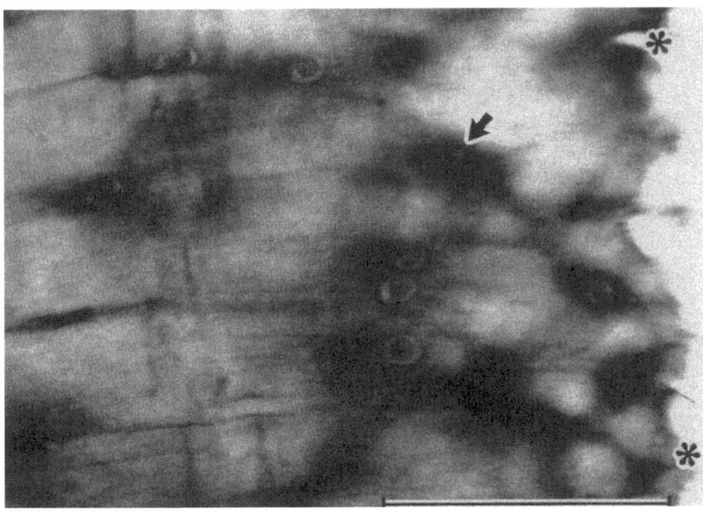

Figure 7: Fibrocartilage ligament insertion, showing zones of cell types from ligament on the left into calcified fibrocartilage on the right, (marked by asterisks). Note the pericellular staining with toluidine blue, indicating the chondroid nature of the intervening zone of fibrocartilage (Matyas 1990).

A second type of insertion involves a slightly different mechanism of attachment to bone, at least temporarily (during growth) involving attachment to periosteum. The tibial insertion of the rabbit MCL represents such a unique attachment, changing in character very dramatically during growth and maturation. The zonal changes of this insertion have been described by Matyas (1990a) with some of the cells present in each of these zones being seen pictorially in Figure 8. It is again clear from this simple histologic appearance that cellular heterogeneity exists in these insertions even in the relatively static adult condition, providing an opportunity for variable cellular responses to any number of environmental stimuli.

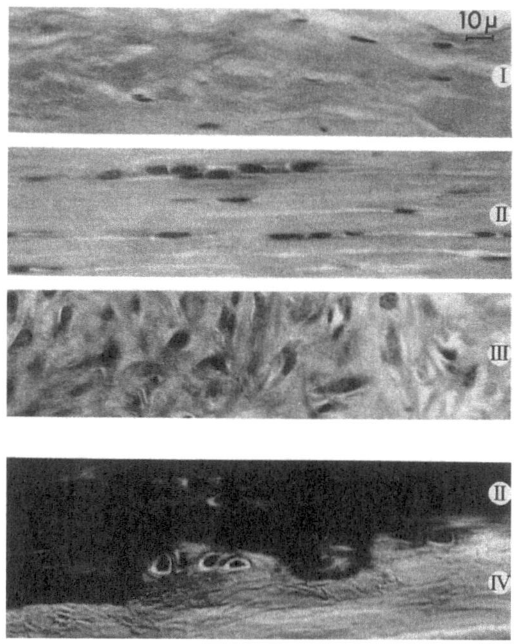

Figure 8: Tibial insertion of immature rabbit MCL showing cellular zones, numbered I though IV. Zone III disappears with maturation of this insertion, with zones II and IV becoming contiguous (bottom frame). Reproduced with permission (Matyas 1990a).

Regulation of Metabolic Activity in Ligaments and Tendons

During growth and maturation of ligaments and tendons, the tissues undergo increases in mass and alterations in biomechanical parameters. Thus, during growth there must be an anabolic environment which is followed by a state in the mature tissue which exhibits a homeostatic balance between matrix synthesis (anabolic activity) and matrix removal and remodelling (catabolic activity). This situation is not unique to these tissues and is a requirement for all differentiated tissues. However, the regulatory mechanisms controlling these processes in different tissues very likely have unique features dependent on the functional needs of the tissues.

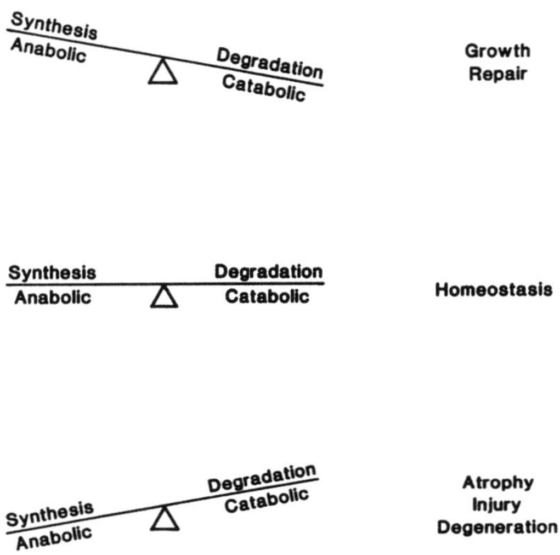

Figure 9: Metabolic regulation in connective tissue states.

The stimuli influencing tissues such as ligaments and tendons must include biochemical signals (growth factors, hormones, nutrients, matrix-cell receptor signals, inflammatory stimuli) as well as biomechanical signals generated through as yet undetermined mechanisms (Frank 1990) either directly to all cells in the matrix or via a subset of "transducer" cells.

REGULATION OF ANABOLIC/ CATABOLIC ACTIVITY

INTERNAL	EXTERNAL
Endogenous Growth Factors	Nutrients
Cell Matrix Interactions	Exogenous Growth Factors
Tissue Loading	Inflammatory Mediators
	Inflammatory Cells

TABLE 1: Stimuli influencing tissue responses.

For a connective tissue to maintain an anabolic or homeostatic state the production of matrix components and enzymes capable of influencing matrix remodelling and turnover must be regulated both qualitatively and quantitatively. Some of the major components of the matrix have been discussed previously (Viidik, this volume) but these elements and the proteolytic enzymes implicated in matrix remodelling and turnover are summarized in Table 2.

CONNECTIVE TISSUE	
SYNTHESIS Anabolic	DEGRADATION Catabolic
MATRIX COMPONENTS	PROTEINASES/INHIBITORS
Collagen	Collagenases
Proteoglycans	Stromelysin
Elastin	Cathepsins
Others	Plasminogen Activators
	TIMP, PAI, Others

TABLE 2: Tissue components contributing to tissue homeostasis.

Expression of Plasminogen Activator and Plasminogen Activator Inhibitor by Rabbit Ligaments

One of the proteinase-proteinase inhibitor systems that has been reported to be involved in tissue remodelling is the plasminogen activator -- plasminogen activator inhibitor system (Sakesela 1985; Hart 1988a; Hart 1989). This system is comprised of two genetically distinct enzymes (tissue plasminogen activator, tPA and urokinase, UK) and several inhibitors (plasminogen activator inhibitor-1, PAI-1; plasminogen activator inhibitor-2, PAI-2; protein C inhibitor; protease nexin types 1-3). These components have been reviewed recently (Hart 1988a; Hart 1989) and will not be discussed in detail here.

The expression of elements of this system by normal rabbit MCL and anterior cruciate ligament (ACL) was determined by *in vitro* culture of segments of tissue followed by activity analysis. Analysis of PA activity derived from tissues from immature and mature animals led to the detection of heterogeneous expression in both the MCL (Figure 10) and the ACL (Figure 11).

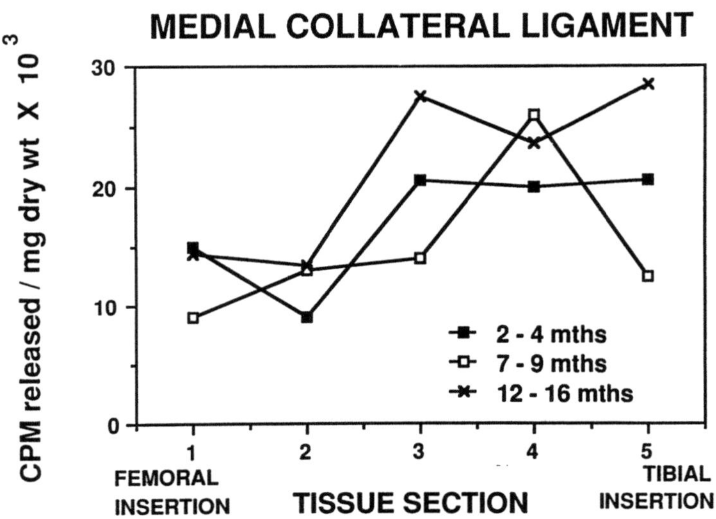

Figure 10: Expression of plasminogen-dependent plasminogen activator activity by medial collateral ligament tissue from rabbits of different ages.

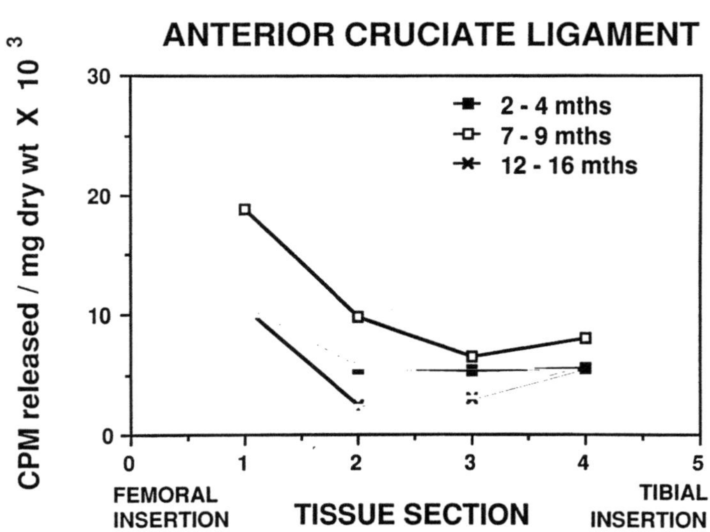

Figure 11: Expression of plasminogen-dependent PA activity by anterior cruciate ligament tissue from rabbits of different ages.

Interestingly, the highest levels of PA activity were released from the femoral end of the ACL and the tibial end of the MCL. The reproducible finding of polarity in the expression of this enzyme activity in ligaments and the opposite polarity between the two ligaments tested, leads to the conclusion that the enzyme serves a specific function within the ligament and therefore different sections of the ligaments are tightly regulated. Histologic analysis of the two ligaments indicated that the heterogeneous expression of PA activity was not due to detectable differences in cell densities in the different segments of the tissue. Analysis of the MCL and ACL PA activity by zymographic and reverse zymographic techniques, revealed the presence of a UK-like enzyme and a complex between this enzyme and an inhibitor (Hart 1988). Preliminary characterization of the inhibitory 40,000 dalton glycoprotein has indicated that it is not of the protease nexin family of inhibitors, but its identity has not been established. The finding of a UK-like enzyme is consistent with the postulated role of this enzyme in tissue remodelling and minimizes the possibility that the enzyme is derived from the vasculature of the tissue, which produces predominately tPA (reviewed in Hart 1988a; Hart 1989). Further analysis of the source of the PA and PAI expressed by both ligaments has revealed that the epiligamentous layer of cells produces PA and PAI and that the tissue remaining after removal of the surface cells still exhibits the polarity of expression observed with the intact tissue. Both enzyme and inhibitor were expressed by the superficial and internal cells. Therefore, the expression and the polarity are intrinsic to the ligament. This conclusion is supported by the observation that the polarity is maintained in immature and mature tissues. In the MCL the only observation that is not consistent with that conclusion was obtained with tissue derived from the tibial insertions of 9 month old animals. Whether this was an anomaly or is due to a change in tissue function at this age remains to be determined. Interestingly, in this time frame the animals are becoming skeletally mature and the observed temporary alteration may reflect changes related to this physiologic transition.

Other investigators have reported that normal rabbit ligaments also secrete the enzyme collagenase (Harper 1988). Rabbit ACL and MCL secreted similar levels of activity as well as similar levels of a collagenase inhibitor. In this study no comparisons were made between different segments of the ligaments so it is not known whether the values obtained by Harper et al (1988) represent the homogeneous expression of enzyme along the length of the tissue or are an average value of the heterogeneous expression of collagenase in the tissue. In addition, Harper et al (1988) used mature rabbits in their study and it would be of interest to determine whether immature animals in a more anabolic state express a different level of activity. In contrast to the plasminogen activator activity discussed earlier, Harper et al (1989) did not detect any obvious polarity in collagen synthetic activity with either MCL or ACL organ cultures. The femoral and tibial halves of either the MCL or the ACL yielded values that were not significantly different from one another. Recently, Wiig et al (1990) reported that the ACL and MCL of mature rabbits are actively synthesizing collagen as detected by *in situ* hybridization. Of the many interesting points raised by this preliminary report, three of them are relevant to the present discussion. The first is that the ACL appeared to be expressing less mRNA for type 1 procollagen than the MCL. The second point is that not all of the cells were labelled. This finding could be a methodological artefact or it could, as with our metabolic studies mentioned earlier, indicate that not all of the cells in the tissue are metabolically active in matrix synthesis at any one point in time. The third point is that the authors used mature animals for their study. Thus, the expression of the procollagen mRNA in this situation is very likely involved in the homeostatic regulation of the tissue rather than a function of an anabolic state within the tissue. Thus, not only is the ligament a biochemically complex tissue, it is a dynamic tissue which operates under a number of metabolic influences during normal growth and maturation.

Response of Rabbit Ligaments to Alterations in Stimuli

From the above discussion it is obvious that ligaments such as the MCL and ACL are complex tissues under normal conditions. Such tissues must also respond to a number of stimuli including disruption of biochemical integrity, inflammatory processes within the joint, immobilization, as well as variations in hormone levels. A considerable literature dealing with the healing process in ligaments has evolved, but is a subject that has been covered elsewhere (Andriacchi 1988) and will not be discussed here.

The metabolic response to immobilization and the subsequent alterations in biomechanical properties of the ligaments has been the subject of a more limited number of studies but they are relevant to the general theme of this discussion. Prolonged immobilization (3 months) of one leg of a mature rabbit leads to a loss of several biomechanical properties of the tissue (Woo 1982, 1987; Akeson 1987). The tissue atrophies, indicating activation of systems which create a catabolic environment and resultant loss of matrix material. In contrast to observations associated with prolonged immobilization, Harper et al (1990) very recently reported that at 4 weeks post-immobilization there is less collagenase activity expressed by the ACL and MCL from the immobilized leg than from the contralateral unhindered leg. Thus, prior to the onset of a catabolic state there appears to be an early response to "unloading" the tissue which results in a lowering of even enzymes that are generally thought to be actively involved in the breakdown of ligament matrix.

These latter findings support earlier studies reported from our laboratory in which immature rabbits were used in immobilization studies (Walsh 1988, 1989, 1989a, 1990). Immobilization of one leg of three month old rabbits led to a decline in both collagen synthesis rates and plasminogen activator secretion rates by 2-4 weeks post-immobilization (Walsh 1988). With more prolonged immobilization times, a shift to a catabolic environment occurred as evidenced by increased expression of PA activity and continued suppression of collagen synthetic rates. Interestingly, the immobilized ligaments did not grow and appeared to be "arrested" at the stage of maturation which existed at the time of initiation of the immobilization (Walsh 1989a). Thus immobilization of the immature ligament provides an environment which overrides growth stimuli and prevents the biomechanical maturation of the tissue (Walsh 1989, 1989a). This finding implies that in the absence of tissue loading, the stimuli creating the anabolic conditions are either not perceived or are not generated. Likewise, the findings of Harper, et al (1989, 1990) also indicate that in the mature tissue, immobilization leads to a loss of metabolic function, again generating the conclusion that regulation is maintained by loading of the tissue and the response to unloading is intrinsic to the ligament.

A further important point was derived from the immobilization studies discussed above. That is, the ligaments of the contralateral leg are in an abnormal metabolic state and can not be considered as normal controls for the results from the immobilized tissues (Walsh 1988, 1989, 1989a). Concurrent weight-bearing studies have revealed that animals with one leg immobilized maintain their activity level but nearly exclusively use the contralateral leg for weight-bearing. Thus, this limb bears more weight than normal. Analysis of collagen synthetic rates and PA secretion rates of such tissues were also found to be altered compared to age-matched nonoperated controls. Thus, the cells in the ligaments can apparently modify their metabolic activity in response to both under- and over-use.

In certain inflammatory states such as rheumatoid arthritis, osteoarthritis, or following trauma, ligaments may be exposed to mediators released from damaged tissues or inflammatory cells such as macrophages or polymorphonuclear leukocytes (reviewed in Hart 1989). This is particularly true of the anterior cruciate ligament which is exposed to synovial fluid. In inflammatory conditions, synovial fluid may contain elevated levels of mediators and cells which could influence the metabolism of ligaments. Recently, we have found that certain ligaments uniquely respond to specific inflammatory mediators, such as IL-1, by elevating their secretion rates for proteinases such as plasminogen activators (unpublished). As the mediators in question are known to interact with cells via receptor-mediated processes, at least some cells in the normal mature ligament must express receptors for such molecules.

Metabolic Activity of Human Ligaments

Human ligaments were obtained from autopsy specimens within 12 hr of death. The specimens were all from mature males and females. Analysis of PA expression along the length of the ACL and the MCL revealed the same polarity and heterogeneity in secretion rates that was detected with the analogous rabbit tissues (as in Figures 10 and 11). Zymographic analysis of the conditioned medium from these specimens, again revealed the presence of a UK-like PA and an enzyme-inhibitor complex. Thus, the human and rabbit ligaments are very similar with regard to PA expression. Further *in vitro* experiments also demonstrated that the level of secretion of this enzyme could be enhanced when the ligament sections were cultured in the presence of inflammatory mediators such as Interleukin-1. Thus, human ligaments must also express receptors for mediators and could be influenced by inflammatory processes occurring in the joint. Interestingly, the basal rate of PA secretion was also found to be inhibited by drugs commonly used to treat inflammatory joint disease. The drugs tested (aspirin, indomethacin and corticosteroids) could therefore potentially disrupt homeostatic mechanisms within the uninvolved ligaments due to bystander effects (Hart 1988). Such disruption could theoretically lead to alterations in the biomechanical integrity of the tissue and contribute to the joint disease.

Biological Regulation in Tendons

As discussed in earlier sections of this chapter, tendons are also morphologically and biochemically hetergeneous. There are a number of reports dealing with the regulation of metabolic activity of tendons from both avian and mammalian sources in the literature. Nearly all of the recent reports indicate that tendons are a metabolically dynamic connective tissue with evidence for tendon-specific differentiation and heterogeneity.

Analysis of patellar tendon and Achilles tendon for PA expression during maturation revealed the presence of PA activity along the length of both tendons (Figures 12 and 13).

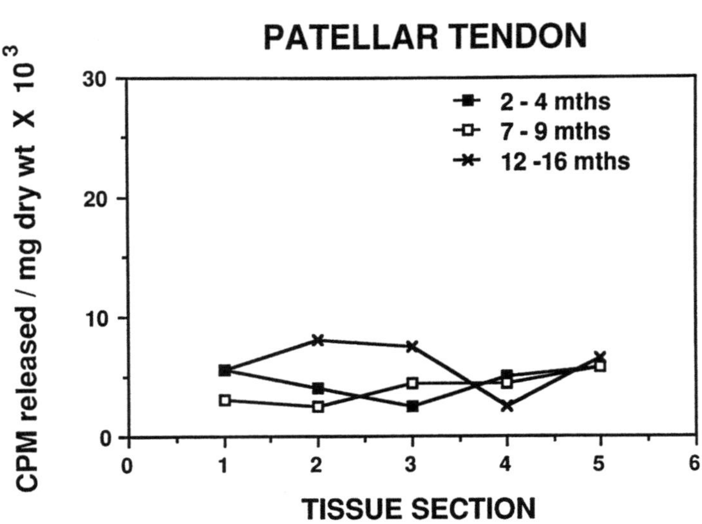

Figure 12: PA expression by rabbit patellar tendon .

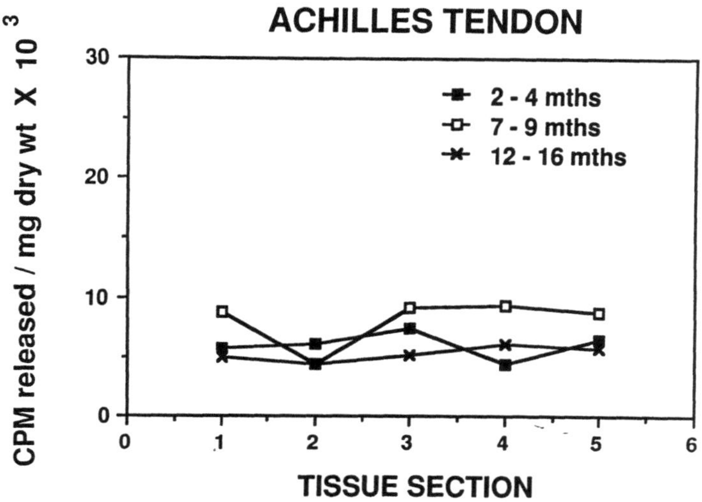

Figure 13: PA expression by rabbit Achille's tendon.

Zymographic analysis of the secretions again demonstrated the presence of a UK-like enzyme and an enzyme-inhibitor complex. Interestingly, the level of activity detected was less than that detected in secretions from cultures of rabbit ligaments. In contrast, Harper, et al (1988) have reported that cultured rabbit patellar tendon secreted higher levels of collagenase than did cultured ligaments. Thus, these two enzymes may be regulated differently in the normal homeostatic state of the two connective tissues.

A number of normal tendons from different locations and sources have been shown to be actively synthesizing matrix components such as collagen and proteoglycans (Vogel 1986; Koob 1987; Banes 1988; Daniel 1988). Recently, Daniel and Mills (1988) have reported that cells derived from biomechanically distinct regions of the rabbit flexor tendon synthesize different matrix molecules. Vogel (1986) and Koob (1987) have reported similar observations with bovine tendons. Such results indicate that cells within tendons are heterogeneous and maintain a differentiated phenotype *in vitro.*

Metabolic Response of Tendons to Stimuli

Like the previously discussed ligaments, the metabolic response of tendons to a variety of stimuli (or lack of stimuli) have been reported. These include injury or trauma (Gelberman 1986; Williams 1986; Russell 1990), exercise (Hansson 1988a; Sommer 1987), immobilization (Harper 1989, 1990) and anabolic steroids (Michna 1986). Harper, et al (1989) have reported that unlike the response of ligaments to immobilization, the level of collagenase secretion was not inhibited in the patellar tendon following pinning of one leg in the rabbit. Michna (1986) has reported that anabolic steroid treatment of mice leads to alterations in the morphology of tendons, which was likely a consequence of metabolic dysregulation. Hansson, et al (1988a) have recently reported that exercise of rats leads to the elevated expression of the anabolic growth factor, insulin-like growth factor (IGF-1, somatomedin C). Using an immunolocalization technique, these authors found that immunoreactivity was detected at very low levels in normal Achilles' and tibialis anterior tendon and the levels increased considerably with exercise, peaking after 7 days. Further exercise did not lead to detectable increases in the level of expression. The highest levels were detected in cells in areas of highest mechanical stress. Cessation of the exercise led to a return to base-line levels within 7 days. Thus, exercise apparently resulted in the induction/expression of this growth factor which is well known to exert positive effects on matrix synthesis (Osborn 1989, Morales 1989). Interestingly, in the normal state, the cells in the paratenon exhibited more immunoreactivity than did the cells within the tendons. The same group of investigators has also reported that ICGF-1 expression can be induced in rat tendons following vibration trauma (Hansson 1988). Other investigators have reported that regulation of matrix secretion is altered in tendons from diabetic rats compared to non-diabetic control rats (Leung 1986). These authors concluded that there is more intracellular degradation of procollagen in the diabetic state, but the mechanism was not elucidated.

Thus tendons are dynamic and metabolically responsive to a variety of environmental conditions. In particular, these tissues respond to loading and unloading situations in a fashion not unlike that found in ligaments.

Can Environment Induce the Biotransformation of a Tendon into a Ligament?

From the above discussion of the biology and biochemistry of ligaments and tendons, it is obvious that both tissues are complex, highly differentiated, and respond to environmental stimuli in a programed fashion. Some differences exist between the two types of tissue, but similarities also exist. The latter have prompted some investigators, to determine whether a tendon can undergo "ligamentization" (Amiel 1986) by placing it in the environment of a ligament. The most common situation in which this has been attempted is to use patellar tendon to replace the anterior cruciate ligament of the knee (discussed in Cabaud 1980; Amiel 1986; Jonsson 1989; Kleiner 1989). Amiel et al (1986) have investigated this phenomenon in a rabbit model. By 30 weeks post-operation, the grafted PT had assumed several of the morphological and biochemical characteristics of the ACL. The cells appeared similar to those found in ligaments and the matrix (collagen type, GAG content, cross-links) had been altered to become more like the ACL phenotype. However, based on the study design, it was not possible to determine whether the "metamorphosis" was due to the plasticity of the endogenous PT cells in the new environment or due to repopulation of the PT matrix by synovial cells or other cells from the new environment. Further experiments (Kleiner 1989) indicated that the cells within the tissue died and were replaced. Additionally, while the grafted PT had assumed an ACL phenotype, it failed to maintain and assume the biomechanical phenotype of the PT or ACL, respectively (Ballock 1989). Thus, this is an interesting approach to investigating the regulatory control of connective tissue biology and function which needs more attention and thorough analysis.

Summary

In this discussion, we have attempted to survey the relationships between ligament and tendon biology, biochemistry, morphology and function. It is obvious that these tissues are extremely complex with regard to these parameters and each experimental approach contributes to our understanding. The concept that such tissues maintain their biomechanical integrity and function through tight regulation of these differentiated, dynamic activities has yielded new insights into the the relationships between biology and biomechanics. The observations that cells within these tissues respond to loading and unloading stimuli should provide renewed impetus to understand how biomechanical stimuli are converted to biological responses. Perhaps the newer *in situ* techniques of molecular and cellular biology and immunolocalization will provide some answers. However, complete understanding will, no doubt, have to rely on a multi-disciplinary approach.

Acknowledgements

The authors thank their colleagues, students (John Matyas, Suzanne Walsh) and resident (Maureen O'Brien) for their helpful discussions and research contributions to this manuscript. We also thank Dr. R. Bray and Mr. D. Bray for contributing some of their Figures. The authors also thank Donna McDonald, Linda Marchuk and Judy Crawford for assistance in the preparation of the manuscript. Research discussed in the chapter has been supported in part by the Canadian Arthritis Society, the Medical Research Council of Canada and the Alberta Heritage Foundation for Medical Research.

References

Akeson W, Woo SL-Y, Amiel D, Frank C: The biology of ligaments, in Funk FJ, Hunter LY (eds): Rehabilitation of the Injured Knee. CV Mosby, St. Louis, 1984, pp 93-148..

Akeson WH, Amiel D, Abel M, Garfin SR, Woo SL-Y: Effects of immobilization on joints. Clin Orthop 1987;219:28-37.

Amiel D, Frank C, Harwood F, Fronek J, Akeson W: Tendons and ligaments -- A morphological and biochemical comparison. J Orthop Res 1983;1:257-265.

Amiel D, Kleiner JB, Roux RD, Harwood FL, Akeson WH: The phenomenon of "ligamentization": Anterior cruciate ligament reconstruction with autogenous patellar tendon. J Orthop Res 1986;4:162-172.

Andriacchi T, Sabiston P, DeHaven K, Dahners L, Woo SL-Y, Oakes B, Frank CB: Ligament: Injury and repair, in Woo SL-Y, Buckwalter JA (eds): Injury and Repair of Musculoskeletal Soft Tissues. Am Acad Orthop Surgeons, 1988, pp 103-132.

Ballock RT, Woo SL-Y, Lyon RM, Hollis JM, Akeson WH: Use of patellar tendon autograft for anterior cruciate ligament reconstruction in the rabbit: A long term histologic and biomechanical study. J Orthop Res 1989;7:474-485.

Banes AJ, Link GW, Bevin AG, Peterson HD, Gillespie Y, Bynum D, Watts S, Dahners L: Tendon synovial cells secrete fibronectin in vivo and in vitro. J Orthop Res 1988;6:73-82.

Berger RA, Blair WF: The radioscapholunate ligament: A gross and histologic description. Anat Rec 1984;210:393-405.

Brand RA: Knee ligaments: A new view. J Biomech Eng 1986;108:106-110.

Bray DF, Frank C, Bray R: Ultrastructure of ligament ground substance after ruthenium red staining. J Orthop Res 1990;8:1-12.

Bray RC, Fisher AWF, Hennenfent BW, Rossler R, Marchuk L, Frank C: Neurovascular anatomy of collateral knee ligaments revealed by metallic impregnation and vascular injection techniques. Trans Orthop Res Soc 1990;15:526,

Bray R, Fisher AWF, Frank C: Fine vascular anatomy of adult rabbit knee ligaments. Br J Anat 1990a;in press.

Cabaud H, Feagin JA, Rodkey W: Acute anterior cruciate ligament injury and augmented repair. Am J Sports Med 1980;8:395-401.

Cooper RR, Misol S: Tendon and ligament insertion: A light and electron microscopic study. J Bone Joint Surg 1970;52A:1-21.

Daniel JC, Mills DK: Proteoglycan synthesis by cells cultured from regions of the rabbit flexor tendon. Connect Tissue Res 1988;17:215-230.

Frank C, Amiel D, Woo SL-Y, Akeson WH: Normal ligament properties and ligament healing. Clin Orthop 1985;196:15-25.

Frank C, Bodie D, Andersen M, Sabiston P: Growth of a ligament. Trans Orthop Res Soc 1987;12:42.

Frank C, Woo SL-Y, Andriacchi T, Brand R, Oakes B, Dahners L, DeHaven K, Lewis J, Sabiston P: Normal ligament: Structure, function and composition, in Woo SL-Y, Buckwalter JA (eds): Injury and Repair of Musculoskeletal Soft Tissues. Am Acad Orthop Surgeons, 1988, pp 45-101.

Frank C, Edwards P, McDonald D, Bodie D, Sabiston P: Viability of ligaments after freezing: An experimental study in a rabbit model. J Orthop Res 1988a;6:95-102.

Frank C, Hart DA: Cellular responses to loading, in Leadbetter WB, Gordon SL (eds): Sports Induced Soft Tissue Inflammation, Am Orthop Soc Sports Med 1990;in press.

Gelberman RH, Manske PR, Akeson WH, Woo SL-Y, Amiel D: Flexor tendon repair. J Orthop Res 1986;4:119-128.

Gelberman R, Goldberg V, An K-N, Banes A: Structure and function of normal tendons, in Woo SL-Y, Buckwalter JA (eds): Injury and Repair of Musculoskeletal Soft Tissues. Am Acad Orthop Surgeons, 1988, pp 5-40.

Hansson HA, Dahlin LB, Lundborg G, Lowenadler B, Paleus S, Skottner A: Transiently increased insulin-like growth factor I immunoreactivity in tendons after vibration trauma. Scand J Plast Reconstr Surg Hand Surg 1988;22:1-6.

Hansson HA, Engstrom AMC, Holm S, Rosenquist A-L: Somatomedin C immunoreactivity in the Achilles tendon varies in a dynamic manner with the mechanical load. Acta Physiol Scand 1988a;134:119-208.

Harper J, Amiel D, Harper E: Collagenase production by rabbit ligaments and tendons. Connect Tissue Res 1988;17:253-259.

Harper J, Amiel D, Harper E: Collagenases from periarticular ligaments and tendon: Enzyme levels during the development of joint contracture. Matrix 1989;9:200-205.

Harper J, Amiel D, Harper E: Immunochemical characterization and determination of collagenase activity in periarticular tendon and ligaments during the early development of stress deprivation. Trans Orthop Res Soc 1990;15:535.

Hart DA, O'Brien MD, Walsh SL, Frank CB: Plasminogen activators and inhibitors in rabbit connective tissues. Fibrinolysis 1988;2:171.

Hart DA, Rehemtulla A: Plasminogen activators and their inhibitors: Regulators of extracellular proteolysis and cell function. Comp Biochem Physiol 1988a;90B:691-708.

Hart DA, Fritzler MJ: Regulation of plasminogen activators and their inhibitors in rheumatic diseases: New understanding and potential for new directions. J Rheumatol 1989;16:1184-1191.

Jackson RW: Anterior cruciate ligament injuries, in Casscells SW (ed): Arthroscopy Diagnostic and Surgical Practice. Lea and Febiger, Philadelphia, 1984, pp52-63.

Jonsson T, Peterson L, Renstrom P, Althoff B, Myrhage R: Augmentation with the long patellar retinaculum in the repair of an anterior cruciate ligament rupture. Am J Sports Med 1989;17:401-408.

Kennedy JC, Weinberg HW, Wilson AS: The anatomy and function of the anterior cruciate ligament. J Bone Joint Surg 1974;56A:223-235.

Kleiner JB, Amiel D, Harwood FL, Akeson W: Early histologic, metabolic and vascular assessment of anterior cruciate ligament autografts. J Orthop Res 1989;7:235-242.

Koob TJ, Vogel KG: Proteoglycan synthesis in organ cultures from regions of bovine tendon subjected to different mechanical forces. Biochem J 1987;246:589-598.

Leung MK, Folkes GA, Ramamurthy NS, Schneir M, Golub LM: Diabetes stimulates procollagen degradation in rat tendon in vitro. Biochim Biophys Acta 1986;880:147-152.

Matyas J: The Structure and Function of the Insertions of the Rabbit Medial Collateral Ligament. Ph.D. Thesis, University of Calgary 1990.

Matyas J, Bodie D, Andersen M, Frank C: The developmental anatomy of a "periosteal" ligament insertion: Growth and maturation of the tibial insertion of the rabbit medial collateral ligament. J Orthop Res 1990a;in press.

Michna H: Organization of collagen fibrils in tendons: Changes induced by an anabolic steroid. Vichows Arch B 1986;52:75-86.

Morales TI, Hascall VC: Factors involved in the regulation of proteoglycan metabolism in articular cartilage. Arth Rheumat 1989;32:1197-1201.

Osborn KD, Trippel SB, Mankin HJ: Growth factor stimulation of adult articular cartilage. J Orthop Res 1989;7:35-42.

Russell JE, Manske PR: Collagen synthesis during primate flexor tendon repair in vitro. J Orthop Res 1990;9:13-20.

Sakesela O: Plasminogen activation and regulation of pericellular proteolysis. Biochim Biophys Acta 1985; 823:35-65.

Schultz RA, Miller DC, Keer CS: Mechanoreceptors in human cruciate ligaments: A histological study. J Bone Joint Surg 1984;66a:1072-1076

Sommer HM: The biomechanical and metabolic effects of a running regime on the Achilles tendon in the rat. Int Orthop 1987;11:71-75.

Vogel KG, Keller EJ, Lenhoff RJ, Campbell K, Koob TJ: Proteoglycan synthesis by fibroblast cultures initiated from regions of adult bovine tendon subjected to different mechanical forces. Eur J Cell Biol 1986;41:102-112.

Walsh SL: Immobilization Effects Growing Ligaments. M.Sc. Thesis, University of Calgary, 1989.

Walsh SL, Frank C, Chimich D, Lam T, Hart D: Immobilization alters biomechanical maturation of growing ligaments. Trans Orthop Res Soc 1989a;14:253.

Walsh SL, Frank CB, Hart DA: Immobilization alters cell metabolism in an immature ligament, submitted 1990.

Wiig M, Amiel D, Ivarsson M, Arfors K: In situ hybridization of type I procollagen mRNA in normal and healing medial collateral ligament (MCL) and anterior cruciate ligament (ACL). Trans Orthop Res Soc 1990;15:522.

Williams IF, Nicholls JS, Goodship AE, Silver IA: Experimental treatment of tendon injury with heparin. Br J Past Surg 1986;39:367-372.

Woo SL-Y, Gomez M, Woo Y-K, Akeson WH: Mechanical properties of tendons and ligaments II. The relationship of immobilization and exercise on tissue remodeling. Biorheology 1982;19:397-408.

Woo SL-Y, Gomez, M, Sites T, Newton PO, Orlando CA, Akeson WH: The biomechanical and morphological changes of the MCL following immobilization and remobilization. J Bone Joint Surg 1987;69A:1200-1211.

Woo SL-Y, Maynard J, Buller D, Lyon R, Torzilli P, Akeson W, Cooper R, Oakes B: Ligament, tendon and joint capsule insertions to bone, in Woo SL-Y, Buckwalter JA (eds): Injury and Repair of Musculoskeletal Soft Tissues. Am Acad Orthop Surgeons, 1988, pp 133-166.

Yahia L-Y, Drouin G: Microscopical investigation of canine anterior cruciate ligament and patellar tendon: Collagen fascicle morphology and architecture. J Orthop Res 1989;7:243-251.

Chapter 3

Biomechanics and Morphology of the Medial Collateral and Anterior Cruciate Ligaments

S.L-Y. Woo, J.A. Weiss, D.A. MacKenna

Introduction

The ligaments of the knee serve to guide normal joint motion and provide stability. They are composed of densely packed collagen fibers, running parallel to the axis of loading. When unloaded, the tissue has a characteristic crimp pattern. As the ligament is stretched, more collagen fibers are recruited to bear load and the collagen crimp pattern disappears (Viidik and Lewin 1966). This gradual recruitment of ligament fibers results in a nonlinear constitutive relation for the ligament as a whole. During normal activity levels, the ligaments maintain normal knee joint kinematics with relatively small loads. When the knee is subjected to large externally applied forces such as those that occur in sporting activities, excessive joint motion is restricted by the increasing stiffness of the ligament.

By definition skeletal ligaments are attached to bone at both ends. The strength and stiffness characteristics of the ligament insertions to bone allow for the dissipation of forces across the joint and for their distribution over an area of bone. Force dissipation is achieved through a gradual transition from ligament to fibrocartilage to bone. Disruption is less likely to occur in this transition region than in the bone or peri-insertional tissue substance (Noyes et al. 1974a). The morphology and strength/stiffness properties of insertion sites have been shown to be affected by animal age, levels of stress and motion, as well as injury and healing (Woo et al. 1986a; Woo et al. 1982b; Woo et al. 1987a; Weiss et al. 1990; Matyas and Frank 1990a, 1990b).

Systemic factors could also play important roles.

The experimental determination of the tensile properties of ligaments poses several unique problems. The simplest approach would be to test the isolated ligament, however this presents the problem of how to clamp the ligament ends. The length/width ratio of most ligaments is too small to achieve a uniform stress distribution during tensile testing. To remedy these problems a bone-ligament-bone complex is used. This preparation provides secure clamping and better approximates *in situ* conditions, but makes it difficult to isolate the properties of the ligament substance from those of the insertions to bone. In our laboratory we have developed a methodology of tensile testing whereby both the *structural properties of the bone-ligament-bone complex* (represented by the load-elongation curve) and the *mechanical properties of the ligament substance* (represented by the stress-strain curve) can be obtained simultaneously (Woo et al. 1983). In this way we can examine the stiffness, energy absorbed at failure, ultimate load and elongation at failure of the entire structure (Figure 1a). These structural properties are affected by the ligament mechanical properties, the geometry of the ligament (i.e. cross-sectional area) and the strength/stiffness characteristics of the ligament insertions to bone. In addition, we can examine the tensile strength, ultimate strain, and modulus. These mechanical properties describe the material characteristics of the ligament substance itself, and are affected in part by the organization, orientation, and type of

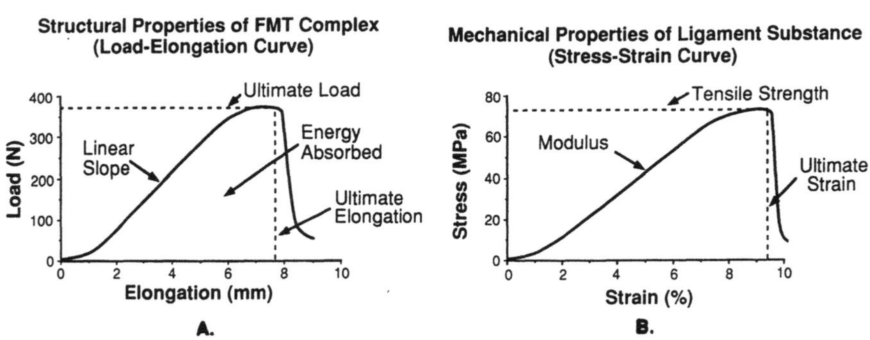

Figure 1: a. Structural properties of the bone-ligament-bone complex. b. Mechanical properties of the ligament substance.

collagen fibers, as well as interactions with other matrix constituents (Figure 1b). These parameters will remain constant for a given tissue, irrespective of any geometric differences (i.e. different cross-sectional areas or initial lengths).

Kinematic measurements are used to assess the contribution of knee ligaments to joint function. Some investigators have measured the force or moment produced by translation or rotation of a joint (Grood et al. 1981; Seering et al. 1980), whereas others have measured joint motion as a result of an externally applied load (Inoue et al. 1987; Nielson et al. 1984; Woo et al. 1987a). The normal knee joint permits 6 degrees of freedom (DOF) of motion: anterior-posterior, proximal-distal, and medial-lateral translations; and varus-valgus, flexion-extension, and internal-external rotations. Therefore, measurement of normal knee motion should incorporate as many DOF as possible. When the knee motion is restricted, such as in the case of 3 DOF (varus-valgus rotation, proximal-distal and medial-lateral translations), the medial collateral ligament (MCL) is the primary restraint to valgus knee rotation. Others have shown that when internal-external tibial rotation and anterior-posterior translation are allowed, the anterior cruciate ligament (ACL) plays an equally or more important role in maintaining valgus knee stability. Additionally, the ACL has been shown to be vital in limiting anterior-posterior translation of the tibia with respect to the femur.

The ligaments of the knee are anatomically and functionally different. In this chapter we will concentrate on the MCL and ACL. The ACL is an intra-articular ligament composed of several discrete fiber portions which change length (and thus tension) independently through the normal range of knee motion. The MCL is an extra-articular ligament with a more uniform geometry. It serves to passively stabilize the knee and restrain the motion of the medial meniscus. A multidisciplinary evaluation reveals the structural and functional similarities and differences between these two ligaments. The normal properties and functions of the MCL and ACL, as well as their response to changing stress levels, are different. These ligaments may remodel differently in response to stress deprivation, stress enhancement or injury. The effects of maturation and aging, as well as sex differences, on the tensile properties of ligaments will be presented. We will address the effects of stress deprivation and stress enhancement on the properties of knee ligaments and offer recent experimental results on ligament healing and postinjury treatment regimens. Some of the similarities and differences between the MCL and ACL will be explained. To conclude this chapter, future directions for ligament research are identified.

Tensile Properties of Knee Ligaments

Tensile Testing of Bone-Ligament-Bone Complexes

The structural properties of the bone-ligament-bone complex, represented by the load-elongation curve, can be determined through direct measurement of the load (using a load cell) and elongation (measured clamp-to-clamp distance). However, determining the mechanical properties, represented by the stress-strain curve, requires measurement of stress and strain of the ligament substance. In order to measure stress in the ligament, the cross-sectional area of the ligament must be known so that the tensile load can be normalized. The determination of ligament strain from elongation of a bone-ligament complex is less straight-forward. The techniques for determining both cross-sectional area and strain are discussed below.

Cross-sectional Area Measurements

Accurate measurement of ligament cross-sectional area is essential for stress measurement, and many different approaches have been implemented. In the 1960's, the gravimetric method, which calculated the cross-sectional area through division of the volume by the length was utilized by many investigators (Abrahams 1967; Elden 1964; Matthews and Ellis 1968; Van Brocklin and Ellis 1965). Conventional length measurement methods, such as vernier calipers, have also been used to measure the width and thickness of ligaments, and the area has been calculated assuming a rectangular cross-section. Alternatively, a different cross-sectional shape can be assumed and critical dimensions can be measured. For example, Haut et al. (1969) assumed the canine ACL to have an elliptical cross-section and measured the major and minor axes using a micrometer. The cross-sectional shape of some ligaments is irregular and geometrically complex. Hence, large errors in measurements can be introduced by such geometric approximations.

An area micrometer system, as described by Ellis (1969) and utilized by several other investigators (Walker et al. 1964; Butler et al. 1986) involves compressing the specimen into a rectangular slot of known width and measuring the specimen height with a micrometer. This method has been shown to give measurements that are dependent on the amount of pressure applied to the specimen (Allard et al. 1979). Unfortunately, contact with the deformable ligament may introduce errors into the area measurements. To avoid this limitation, many investigators have turned towards non-contact methods. Ellis (1968) used a "shadow amplitude method" to determine the radius of specimen profiles in order to reconstruct the specimen cross-section. Gupta et al. (1971) used a rotating microscope while Njus and Njus (1986) used a video dimension analyzer to determine the ligament profiles.

The laser micrometer system is a non-contact method recently developed in our laboratory for ligament cross-sectional area and shape measurement (Lee and Woo 1988). The specimen is placed perpendicular to a 46 mm wide collimated laser beam and is rotated through 180° (in 3° increments) by a computer controlled drive system. For each increment, the width and location of the shadow is recorded by a computer. The center of rotation and object boundaries are determined for each incremental rotation, and the ligament cross-sectional shape and area can be determined. An important limitation of this system is its inability to measure concavities. However, most ligaments and tendons have few concavities, and thus the error introduced by this method of measurement is minimal. The laser micrometer has proven to be both highly accurate an reproducible in its reconstruction of the complex ligament geometry of the ACL, as verified by histological sections. In addition, this technique has been used to measure the variation in shape and cross-sectional area along the length of a ligament (Danto et al. 1989). It would be difficult for conventional methods to accomplish these tasks.

Strain Measurements

To obtain the displacement properties of the ligament substance instead of the entire bone-ligament-bone complex, it is necessary to examine the strain of the ligament substance. Strain is defined as the elongation of the ligament substance normalized by the initial length. Ligament strain has been estimated by a wide variety of methods (Arms et al. 1982; Butler et al. 1986; Dorlot et al. 1980; Lewis and Shybut 1981; Meglan et al. 1986; Monahan et al. 1984; Trent et al. 1976; Warren et al. 1974). A common approach is to use a strain transducer sutured to or in contact with the ligament substance. Kennedy et al. (1977) performed one of the first studies of knee ligament strain using a liquid mercury strain gauge. Additionally, Hall effect transducers have been used to estimate ligament strain (Arms et al. 1982). These methods involve direct contact with the ligament, and this introduces systematic errors in strain measurement.

A non-contact method to measure ligament strain was developed in our laboratory (Woo et al. 1983). The video dimension analyzer (VDA) system uses a recorded video image of the test specimen. Prior to testing, two or more reference lines are placed on the specimen perpendicular to the loading axis using Verhoeff's elastin stain. These markers define a gauge length for strain measurement. A taped image of the tensile test is played back and the VDA system superimposes two electronic "windows" on the screen. The windows automatically track the movement of the reference lines and convert the horizontal scan time between the lines into an output voltage, which can be calibrated to correspond to percent strain of the ligament tissue. The frequency response of the VDA system is as high as 120 Hz and errors in linearity and accuracy are less than 0.5%. This method of determining strain has certain advantages including: a) no physical contact with the specimen during testing; b) midsubstance strains can be measured independent of the insertions to bone; c) different regional strains can be obtained from a single test based on selective placement of reference lines; and d) video recording of testing permits the data to be analyzed after the test, as well as providing a permanent record. The technique has recently been adopted by several other laboratories for strain measurements of soft tissues such as knee ligaments, articular cartilage and shoulder tendons and ligaments (Sabiston et al. 1990; Butler et al. 1984; Pollock et al. 1990). We have also used this system in conjunction with a high-speed video recorder to tape high strain rate tests. (Woo et al. 1990c).

Tensile Properties of the MCL and ACL

The MCL of most animal models has a relatively uniform geometry which is composed of parallel fibers. Consequently the stress distribution in the ligament during tensile testing is uniform. In this case, both the structural properties of the femur-MCL-tibia complex (FMTC) and mechanical properties of the MCL substance can be obtained from one testing configuration (Woo et al. 1983). The ACL, however, is more problematic due to the complex geometric arrangement of the fibers that twist along the length of the ligament. It is not possible to determine the tensile stress of the whole ACL because the entire ligament cannot be loaded uniformly. To alleviate this problem, several investigators have chosen to test individual bundles (or functional bands) to determine mechanical properties (Butler et al. 1986, Hollis et al. 1989). In this case, the structural properties of the femur-ACL Bundle-tibia complex have little or no meaning.

Studies have been performed both in our laboratory and others to examine the tensile behavior of the MCL and ACL from both animal and cadaveric models. However, few have directly compared the MCL and ACL from the same animal. A recent study in our laboratory directly compared the mechanical properties of the normal rabbit MCL and ACL (Newton et al. 1990a). It was necessary to divide the ACL into two portions (the medial and lateral) so that a uniform stress distribution could be achieved. Distinct differences in the tensile stress-strain behavior of the two ligaments were found. The modulus of the MCL was nearly twice that of the ACL, while the two portions of the ACL had similar moduli. This is in contrast to a study of human knee ligaments by Butler et al. (1986), in which differences between the mechanical properties of the anterior cruciate, posterior cruciate and lateral collateral ligaments could not be demonstrated. However, the patellar tendon was found to have a higher stiffness than all ligaments examined.

In an attempt to explain the differences in the mechanical properties of the MCL and ACL, the ultrastructure of these ligaments was examined (Newton et al. 1990a). Using both scanning and transmission electron microscopy, the MCL cross-section appeared to have a higher density of collagen fibers (oriented along the long axis of the ligament), while the ACL had a larger amount of interfascicular space and transversely oriented collagen (Figures 2a and b). This difference in cross-sectional collagen density could explain the lower modulus of the ACL. The smaller amount of effective load bearing collagen would lead to a lower stress for a given strain in comparison to the MCL.

The specimen orientation with respect to the axis of the applied load has been shown to affect the tensile properties of the bone-ACL-bone complex of rabbit and porcine knees (Woo et al. 1987d; Lyon et al. 1989).

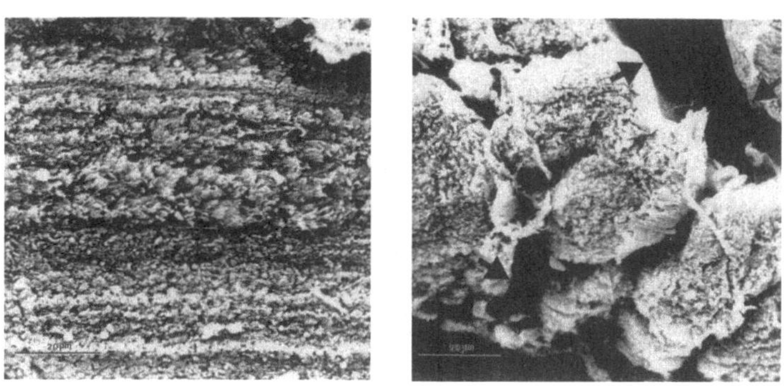

A B

Figure 2: Scanning electron microscope cross-section of ligaments. a. rabbit MCL. b. rabbit ACL. Arrows point to interfascicular space.

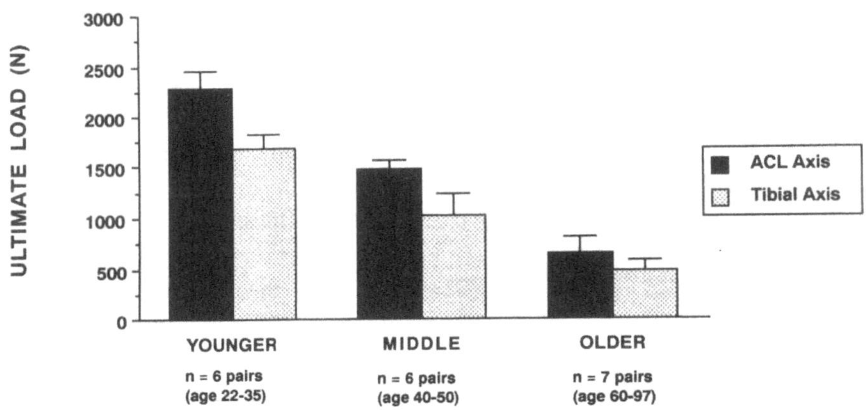

Figure 3: Changes in the ultimate load of the human FATC with loading axis.

Studies of human cadaver knees also have demonstrated a higher ultimate load and stiffness when the ACL is loaded along its own axis (without altering the angles of the ACL insertions to bone) as opposed to the tibial axis (Figure 3) (Hollis et al. 1988).

Other factors that may affect the mechanical properties of ligaments have also been examined in our laboratory, using the MCL as a model. While environmental temperature had an inverse effect on the modulus of the MCL (Woo et al. 1987c), freezing at -20°C for up to three months had no effect on the ligament properties (Woo et al. 1986b). Strain rate has been shown to affect the structural properties of the FMTC, but not the mechanical properties of the ligament substance (Woo et al. 1990c). Also, the effects of aging and sex on the biomechanical properties of the rabbit MCL have been investigated (Ohland et al. 1989). It was found that the rate of skeletal maturation contributed in part to the differences in tensile properties of both male and female rabbits. These differences will be discussed in more detail below.

Viscoelastic Properties of Ligaments

Ligaments are viscoelastic materials and their nonlinear time- and history-dependent properties have been described in the literature (Lin et al. 1987; Woo et al. 1981; Woo et al. 1982). These properties are the result of complex interactions between collagen and surrounding proteins, ground substance as well as interstitial fluid. Ligaments demonstrate creep (an increase in elongation over time under a constant load) and stress relaxation (a decline in stress over time under a constant elongation). The loading and unloading curves do not follow the same path, forming a hysteresis loop due to energy dissipation.

The viscoelastic behavior of ligaments has important physiological significance. Stress relaxation becomes important during walking or jogging, in which the applied strains are repetitive. Cyclic stress relaxation effectively reduces the stress in the tissue substance, possibly helping to prevent fatigue failure of ligaments following prolonged use. On the other hand, repetitious loading to a constant load results in a gradual increase in elongation, as demonstrated by increased joint laxity following prolonged exercise or stretching. After a period of recovery, however, the ligaments return to their original length and a return of normal joint laxity is noted.

The viscoelastic behavior of ligaments can be described mathematically by a theoretical relationship for soft tissues first proposed by Fung (1972). Known as the quasi-linear viscoelastic (QLV) theory, this relationship assumes that the stress response $\sigma(t)$ for an applied strain history $\varepsilon(t)$ can be expressed as an integral sum of responses to a series of infinitesimal step increases in strain, in terms of a *reduced relaxation function* G(t) and the elastic response of the tissue $\sigma^e(\varepsilon)$:

$$\sigma(t) = \int_0^t G(t-\tau)\,\frac{\partial \sigma'(\varepsilon)}{\partial \varepsilon}\,\frac{\partial \varepsilon}{\partial \tau}\,d\tau$$

The reduced relaxation function is defined as $G(t) = \sigma(t)/\sigma(0)$ and has the property that $G(0) = 1$. The common expressions chosen for G(t) and $\sigma^e(\varepsilon)$ are

$$G(t) = \frac{1 + C\left[E_1\left(\frac{t}{\tau_2}\right) - E_2\left(\frac{t}{\tau_1}\right)\right]}{1 + C\ln\left(\frac{\tau_2}{\tau_1}\right)}$$

$$\sigma^e(\varepsilon) = A\,(e^{B\varepsilon} - 1)$$

These expressions contain the material constants C, τ_1, τ_2, A, and B which describe the viscoelastic properties of the tissue. They can be determined from experimental data by using a nonlinear least-square curve fitting procedure. Recently, the QLV theory has been further refined to apply to a ramp loading condition, since a true step load cannot be achieved experimentally. This refined theory has been successfully used to determine the viscoelastic constants for the anteromedial bundles of porcine ACL (Lin et al. 1987). The constants were determined from the results of an experimental stress relaxation test. The QLV theory agreed well with the experimental data. Using the experimentally determined constants, the reduced relaxation function and the elastic response (for porcine ACL anteromedial bundles) were found to be

$$G(t) = 0.858 - 0.049\ \ln(t)$$

$$\sigma^e(\varepsilon) = 210(e^{0.63\ \varepsilon} - 1)$$

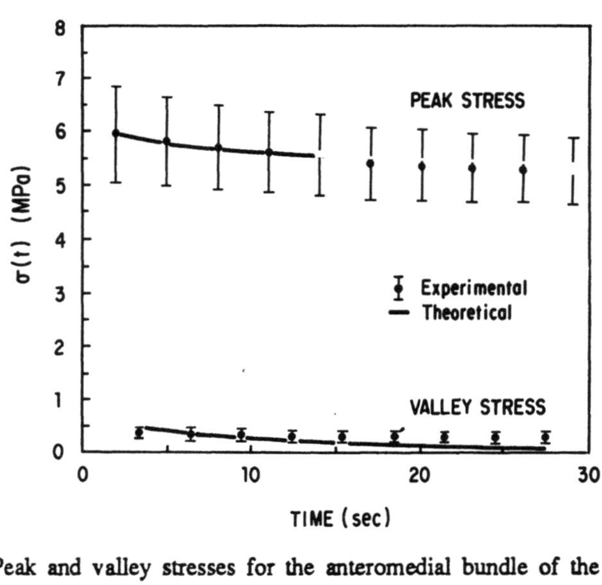

Figure 4: Peak and valley stresses for the anteromedial bundle of the porcine ACL under cyclic loading.

The expressions for G(t) and $\sigma^e(\varepsilon)$ were validated by a second experiment in which these equations were used to predict the behavior of the tissue under cyclic loading between 1% and 5% strain. The predicted peak and valley stresses matched well with experimental data (Figure 4). Thus, we believe the QLV theory provides an accurate mathematical description of the time- and history-dependent viscoelastic properties of ligaments within the range of strains considered.

Effects of Aging and Sex

Investigators have long been aware of the anatomical, morphological, biochemical and biomechanical changes that ligaments undergo with growth (Booth and Tipton 1970; Brown and Consden 1958; Cannon and Davison 1973; Frank et al. 1983, 1988; Hall 1976; Mays et al. 1988; Muller and Dahners 1988; Viidik 1968a). The majority of the data available are from the rat. However, as closure of the epiphyses (an indication of skeletal maturity) does not occur until senescence in the rat, tensile testing of these specimens frequently results in failure by avulsion at the tibial insertion to bone, and the tensile strength of the ligament cannot be obtained. Therefore, other animal models have been used. Blanton and Biggs (1970) investigated the strength of fetal and adult human tendons and found that the latter had a slightly higher tensile strength. Wang et al. (1990) examined the biomechanical properties of the MCL in 1 and 10 year old beagles and found changes in the tensile strength of the ligament substance but not in the ultimate load of the FMTC. Several investigators have assessed changes in tensile properties of the human bone-ACL-bone complex with age and have found that ligaments from older donors failed at a significantly lower ultimate load than those from younger donors (Hollis et al. 1988; Noyes and Grood 1976; Rauch et al. 1988; Trent et al. 1976). Hollis et al. (1988) showed that there was a drastic decrease in the stiffness and ultimate load of the human FATC with age (Figure 5), however there was little change in the anterior-posterior translation of the knee with age. Although these studies have documented changes in structural properties with age, limited data exist regarding changes in the mechanical properties of ligament substance with age.

Changes in the tensile properties of the male rabbit MCL from 1.5 to 15 months of age have been reported by our laboratory (Woo et al. 1986a). Increases in both body mass and cross-sectional area of the MCL were observed as the animals matured, with the largest changes noted between 1.5

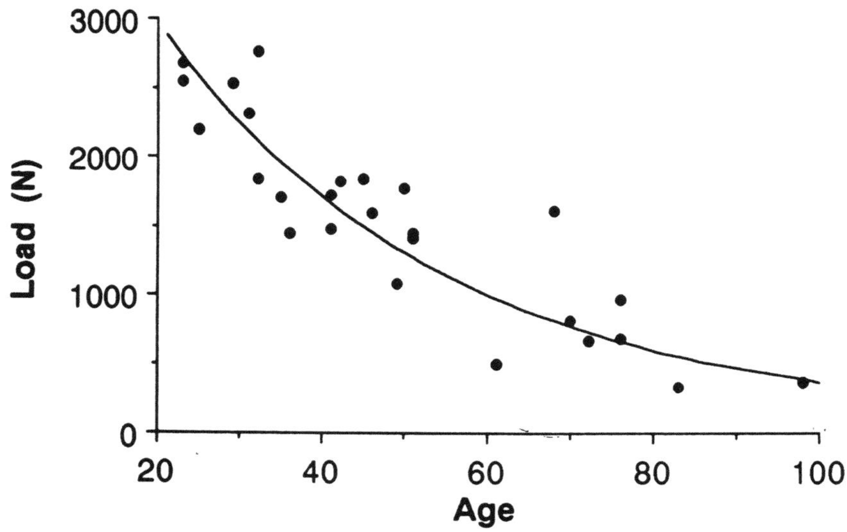

Figure 5: Ultimate load of the human FATC as a function of age.

and 5 months of age. The stiffness and ultimate load of the FMTC increased with age and reached a plateau at 7 months. Animal with open epiphyses failed by tibial avulsion, whereas those with closed epiphyses failed in the MCL midsubstance. The age-related changes in the mechanical properties of the MCL substance were found to be smaller, especially after 4-5 months of age. These results suggested that there was a rapid increase in the strength of the MCL-tibial junction as the animals reached skeletal maturity.

Recent studies have found that there are differences in the structure and function of collagen between male and female animals (Booth and Tipton 1970; Hama et al. 1976; Shikata et al. 1979; Tipton et al. 1978). Other investigators have also described the effects of sex hormones on ligamentous tissue. Rundgren and Viidik (1972) showed that the stiffness of the ACL was reduced immediately after parturition, but the ultimate load of the bone-ligament complex was not affected. Hama et al. (1976) reported that the collagen content of connective tissue from sexually mature male rats was higher than that from sexually mature female rats.

Our laboratory recently completed a comprehensive study which examined the biomechanical properties of the rabbit FMTC in male and female animals up to 4 years of age, i.e near senescence (Ohland et al.

1989). The age groups studied were: 3.5, 6, 12, and 36 months. Only females (retired breeders) were examined at 48 months, as males of a similar age could not be obtained.

Rapid increases in body mass and MCL cross-sectional area occurred between the ages of 3.5 and 6 months, but afterwards remained relatively constant even for the older age groups. The body mass of the females was greater at each age. In general, these findings agree with those of Masoud et al. (1986).

Typical load-elongation curves for the FMTCs of selected animals from different age groups of male and female rabbits are shown in Figure 6. The stiffness was found to change with age for both male and female animals. In males, the stiffness increased until 12 months but had declined by 36 months. The highest value for the females was reached at 36 months. In general, the stiffness for the male specimens was higher. The ultimate load also increased with age for both male and female animals. In males it more than tripled between 3.5 and 12 months of age. A similar trend was seen in females. These results are similar in trend to those found by Tipton et al. (1978) for the rat.

The status of the proximal tibial epiphyses correlated well with the failure mode of the FMTC. Both male and female rabbits at 3.5 months of age had open epiphyses and failed by tibial avulsion. Similarly, females at 6 months were skeletally immature and failed by tibial avulsion. However, the proximal tibial epiphysis was closed in 33% of the males at 6 months, and there was a mixture of failure modes. These findings suggest that the rates of skeletal maturation may be different between males and females. At 12 months and thereafter, the epiphyses of all animals were closed, and all failures occurred in the MCL substance.

Typical stress-strain curves for the MCL substance illustrate the changes that occur as a function of age (Figure 7). There was a significant effect of age on the modulus ($p<0.001$), but no effect of sex ($p>0.50$). The modulus peaked at 12 months and declined at 36 months and 48 months. The tensile strength of the MCL substance was only obtained for the skeletally mature animals, as the FMTC of the immature animals failed by tibial avulsion. In males the tensile strength was highest at 12 months and only declined slightly by 36 months. The trend was similar for both males and females, and the tensile strength of the females had decreased further by 48 months. There was no significant effect of age or sex on the tensile strength ($p>0.1$ in both cases).

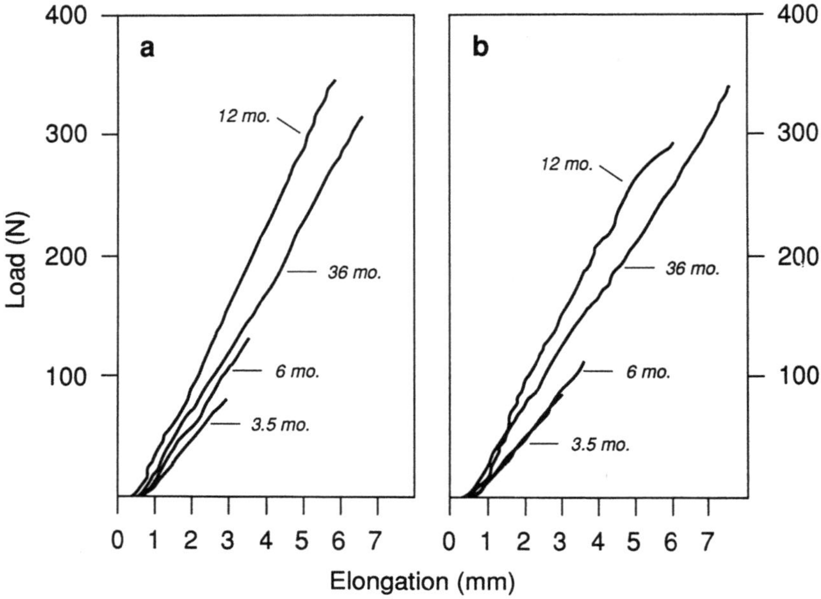

Figure 6: Typical load-elongation curves for the (a) male and (b) female rabbit FMTC as a function of age.

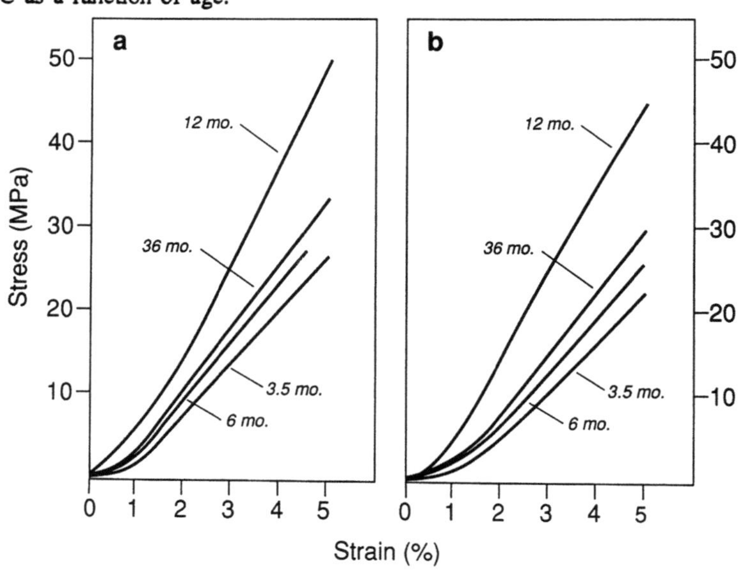

Figure 7: Typical stress-strain curves for the (a) male and (b) female rabbit MCL substance as a function of age.

The lack of major changes in structural properties following skeletal maturation was also observed in a canine model in our laboratory (Wang et al. 1990). Also, it seems that establishment of the structural integrity of the tibial insertion site can explain the change in the failure mode, as well as changes in structural properties observed during maturation. Figure 8 is a schematic representing our findings on the effects of age. Prior to skeletal maturity, the MCL substance was stronger, and the FMTC failed by tibial avulsion. Once skeletal maturity was reached, the tibial insertion was stronger, and the FMTC failed in the MCL substance. The histological changes at the proximal tibial insertion site during maturation have been documented (Woo et al. 1990c). During the aging process, there was no significant reduction in the MCL cross-sectional area, and the changes in the mechanical properties were also small. As a result, there were minimal changes in the structural properties of the FMTC.

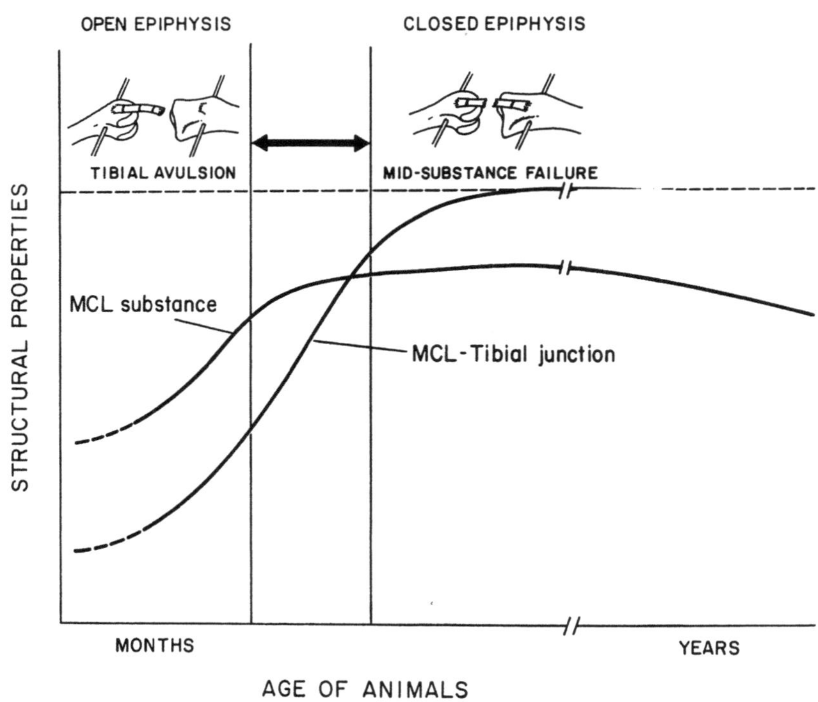

Figure 8: Changes in the properties of the MCL-tibial junction and MCL substance that occur as a result of maturation and aging.

The age-related changes in the tensile properties and failure mechanism of the rat, rabbit, and canine are similar, but do not parallel changes observed for other knee ligaments, particularly the human femur-ACL-tibia complex (FATC). Significant decreases in the stiffness and ultimate load as a function of age have been reported (Hollis et al. 1988; Noyes and Grood 1976; Rauch et al. 1988). Whether these differences are related to anatomic location (intra-articular vs. extra-articular) or other factors, such as stress and strain levels, remains to be determined.

Stress Deprivation and Stress Enhancement

Ligaments, like other tissues of the body, have the ability to respond to environmental demands. The homeostatic response appears to be stress dependant, with the ligament adapting positively to limited levels of increased stress and negatively to decreased stress. The biomechanical properties of ligaments have been studied extensively in situations of both stress deprivation and stress enhancement.

Immobilization (Stress and Motion Deprivation)

Immobilization is often used as part of the treatment of musculoskeletal injuries to protect the injured tissue from the disruptive forces during the early healing period. The increases in joint stiffness that are often seen clinically can be associated with a proliferation of fibro-fatty connective tissue. This can eventually obliterate the joint space after long-term immobilization (Enneking and Horowitz 1972). Resulting synovial adhesions may lead to tearing of the articular surface during forced manipulation. Evans et al. (1960) examined rat knees which had been immobilized for 15 to 90 days. They observed well established adhesions by 30 days which were felt to contribute substantially to joint stiffness. Similarly, Langenskoild et al. (1979) reported a thickening of the periarticular soft tissues of the rabbit knee after only two weeks of immobilization. The corresponding joint stiffness restricted knee motion to only 20-40° after 2-14 weeks of immobilization.

In our laboratory, knee stiffness following immobilization was measured using a device called an arthrograph. This device measures the torque and energy required to cycle a knee through a specific range of motion (Akeson et al. 1974). After nine weeks of immobilization, a substantial increase in torque and energy was required to extend the rabbit knee joint. This was attributed to adhesions of the periarticular connective tissues (Akeson et al. 1980; Woo et al. 1987b). It was hypothesized that the new collagen fibrils synthesized during the immobilization period formed interfibrillar contacts and thus restricted normal sliding of fibers in the extensible structures of the joint capsule.

The tensile properties of the bone-ligament-bone complex also change significantly following immobilization. A study in our laboratory demonstrated that the FMTC failed at only 29% of the ultimate load observed for the contralateral non-immobilized knee. Similarly, the energy absorbed at failure was only 16% of the control (Woo et al. 1987b). These results agree with those of Tipton et al. (1975b), who found a 28% decrease in the ultimate load of the rat FMTC following six weeks of immobilization in a plaster cast. Studies involving the structural properties of the FATC have had similar results. For example, Larsen et al. (1987) found a 25% decrease in the ultimate load and linear stiffness of the FATC of rats after 4 weeks of immobilization. Similarly, Noyes (1977) found decreases in the structural properties of the FATC of the rhesus monkey after 8 weeks of total body cast immobilization.

These changes in the structural properties may be the results of changes in the insertion sites. At the tibial insertion of the MCL, an increase in the number of osteoclasts was noted following immobilization, leading to resorption of sub-periosteal bone and disruption of the attachment of collagen fibers. These changes correlated well with the decreases seen in ultimate loads of the FMTC, especially considering that the failure mode was exclusively avulsion of the MCL at the tibial insertion (Woo et al. 1987b). The correlation between tibial avulsion and osteoclastic activity was also seen by Laros et al. (1971).

Noyes (1977) demonstrated a similar but less dramatic effect of immobilization on the insertion sites of the ACL. While the percentage of failures of the FATC by avulsion increased slightly, they found sub-periosteal resorption in the tibia and femur of immobilized primate knees and concluded that the loss of cortex immediately beneath the ligament insertion was responsible for decreasing the integrity of the insertion. The less dramatic effects on the insertion sites of the ACL following immobilization may be due in part to the type of insertions of the ACL into both the femur and tibia.

There were corresponding changes in the mechanical properties of the ligament substance and the cross-sectional area of the ligament following immobilization. Following 9 weeks of immobilization, we measured changes in the mechanical properties of the rabbit MCL and ACL (Figures 9a and b).

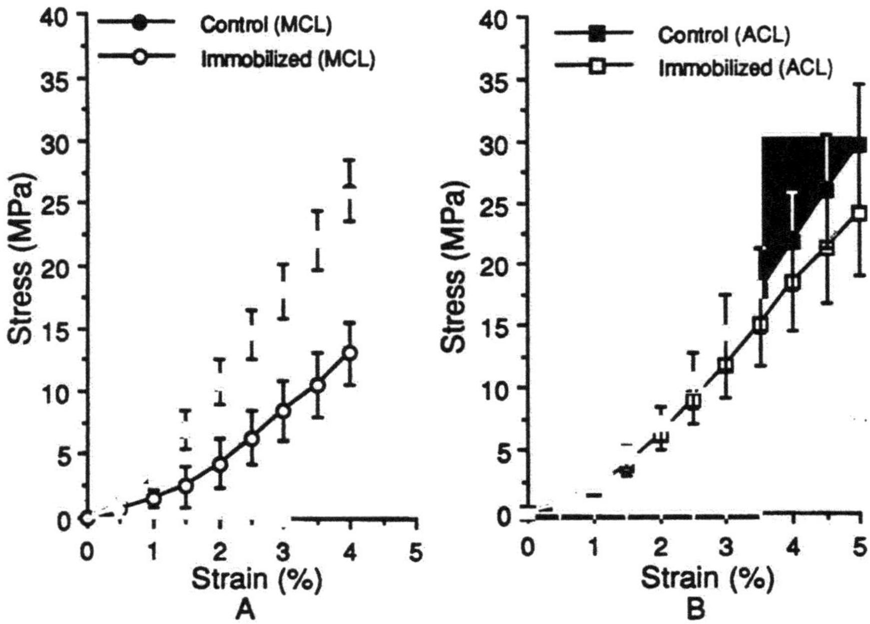

Figure 9: Changes in the mechanical properties of the (a) MCL and (b) ACL following 9 weeks immobilization.

The modulus of the MCL substance decreased by approximately 50% (Woo et al. 1987b). The modulus of the ACL dropped only 25% (Newton et al. 1990b). Although the effects of immobilization on the mechanical properties of the ligament substance are greater for the MCL than the ACL, the histological changes in the ligament substance are more noticeable for the ACL. Following immobilization, the shape of fibroblasts of the ACL changed from oval without long processes extending into the collagen matrix to a more elongated cell with long processes extending into the collagen matrix. In addition, the cross-sectional area of both ligaments decreased. Binkley and Peat (1986) also demonstrated decreases in the properties of the rat MCL after immobilization. They also noted significant decreases in the proportion of small collagen fibers, which they attributed to decreased synthesis and degradation. The decreases seen in both cross-sectional area and mechanical properties, when combined with changes in the insertion sites, would explain the substantial decreases seen in the stiffness and strength of the bone-ligament-bone complexes.

Remobilization

Several studies have shown that remobilization leads to a slow reversal of the changes to the structural properties of the bone-ligament-bone complex. Noyes et al. (1983) subjected primates to eight weeks of body cast immobilization and demonstrated that a 12 month period of remobilization was required for the structural properties of the FATC to approach normal control values. Laros et al. (1971) found that after six weeks of immobilization, the canine knee required 18 weeks of remobilization for the structural properties of the FMTC to return to normal. New bone formation was seen at the recovering insertion sites. Shorter periods of immobilization, as in the case of Larsen et al. (1987) who immobilized rats for only four weeks, required a shorter remobilization period (6 weeks) for the strength and stiffness characteristics to return to a normal level.

In addition to the structural properties of the FMTC, it was found that the mechanical properties of the rabbit MCL rapidly returned to a normal level (Woo et al. 1987b). This return occurred after only nine weeks of remobilization following nine weeks of immobilization. The structural properties of the FMTC of the remobilized specimens, on the other hand, were still substantially different from the controls. Failure of the experimental FMTC continued to occur at the tibial insertion after remobilization, and histological examination of the insertion revealed incomplete reorganization. A fifty-two week period of remobilization was required for the integrity of distal insertion site to be reestablished. These results demonstrate a differential rate of recovery of the ligament substance and its insertions to bone. While the ligament substance appears to recover relatively quickly, the bone-ligament-bone complex remains weak for a significant period of time. A remobilization period substantially longer than the time of immobilization may be required for recovery.

Increased Tension

Based on the hypothesis that increased stress levels could profoundly improve the biomechanical properties of ligaments, an *in vivo* study of the effect of increased tension on the properties of ligaments was undertaken in our laboratory (Gomez et al. 1988). A stainless steel pin (9.5 mm in length, 1.6 mm in diameter) was surgically inserted beneath the left rabbit MCL perpendicular to the distal attachment. To quantitatively evaluate any effects of the addition of the pin, it was necessary to first obtain the *in situ* ligament tension. To do this, our laboratory developed a methodology to indirectly determine ligament *in situ* load based upon *in situ* strain (Woo et al. 1990a). The *in situ* strain of the MCL was shown to be most uniform across the MCL when the knee was positioned at 90° flexion, while the *in situ* strain varied across the ligament from anterior to posterior when the knee was in either 60° or 120° of flexion. Insertion of the tension pin beneath the MCL increased the strain levels from 2.5% to 4.0% at 90° of knee flexion. The MCL *in situ* load and stress were also elevated from 5.8 to 18.0 N and from 0.5 to 1.6 MPa, respectively. Significant increases in load were found at other knee flexion angles as well. These measurements quantified the initial increases in ligament tension that occurred following application of the pin.

An *in vivo* study was then carried out to assess the effects of increased tension on normal and healing rabbit ligaments. The pin was surgically placed beneath the contralateral MCL of the left knee near the tibial insertion site, while the MCL was simply exposed to serve as a sham operated control. Animals were allowed free cage activity until their sacrifice at either 6 or 12 weeks postoperatively. At 6 weeks postoperatively, load-elongation curves of the FMTC were found to be similar up to 4 mm of elongation between the normal ligaments and those with increased tension. Beyond this point the structural behavior began to diverge. The FMTCs with increased tension failed at a 26% higher ultimate load and a 33% higher ultimate elongation than the controls. However, by 12 weeks these differences diminished, and the load-elongation curves became similar for both groups. Histologically, there was an initial reaction to the pin, as noted by surrounding increased cellularity in the MCL substance. The increased tension also induced regional changes in fiber alignment and a decreased periodicity in the crimp pattern.

Comparison of the stress-strain curves of the MCL substance at 6 weeks showed that for a given strain level, the stress was lower for the groups with increased tension (i.e. a lower modulus). However, by 12 weeks this trend had reversed; the group with increased tension exhibited a higher modulus than the controls. This is the first study of its kind in which positive effects of measured increased stress levels on the mechanical properties of ligament were determined. Future studies should consider longer durations of increased tension, comparable to the studies of exercise training regimens.

Exercise/Training

Many experimental studies have suggested that exercise and training can strengthen ligament structures. Biomechanical properties of the ligament substance and the insertion sites are affected by exercise, and some histological changes have been documented as well. Laros et al. (1971) examined the effect of various activity levels on the strength of the canine MCL and on the morphological changes in the insertion sites. The ultimate load, normalized to body weight, was found to increase with the level of activity. Interestingly, limited activity resulting from cage confinement for more than 6 weeks induced bone resorption at the MCL tibial insertion. Tipton et al. (1979) and Vailas et al. (1981) also examined the effects of exercise on knee structures. Primates were trained on a treadmill for 20 weeks (Vailas et al. 1981). The MCL weight/lengths ratio (an indirect method for determining cross-sectional area) increased significantly by 26%. Tensile strength measurements revealed no change in the MCL, and the ultimate load of the FMTC *in situ* was not found to be affected by exercise.

Noyes (1974b) examined the effects of isolated lower limb exercise on the properties of the primate ACL while the rest of the body was immobilized in a cast. The active exercise was found to be ineffective in preventing the detrimental effects of immobilization, as load-elongation curves for the experimental FATCs were similar to those for limbs immobilized in casts. In contrast, Viidik (1968b) demonstrated positive effects of training on the structural properties of the rabbit ACL. The ultimate load, ultimate elongation and energy absorbed at failure of the FATC were elevated significantly above control levels in response to 40 weeks of daily training. Increases in the stress relaxation rate of the ligament substance were also measured following the exercise regimen.

The type and duration of training regimens have been reported to effect the properties of ligaments. Zuckerman and Stull (1969) subjected rats to 9 weeks of swimming or running (15 min/day, 5 days/week). This forced physical activity accompanied by ad lib cage activity increased the ultimate load of the FMTC by more than 35% over those of untrained controls. Similarly, Tipton et al. (1975b) demonstrated that 10 weeks of endurance treadmill training significantly increased the ultimate load of the rat FMTC and the ultimate load/body weight ratio by 10%. In contrast, sprint training had no effect on the strength of the FMTC, but did produce heavier ligaments. The response of a single exercise bout was found to have no effect of any of the biomechanical parameters. The properties of the ligament were enhanced only when the animals were subjected to endurance exercise. Further studies by Tipton et al. (1977) demonstrated that running on an inclined treadmill produced a 12% increase in the ultimate load of the FMTC, but level running produced no significant effects. This was attributed to the lack of stress on knee structures when running on level ground. Cabaud et al. (1980) examined the effects of frequency and duration of treadmill exercise on the tensile properties of the rat ACL. Exercising 6 days/week proved to be more effective than 3 days/week on improving both the structural and mechanical properties. Interestingly, exercise periods of 30 min/day enhanced the stiffness, ultimate load, modulus and tensile strength more than 60 min/day. Age and sex have also been shown to have an influence on the response of ligaments to exercise (Tipton et al. 1975a, 1986).

Changes induced by long-term exercise are equally important, but only limited data are available. Our laboratory studied the effects of prolonged exercise on the biomechanical properties of the swine FMTC (Woo et al. 1979). One-year-old swine were trained for 12 months for 1 hr/day at 1.6 m/sec plus 0.5 hr every other day at 2.2 m/sec, based on a 5-day/week regimen. Age-matched control swine were allowed ad lib activity during this time. At sacrifice the average body masses of the two groups were significantly different from each other; the mass of exercised swine was 66±6 kg, while that of controls was 77±16 kg. Tensile testing showed that this long-term exercise induced some increases in the structural properties of the FMTC. The ultimate load/body weight increased by 38%, and there was a 14% increase in the stiffness. The mechanical properties of the MCL substance were also affected by the exercise regimen, but to a lesser extent. The modulus increased slightly, and there was a 20% increase in tensile strength and a 10% increase in ultimate strain.

The effects of lifelong exercise on the properties of the canine FMTC have recently been examined by our laboratory. In a collaborative study with the University of Iowa, beagles were exercised on a treadmill (3 km/hr, 75 min/day, 5 days/wk) for most of their life span (Wang et al. 1990). This exercise regimen did not induce changes in the structural properties of the FMTC or the mechanical properties of the MCL substance. No statistical differences in the stiffness, ultimate load, ultimate elongation or energy absorbed between the 'trained' and age-matched 'old' groups could be measured. The modulus of the MCL substance was elevated over 20% in the trained group; however this value, as well as the tensile strength, was not significantly different between the two groups. The lack of effect of exercise was attributed to aging effects, which may have masked any potential gains of exercise training. It is possible that shorter exercise periods (i.e. 2-3 years) would produce more pronounced changes in the tensile properties of the FMTC.

From these studies it is clear that differing levels of stress can produce different effects on the biomechanical properties of knee ligaments. Examining the results of these studies, a general trend of the responses of

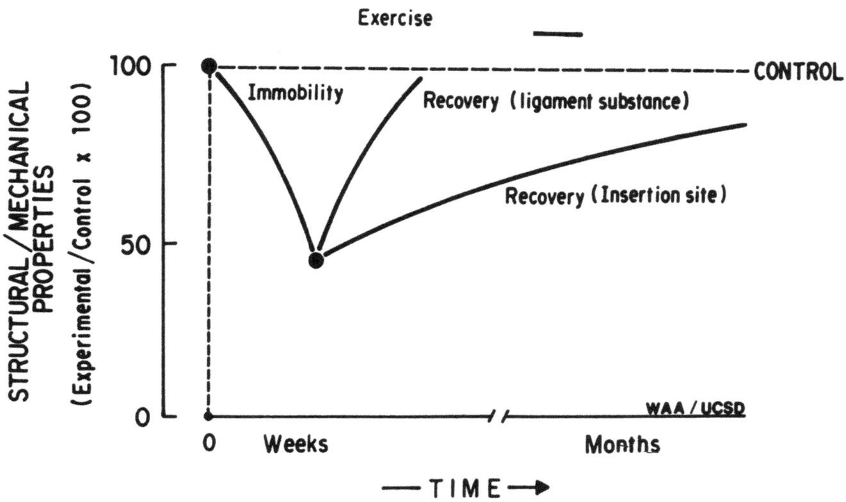

Figure 10: A schematic representation of the time course and magnitude of the effects of various stress levels on the tensile properties of ligaments.

ligaments and their insertions to bone to stress deprivation and stress enhancement emerges (Figure 10). In general, immobilization quickly compromises the stiffness and strength of the bone-ligament-bone complex, and the weakening occurs most notably at the insertion sites. This is illustrated by the fact that the FMTCs of immobilized knees fail in tension most frequently at the tibial insertion. Histological findings suggest that bony resorption by increased osteoclastic activity is the cause of the loss of integrity of the insertion following immobilization. Following remobilization, the biomechanical properties of the bone-ligament-bone complex may return to normal after a retraining period. However, there is an asynchronous rate of recovery of the ligament substance and its insertions to bone. Increased tension or exercise produce much less dramatic changes in the biomechanical properties. While the biomechanical properties of the ligament were enhanced in response to increased tension, there were only mild improvements. In the case of exercise training, the effects on ligaments are less straightforward. The important parameters include age, species, sex, exercise type and duration. However, cumulated data indicate that increased stress levels enhance the structural and mechanical properties of ligaments. The effects are small, and long durations of increased stress are required.

Injury and Healing

Medial Collateral Ligament

Generally, isolated collateral ligament tears heal even when treated nonoperatively. However, factors such as the location and extent of injury can affect the end result of healing. To determine the most appropriate treatment regimen, one must obtain an understanding of the injury mechanism, location of injury and the natural course of unaided ligament healing.

Mechanism and Location of Injury

Study of the injury mechanisms of the knee ligaments has yielded information on the types and frequency of MCL injuries. In Palmer's study (1938) of the response of cadaver knees to abduction-flexion-supination, there was complete rupture of the superior insertion of the MCL in one instance, while the rest had what were described as "dissociated ruptures in the body with shifting of the sections in relation to each other". He emphasized that injuries produced in cadaver knees do not represent the same injuries that are seen clinically, due to the lack of pressures on the joint from stance and muscle action. Both Palmer and Hultén (1929) felt that one of the most common injuries to the MCL seen clinically was at the femoral insertion. Other types of injuries reported were complete rupture near or in the inferior insertion, multiple ruptures in the superficial MCL with associated tears of the meniscal anchorages, and "overstretching" of the superficial MCL without loss of continuity. Kennedy and Fowler (1970) found that following application of a valgus moment at 20° knee flexion the oblique ligament was torn first, followed by the medial collateral ligament. Price and Allen (1978) reported that the most commonly seen MCL injury was distal avulsion of the ligament with central disruption of the oblique MCL as well. They emphasized that usually both the superficial and deep layers of the MCL are injured, with all combinations of proximal, central and distal rupture of these two structures occurring.

Early experimental studies examined the mechanisms of MCL injury and the natural course of healing. Miltner et al. (1937) used manual force to produce both mild and severe knee sprains in rabbits. Damage to both the ligament substance and its insertions to bone was identified histologically. Fibroblastic proliferation was present in both groups at one week postoperatively. Horwitz (1939) studied ligament healing using the surgically transected rabbit MCL as the experimental injury model. Healing was noted to occur even when a large gap existed between the ligament ends. Edema and hematoma formed the scaffold of the early scar, which was penetrated by young fibroblasts and vascular endothelial buds. Jack (1950) used manual knee abduction to produce both minor and severe ruptures of the feline MCL. He reported that tears at the insertions and in the ligament substance were equally common. During the early stages of healing, the ligament had numerous fibroblasts and blood vessels along the entire length of the structure. At two weeks postoperatively, the torn ends of the ligament were almost indistinguishable from the surrounding scar mass. However, the number of cells and blood vessels remained elevated for many weeks after injury. When the injury occurred at the femoral insertion, poor healing occurred, probably due to disruption of the blood supply from the areolar covering and synovial membrane.

Recently, our laboratory used a braided wire suture to produce a consistent midsubstance defect in the MCL of rabbits (Frank et al. 1983). Animals were evaluated up to 40 weeks postoperatively. The gap was filled with vascular inflammatory tissue at 10 days, but by 3 weeks the healing zone was dominated by fibroblasts. A decrease in cell number and some improvement in collagen organization was noted by 6 weeks. A further decrease in cell number occurred by 14 weeks, but between 14 and 40 weeks histological appearance did not change notably. The cross-sectional area of the ligament was over three times that of the sham-operated control at 3 weeks postoperatively. The area decreased over time but was still 1.7 times larger than the sham at 40 weeks. The ultimate load of the experimental FMTCs increased over time, but only reached 60% of that of the sham-operated controls. The mechanical properties of the healing MCL substance were also found to be inferior to those of the sham at 40 weeks postoperatively. It was observed that all ligaments healed by scar formation, with large amounts of type III collagen present up to 40 weeks postinjury. From these findings it was concluded that the increased ligament area could not restore normal structural properties due to the mechanically inferior scar tissue.

It is well-known that surgical transection cannot produce a MCL injury similar to those seen clinically. Walsh and Frank (1988) demonstrated that both the scalpel and wire suture methods of injury produce relatively localized damage to the ligament substance with virtually no damage to the insertions to bone. In our laboratory we recently developed a combined injury model which includes damage to both the MCL substance and its

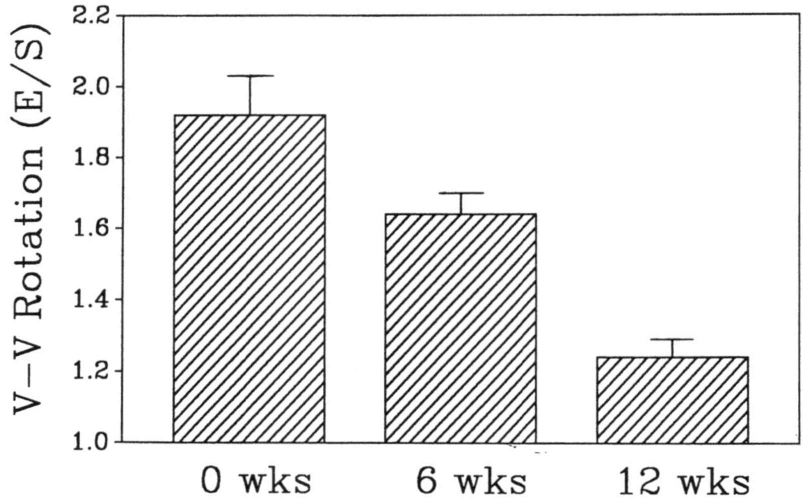

Figure 11: Varus-valgus rotation of healing rabbit knees as a function of postoperative time.

insertions to bone (Weiss et al. 1990). A stainless steel rod (2.3 mm dia.) was passed transversely beneath the MCL of skeletally mature rabbits at the joint line. Two small nicks were placed in the ligament at the level of the pin, and the rod was then pulled medially until the MCL ruptured.

Histological examination of the ligament and its insertions to bone at 10 days postoperatively showed evidence of a tearing injury with increased vascularity at the tibial insertion. The varus-valgus knee rotation was increased almost twofold immediately following injury (Figure 11). There was a recovery of the joint stability over time, but by 12 weeks the varus-valgus rotation was still significantly larger than the sham-operated contralateral controls. ($p<0.001$). Tensile testing of the FMTCs revealed a significant increase in all structural properties (ultimate load, ultimate elongation, and energy absorbed) from 6 to 12 weeks, but even at 12 weeks postoperatively these properties of the healing ligaments were far inferior to the shams (Figure 12a). All sham operated controls failed in the MCL midsubstance. At 6 weeks, all experimental MCLs failed by avulsion at the tibial insertion, indicating that this was the weakest structural link. By 12 weeks, over 70% of the experimental MCLs failed in the ligament substance. These failure modes are different from those found in a previous study from our laboratory using simple scalpel transection as the injury model, in which

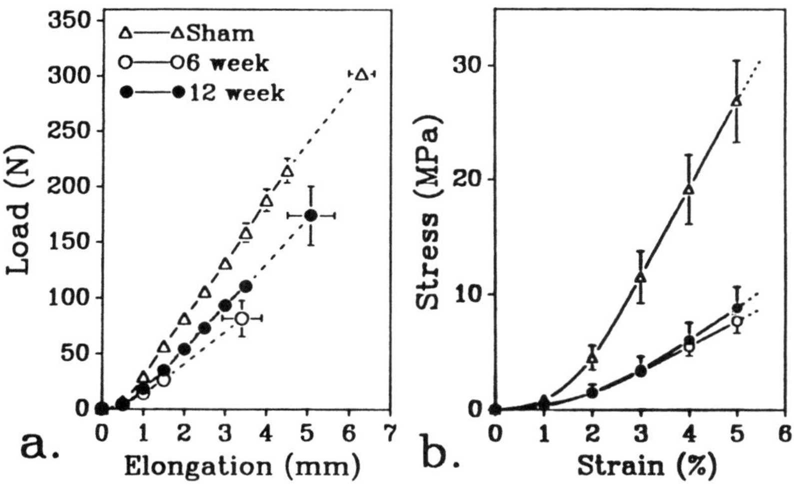

Figure 12: (a) Load-Elongation and (b) stress-strain curves of healing rabbit MCL-bone complexes.

all failures occurred in the MCL midsubstance (Gomez et al. 1988). This suggests that the tibial insertion was damaged during the MCL injury.

It is also interesting to note that there was little or no change in the mechanical properties of the MCL substance from 6 to 12 weeks, but at both time periods the modulus was significantly less than the shams (Figure 12b). The cross-sectional area of healing ligaments was elevated and did not change between 6 and 12 weeks postoperatively. From these results, we can surmise that there was a differential rate of healing of the MCL substance and the tibial insertion, i.e. the MCL substance healed faster than the tibial insertion. Further, the healing MCL had a larger cross-sectional area, but the properties of the material (mechanical properties) were inferior to those of normal tissue. Preliminary data on long-term healing suggest that at 52 weeks postoperatively, the structural properties of the FMTC are similar to the shams, but the mechanical properties of the MCL substance are still inferior.

Treatment Regimen

Clinical studies of the effect of different treatment regimens on MCL healing have produced conflicting results. O'Donoghue (1955) recommended the surgical repair and subsequent immobilization of MCL injuries to afford the best outcome in the least time. Other investigators have also advocated these surgical techniques (Price and Allen 1978; Ginsburg and Elsasser 1978). In the last ten to fifteen years, many have found that patients respond equally well (or better) to nonoperative treatment of MCL injury (Fetto and Marshall 1978; Holden et al. 1983; Indelicato 1983; Warren and Marshall 1978). These studies have suggested that immobilization is not necessary, and that early motion and exercise accelerates recovery. Still others felt that treatment regimen should be based on the type or degree of MCL injury (Ellsasser et al. 1974; Hastings 1980; Kannus 1988; Weaver et al. 1985). Clearly the treatment of choice following MCL injury is highly debated, in part due to the subjective and widely divergent nature of grouping and evaluation techniques, as well as diagnostic inaccuracies.

Experimental studies have also examined the efficacy of primary repair of the torn MCL vs. nonoperative treatment. Clayton and Weir (1959) evaluated the effect of primary repair on healing of the surgically transected canine MCL. Both limbs were immobilized. Repaired ligaments were found to have a higher ultimate load at all time intervals up to 9 weeks postoperatively and better collagen fiber organization. Kappakas et al. (1978) examined the effect of immediate and delayed repair on healing of the surgically transected rabbit MCL, and reported that repair carried out within 3 days of injury improved the ultimate load of the FMTC. However, a delay in repair of more than 10 days produced results no different from those obtained following nonoperative treatment. Vailas et al. (1981) found that surgical repair of the rat MCL followed by brief immobilization produced MCLs with a higher ultimate load than that of nonrepaired, nonimmobilized animals. Conversely, Hart and Dahners (1987) reported that surgically transected and repaired rat MCLs were not stronger than nonrepaired ligaments. Again, the literature on experimental animal studies does not agree as to the effect of repair on MCL healing. This could be due to differences in injury model, healing time and other treatment factors such as immobilization.

Our laboratory recently performed a comparative study in which healing of the transected canine MCL was examined histologically, biomechanically and biochemically at 6, 12 and 48 weeks postoperatively (Woo et al. 1987a). Ligament injuries received either (a) conservative treatment with no repair or (b) surgical treatment with repair and 6 weeks of immobilization. The biomechanical properties of the nonrepaired ligaments exhibited the best results at all time periods. At 6 weeks, both groups showed higher V-V rotation than their controls, but there was no significant difference between them. At 12 weeks, the V-V rotation values of the nonrepaired group returned to normal, but the values of the repaired knees were still more than two times those of the controls. This trend persisted at 48 weeks.

The structural properties of the FMTC were found to be similar for the repaired and nonrepaired groups at 6 weeks postoperatively. Both load-elongation curves were below the curve for the controls (Figure 13). At 48 weeks the nonrepaired group had a load-elongation curve that more closely resembled the control curve. The ultimate load of the nonrepaired group was similar to the controls, but that of the repaired group was well below the controls. The mechanical properties of the healing ligaments did not improve as rapidly or as completely as the structural properties of the FMTCs. At 6 weeks, the moduli of the experimental groups were far less than that of the control group. At 48 weeks, the tensile strength of the MCL of the nonrepaired group was still only 63% of the control group.

Histologic findings showed that by 48 weeks postoperatively, the healing tissues from both the repaired and nonrepaired groups had appearances similar to those of normal MCL. Examination under polarized light microscopy, however, revealed that the orientation of the collagen fibers remained irregular.

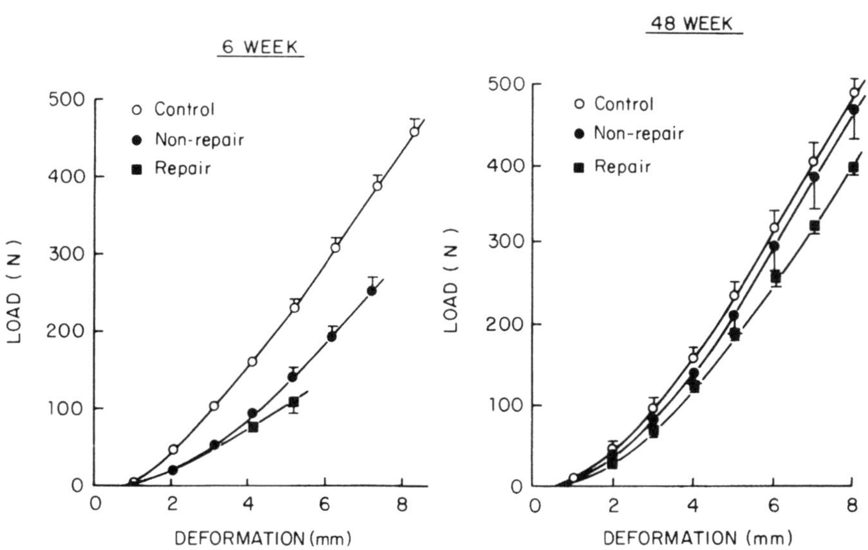

Figure 13: Structural properties of the repaired and nonrepaired canine FMTC at 6 and 48 weeks postoperatively.

Associated ACL Injury

The prognosis for healing of combined MCL-ACL injuries is generally worse than that for the isolated MCL injury, regardless of the treatment regimen used (Fetto and Marshall 1978). However, Jokl et al. (1984) reported favorable results following nonoperative treatment of combined MCL-ACL injuries in young and active patients. Our laboratory has examined the effect of partial and total transection of the canine ACL on MCL healing (Woo et al. 1990b). At 6 weeks postoperatively, the V-V rotation of experimental knees from both groups was significantly higher than that of the sham-operated controls. The V-V rotation of the coomplete ACL transection group was 3.5 times as large as the controls, but that of the partial ACL transection group was only twice that of the controls. At 12 weeks, however, the V-V rotation for knees with partial transection of the ACL was similar to the control values, whereas that of the complete ACL transection group was still over 3.5 times as large as the controls (Figure 14). These results are in agreement with those obtained by Forbes et al. (1988). The structural properties of the FMTC from the experimental groups changed differentially with healing time. The ultimate load of the partial ACL transection group was equivalent to that of the controls by 12 weeks postoperatively, but that of the total ACL transection group was only 80% of control values at this time. The mechanical properties of the healed MCL of both groups remained significantly inferior to those of control ligaments. At 12 weeks postoperatively. the tensile strength of the partial transection group was 45% of control values, while that of the total transection group was only 14%. The detrimental effects of ACL deficiency on MCL healing have been clearly demonstrated.

Anterior Cruciate Ligament

Mechanism of Injury

Injury to the ACL can occur through several different mechanisms. A rotational stress on the knee, often incurred while turning and cutting during sports activities, has been observed by several clinical investigators to be the most common mode of injury (Arnold et al. 1979; Feagin 1979; Feagin et al. 1982; Sandberg et al. 1987; Straub and Hunter 1988). A valgus stress, in addition to causing injury to the MCL, can also damage the ACL (Straub and Hunter 1988). The ACL is considered the primary restraint to anterior

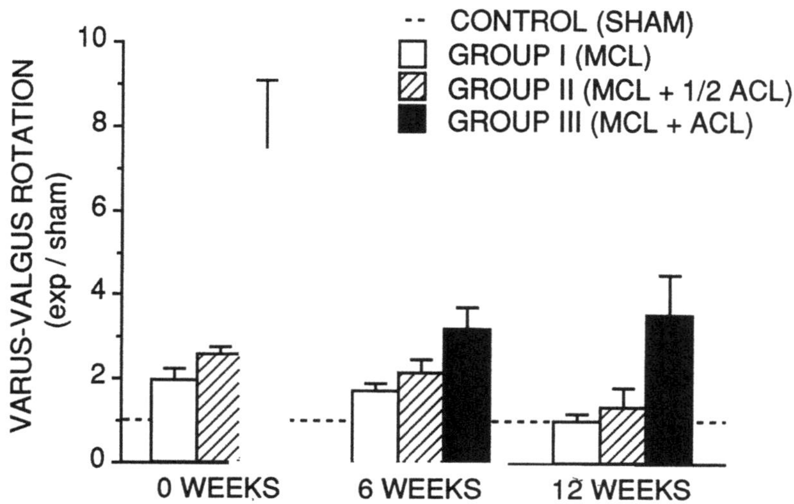

Figure 14: Varus-valgus rotation for canine knees. The groups are: I) MCL transection; II) MCL transection with partial ACL transection; III) both MCL and ACL transection.

tibial translation, hence an anterior force applied to the posterior of the tibia can also tear the ACL. Finally, hyperextension of the knee can injure this ligament as well (Straub and Hunter 1988). Although isolated injury to the ACL is relatively rare (Arnold et al. 1979; Johnson 1983), concomitant injuries to the meniscus, MCL, PCL, or other soft tissue structures around the knee occur frequently (Noyes et al. 1983; Feagin 1979; Johnson 1983; Arnold et al. 1979).

Unlike the MCL, the untreated ACL injury in the midsubstance cannot heal (Arnold et al. 1979; Sandberg et al. 1987; McDaniel and Dameron 1980; Johnson 1983; Kennedy et al. 1974). When the ACL is torn, it is often resorbed (O'Donoghue et al. 1966). It has been hypothesized that the presence of blood and enzymatic action by collagenase in the synovial fluid may be the cause (Ishizue et al. 1990, Pforringer 1982). If these enzymes are indeed responsible for the degradation, then the question arises as to what protects the intact ACL.

The biosynthetic activity of the fibroblasts as well as the intrinsic differences in the morphological structure may also explain the differences in healing between the MCL and ACL. Histologically, fibroblasts of the ACL have a different appearance when compared to those of the MCL (Lyon et al. 1989). The ACL cells are more oval and arranged in distinct columns between the collagen fibrils, while the fibroblasts of the MCL are more elongated and interspersed more randomly throughout the collagen. The MCL fibroblasts have long processes that extend out into the collagen matrix and abut directly against the collagen fibrils. In contrast, the ACL fibroblasts do not possess any long processes, and ground substance exists between the collagen fibrils and the cell wall. In both cases the long axis of the cells are aligned with the loading axis of the ligaments.

Perhaps the most widely accepted explanation for the lack of healing of the ACL is the disruption of the ligament's blood supply following injury. While all ligaments are relatively avascular tissues, the MCL appears to have a better vascular supply. The primary blood supply to the ACL is from the middle geniculate artery which enters at the posterior intercondylar notch with some collateral vessels extending from the infrapatellar fat pad (Kennedy et al. 1974). However, vessels do not enter the ligament from insertions to bone or through the mineralized fibrocartilage zone of the insertion (Whiteside and Sweeney 1980). It is possible that upon injury the torn ends of the ligament are not able to obtain the nutrients necessary for healing to take place. Arnoczky et al. (1979) examined changes in the blood supply due to partial laceration of the ACL. Although a "vigorous and extensive" vascular response was reported, "spontaneous healing of the defect had not occurred ... by eight weeks." They also noted that the vascular response was reduced by removal of the infrapatellar fat pad and synovial membrane at the time of transection.

Treatment Regimen

Treatment of the ACL injury has been a subject of controversy for many years. For young and active patients, reconstruction of the ACL using either an autograft or allograft is widely performed, and clinical studies have generally claimed good to excellent results. The appropriate choice of the ligament graft, graft placement, and surgical technique are highly debated. Experimental animal studies have reported less optimistic results using the patellar tendon autograft. In general, the strength and stiffness obtained during tensile testing of the femur-graft-tibia complexes have been substantially lower in comparison to the control FATC up to two years postoperatively (Butler et al. 1983; McPherson et al. 1985). In a rabbit model using the medial third of the patellar tendon as an autograft, very results were reported (Ballock et al. 1989). The stiffness and load of the femur-graft-tibia complex were only 13% and 11% of the control FATC. The different results from this study, in comparison to others may be due in part to differences in the methods of testing. A more sophisticated clamping device for tensile testing was used so that the specimen can be aligned in favorable orientations, without altering the angles of ligament insertions to bone. This yielded a much higher stiffness and strength data for the control specimens.

ACL/Knee Kinematics

Since the anatomy and function of the ACL is rather complex, it is necessary to study and develop a better understanding of knee kinematics and *in-situ* length and *in-situ* loads of various fiber bundles of the ACL. Additionally, kinematic measurements are necessary to evaluate the functional success of ACL replacements. These data can be further utilized for replacement design and selection. There are numerous published reports on this topic and the details can be found in this book in the chapter by Butler and associates. Note, however, that the majority of studies have not considered the effects of muscle forces. Recently, we have examined the 6 DOF motion of intact and ACL deficient human cadaver knees using a device called an Oxford Rig (O'Connor et al. 1988) in which specimens are tested in a simulated vertical stance with and without simulated quadriceps stabilization (Figure 15).
In the absence of quadriceps force, the tibia translated anteriorly 24.8±1.8 mm with respect to the femur as the intact knee was extended from 100 to 0° flexion. When a quadriceps load was applied, the translation increased anteriorly throughout the range of knee flexion (Adams et al. 1990). Sectioning the ACL led to increased anterior tibial translation at all flexion angles over the intact state, independent of quadriceps force. In quadriceps stabilized knees, the change in translation was small as the knee was extended from 100° to 70° flexion. The change in tibial translation gradually increased to a maximum at 20° and decreased again at full flexion (Figure 16).

Using the same testing device, we further examined the load experienced by a patellar tendon allograft in two different reconstruction models (Takai et al. 1989). A patellar tendon allograft was either placed in an isometric double bone tunnel position or in the "over the top" position. The graft load was measured in either the quadriceps stabilized or quadriceps absent state. For both states, the over the top method showed increases increases from ~5N to ~70N as the knee was extended from 100° to 0° flexion. The double bone tunnel reconstruction showed less variation in the graft loads through the arc of flexion, it must be pointed out, however, that no true isometry of the graft could be demonstrated.

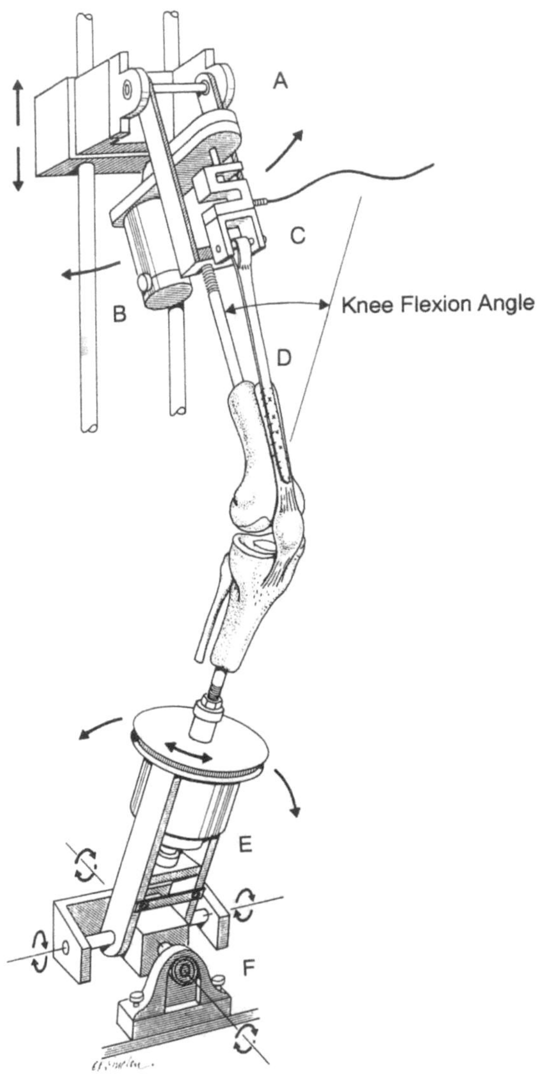

Figure 15: Schematic of Oxford Rig allowing 6 degrees of freedom.

In the quadriceps absent state, the load started at ~40N at 100° flexion, decreased to ~25N at 30° and then returned to ~40N at 0° flexion. Quadriceps stabilized knees had consistently higher graft loads which increased from 100°-60° and then decreased to approximately the same level at 0° flexion.

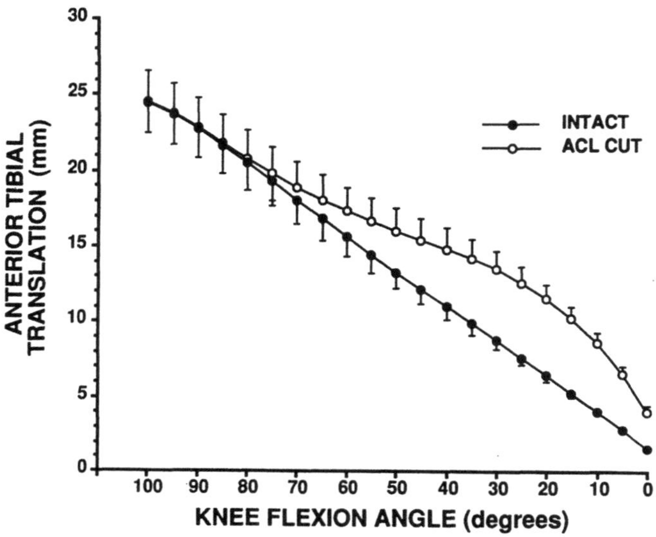

Figure 16: Anterior tibial translation of intact and ACL deficient human knees as a function of knee flexion angle.

Future Studies

This chapter has reviewed some of our recent findings on the biomechanics and morphology of the medial collateral and anterior cruciate ligaments. The development of new measurement and analysis techniques has proivided data to further understand the structure and function relationship of these knee ligaments. Accurate experimental techniques have allowed us to evaluate the effects of factors such as aging, stress level, injury and treatment regimen on the biomechanical propterties of normal and repaired ligaments. Sophisticated technology has also allowed the observation of details of the ligament and insertion sites.

In the furture we hope to use our MCL injury model that more closely approximates clinical injury to examine healing following concomitant injury to the ACL and the medial meniscus. Once these baseline data are obtained, the effect of ACL reconstruction on the healing of this "triad" injury will be evaluated. Furthermore, we are currently developing new methodologies to determine the *in situ* forces in ligaments and the effects of these forces on the healing and remodeling of the tissue.

Abrahams M: Mechanical behavior of tendon *in vitro*. Med Biol Eng 1967;5:433-443.

Adams DJ, Shoemaker SC, Harris SL, Daniel D, Woo SL-Y: Trans of 36th annual ORS, 1990;15(2):508.

Akeson WH, Amiel D, Woo SL-Y: Immobility effects on synovial joints. The pathomechanics of joint contracture. Biorheology 1980;17:95-110.

Akeson WH, Woo SL-y, Amiel D, Matthews JV: Biomechanical and biochemical changes in the periarticular connective tissue during contracture development in the immobilized rabbit knee. Connect Tissue Res. 1974;2:315-323.

Allard P, Thirty PS, Bourgault A, Drouin G: Pressure dependence of the "area micrometer" method in evaluation of cruciate ligament cross-section. J Biomed Eng 1979;1:265-267.

Arms SW, Pope MH, Boyle JB, Davignon PJ, Johnson RJ: Knee medial collateral ligament strain. Trans of 28th annual ORS 1982;7:47.

Arnoczky SP, Rubin RM, Marshall JL: Microvasculature of the cruciate ligaments and its response to injury. An experimental study in the dog. J Bone Joint Surg [Am] 1979;61A:1221-1229.

Arnold JA, Coker TP, Heaton LM, Park JM, Harris WD: Natural history of anteroir cruciate tears. Am J Sports Med 1979;7:305-313.

Ballock RT, Woo SL-Y, Lyon RM, Hollis JM, Akeson WH: Use of patellar tendon autograft for anterior cruciate ligament reconstruction in the rabbit - A long-term histological and biomechanical study. J Orthop Res 1989;7(4):474-485.

Binkley JM, Peat M: The effects of immobilization on the ultrastructure and mechanical properties of the medial collateral ligament of rats. Clin Orthop 1986;203:301-308.

Blanton PL and Biggs NL: Ultimate tensile strength of fetal and adult human tendons. J Biomech 1970;3:181-189.

Booth FW and Tipton CM: Ligamentous strength measurements in pre-pubescent and pubescent rats. Growth 1970;34:177-185.

Brown PC and Consden R: Variation with age of shrinkage temperature of human collagen. Nature 1958;181:349-350.

Butler DL, Grood ES, Noyes FR, Zernicke RJ, Brackett K: Effects of structure and strain measurement technique on the material properties of young human tendons and fascia. J Biomech 1984;17:579-596.

Butler DL, Hulse DA, Kay MD, Grood ES, Shires PK, D'Ambrosia R, Shoji H: Biomechanics of cranial cruciate ligament reconstruction in the dog. II. Mechanical properties. Vet Surg 1983;12:113-118.

Butler DL, Kay MD, Stouffer DC: Comparison of material properties in fascicle-bone units from human patellar tendon and knee ligaments. J Biomech 1986;19:425-432.

Cabaud HE, Chatty A, Gildengorin V, Feltman RJ: Exercise effects on the strength of the rat anterior cruiciate ligament. Am J Sports Med 1980;8(2):79-86.

Cannon DJ and Davison PF: Cross-linking and aging in rat tendon collagen. Exp Geront 1973;8:51-62.

Clayton ML and Weir GJ: Experimental investigations of ligamentous healing. Am J Surg 1959;98:373-378.

Danto MI, Marcin JP, Schultz EP, Ohland KJ, Newton PO, and Woo SL-Y: Comparison of three methods for measuring the cross-sectional area along the rabbit medial collateral ligament. ASME Biomech Symp AMD 1989;98:97-100.

Dorlot JM, Ait ba Sidi M, Gremblay GM, Drouin G: Load-elongaton behavior of the canine anterior cruciate ligament. J Biomech Eng 1980;102:190-193.

Elden HR: Aging of rat tail tendon. J Gerontol 1964;19:173-178.

Ellis DG: A shadow amplitude method for measuring cross-sectional areas of

biological specimens. 21st Annu Conf Eng Med Biol 1968;51:6.
Ellis DG: Cross-sectional area measurements for tendon specimens: A comparison of several methods. J Biomech 1969;2:175-186.
Elsasser JC, Reynolds FC, Omohundro JR: The non-operative treatment of collateral ligament injuries of the knee in professional football players: An analysis of seventy-four injuries treated non-operatively and twenty-four injuries treated surgically. J Bone Joint Surg 1974;56A(6):1185-1190.
Enneking WF, Horowitz M: The intra-articular effects of immobilization on the human knee. J Bone Joint Surg [Am] 1972;54A:973-985.
Evans EB, Eggers GWN, Butler JK, Blumel J: Experimental immobilization and remobilization of rat knee joints. J Bone Joint Surg [Am] 1960;42A:737-758.
Feagin JA: The syndrome of the tornb anterior cruciate ligament. Orthop Clin of N America 1979;10:81-90.
Feagin JA, Cabaud HE, Curl WW: The anterior cruciate ligament: Radiographic and clinical signs of successful and unsuccessful repairs. Clin Orthop 1982;164:54-58.
Fetto JF and Marshall JL: Medial collateral ligament injuries of the knee: A rationale for treatment. Clin Orthop 1978;132:206.
Forbes J, Frank C, Lam T, Shrive N: The biomechanical effects of combined ligament injuries on the medial collateral ligament. Trans Orthop Res Soc 1988;13:196.
Frank C, McDonald D, Lieber R, Sabiston P: Biochemical heterogeneity within the maturing rabbit medial collateral ligament. Clin Orthop 1988;236:279-285.
Frank C, Woo SL-Y, Amiel D, Harwood FL, Gomez M, Akeson W: Medial collateral ligament healing: A multidisciplinary assessment in rabbits. Am J Sports Med 1983;11(6):379-389.
Fung YC: Stress-strain-history relations of soft tissues in simple elongation, in Fung YC, Perrone N, Anliker M (eds): Biomechanics: Its Foundations and Objectives. Englewood Cliffs, New Jersey, Prentice Hall 1972;181-208.
Ginsburg JH and Elsasser JC: Problem areas in the diagnosis and treatment of ligament injuries of the knee. Clin Orthop 1978;132:201-205.
Gomez MA: The effect of tension on normal and healing medial collateral ligaments. PhD thesis, University of California, San Diego, 1988.
Gomez MA, Ishizue KK, Lyon RM, Kwan MK-W, Wayne JS, Furniss MA, Woo SL-Y: The effects of increased stress on medial collateral ligaments: an experimental and analytical approach. Trans of 34th annual ORS 1988;13:194.
Grood ES, Noyes FR, Butler DL, Suntay WJ: Ligamentous and capsular restraints preventing straight medial and lateral laxity in intact human cadaver knees. J Bone Joint Surg 1981;63A:1257-1269.
Gupta BN, Subraminian KN, Brinker WO, Gupta AN: Tensile strength of canine cranial cruciate ligaments. Am J Vet Res 1971;32:183-190.
Hall DA: The ageing of connective tissue, Academic Press, London, 1976.
Hama H, Yamamuro T, Takeda T: Experimental studies on connective tissue of the capsular ligament. Influences of aging and sex hormones. Acta Orthop Scand 1976;47:473-479.
Hart DP and Dahners LE: Healing of the medial collateral ligament in rats: The effects of repair, motion, and secondary stabilizing ligaments. J Bone Joint Surg 1987;69A:1194-1199.
Hastings DE: The non-operative management of collateral ligament injuries of the knee joint. Clin Orthop 1980;147:22-28.
Haut RC, Little RW: Rheological properties of canine anterior cruciate ligaments. J Biomech 1969;2:289-298.
Holden DL, Eggert AW, Butler JE: The nonoperative treatment of Grade I and II medial collateral ligament injuries to the knee. Am J Sports Med 1983;11:340-

344.
Hollis JM, Horibe S, Adams DJ, Marcin JP, Woo SL-Y: Force distribuion in the anterior cruciate ligament as a function of flexion angle. Biomech Symp AMD 1989;98:41-44.
Hollis JM, Lyon RM, Marcin JP, Horibe S, Lee EB, Woo SL-Y: Effect of age and loading axis on the failure properties of the human ACL. Trans of 34th annual ORS 1988;13:81.
Horwitz MT: Injuries of ligaments of knee joint: An experimental study. Arch Surg 1939;38:946-954.
Hultèn: Ueber die indireckten Brücke des Tibiakopfes nebst Beiträgen zur Röntgenologie des Kniegelenks. Acta Chir Scand (Supp. 15) 1929;66:1-167.
Indelicato PA: Non-operative treatment of complete tears of the medial collateral ligament of the knee. J Bone Joint Surg 1983;65A(3):323-329.
Inoue M, McGurk-Burleson E, Hollis JM: Treatment of the medial collateral ligament injury. 1. The importance of anterior cruciate ligament on the varus-valgus knee laxity. Am J Sports Med 1987;15:15-21.
Ishizue KK, Amiel D, Lyon RM, Woo SL-Y: Acute Hemarthrosis: A histological, biochemical and biomechanical correlation of effects on the anterior cruciate ligament in a rabbit model. J Orthop Res, In Press 1990.
Jack EA: Experimental rupture of the medial collateral ligament of the knee. J Bone Joint Surg [Br] 1950;32B:396-402.
Johnson RJ: The anterior cruciate ligament problem. Clin Orthop 1983;172:14-18.
Kannus P: Long-term results of conservatively treated medial collateral ligament injuries of the knee joint. Clin Orthop 1988;226:103-111.
Kappakas GS, Brown TD, Goodman MA, Kikuike A, McMaster JH: Delayed surgical repair of ruptured ligaments. Clin Orthop 1978;135:281-296.
Kennedy JC and Fowler PJ: Medial and anterior instability of the knee. An anatomical and clinical study using stress machines. J Bone Joint Surg 1970;53A:1257-1270.
Kennedy JC, Hawkins RJ, Willis RB: Strain gauge analysis of knee ligaments. Clin Orthop 1977;129:225-229.
Kennedy JC, Weinberg HW, Wilson AS: The anatomy and function of the anterior cruciate ligament. As determined by clinical and morphological studies. J Bone Joint Surg [Am] 1974;56A:223.
Langenskoid A, Michelsson JE, Videman T: Osteroarthritis of the knee in the rabbit produced by immobilization. Acta Orthop Scan 1979;50:1-14.
Laros GS, Tipton CM, Cooper RR: Influence of physical activity on ligament insertions in the knees of dogs. J Bone Joint Surg [Am} 1971;53A(2):275-286.
Larsen NP, Forwood MR, Parker AW: Immobilization and retraining of cruciate ligaments in the rat. Acta Orthop Scand 1987;58:260-264.
Lee TQ and Woo SL-Y: A new method for determining cross-sectional shape and area of soft tissues. J Biomech Eng 1988;110:110-114.
Lin H-C, Kwan MK-W, Woo SL-Y: On the stress relaxation properties of anterior cruciate ligament (ACL). Adv. Bioeng [WAM/ASME BED] 1987;3:5-6.
Lyon RM, Billings E Jr, Woo SL-Y, Ishizue KK, Kitabayshi LR, Amiel D, Akeson WH: The ACL: A fibrocartilagenous structure. Trans. of 35th annual ORS. 1987;14:189.
Lyon RM, Woo SL-Y, Hollis JM, Marcin JP, Lee EB: A new device to measure the structural properties of the femur-anterior cruciate ligament-tibia complex. J Biom. Engrg 1989;111:350-354.
Masoud I, Shapiro F, Kent R, Moses A: A longitudinal study of the growth of the New Zealand White rabbit: Cumulative and biweekly incremental growth rates for body length, body weight, femoral length, and tibial length. J Orthop Res

1986;4:221-231.

Matthews LS and Ellis D: Viscoelastic properties of cat tendon: Effects of time after death and preservation by freezing. J Biomech 1968;1:65-71.

Matyas JR, Frank C: Midsubstance injury of the rabbit MCL affects the tissue architecture of the femoral insertion. Trans. of 36th annual ORS, 1990a;15(1):34.

Matyas JR, Frank C: Midsubstance injury to the rabbit MCL causes changes similar to immobilization at the tibial insertion. Trans. of 36th annual ORS, 1990b;15(2):525.

Mays PK, Bishop JE, Jaurent GJ: Age-related changes in the proportion of types I and III collagen. Mech Ageing and Dev 1988;45:203-212.

McDaniel WJ and Dameron TB: Untreated ruptures of the anterior cruciate ligament: A follow-up study. J Bone Joint Surg [Am] 1980;62A:696-705.

McDaniel WJ and Dameron TB: The untreated anterior cruciate ligament rupture. Clin Orthop 1983;172:158-163.

McPherson GK, Mendenhall HV, Gibbons DF, et al.: Experimental, mechanical and histologic evaluation of the Kennedy ligament augmentation device. Clin Otrhop 1985;196:186-195.

Meglan D, Zuelzer W, Buck W, Berme N: The effects of quadriceps force upon strain in the anterior cruciate ligament. Trans of 32nd annual ORS 1986;11:55.

Miltner LJ, Hu CH, Fang HC: Experimental reproduction of joint sprain. Arch Surg 1937;35:234-240.

Monohan JJ, Grigg P, Pappas AM, et al.: In vivo strain patterns in the four major canine knee ligaments. J Orthop Res 1984;2:408-418.

Muller P and Dahners LE: A study of ligamentous growth. Clin Orthop 1988;229:272-277.

Newton PO, MacKenna DA, Danto MI, Kitabayashi LR, Woo SL-Y: Improved methodologies to differentiate the mechanical properties of the rabbit anterior cruciate ligament (ACL) and medial collateral ligament (MCL). Trans of 36th annual ORS 1990a;15(2):509.

Newton PO, MacKenna DA, Kitabayashi LR, Akeson WH, Woo SL-Y: Biomechanical and ultrastructural changes in the rabbit anterior cruciate ligament (ACL) following immobilization. Trans of 36th annual ORS 1990b;15(1):35.

Nielson S, Andersen CK, Rasmussen O, Andersen A: Instability of cadaver knees after transection of capsule and ligaments. Acta Orthop Scan 1984;55:30-34.

Njus GO and Njus NM: A non-contact method for determining cross-sectional area of soft tissues. Trans Orthop Res Soc 1986;32:126.

Noyes FR: Functional properties of knee ligaments and alterations induced by immobilization. A corresative biomechanical and histologial study in primates. Clin Orthop 1977;123:210-242.

Noyes FR, DeLucas JL, Torvik PJ: Biomechanics of anterior cruciate ligament failure: an analysis of strain rate sensitivity and mechanisms of failure in primates. J Bone Joint Surg 1974a;56A:236-253.

Noyes FR and Grood ES: The strength of the anterior cruciate ligament in humans and rhesus monkeys. Age-related and species changes. J Bone Joint Surg 1976;58A:1074-1082.

Noyes FR, Mooar PA, Matthews DS, Butler DL: The symptomatic anterior cruciate deficient knee - Part I: The long-term functional disability in athletically active individuals. J Bone Joint Surg 1983;65A:154-162.

Noyes FR, Torvik PJ, Hyde WB, DeLucas JL: Biomechanics of ligament failure. J Bone Joint Surg 1974b;56A(7):1406-1418.

O'Connor JJ, Goodfellow JW, Bradley JA: Quadriceps forces following mensical knee arthoplasty - an in vitro study. Trans of 34th annual ORS 1988;13:357.

O'Donoghue DH: An analysis of end results of surgical treatment of major injuries to

the ligaments of the knee. J Bone Joint Surg 1955;37A:1-13.
O'Donoghue DH, Rockwood CA, Jack SC, Kenyon R: Repair of the anterior cruciate ligament in dogs. J Bone Joint Surg [Am] 1966;48A:503-519.
Ohland KJ, Weiss JA, Wang CW, Woo SL-Y: The effects of age and sex on the biomechanical properties of the medial collateral ligament. ASME Biomech Symp BED 1989;15:113-114.
Palmer I: On the injuries to the ligaments of the knee joint. Acta Chir Scan (Supp) 1938;81:3-282.
Pforringer W: Hamarthros and Kreuzbander - tiel 1. biomechanische untersuchangen. Unfallchirugie 1982;8:353-367.
Pollock RG, Soslowsky LJ, Bigliani LU, Flatow EL, Pawluk RJ, Mow VC: The mechanical properties of the inferior glenohumeral ligament. Trans. of 36th annual ORS 1990;15(2):510.
Price CT and Allen WC: Ligament repair of the knee with preservation of the meniscus. J Bone Joint Surg 1978;60A:61-65.
Rauch G, Allzeit B, Gotzen L: Biomechanical studies on the tensile strength of the anterior cruciate ligament, with special reference to age-dependence. Unfallchirugie 1988;91:437-443.
Robins SP, Shimokomaki M, Bailey AJ: The chemistry of the collagen cross-links: Age-related changes in the reducible components of intact bovine collagen fibres. Biochem J 1973;131:771-780.
Rundgren A and Viidik A: Graviditetens inverkan pà ledkomponenters mekaniska egenskaper. Nord Med 1972;86:1091.
Sabiston P, Frank C, Lam T, Shrive N: Transplantation of the rabbit medial collateral ligament I. Biomechanical evaluation of fresh autografts. J Orthop Res 1990a;8(1):35-45.
Sabiston P, Frank C, Lam T, Shrive N: Transplantation of the rabbit medial collateral ligament II. Biomechanical evaluation of frozen/thawed allografts. J Orthop Res 1990b;8(1):46-56.
Sandberg R, Balkfors B, Nilsson B, Westlin N: Operative versus non-operative treatment of recent injuries to the ligaments of the knee. J Bone Joint Surg 1987;69A:1120-1126.
Seering WP, Piziali RL, Nagel DA, Schurman DJ: The function of the primary ligaments of the knee in varus-valgus and axial rotation. J Biomech 1980;13:785-794.
Shikata J, Sanada H, Yamamuro T, Takeda T: Experimental studies of the elastic fiber of the capsular ligament: Influence of ageing and sex hormones on the hip joint capsule of rats. Conn Tissue Res 1979;7:21-27.
Straub T and Hunter RE: Acute anterior cruciate ligament repair. Clin Orthop 1988;227:238-250.
Takai S, Adams DJ, Shoemaker DM, Woo SL-Y: Use of patellar tendon autografts for anterior cruciate ligament (ACL) reconstruction: A tissue engineering perspective. ASME Tissue Eng Symp 1989;107-110.
Tipton CM, Martin RK, Matthes RD, Carey RA: Hydroxyproline concentrations in ligaments from trained and nontrained rats, in Poortmans HJ JR (ed): Metabolic Adaptation to Prolonged Physical Exercise. Basel, Birkhauser Verlag, 1975a;262-267.
Tipton CM, Matthes RD, Martin RK: Influence of age and sex on the strength of bone-ligament junctions in knee joints of rats. J Bone Joint Surg 1978;60A:230-234.
Tipton CM, Matthes RD, Maynard JA, Carey RA: The influence of physical activity on ligaments and tendons. Med Sci Sports 1975b;7(3):165-175.
Tipton CM, Matthes RD, Vailas AC: Influences de l'exercise sur les structures

ligamentaires. In: Lacour J. ed. Facteurs limitant l'endurance humaine. Saint-Etienne Conference, 1977;103-114.

Tipton CM, Matthes RD, Vailas AC, Schnoebelen CL: The response of the Galago senegalensis to physical training. Comp Biochem Physiol 1979;63A:29-36.

Tipton CM, Vailas AC, Matthes RD: Experimental studies on the influences of physical activity on ligaments, tendons and joints: a brief review. Acta Med Scand [Suppl] 1986;711:157-168.

Trent PS, Walker PS, Wolf B: Ligament length patterns, strength, and rotational axes of the knee joint. Clin Orthop 1976;117:263-270.

Vailas AC, Tipton CM, Matthes RD, Gart M: Physical activity and its influence on the repair process of medial collateral ligaments. Connect Tissue Res 1981;9:25-31.

VanBrocklin JD and Ellis DG: A study of the mechanical behavior of toe extensor tendons under applied stress. Arch Phys Med 1965;46:369-373.

Viidik A: The aging of collagen as reflected in its physical properties. In Engel A and Larsson T (eds): Aging of Connective and Skeletal Tissue. Thule International Symposia, Nordiska Bokhandelns Forlag, Stockholm, 1968a, pp. 125-148.

Viidik A: Elasticity and tensile strength of the anterior cruciate ligament in rabbits as influenced by training. Acta Physiol Scand 1968b;74:372-330.

Viidik A, Lewin T: Changes in tensile strength characteristics and histology of rabbit ligaments induced by different modes of postmortem storage. Acta Orthop Scand [Suppl] 1966;37:141-155.

Walker LB, Harris EH, Benedict JV: Stress-strain relationship in human cadaveric plantaris tendon: A preliminary study. Med Electron Biol Eng 1964;2:31-38.

Walsh S and Frank C: Two methods of ligament injury: A morphological comparison in a rabbit model. J Surg Res 1988;45:159-166.

Wang CW, Weiss JA, Albright J, Buckwalter JA, Martin R, Woo SL-Y: Life-long exercise and aging effects on the canine medial collateral ligament. Trans of 36th annual ORS, 1990;15(2):518.

Warren RF and Marshall JL: Injuries of the anterior cruciate and medial collateral ligaments of the knee: A long term follow-up of 86 cases. Clin Orthop 1978;136:198-211.

Warren RF, Marshall JL, Girgis F: The prime static stabilizers of the medial side of the knee. J Bone Joint Surg [Am] 1974;56A:665-674.

Weaver JK, Derkash RS, Freeman JR, Kirk RE, Oden RR, Matyas J: Primary ligament repair - Revisited. Clin Orthop 1985;199:185-191.

Weiss JA, Ohland KJ, Newton PO, Danto MI, Horibe S, Young EP, Woo SL-Y: A new injury model to study medial collateral ligament healing. Trans of 36th annual ORS, 1990;15(1):60.

Whiteside LA and Sweeney RE: Nutrient pathways of the cruciate ligaments. An experimental study using the hydrogen washout technique. J Bone Joint Surg [Am] 1980;62A:1176.

Woo SL-Y, Kuei SC, Gomez MA, Winters JM, Amiel D, Akeson WH: The effect of immobilization and exercise on the strength characteristics of bone-medial collateral ligament-bone complex. 1979 ASME biomech Symp AMD 1979;32:67-70.

Woo SL-Y, Gomez MA, Akeson WH: The time and history dependent viscoelastic properties of the canine medial collateral ligament. J. Biomech. Engrg. 1981;103:293-298.

Woo SL-Y: Mechanical properties of tendons and ligaments I: static and nonlinear viscoelastic properties. Biorheology 1982a;19:385-396.

Woo SL-Y, Gomez MA, Woo YK, Akeson WH: Mechanical properties of tendons and ligaments. II. The relationships of immobilization and exercise on tissue remodeling. Biorheology 1982b;19:397-408.

Woo SL-Y, Gomez MA, Seguchi Y, Endo C, Akeson WH: Measurement of mechanical properties of ligament substance from a bone-ligament-bone preparation. J Orthop Res 1983;1:22-29.

Woo SL-Y, Orlando CA, Frank CB, Gomez MA, Akeson WH: Tensile properties of the medial collateral ligament as a function of age. J Orthop Res 1986a;4:133-141.

Woo SL-Y, Orlando CA, Camp JF, Akeson WH: Effects of post-mortem storage by freezing on ligament tensile behavior. J Biomech 1986b; 19:399-404.

Woo SL-Y, Gomez MA, Inoue M, Akeson WH: New experimental procedures to evaluate the properties of healing medial collateral ligaments. J Orthop Res 1987a;5:425-432.

Woo SL-Y, Gomez MA, Sites TJ, Newton PO, Orlando CA, Akeson WH: The biomechanical and morphological changes in the medial collateral ligament of the rabbit after immobilization and remobilization. J Bone Joint Surg [Am] 1987b;69A(8):1200-1211.

Woo SL-Y, Lee TQ, Gomez MA, Sato S, Field FP: Temperature dependent behavior of the canine medial collateral ligament. J Biomech Eng 1987c;109:68-71.

Woo SL-Y, Hollis JM, Roux RD, Gomez MA, Inoue M, Kleiner JB, Akeson WH: Effects of knee flexion on the structural properties of the rabbit femur-anterior cruciate ligament-tibia complex (FATC). J. Biomech 1987d;20(6):557-563.

Woo SL-Y, Weiss JA, Gomez MA, Hawkins DA: Measurement of changes in ligament tension with knee motion and skeletal maturation. J Biomech Engrg 1990a;112:46-51.

Woo SL-Y, Young EP, Ohland K, Marcin J, Horibe S, Lin HC: The effects of anterior cruciate ligament transection on medial collateral ligament healing: An experimental study of the canine knee. J Bone Joint Surg 1990b;72A:382-392.

Woo SL-Y, Peterson RH, Ohland KJ, Sites TJ, Danto MI: The effects of strain rate on the properties of the medial collateral ligaments in skeletally immature and mature rabbits: A biomechanical and histological study. J Orthop Res, 1990c; In Press.

Zuckerman J, Stull GA: Effects of exercise on knee ligament separation force in rats. J Appl Physiol 1969;26(6):716-719.

Chapter 4

Biomechanics of the Anterior Cruciate Ligament and its Replacements

D.L. Butler, Y. Guan

Introduction

The knee remains one of the most frequently injured joints in the body and the anterior cruciate (ACL), one of its most often ruptured ligaments (DeHaven, 1980, 1988; Noyes et al, 1980). In fact, the ACL is probably *the* most commonly, and totally disrupted knee ligament (England, 1976; Eriksson, 1976; Feagin et al, 1976; Marshall and Rubin, 1977; Torg et al, 1976). ACL ruptures can also lead to meniscal tears (Noyes et al, 1983b), and in many patients, evidence of osteoarthrosis on X-ray (McDaniel and Dameron, 1980; McDaniel and Dameron, 1983).

The primary function of ligaments like the anterior cruciate continues to be debated. Based partly on the presence of mechanoreceptors near its insertions (Schultz et al, 1984, Shutte et al, 1987; Zimny et al, 1986) and their presumed role in influencing joint motions (Solomonow et al, 1987), Brand (1986) and Wroble and Brand (1988) recently postulated the anterior cruciate might function more in a neurosensory mode than a mechanical one. Other arguments they proposed to support this hypothesis were that, i) in animal studies conducted by Brand (1986) and Lewis et al (1985), in vivo knee ligament forces were small during normal jumping and cutting activities, and far below the forces supported by ligaments during a clinical examination, and ii) many patients without an anterior cruciate continue to function well, without any gross signs of joint degeneration. While his hypothesis could ultimately be supported, the anterior cruciate ligament probably has, as Lewis et al (1985) contends, both "low load" and "high load" functions, the latter arising during moderate to vigorous daily activities. Regardless, the mechanical restraining action of the anterior cruciate, based on injury frequency alone, cannot be ignored.

If the ACL indeed has an important mechanical function, it is rather surprising how much we do not know about, 1) its function during various knee motions, 2) it's anatomical structure, 3) how its structure confers its mechanical properties, and 4) the relationship between its mechanical properties and its biology. This paper will address some of these mechanically-related issues.

Once an injury occurs, orthopaedic surgeons have had available several treatment options. Unfortunately, primary repair of the ACL has not been one of them (Cabaud, 1979, 1980) because of the significant collagen disruption which occurs, and because of the tissue's modest blood supply, thought to be necessary for extrinsic repair to occur. Instead surgeons now routinely replace the ruptured anterior cruciate ligament with an *autograft*, a tissue taken from another site in the same patient (Johnson and co-workers, 1982,1984). Although this approach has been used with varied success for the last 75 years (eg Hey Groves, 1917; Campbell, 1939; Jones, 1963), mechanically-driven questions persist about which tissue to use, where it should be fixed in the knee, what tension and initial flexion angle should be selected, and what effects removal of the normal graft tissue might have on knee and limb function. These uncertainties have led surgeons to use other biological replacements including *allografts* and *xenografts*. While xenografts have had little impact in this area due to potential rejection problems, allografts have been used clinically and studied in the laboratory. As with autografts, the success of these replacements hinges on many factors, not the least of which are mechanical.

Despite the importance of mechanical factors in graft replacement of the anterior cruciate, much research is still needed. While cadaveric studies have helped educate the field about the "initial conditions" necessary to achieve proper knee kinematics and ligament load-sharing, how these conditions affect the outcome *after* surgery is still in question. Further the influence of other surgical factors (eg maintaining vascularity, inducing passive motion, and allograft preservation and sterilization) on graft mechanics are not well understood. Yet nearly all of these factors can be studied using a biomechanical approach.

The objectives of this report are to: i) review selected studies which have investigated the mechanical properties of the anterior cruciate ligament and its functions in the knee; and ii) review work which has explored mechanical factors in anterior cruciate ligament replacement. As part of this effort we will describe how our research on the normal and reconstructed ACL has contributed to these studies. While this paper will attempt to provide a broad overview of ACL and replacement biomechanics, it cannot hope to describe all the important work which has been done to date.

The Mechanical Response of the Anterior Cruciate Ligament

Studies of the "normal" anterior cruciate ligament will be described under two major headings. These are, 1) the mechanical function of the ligament as a structural element in the knee, and 2) the mechanical properties of the anterior cruciate-bone unit as a tensile-load-bearing element.

Mechanical Function of the ACL in the Knee

The functions of the anterior cruciate ligament during selected knee motions are considered. For each motion, qualitative studies involving uncontrolled manual forces will first be described. These will be followed by a summary of more quantitative studies where joint forces (flexibility approach) and joint displacements (stiffness approach) are controlled.

ACL Function during Flexion-Extension of the Knee

Observations

Much of what we know about ACL behavior during flexion-extension motions has come from early qualitative studies using cadaveric preparations. The presence or absence of ACL forces was estimated by observing whether the tissue was taut or relaxed. The Weber brothers (1836) first distinguished anterior and posterior bundles in the ACL, the former taut in extension but relaxed in flexion, and the latter having reciprocal functions. They concluded the ACL was most important near full extension and if ruptured would produce a small amount of hyperextension in the knee. Honigschmied (1893) confirmed that hyperextension resulted in rupture to the cruciates. Fick

(1904) subdivided the tissue into anteromedial (AMB) and posterolateral (PLB) bands but reached the same conclusions about their degree of tension at different flexion angles. In Palmer's classic study (1938), the ACL developed larger tensions in extension but was also tense throughout flexion. Further, once flexion was initiated, the ACL first relaxed slightly and then retightened after about 20 degrees flexion. While Abbott et al (1944) also observed a small relaxation of the tissue with early flexion, they found no subsequent retightening. In fact, their results were contrary to Fick's (1904); the anteromedial band tightened with flexion and the posterolateral band tightened in extension. Brantigan and Voshell (1941) also noted increasing tension of the ACL with flexion, but did not distinguish the roles of the two parts.

These early reports, which showed contradictory roles for the anterior cruciate ligament and its bands, were essentially repeated by clinicians in the 1970's. Hughston and coworkers (1969,1976) concluded that during flexion and extension, the anterior cruciate ligament only provided significant restraint in hyperextension. Kennedy (1974) also assigned an important function to the ligament in extension, and like others before him, noted a "relaxation" of the tissue in midflexion. However he then found a retightening phenomena with flexion to 70-90 degrees. In a pair of reports by Marshall and coworkers, anteromedial and posterolateral bundles were again identified and their tautness estimated. Girgis et al (1975) found the AMB to tighten with flexion, whereas the PLB portion tightened with extension. Furman et al (1976) concluded this increasing tension in the PLB with extension was a mechanism by which the ligament resisted hyperextension.

Length Patterns

While obviously important in their time, these studies lacked the technical sophistication necessary to quantitate the actual function of the anterior cruciate ligament during flexion-extension motions. Part of assigning such a "function" is knowing the force state in the ligament and its components. Unfortunately, direct measurement of these forces has been difficult (see below). An alternative has been to try and quantitate the length patterns between the bundle ends. Then, by measuring the constitutive properties of these components, the original forces could be estimated. These are now described.

Wang and Walker (1973) studied length changes in the cruciate ligament bands during knee flexion. Pins were inserted into the attachments of the ligament's fiber bundles and the distance between the pin tips computed to provide bundle end-to-end lengths. From full extension to 120 degrees flexion, the ACL as a whole gradually increased in length by 10%. They also found a distinct difference between the behavior of the anterior, central and posterior groups of fibers in the cruciates. The posterior and anterior fibers tended to perform reciprocal functions. The percentages were comparable with the length pattern of the central fibers, so that at all angles of flexion, some portion of the ligament would be in a lengthened position.

Van Dijk (1983) used a roentgen stereophotogrammetric method developed by Selvik (1974) to compute ACL band lengths with flexion. By embedding small radiopaque beads in the bones and in the bundle insertions, he found the anteromedial band of the ACL increased in length during flexion. These length changes exceeded those produced by rotation of the tibia. Van Dijk made no attempt, however, to determine the material properties of these bundles; hence stress and force were not estimated.

Other investigators have attempted to measure anterior cruciate ligament length changes by attaching liquid metal strain gages (eg Brand et al, 1986; Edwards et al, 1970; Kennedy et al, 1977) and Hall effect strain transducers or HESTs (eg Arms et al, 1983, 1984; Beynnon et al, 1990;Fleming et al, 1990; Renstrom et al, 1986) to the ligament surface. These studies showed the anterior surface of the ACL lengthens as the knee extends and as anterior forces (either manual or via the quadriceps mechanism) are applied to the tibia. Unfortunately, the liquid metal gage uses mercury and can leak, precluding its in vivo use. The HEST device has proved more successful in vivo. For example, changes in ligament band length after application of a knee brace have been examined (Beynnon et al, 1990). However, strains are difficult to compute using the HEST since the "just unloaded" length of the tissue is not readily measured. Without these strains and the associated material properties of the tissue, forces can only be determined through careful post-test calibration, obviously not possible in patients. Surrounding soft tissues and bone can also impinge upon both types of devices.

Still other approaches to measuring ACL deformations have been tried by Santora and coworkers (1984) and Henning et al (1985). Santora bonded strain gages adjacent to the ligament attachment in cadaveric knees and attempted to infer ACL force from bone deformation. The difficulty with such approaches in vivo is that force in the cruciate can be difficult to distinguish from forces produced in surrounding tissues and due to weight-bearing. Henning et al (1985) applied an in-line transducer immediately beneath the tibial insertion in two patients. They found that minimal elongations occurred for walking with crutches, but that increasingly greater elongations resulted for walking, anterior drawer tests, jogging, and running downhill. These results would suggest that the deformations (and presumably forces) in the tissue would be small for passive flexion-extension motions.

Force Measurements

Investigators have also attempted to measure anterior cruciate ligament force in vitro using buckle gages (Ahmed et al, 1987; Lewis et al, 1980, 1982) and instrumented washers (Grood et al, 1984; Paulos et al, 1981). Ligament tension remained negligible with extension until approximately 30 degrees after which it increased sharply up to full extension. Application of quadriceps forces also dramatically increased ACL tension, especially near full extension (Paulos et al, 1981). While both methods provide more direct indications of tissue force, only the buckle gage might be useful for in vivo measurements. However, the buckle has been criticized as possibly preloading shorter ligaments like the ACL and as inpinging with the femur when installed on the anteromedial band.

ACL Function during Anterior-Posterior Drawer

Observations

Numerous reports describe the restraining action of the cruciate ligaments in anterior-posterior drawer. Weber and Weber (1836) showed that loss of the cruciate ligaments increased A-P drawer. Pagenstecher (1903) found the ACL and PCL failed when the tibia was impacted in anterior and posterior directions, respectively. Abbott et al (1944) observed that while the cruciate ligaments resisted drawer in flexion, the cruciates and collateral ligaments acted in tandem to resist drawer in full extension. Lenggenhager (1940) concluded that the medial joint capsule resisted anterior drawer, not the anterior cruciate ligament. Wheeler Haines (1941) suggested the cruciate ligaments must be under similar tensions since excessive tension in one produced either an anterior or posterior displacement to restore neutral joint position.

More recent studies have reevaluated the function of the anterior cruciate in A-P drawer. In 1972, Castaing performed a study to investigate the restraints to anterior drawer in neutral, internal, and external rotations. He found the ACL resisted anterior drawer in neutral rotation, the ACL and anterolateral capsule restrained drawer in internal rotation, and only the medial structures resisted drawer in external rotation. From their clinical observations and cadaveric dissection studies, Hughston et al (1976) concluded the PCL, not the ACL, resisted anterior drawer. Furman et al (1976), by contrast, found a complimentary role for the two parts of the ACL in resisting anterior tibial displacement. Specifically, the posterolateral band blocked manually-applied anterior drawer forces in extension whereas the anteromedial band inhibited drawer in flexion. Van Dijk (1983) reached a similar conclusion concerning the anterior most bundle; ie. the AMB was the first bundle to tense in anterior drawer with the knee flexed.

In vivo, Rosenberg et al (1984) subjected the knee to anterior drawer at 90 degrees flexion. The ACL was classified into anteromedial, central and posterolateral portions. The relative tension was determined by a specifically designed probe. During the test, the anteromedial portion developed highest tension, and posterolateral portion developed lowest. Such studies have helped identify ligamentous restraints to anterior drawer, but have been confusing, possibly due to the uncertainties in the loads applied to produce drawer and the difficulty in controlling precise loading direction (eg anterior drawer vs coupled drawer and tibial rotations). Two approaches have been advocated to overcome these problems.

Flexibility Approach

Many investigators have used a flexibility approach to study the role of the anterior cruciate ligament in the human knee during anterior-posterior drawer (Grood and Noyes, 1988). With this approach, controlled anterior or posterior tibial forces are applied to the intact knee, the ACL transected, and the test repeated. Fukubayashi et al (1982), found that without affecting posterior drawer, anterior displacement more than doubled for all seven flexion angles studied. Torzilli et al (1982) then confirmed the increased anterior motion of the tibia in ACL-deficient patients. Markolf et al (1976) concluded that, compared to uninjured knees, specimens without the ACL demonstrated significantly increased total anterior - posterior laxity and decreased anterior stiffness for all positions of the foot and knee studied. For example, with 20N applied anterior force, the mean increased anterior - posterior laxity was 39% at full extension, and 57% at 20 degrees flexion. Sullivan et al (1984) also found from motion studies of cadaveric knees that the contribution of medial-side restraints to anterior displacement depended on the integrity of the ACL. When the ACL was intact, progressive cutting of other tissues had no effect on anterior or posterior displacement of the tibia. However, when the ACL was cut before the medial structures, anterior displacement exceeded that seen after isolated section of the ACL. These differences reflect the "cutting-order" nature of the flexibility approach.

Structural Mechanics Approach

Butler et al (1980) also recognized inherent problems of past selective cutting studies which used a flexibility approach. Typically, an anterior force was applied to the tibia of the intact knee, a ligament was cut, the force reapplied, and the increase in tibial translation measured. While more closely simulating the clinical laxity examination, one problem with this approach was that the increased translation depended on the order of ligament cutting; if the cutting order changed, the measured translation changed. It was thus impossible to precisely define the function of a single ligament.

Instead Butler et al (1980) applied a precise anterior or posterior *displacement* to the tibia while recording the knee's restraining force. The contribution of each ligament was defined separately by the reduction in restraining force which occurred after the structure was cut. If its role was a principal one for that displacement, it was classified as a *primary* restraint; otherwise, it was classified as a *secondary restraint*.

Butler and coworkers (1980) studied the restraints to anterior-posterior displacement under both clinical forces (drawer test) and higher, functional forces, typical of in vivo activities. Shown in Figure 1 is a force-displacement curve for anterior-posterior drawer in an intact cadaveric knee and after cutting the anterior cruciate ligament. Arrows indicate the direction of applied displacement. After cutting the ACL, the restraining force significantly dropped for anterior drawer but did not change for posterior drawer.

The anterior cruciate ligament was the primary restraint to anterior tibial displacement up to 5 millimeters for both 90 and 30 degrees of knee flexion (Butler et al, 1980). The ACL provided 85-87 percent of the total restraining force at 5 mm anterior drawer for the two flexion angles. All other structures provided only a small secondary restraint. Similarly, the posterior cruciate ligament was the primary restraint to posterior drawer up to 5 mm. Besides establishing the primary importance of the anterior cruciate ligament, this data also helped explain the clinical paradox of a negative anterior drawer sign after an acute ACL injury (Butler et al, 1980). With loss of the ACL, clinicians still noted a moderate anterior restraint during the clinical laxity exam (similar to Figure 1). The group postulated the secondary restraints could block the anterior motions produced by small clinical forces and when effusion and muscle spasm were present. Under higher *in vivo* functional loads, anterior translation of the joint would increase, however.

Other investigators have studied the contribution of the ACL using this controlled-displacement or structural mechanics method. Piziali and coworkers (1980) evaluated the response of the human cadaveric knee to +/- 7.5 mm anterior-posterior displacement with the knee at 30 and 90 degrees flexion. All three resultant orthogonal components of force and moment were measured. The load - displacement characteristics of the ACL were measured by determining the difference from before and after cutting the ligament. The ACL carried 73-87% of the load during anterior tibial displacement at 30 degrees flexion. At full extension, the cruciates also carried a large fraction of the entire anterior - posterior load (Figure 2), the anterior load being resisted by the ACL (75%) and the posterior load resisted by the PCL.

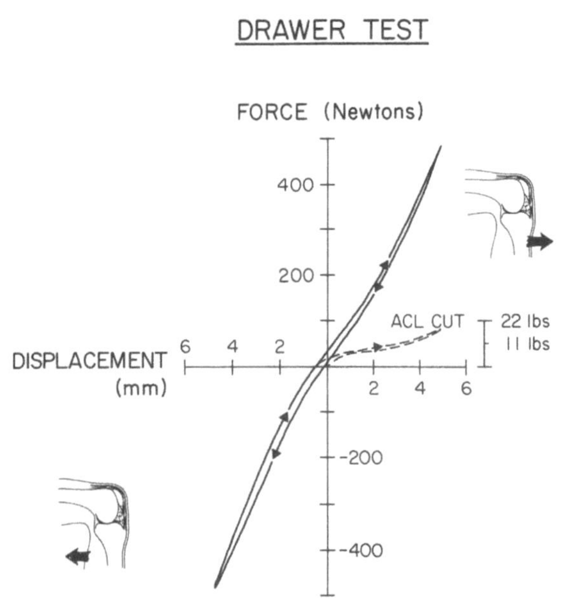

FIGURE 1. A typical force - displacement curve for anterior - posterior drawer in an intact joint (solid line) and after cutting the anterior cruciate ligament (ACL) (broken line). The arrows indicate the direction of motion. (reproduced with permission from Butler DL et al, The Journal of Bone and Joint Surgery, Vol 62-A, 1980, p. 262)

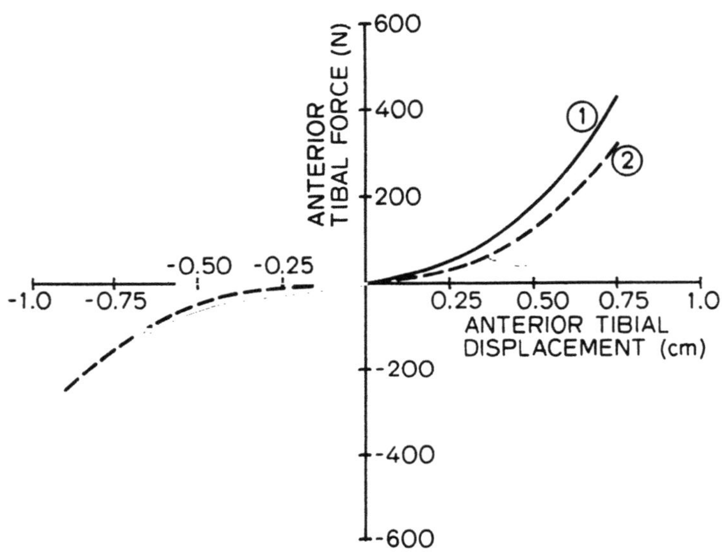

FIGURE 2. Contribution of the cruciate to the anterior - posterior load at 0 deg of flexion - 1 intact knee, 2 knee with only the cruciate ligaments intact (no condylar interference was present); knee specimen no. 4. (reproduced with permission from Piziali RL et al, Journal of Biomechanical Engineering, Vol. 102, 1980, p. 279)

ACL Function during Tibial Rotation

The ACL also plays an important role in resisting internal rotation (Grood and Noyes, 1988). Both cruciate ligaments wind upon each other during the rotation. Kennedy et al (1974) observed that the ACL consistently increased its tension during internal tibial rotation for all flexion angles studied. Piziali et al (1980) and Seering et al (1980) could not separate the function of the ACL and PCL in rotation. Thus they studied the roles of both cruciates and used a structural mechanics approach in a small group of specimens to determine their percentage contributions to knee torque. At full extension and at 30 degrees flexion, the cruciates carried 30%-42% of the total torque transmitted at 19 degrees internal rotation. The medial collateral ligament was equally important in its restraining action. However, the cruciates did not interfere with each other during external rotation of the tibia and, thus, supported only 12% of total external torque at full extension. The contribution decreased to only 3% at 30 degrees flexion.

The ACL was shown to be one of the major soft tissue restraints to the rotational "laxity" of the knee. Comparing displacements from intact and ACL-deficient knees, Markolf et al (1984) reported that at +/- 10 N-m of applied torque, the torsional laxity increased by an average of 10% in knees without an ACL. Internal rotational stiffness also decreased 16% at +/- 5 N-m torque. In their tests, no significant differences were found between injured and normal knees as far as maximum internal and external torques were concerned.

The cruciate ligaments are not only primary restraints to anterior-posterior tibial displacement, but also constitute a primary mechanism controlling internal and external rotation during anterior - posterior drawer. Fukubayashi et al (1982) observed in their tests that internal and external tibial torques were produced in the rotationally constrained knee during application of both anterior and posterior drawer force. After sectioning either cruciate ligament, the average torque decreased markedly (Figure 3).

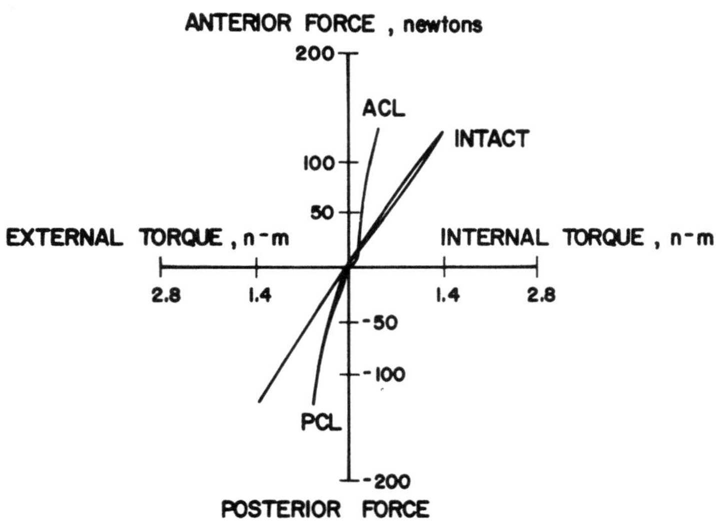

FIGURE 3. A typical recording of tibial torque generated from application of anterior - posterior force at 30 degrees of flexion in intact knee and after isolated section of either cruciate ligament. ACL = anterior cruciate ligament and PCL = posterior cruciate ligament. (reproduced with permission from Fukubayashi T et al, The Journal of Bone and Joint Surgery, Vol.64-A, 1982, p.263)

ACL Function during Varus-Valgus Rotations

In varus - valgus rotation, the ACL contributes to the knee's rotational stiffness. Markolf et al (1984) tested intact and ACL-deficient patients using a flexibility approach (ie by controlling applied moments). They showed that at full extension, under 20 N-m moment, mean varus - valgus laxity increased 36% compared to the knee with the ACL. The associated varus and valgus stiffnesses decreased 21% and 24%, respectively. For 20 degrees flexion, the increase in mean varus - valgus laxity was 19% for the injured knees, but the stiffnesses were not significantly affected by ACL loss.

During controlled varus-valgus rotations, the ACL appears to function with the PCL, carrying a small, but not insignificant percentage of the restraining moment. Piziali et al (1980) evaluated intact knees, and knees devoid of all soft tissues except the cruciates. In full extension and at 6 degrees of varus rotation, the dissected soft tissues carried 73% of the moment while at 6 degrees of valgus, they carried over 82%. The percentage of total restraining moment also varied with the flexion angle selected. The contribution decreased at 15 degrees flexion, then increased again for flexion angles up to 45 degrees.

Seering et al (1980), using a similar selective cutting methodology, investigated the function of the primary ligaments of the knee in varus and valgus rotation at full extension and 30 degrees flexion. They suggested a correlation between the anterior and posterior loads applied to the tibia by the cruciate ligaments and their ability to resist varus - valgus moments. During the rotations, the PCL pulled anteriorly on the tibia while the ACL pulled posteriorly on the tibia. Seering conceded, however, that the ACL was probably not very important in restraining the rotation.

Grood and coworkers (1981) also studied the role of the cruciate ligaments during varus and valgus rotations of the knee. In 16 cadaveric knees tested at both 5 and 25 degrees of flexion (from hyperextension), Grood found that the cruciate ligaments acted together to resist the rotations. As medial restraints (ie to valgus rotations), the cruciates provided about 14-15% of total restraining moment at 5 (Figure 4a) and 25 degrees flexion. The only changes which occurred in relative contribution were an increase in MCL percentage and decrease in capsular percentage as flexion angle increased. In varus, the cruciates were again secondary restraints and the LCL assumed a primary role. The cruciate percentages decreased from 22% of total moment at 5 degrees flexion (Figure 4b) to 14% at 25 degrees flexion.

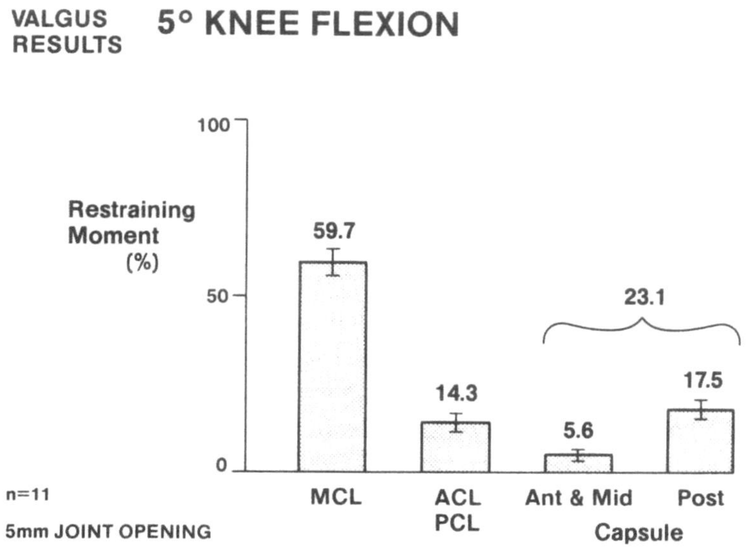

FIGURE 4a. The average per cent contribution to the medial restraints by the ligaments and capsule at five millimeters of medial joint opening and 5 degrees of flexion. The error bars represent +/- one standard error of the mean. (adopted with permission from Grood ES et al, The Journal of Bone and Joint Surgery, Vol. 63-A, 1981, p. 1261)

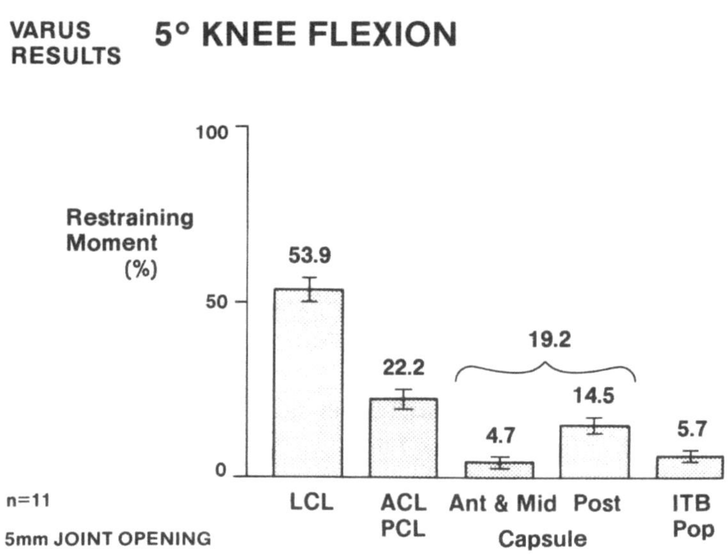

FIGURE 4b. The average per cent contributions to the lateral restraints by the ligaments and capsule at five millimeters of lateral joint opening and 5 degrees of flexion. The error bars represent +/- one standard error of the mean. There was no tension on the iliotibial band proximal to the lateral femoral condyle in these preparations. (adopted with permission from Grood ES et al, The Journal of Bone and Joint Surgery, Vol. 63-A, 1981, p. 1263)

Mechanical Properties of the ACL

Force - Elongation Behavior

The force-elongation behavior of the anterior cruciate ligament has been extensively studied and reviewed (Butler et al, 1978a,b; Kennedy et al, 1976; Noyes et al, 1974a,b, 1977a,b; Noyes and Grood, 1976; Trent et al, 1976; Woo et al, 1987). It is generally now agreed that the ligament must be tested with its bone ends to avoid directly gripping the tissue ends. An example of a force vs time record for a failure test of a femur-anterior cruciate ligament-tibia preparation from the rhesus monkey is shown in Figure 5 (Butler et al, 1978b; Noyes et al, 1974a). Also shown are high-speed films correlated to the loading curve.

The curve typically exhibits four regions (Butler et al, 1978a,b; Noyes et al, 1974a). The initial concave part of the curve, Region I, is called the *nonlinear toe region* where unfolding and progressive recruitment of fibers occurs. In Region II, the nearly *linear region*, collagen fibers are further elongated until first significant failure occurs at the linear load point. In Region III, a *serial failure process and maximum loading* occurs. This is characterized by a series of small, sudden force drops and fiber separation until maximum force when catastrophic failure begins. Finally in Region IV, the *post-failure region*, the tissue loses its load-carrying ability, although the fibers may still appear to be in continuity (Butler et al, 1978a,b; Noyes et al, 1974a,1976).

ACL Failure Mechanisms

The anterior cruciate fails by three primary mechanisms (Noyes et al, 1974a):
1) ligamentous failure: fibers of the ligament pull apart in the tissue midsubstance;
2) ligament-bone interface failure: fibers fail through the zonal insertion without fracture of the underlying bone;
3) tibial or femoral avulsion fracture: fracture of the bone beneath the zonal insertion site of the ligament.

At surgery, clinicians generally find the anterior cruciate has sustained a midsubstance failure, especially in the young adult patient. However, failure mechanism can change, depending upon both testing-related and biological factors. The effects of these factors on mechanical properties and failure mechanisms of the anterior cruciate will now be discussed.

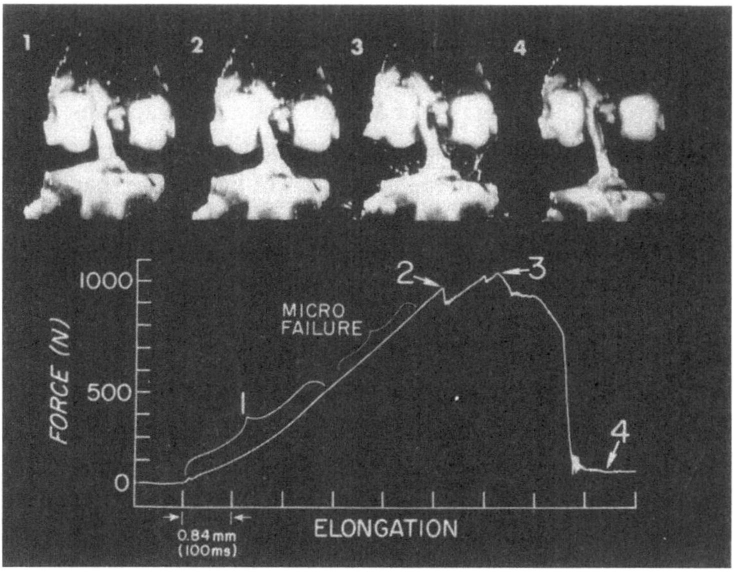

FIGURE 5. Oscillograph record of force vs time for a tension test to failure of a rhesus femur-anterior-cruciate-tibia preparation. A constant distraction rate was used so that the time axis was proportional to specimen elongation. The photographs, obtained from high-speed movies taken during the test, show the preparation at four stages in the test (reproduced with permission from Butler et al, ESSR reviews, Vol 6, 1978; p. 153.

Testing-Related Factors Affecting ACL Mechanical Properties

Among the many testing-related variables which can affect ligament properties, three have been most studied in the anterior cruciate ligament. These are post-mortem storage medium and temperature, strain rate, and knee position and direction of loading on the tissue.

Storage Medium and Temperature

Viidik et al (1965,1966) were among the first to study how mechanical properties of the anterior cruciate ligament would be influenced by post-mortem storage. They stored rabbit ACLs in four ways (saline, 20 degrees C; formaldehyde; saline, 4 degrees C; and deep-freezing). Viidik found the mechanical properties of specimens subjected to all four media differed from properties for fresh rabbit ACLs and recommended specimens be tested immediately postmortem in either synovial fluid or blood plasma.

Noyes and Grood (1976), as part of a larger study, evaluated how freezing to -15 degrees C would affect the mechanical properties of the rhesus monkey ACL-bone preparation. Using 10 matched pairs of limbs, one specimen was tested fresh while the other was immediately frozen for 4 weeks. By contrast to Viidik et al (1965, 1966) they found no significant differences in mechanical properties or cross-sectional area due to the freezing process.

Strain Rate

In one of the earlier reports on cruciate ligament mechanical properties, Haut and Little (1969) performed subfailure tests on canine femur-ACL-tibia preparations near full extension in several environments (in air, and in saline at room and body temperatures) and over a range of strain rates (up to about 1%/s). Peak strain levels did not exceed 10%. For all temperatures, the general shape of the stress - strain curves was not affected by variations in strain rate, except for the higher rates where the toe region ended at an earlier strain level. Toe region slope increased with increasing rate as did the apparent Young's modulus in the nearly linear region of loading. Increasing temperature affected Young's modulus, producing lower values at low strain rates, and much higher moduli at higher rates. The reported strain rates were low, however, compared to the expected strain rates encountered when an ACL sustains injury.

Noyes and coworkers (1974a) studied how larger variations in strain rate influence tissue stiffness, and failure mechanical properties and modes. They found that stiffness of the rhesus monkey ACL-bone unit was relatively unaffected by a two-fold increase in rate (0.66%/s to 66%/s). However, the ligament tested at the faster strain rate failed at higher maximum load and maximum strain, and absorbed more energy, prior to failure. At the faster deformation rate, the ligament-bone unit also typically failed through its midsubstance. At the slower rate, the most common type of failure was tibial avulsion fracture. After analyzing failure mode mechanics, they concluded that geometrical arrangement of collagen fibers, surrounding ground substance effects, and osseous insertion site effects were also important factors affecting failure properties of the tissue.

Knee Position and Direction of Loading Relative to Ligament Orientation

Because of its nonparallel bundles of unequal length, the ACL exhibits different force -deformation relationships at different flexion angles. Figgie et al (1986) tested canine femur-ACL-tibia complexes in tension with axial tibial orientation and three femoral orientations with respect to load direction. The ultimate load, total energy absorbed, and stiffness at 45 and 90 degrees flexion were less than 50 percent of the values obtained with the knee at full extension. The modes of failure also differed for the three cases. They concluded that ligaments should not be considered as one dimensional structures and loading conditions should be specified.

The recent study by Woo et al (1987) on the femur-ACL-tibia complex (FATC) of rabbits also found that several factors (method of holding the specimen, strain rate applied, angle of knee flexion, and direction of the applied loading) affected the mechanical response of the tissue. Maximum force (as well as other structural properties) decreased with increasing knee flexion for specimens loaded along the tibial axis, but was unchanged when loading occurred along the ligament axis. These differences in load-deformation behavior were particularly obvious at 90 degrees flexion (Figure 6). They recommended that future studies control and specify the direction of loading with respect to the ligament axis.

With extension from 90 degrees, the ACL, as a structure, develops little tension until about 30 degrees flexion, where it develops increasing force (Paulos et al, 1981, Grood et al, 1984). Factors which greatly affected the tissue force levels were the presence of weight at the foot and the direction of loading relative to the ligament axis. Both studies showed that adding only seven pounds to the foot during a simulated progressive resistance exercise approximately doubled the quadriceps force needed to extend the leg. ACL force increased by over 30% at full extension (Paulos et al, 1981). Clearly the change in direction and magnitude of loading during this exercise affected anterior cruciate ligament forces.

Biological Factors Affecting ACL Mechanical Properties

Species-Related Differences

Noyes et al (1974a,b;1976) extensively studied ACL-bone preparations from human and non-human primates. Material properties were determined with specimens mounted in 45 degrees flexion, and then failed at high strain rates (66-100%/s). They found that ACL specimens from young human cadaveric ACL-bone units had elastic moduli and maximum stresses which were only 60% of respective values from rhesus monkeys (Figure 7). The strains at complete failure were comparable for the two species, however, and both groups failed predominantly by a ligamentous mode. The average modulus of young human ACL-bone units in the linear portion was measured as 111 MPa. The maximum stress was about 37 MPa, and the strains at maximum stress and failure were 44% and 60%, respectively (Noyes and Grood, 1976).

Bain (1989) recently tested anterior cruciate ligament-bone units from a large number of mammals. He tested all preparations to failure at 45 degrees flexion. He determined that the maximum force in the ACL was related to

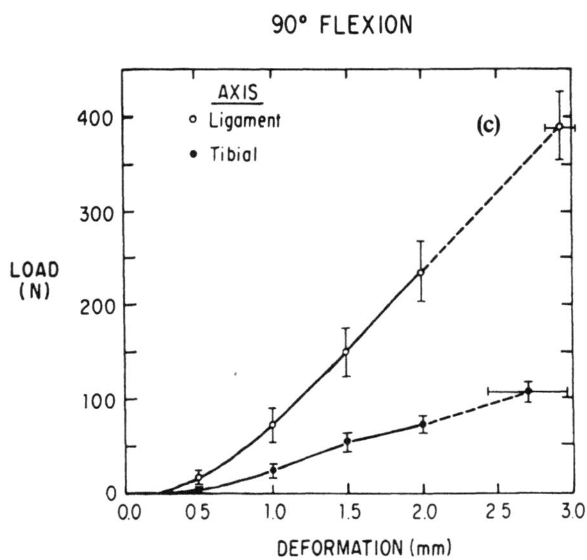

FIGURE 6. Average load - deformation curves for rabbit FATC tested along tibial axis or ligament axis at 90° of knee flexion (mean +/- S.E.) (reproduced with permission from Woo SLY et al, Journal of Biomechanics, Vol. 20, 1987, p.561)

body mass through a scaling law of the form, $F = 157\,m^{0.65}$. This result did not apply within species and the exponent was similar to the results of Noyes and Grood (1976).

Age

Noyes and Grood (1976) also compared the mechanical properties of human cadaveric ACL-bone units from younger and older human donors. They categorized the specimens into two age groups, 16 to 26 years and 48 to 83 years, and showed that the force carried by the ACL decreased markedly with increasing age. The ACLs failed at an average 1730N for the younger humans and only 734N for the older group. Selected material properties also decreased with increasing age. Between 20 and 50 years, elastic modulus significantly decreased two-fold (Figure 8a) and maximum stress (Figure 8b) and strain energy density to maximum stress significantly declined three-fold. After the age of 50, the declines continued in these parameters but were not significant. Failure modes also converted from exclusively ligamentous in the younger group to bone avulsion in the older group.

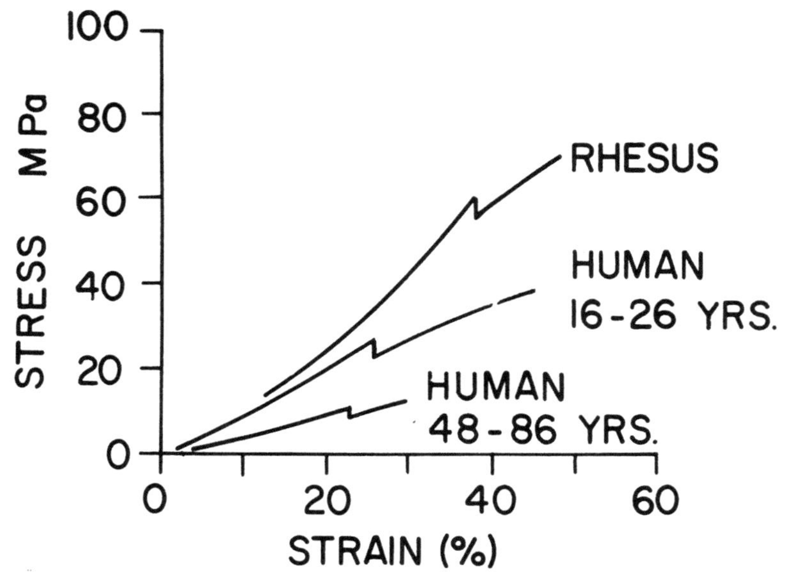

FIGURE 7. Summary of stress - strain behavior for the ligament preparation from the rhesus monkey, younger human donors and older human donors. (reproduced with permission from Noyes FR et al, The Journal of Bone and Joint Surgery, Vol. 58-A, 1976, 1079)

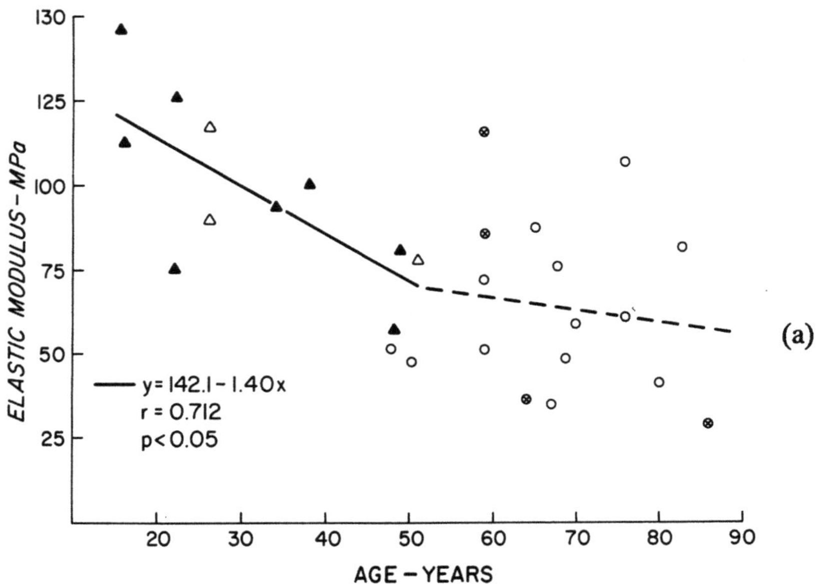

FIGURE 8. Correlation of ligament a) elastic modulus and b) maximum stress with age. The solid line represents the statistically significant correlation with age found in the trauma specimens (solid triangle) and younger cadaver preparations (hollow triangle), all of which failed through the body of the ligament. The interrupted line represents the correction (not statistically significant) found in the amputation (hollow circle) and older cadaver (crossed circle) preparations, which failed by avulsion fracture of the bone underneath the ligament insertion site. (reproduced with permission from Noyes FR et al, The Journal of Bone and Joint Surgery, Vol. 58-A, 1976, p. 1079)

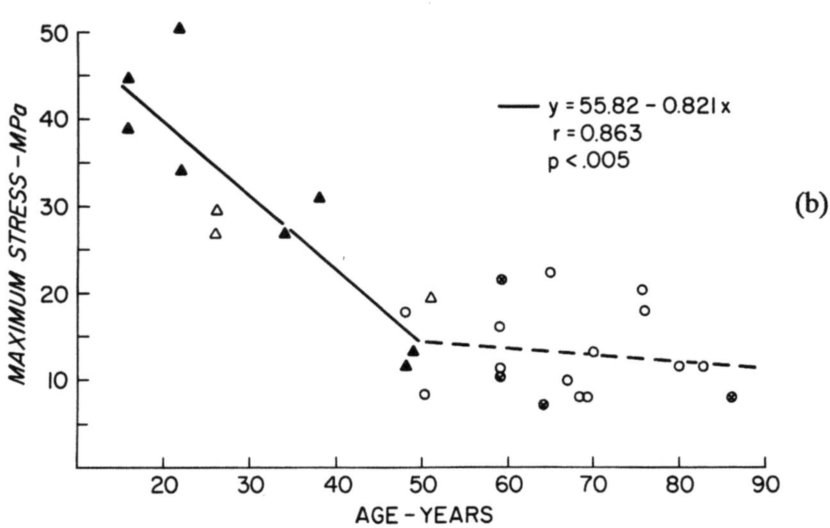

Immobility/Reconditioning

The effects of altered levels of activity on the failure properties of the ACL of primates were investigated (Noyes, 1977; Noyes et al, 1974a). After eight weeks of whole-body immobilization (Figure 9), tension tests of femur-ACL-tibia units showed significant decreases in maximum load (39%) and energy absorbed to failure (32%). Ligament stiffness also showed a moderate, but not significant decrease. These changes indicated an altered functional capacity of the ligament unit. Twenty weeks after resuming activity, ligament stiffness was nearly back to normal but strength had only partially recovered. One full year of activity was required to restore the tissue's maximum force levels. As a result of immobilization, the failure modes also changed from primarily ligamentous to bone avulsion.

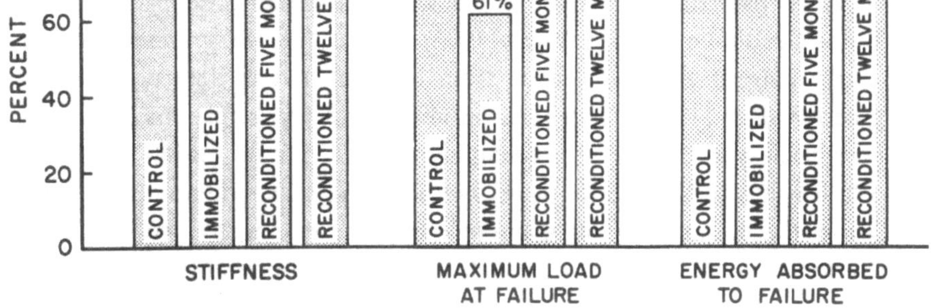

FIGURE 9. Summary of results for stiffness, maximum failure load, and energy to failure. The control group is taken as 100%. Statistically significant decreases occur in all three parameters after 8 weeks immobilization. Only partial recovery occurred after 5 months reconditioning. (reproduced with permission Noyes, FR CORR, Vol 123, 1977, p. 164.)

In Vivo Force Estimates

One of the major challenges facing those investigating ACL function is the level of forces it withstands during daily activities. Morrison (1968,1969,1970) estimated the maximum forces in the ACL and other knee structures for a number of typical daily activities. Using force plate analysis and mathematical modeling, he assumed: i) all anterior-posterior passive restraining forces were controlled by the cruciates; ii) the cruciates lay in the sagittal plane; and iii) they only controlled anterior - posterior motions. The force levels in the ACL were estimated to be 169N for level working, only 27N for ascending stairs, 93N for descending stairs, 67N for ascending a ramp, and as much as 445N for descending a ramp. He also estimated that friction would add or subtract a maximum of 40N from the forces he presented (Morrison, 1970).

Noyes and Grood (1976) estimated forces in the ACL in vivo using two methods. First, by assuming that the normal forces in the tissue were up to one-fifth of the maximum loads, they calculated values of 200 - 400 N for younger humans and 80 - 160 N for older humans. They also approximated the in vivo forces by measuring the forces necessary to elongate the ACL by 10%. These estimates were 160N for younger individuals and 249N for older humans.

In 1980, while investigating prosthetic ACL design, Chen and Black (1980) developed a model to estimate the forces in the ACL for younger (16-34 yrs), middle aged (35-48 yrs), and older humans (49-65 yrs). Modulus was calculated using two methods. One utilized the relationship calculated by Noyes and Grood (1980) between modulus and age. In the other method, flexion angle patterns for the different activities investigated by Morrison (1969) and Seedholm and Terayama (1976) were used. Maximum strains for each angle pattern were also taken from ligament length data obtained by Wang and Walker (1973). The linear moduli for three age groups calculated using method I were 3.8 MPa for young human, 3.0 MPa for middle aged, and 1.8 MPa for elders. Calculation using method II yielded similar results. We now know these estimates of ligament modulus are one to two orders of magnitude too small and hence predicted forces were probably too low.

Correlation of Tissue Mechanical Properties and Structure

The ACL thus functions in many ways, acting as an important restraint to certain varus-valgus and tibial rotations (Piziali et al, 1980; Seering et al, 1980; Grood et al, 1981) as well as anterior-posterior translations (Butler et al,

1980; Piziali et al, 1980; Fukubayashi and coworkers, 1982). To restrain the knee under such varied external loading conditions, it is not surprising that the ACL has such a complex structure. Its structural characterization and correlation with mechanical properties will now be considered.

While the ligament's fiber bundles appear parallel and equally tensed at full extension (Figure 10), the changes in the bundle tensions and orientations can be significant with flexion and rotation (Bradley et al, 1988; Fuss, 1989). Research indicates that the ligament's bundles vary not only in length but in orientation and in material properties as well. These spatial variations in structure and mechanical response exist in the cross-section and along the tissue length (see below). Such variations can also lead to a variety of functions for the anterior cruciate ligament.

Ligament Torque and Rotation

Alm and Stromberg (1974) originally described how the axial strength of the canine ACL was largest in neutral tibial rotation and decreased with internal and external rotation. Stouffer et al (1983) and Butler and Stouffer (1983) observed that the fiber bundles or fascicles of the tissue did not follow a straight path between the tibial and femoral attachment sites, but a rather helical path about the ligament axis. Observation of this geometrical configuration enabled the investigators to develop a simple mathematical cable model for the mechanical response of the canine ACL (Stouffer et al, 1983). The principal conclusion from the modeling work was that a small torque must always accompany the force during axial elongation of the tissue. An experimental program was devised to determine whether the ACL, with this apparent twist of almost 180 degrees, could support a torque (Butler and Stouffer, 1983). The ligament was aligned along the loading axis, tissue deformation measured from one bone end to the other, and the generated axial force and torque simultaneously recorded. At first significant failure, the ACL developed an average maximum torque of 122N-mm and an average force of about 700N. A nearly linear axial force-torque curve was also noted. The cable model predicted both the force and associated torque reasonably 3well (Butler and Stouffer, 1983).

The presence of this ligament torque during axial loading was predicted primarily from the tissue's gross macrostructure. More refined experiments were then needed to relate the mechanical properties of a human cruciate ligament to its detailed macrostructure and insertion site geometries.

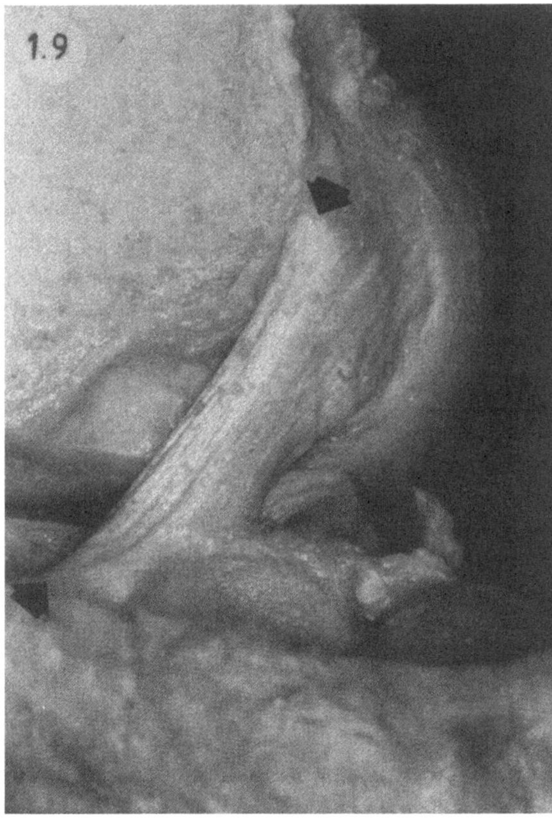

FIGURE 10. Medial view of the ACL, with the antero - medial bundle between the arrows (reproduced with permission from Van Dijk R, in The Behavior of the Cruciate Ligaments in the Human Knee, p. 23)

To develop this more comprehensive, structurally-based mathematical model for the human ACL, Butler et al (1988) measured how the fiber bundles were organized in the tissue and their relative material properties.

Fiber Bundle Organization

Fiber bundle organization was measured in one anterior and one posterior cruciate ligament from a young human donor (Butler, et al, 1988, Martin, et al, 1987). The knee ligaments and capsular structures were maintained. Using methacrylate casts and Steinmann pins, the femur and tibia were rigidly fixed in different flexion angles (0, 30, 60 and 90 degrees) and in various amounts of internal (10 and 20 degrees), neutral, and external (10, 20 and 30 degrees) tibial rotation. The femur was split between the ligaments, in a sagittal plane, to better visualize each tissue structure. Bundle lengths, orientations in space, attachment site locations, and deviations from linearity were measured for 15 - 18 fiber bundles, located at superficial, middle, and deep levels in each tissue. Using an instrumented spatial linkage, each bundle was digitized at five points along its length, each ligament insertion outlined, and selected femoral and tibial landmarks digitized.

Two lengths were measured for each bundle. End-to-end (ETE) length was computed as the straight-line distance between the proximal and distal insertions of each bundle. Point-to-point length (PTP) was also calculated as the sum of the suture-to-suture distances along each bundle to provide an estimate of the actual bundle arc length.

PTP lengths for all observed bundles of the anterior cruciate ligament are shown in Figure 11. Bundle locations are referenced to the tibia, and data is for neutral tibial rotation. Anterior bundles were the longest at each flexion angle, and the posterolateral bundles were the shortest. PTP lengths remained constant as flexion angle was changed. Similar patterns were found for the other five tibial rotations.

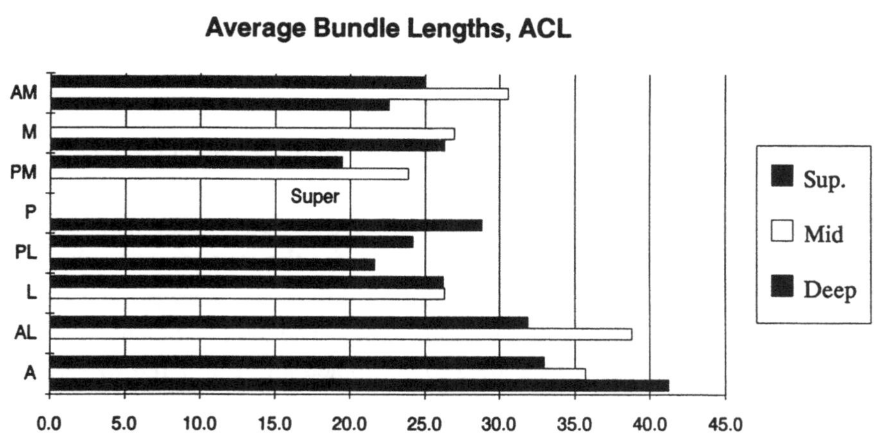

FIGURE 11. Average point-to-point bundle lengths for different locations in one human cadaveric anterior cruciate ligament. A = anterior bundle, AM = anteromedial bundle, M = medial bundle, AL = anterolateral bundle, L= lateral bundle, PM = posteromedial bundle, PL = posterolateral bundle, P = posterior bundle. Sup., Mid. and Deep indicate the relative depth of the bundles.

The orientations of these surface bundles varied dramatically for a given flexion angle and tibial rotation. In general, the posterior and lateral bundles of the tissue were more vertically inclined compared to the anterior and medial bundles.

Because the ACL is clearly composed of bundles which vary in length, curvature, and orientation, the whole ligament's mechanical properties greatly depend upon how the tissue and its bone ends are oriented before testing. Whether such variability could be reduced if bundles from the ligament were tested, has also been investigated.

Subunit Material Properties

The material properties of selected groups of fiber bundles from the human ACL were measured (Butler et al, 1986). They also compared these bundle material properties with similar parameters for subunits from the posterior cruciate (PCL) and lateral collateral ligaments (LCL) and from the patellar tendon (PT) of the same knees. The three *subunits* or groups of ACL fascicles were prepared by cutting along primary fiber directions and then sectioning the femoral bone ends without disturbing the insertions. The tibial ends were maintained. All bone blocks were embedded in methacrylate (Figure 12). The specimens were mounted and failed in tension at a strain rate of 100%/sec. Three load-related material properties were computed (linear modulus, maximum stress, and energy density to maximum stress), as well as the strains to maximum stress and failure using local and end-to-end deformations.

Figure 13 presents typical stress-strain curves for subunits from the four tissues (Butler et al, 1986). Note the responses for the ligament specimens are similar, but the stresses measured for the tendon were much higher. In each knee tested, the load-related material properties for the patellar tendon were significantly larger than corresponding values for the cruciate and collateral ligament specimens. However, no significant differences were present in the maximum strains among the four tissue types. The similar behavior of the ligament subunits permitted the data to be pooled and compared to patellar tendon subunit results (Butler, et al, 1986). Of particular interest, all ligament subunits had an average maximum strain of only 15%. This value is much smaller than the 44% maximum strain reported for the entire ACL (Noyes and Grood, 1976), reflecting better control of loading direction, fiber bundle orientation, and initial length and cross-sectional area.

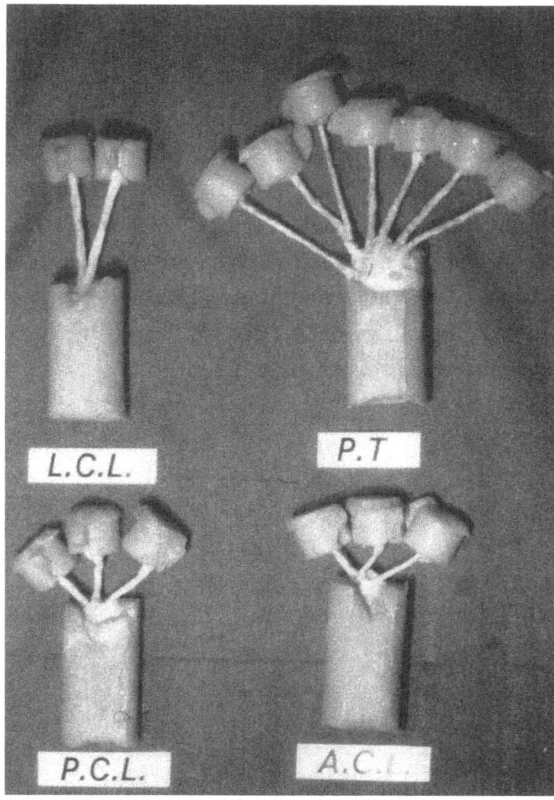

FIGURE 12. Subunits from the lateral collateral ligament (LCL), patellar tendon (PT), posterior cruciate ligament (PCL), and anterior cruciate ligament (ACL). The bone ends have been potted in methylmethacrylate. (reproduced with permission from Butler DL et al, Journal of Biomechanics, Vol. 19, 1986, p. 427)

Surface strains are not uniform along the subunit, however. Local optical surface strains were computed and correlated with the strains between bone insertions (Butler et al, 1985, 1990; Sheh et al, 1985). As time increased during the test, the ACL midsubstance strains were smaller than the strains near the attachment sites. This trend was noted in most subunits and in whole tissues with bone ends (Butler et al, 1984; Noyes et al, 1984; Zernicke et al, 1984). The data indicated that ligaments, like the anterior cruciate ligament, as well as the patellar tendon, are more compliant near the bone insertions. This pattern of larger end strains, which has also been seen in the medial collateral ligament (Woo et al, 1982, 1983), may serve to protect these tissues where abrupt changes occur in stiffness. While mechanisms contributing to these strain variations are not fully known, axial variations in crimp period and angle have been implicated (Butler et al, 1990; Sheh et al, 1985; Stouffer et al, 1985).

Others have also examined the mechanical properties of ACL subunits to determine load distribution in the tissue (Hollis et al, 1988, 1989). Hollis et al (1988) removed and tested four subunits from each ACL after performing subfailure tests on the intact knees. They showed, after accounting for bundle location and orientation, that the anteromedial fibers are primary restraints to anterior tibial translation of the knee at 20 degrees flexion. They also constructed a ligament model to predict forces in the ligament under other loading conditions (Hollis et al, 1989).

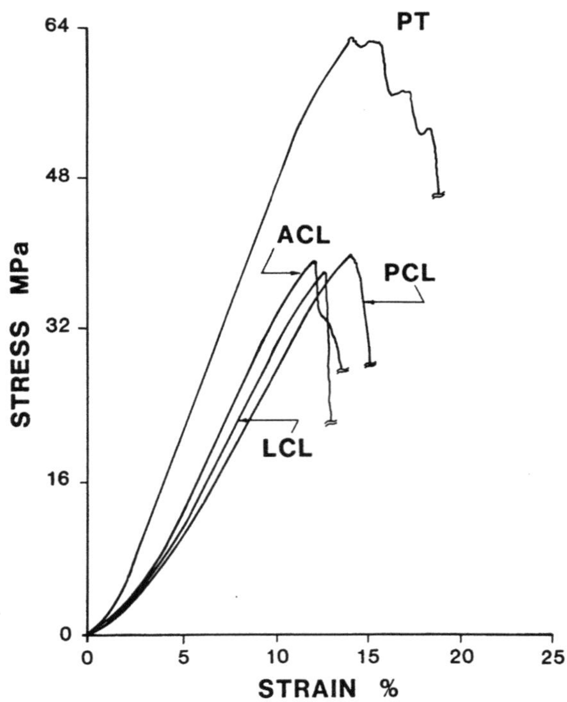

FIGURE 13. Typical stress - strain curves for the PT, ACL, PCL and LCL fascicle - bone units. Note the much larger modulus and maximum stress for the PT specimen. The strains at maximum stress are similar for all four tissues, however. The portions of the curves beyond maximum stress are not shown for clarity. (reproduced with permission from Butler DL et al, Journal of Biomechanics, Vol. 19, 1986, p.429)

The results of these material property studies emphasize the similarities of surface structures and material properties in knee ligaments. Ligament subunits develop smaller stresses than tendon subunits, but they surprisingly fail at similar strain levels. The data also suggest that a tendon, such as the patellar tendon, might have initial mechanical properties which would make it suitable as an anterior cruciate ligament replacement. However, the variations in ACL bundle lengths, curvatures, and orientations would also make this tissue a structure not easy to duplicate with a parallel-fibered tendon. Comparing the structural mechanical properties of ligaments and potential graft replacements will thus be discussed.

Mechanical Behavior of ACL Autografts

Initial Mechanical Properties of Autografts

Initial Tissue Strength

Many approaches have been used to treat the ACL-deficient knee. These include primary direct repair, extra-articular lateral repair, ligament augmentation, and ligament replacement using autografts, allografts, xenografts, and synthetic materials (Cabaud et al, 1979, 1980; Clancy et al, 1981; Curtis et al, 1985; Feagin et al, 1982; Kennedy, 1978; Liljedahl et al, 1965; Marshall et al, 1982; Nikolaou et al, 1986; O'Donoghue et al, 1966, 1971; Roth and Kennedy, 1980; Ryan and Drompp, 1966; Shino et al, 1984; Webster and Werner, 1983) As stated earlier, autograft tissues remain a frequent option (Johnson et al, 1982, 1984). Since the early 1900's, many collagenous tissues (tendons, fascia, menisci) have been transferred in and around the knee as autogenous ACL replacements. Until the late 1970's, however, the mechanical properties (in particular, strength) of such grafts had not been determined. Butler et al (1979, 1984) and Noyes et al (1984) compared subfailure and failure mechanical properties of nine commonly-used autografts from young donors since patients in this age range typically receive these tissues and since age and disuse-related factors cause significant reductions in ACL material properties (Butler et al, 1985; Noyes and Grood, 1976; Noyes et al, 1974b). They failed the tissues at high strain rates to induce soft tissue failures (Noyes et al, 1974a), so commonly seen in patients; and compared the results to earlier mechanical property data for ACL-bone units from young donors (Noyes and Grood, 1976). In this way, tissues with the best initial properties could be identified.

The tissues tested included bone-patellar tendon-bone units (central and medial portions, each 14 mm wide), semitendinosus and gracilis tendons, quadriceps tendon-patellar retinaculum-patellar tendon (medial, central and lateral thirds), fascia lata, and distal iliotibial band. Each tissue was loaded to failure in tension at 100% of initial length per second. The bone-patellar tendon-bone specimens developed the highest maximum force (about 160 percent the strength of the anterior cruciate ligament). These tendons were the only tissues having strengths greater than those of the ligament being replaced. Semitendinosus and gracilis tendons developed 70% and 49% of ACL strength, respectively. Fascia lata (16mm wide) and iliotibial band (18mm wide) followed (36 and 38 percent, respectively). Patellar retinacular tissues were the weakest, bearing only 14-21 percent of the average anterior cruciate maximum load (Noyes et al, 1984). The central and medial patellar tendons also generated three times the stiffness of the ACL and equivalent failure energies.

Noyes et al (1984) indicated the width of patellar tendon they tested (33-40% of total width) was comparable to that used at surgery. On a mechanical basis, other tissues could be acceptable ACL grafts, however. Semitendinosus and gracilis tendon would be suitable if tissues could be adequately fixed to bone and if the forces could be kept below 50% of maximum ACL force of the ligament. If fascia or iliotibial band were used, it would have to be alomost full width to match the initial properties of the ACL. This extreme width could compromise important lateral knee restraints, however. The authors recommended the surgeon not use the retinacular tissues (Noyes et al, 1984).

Other mechanically-related factors in ligament replacements have also been studied. These include attachment site location (Hefzy and Grood, 1986; Sidles et al, 1986), graft pretension and flexion angle at installation (Bylski-Austrow et al, 1990), and the fixation technique used (Kurosaka et al, 1987). These will be briefly addressed.

Attachment Site Location, Graft Tension and Joint Position at Tensioning

Concerns have been raised recently that the function of the anterior cruciate ligament, with its complex macrostructure, would be difficult if not impossible to replace with a parallel-fibered tendon. As a result, several investigators have sought "isometric attachment points". At these ideal attachment locations, the graft would neither overtighten and constrain the knee (and possibly stretch or fail) nor become lax and nonfunctional. Among the studies which have been conducted, Bylski-Austrow, Grood and coworkers (1990), Hefzy and Grood (1986), and Sidles et al (1988) are some of the most comprehensive. Sidles et al (1988) examined over-the-top placement of grafts on the femur. They found that while these repairs provide stability in extension, they are less effective in flexion. Bylski-Austrow et al (1990) found similar results for over-the-top placement with anterior translation being underconstrained. However, they also found that the force in the ACL substitute and the anterior limits of translation in the knee were very sensitive to femoral hole location. Also increasing either flexion angle at tensioning or magnitude of tension increased graft force and moved the tibia posteriorly.

Penner and coworkers (1988) also studied placement and isometry in cadaveric knees. They used a braided material to replace the ACL. While femoral attachment site location was again found critical to graft isometry, tibial hole position was also important to isometric tracking. Anteriorly placed tibial holes yielded the most isometric grafts.

Yoshiya et al (1987) examined how variation in initial graft tensioning would influence the outcome after ACL reconstruction in dogs. Medial patellar tendon grafts were implanted in both knees of one group under two extreme tension levels. Ligament augmentations were used to adjust graft tension in another group. At 3 months postop they found the greatest stiffness and strength occurred when low forces were placed on the patellar tendon graft and augmentation.

Mechanical Properties of Autografts after Implantation

Autogenous replacement of the ACL has been studied by several research groups using rabbits, canines, and primates. The biological and mechanical changes which occur have been well summarized by Grood et al (1985). Unlike primary repair, the graft must heal at its attachments. This can mean reattachment of soft tissue to soft tissue, soft tissue to bone, or bone to bone depending on the method employed. While the graft is mechanically intact at surgery unlike the failed ends of the primary repair, it must heal at its attachments as well as sustain the forces during the expected remodeling of the tissue midsubstance.

The biological remodeling which occurs in the graft substance can be substantial. O'Donoghue et al (1971) replaced the anterior cruciate ligament in the dog with iliotibial band. They noted a marked revascularization process. Other authors have also reported extensive revascularization of rabbit, canine and primate patellar tendon (Alm and Stromberg; 1974; Amiel et al, 1986; Arnoczky et al, 1982; Butler et al, 1983b; Clancy et al, 1981) and rabbit semitendinosus tendon (Roth and Kennedy, 1980). Amiel et al (1986) described a "ligamentization" of the rabbit patellar tendon autograft, whereby the tendon's cellularity, collagen microstructure, and reducible crosslinks began to assume characteristics of the anterior cruciate ligament it was replacing. This extensive remodeling suggests that, in combination with the biological changes occurring at the attachment sites, significant reductions must also be occurring in the strength and stiffness of the tissue's midsubstance.

Numerous investigators have studied the mechanical changes in anterior cruciate ligament reconstructions over time. Ryan and Drompp (1966), for example, found that canine patellar tendon grafts of the ACL developed only 20% of control ligament strength six months postop. O'Donoghue and coworkers (1971) did not report much better results. Their iliotibial band grafts in dogs were only 35% of control strength three and one half years after transplantation. Clancy et al (1981) replaced the anterior cruciate ligament in primates with the central third patellar tendon using eccentrically-placed drill holes to try and align the graft axis with the centroid of the original ACL insertions. They found the grafts had returned to 50% of the maximum force of the contralateral ACL. However their results were based on very small sample sizes. Roth and Kennedy (1980), using the semitendinosus tendon, also found the grafts to be very weak (15% of control) six months post surgery.

Butler et al (1983a) and Hulse et al (1983) were among the first investigators to measure the alterations in anterior-posterior drawer after replacement as well as the mechanical changes to the graft itself. They reconstructed the cranial (anterior) cruciate ligament using fascia lata and the lateral one-third of the patellar tendon. The tendon was left attached distally, but was taken without bone proximally (Hulse et al, 1983). The combined graft was secured "over-the-top" on the femur with a spiked washer and screw and then sutured to the femoral-fabellar ligament. The animals were sacrificed at 0, 4, 12, and 26 weeks post-op. Unrestricted activity was permitted on a farm in the 4, 12, and 26 week groups. Total A-P knee translations were measured immediately after sacrifice. The lengths and cross-sectional areas of the grafts and contralateral ACLs were measured, after which both grafts were tested to failure in anterior drawer (Butler et al, 1983a).

The total anterior-posterior drawer was 154% of the opposite control side immediately after implantation. By four weeks, drawer had increased to over 300% of control (Hulse et al, 1983). Drawer then decreased, returning to approximately zero week values 26 weeks after surgery. This increase and subsequent decrease in translations does not pattern the results in humans, which show a progressive increase in drawer over time.

The cross-sectional areas and structural mechanical and material properties of the grafts also changed dramatically (Butler et al, 1983a). At zero weeks, the graft area was 135% of control ACL area, increasing to 255% at 12 weeks, and then declining to 234% at 26 weeks. Immediately following surgery, stiffness of the graft was only 9 percent of the control side. Stiffness increased with time, reaching 31% of ligament control at 26 weeks. Whether the increasing stiffness contributed to the eventual decrease in anterior translation of the knee was not addressed. The corresponding material property, modulus, was only 14% of control immediately after surgery, increasing to 28% by 12 weeks. Maximum force was 14% of control value immediately after surgery, and increased to 28% at 26 weeks (Figure 14). The maximum stress of the grafts immediately following surgery was 10% of control, decreasing slightly at both 4 and 12 weeks, and then increasing to only 13% at 26 weeks. These results indicate that the graft's structural properties improve faster than their material properties, i.e., the tissues increase strength and stiffness by increasing their cross-sectional area rather than by improving their quality (material properties).

Butler et al (1989) continued these studies in the primate. They sought to improve early fixation strength and prevent large declines in material properties associated with remodeling. Using a bone-patellar tendon-bone graft (for better fixation), they tested the hypothesis that the extent of remodeling and thus loss in mechanical properties would be reduced by using vascularized grafts, grafts in which the blood supply could be maintained (Noyes et al, 1983a; Solomen et al, 1968). While some some loss in strength would be expected, the amount of cell death and tissue necrosis would be less severe than with nonvascularized free grafts. In the first study, cynomolgus monkey vascularized PT grafts (VG) were directly compared with contralateral free grafts (FG) at four times post surgery (7, 14, 29, and 53 weeks). Postoperative care consisted of casting the limbs in 15 degrees knee flexion for six weeks. At sacrifice, the left and right knees were tested in anterior-

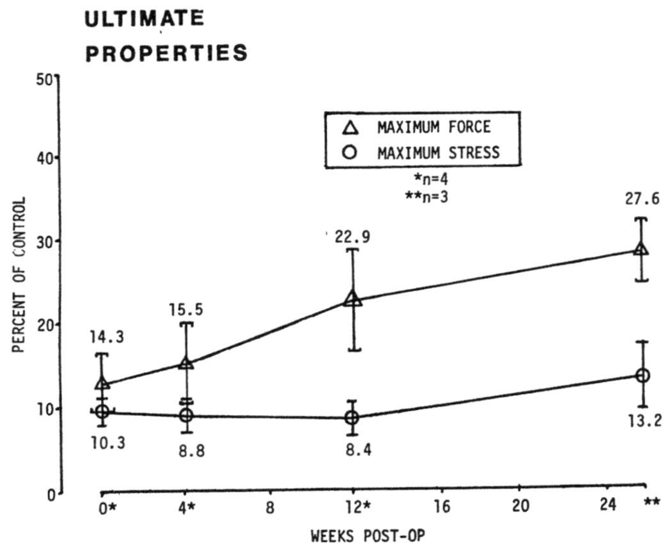

FIGURE 14. Maximum force and maximum stress of the canine cranial cruciate ligament grafts compared to the contralateral control ligament. (reproduced with permission from Butler DL et al, Veterinary Surgery, 12(3), 1983a, p. 117)

posterior drawer after which tissue mechanical properties were measured. Histological changes over time were also described.

The major finding of this study (Butler et al, 1989) was that no significant differences were observed in any measured variable between vascularized and free grafts. That is, no significant improvement in joint resistance to anterior drawer or in mechanical properties were found as a result of maintaining the vascularity to the graft. Thus, the results were pooled to reflect the properties of all grafts at each time period.

The total anterior-posterior translation results for the primate knees are shown in Figure 15. As with the canine reconstructions, (Hulse et al, 1983) total drawer was greater than control early after surgery (160% at 7 weeks), but then decreased over time. Translations in operated knees were actually less than control values at one year.

The stiffness and maximum force results for the VG's and FG's appear in Figure 16. Stiffness was 24% of ACL control at 7 weeks and maximum force 16% (Butler et al, 1989). Both parameters increased at about the same rate up to 29 weeks postop. By one year, stiffness reached 57% of control while maximum force achieved 39%. These results were consistent with the prior canine study (Butler et al, 1983a) up to six months after surgery.

The moduli and maximum stresses were also reported (Butler et al, 1989). Graft modulus tripled between 7 and 53 weeks. The modulus at one year was significantly greater than the values at 7 and 14 weeks ($p < 0.05$). Maximum stress followed a similar pattern, achieving 25% of the maximum stress for the control anterior cruciate ligament at one year. As in their canine study (Butler et al, 1983a), the material properties, indicative of tissue quality, improved at a slower rate than did the structural mechanical properties.

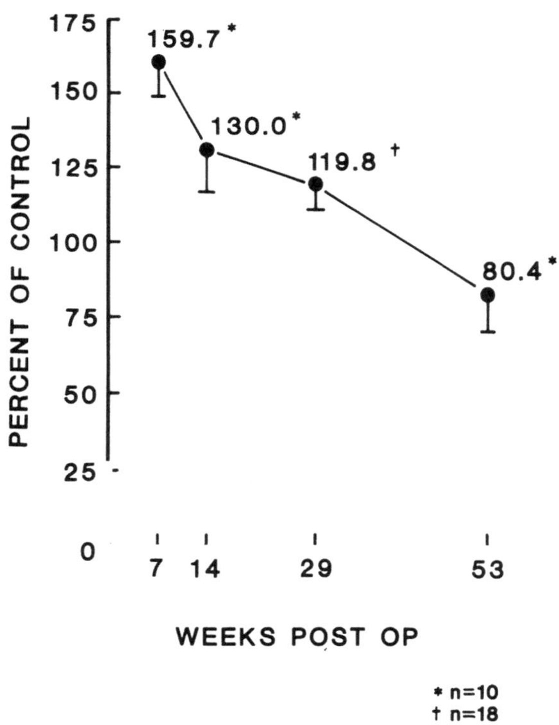

FIGURE 15. Total anterior posterior translation of the primate knee at ±25N. Translation, as a percent of control, decreases over time from 7 to 53 weeks.

The authors, in evaluating possible reasons for these findings, wondered what effect cast immobilization might have had on the knee joints and grafts. One frequent finding they observed in the casted knees was cartilage degeneration; i.e. pannus formation over portions of the medial and lateral femoral condyles, and pitting on the most anterior surfaces of both condyles and in the femoral sulcus. These changes were sometimes accompanied by significant restrictions to full knee extension (Butler et al, 1983b).

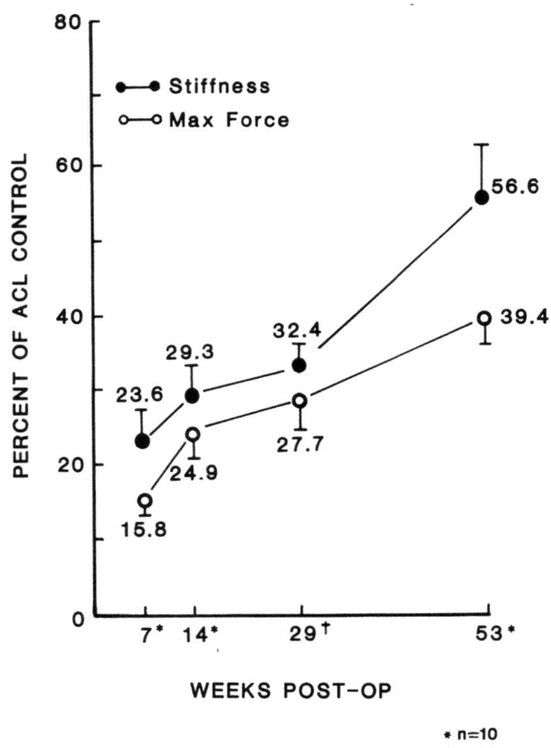

FIGURE 16. Normalized graft stiffness and maximum force (± SEM) are plotted against weeks postoperation. Note the more rapid increase in the stiffness values over time. By 1 year, stiffness and maximum force were 57% and 39% of control, respectively. (reproduced with permission from Butler DL et al, Journal of Orthopaedic Research, Vol. 7, 1989, P. 76)

To eliminate this potentially deleterious effect to the graft and knee, they again compared vascularized and free PT grafts using another postoperative treatment, intermittent passive motion or IPM (Butler et al,1983b). Animals were placed in specially-designed restraint chairs immediately after both surgeries. Motion was applied at one cycle every minute for 16 hours per day for 21 days. Every four days, animals were removed from the chairs overnight to reduce the risk of pressure sores. For one week prior to surgery, animals were acclimated to the chairs.

They compared the VGs and FGs in the presence of IPM at 13 and 26 weeks post-op. All knees showed greater range of motion than in the casted groups (Butler et al, 1989), and at sacrifice, the cartilage surfaces appeared normal by visual inspection (Butler et al, 1983b). However, no significant differences were found in the structural mechanical properties (eg stiffness and maximum force) or material properties (e.g. modulus and maximum stress) between the vascularized and contralateral free grafts. The mechanical properties of these grafts were also no better than values measured in the previous primate study (Butler et al, 1983b, 1989). Thus, neither intermittent passive motion nor maintaining graft vascularity improved the mechanical properties of the tissues, using the animal model, tissue model, and experimental design described.

In another study of autograft mechanical property changes over time, Ballock et al (1989) reconstructed the rabbit anterior cruciate ligament with a medial one-third of the patellar tendon. The grafts were examined immediately postop and at 6, 30, and 52 weeks after surgery. By gross observation, the grafts were unlike the ACL. Histologically they became less hypercellular and more parallel in fibrous structure with time. Mechanically, however, graft stiffness and maximum load were quite low up to six weeks, rising to 24% and 15% of control stiffness and strength by 26 weeks, but then declining in both parameters at one year. This decrease between 6 and 12 months has not previously been reported and may represent results unique to the rabbit or the difficulty of controlling graft attachment site locations and initial tension in the small rabbit knee.

Mechanical Behavior of ACL Allografts

Although autogenous grafts have been the most commonly used replacements for the torn anterior cruciate ligament (ACL) (Johnson et al, 1982), allografts have received increasing attention. Clinically, allografts have several advantages: decreased surgical time and morbidity, unaltered patella-femoral tracking, and a wider graft selection.

Numerous commercial tissue banks now process allografts prior to their clinical use. This processing includes preservation by either freezing or freeze-drying and sterilization by using sterile procurement and careful donor screening or clean procurement and secondary sterilization. Early studies showed that even under the best conditions, up to 20% of grafts procured under sterile conditions became contaminated (Turner et al, 1956). Recently, surgeons and tissue bank personnel have become concerned that grafts procured by sterile means may harbor viruses which can transmit infectious diseases such as AIDS or hepatitis. Even with careful donor screening, it is impossible to be sure that a graft is not infected (CDC, 1988). To alleviate these concerns, allografts have been secondarily sterilized using either ethylene oxide (EtO) or Cobalt^{60} gamma irradiation. Irradiation may be preferable because it is a safe and effective sterilant (Christensen et al, 1982; Darmady et al, 1961; Sommer, 1973; Spire et al, 1985), while the byproducts of ethylene oxide sterilization (e.g., ethylene chlorhydrin and ethylene glycol) are toxic (Lawrence et al, 1971) and not easily removed from grafts during the post-treatment aeration process.

Initial Mechanical Properties of ACL Allografts

A persistent question which remains is whether the processing of allografts adversely affects their mechanical properties. It has been well established that preservation by deep freezing to -15 to -196 degrees C for 1 week to 3 months produces little or no changes in the mechanical properties of tendon, ligament, or bone (Barad et al, 1982; Komender, 1976; Noyes and Grood, 1976; Pelker et al, 1983, 1984; Tkaczuk, 1968; Viidik and Lewin, 1966; Woo et al, 1986). The effects of gamma irradiation on mechanical properties are less clear, however. Most studies have been conducted using bone which is only one of the components of the bone-patellar tendon-bone allograft. The compressive, torsional, and bending strengths of frozen bone are not significantly reduced by gamma irradiation if the dose is maintained below 3 Mrads (Bright and Burstein, 1978; Komender, 1976; Triantafyllou et al, 1975;). Similar results have been reported for bone-patellar tendon-bone units (Butler et al, 1987, Haut, 1987; Paulos et al, 1987); however, each of these reports was preliminary with small sample sizes.

Gibbons et al (1989) compared the initial material properties of two types of goat bone-patellar tendon-bone allograft preparations. Measurements were made on fresh frozen preparations and on their contralateral specimens that were fresh frozen, then exposed to either 2 or 3 Mrads of gamma irradiation. The maximum stress and strain energy density to maximum stress (based on grip-to-grip measurements) were significantly reduced 15% and 26%, respectively, after 3 Mrads of irradiation. Material properties were not significantly altered following irradiation to 2 Mrads. The dose-dependent reductions occurred in both the entire bone-patellar tendon-bone unit and in the tendon midsubstance. These results provide important "time-zero" material property data which will be useful for later anterior cruciate ligament reconstruction studies using irradiated allograft patellar tendons in the goat and other models.

The absence of irradiation effects at the low dosage level is consistent with the report from Haut (1987). In a subsequent study using human patellar tendons, however, Haut and Powlison (1989) found significant effects on material properties following irradiation to 2 Mrads. The significant reductions which occurred in maximum stress and strain energy density following 3 Mrads of irradiation were still not as large as those reported by Paulos et al (1987) who exposed freeze-dried human patellar tendon-bone units to 3 Mrads of gamma irradiation. The difference might be due to the fact that Paulos used freeze-dried tissue while Gibbons et al (1989) used fresh frozen tissue. Freeze drying and irradiation have been shown to produce a synergistic, deleterious effect in bone (Bright and Burchardt, 1983; Bright and Burstein, 1978; Komender, 1976; Triantafyllou et al, 1975). Also important to note is the previous report by Butler et al (1987) which showed that dosage levels of 3.7-3.9 Mrads supplied to frozen patellar tendon-bone units would produce still more significant reductions in the material properties of these specimens.

Successful allograft reconstruction of the anterior cruciate ligament depends on many of the same factors which autografts do, namely graft tissue used, graft placement and tensioning methods, and the post-operative rehabilitation program. Selection of the appropriate graft for any orthopaedic procedure should be based on both its initial mechanical properties and its capacity to withstand the stresses to which it will be subjected after implantation. Since the actual forces on the ACL are unknown, the general rule has been to select a graft that has structural properties as least as great as the anterior cruciate ligament itself. Human patellar tendon-bone units, with widths 40% that of the entire tissue, are the only biological grafts with initial strength greater than the anterior cruciate ligament (Noyes et al, 1984).

Mechanical Properties of Allografts after Implantation

Numerous animal studies have been published indicating the fate of allograft replacement of the ACL. Two types of allografts have primarily been studied-fresh frozen and freeze-dried. Arnoczky et al (1986) showed that unlike fresh patellar tendon allografts which produced a significant inflammatory and rejection response, deep frozen patellar tendon allografts appeared benign in the canine knee, similar to those observed in autogenous replacement. Shino and coworkers (1984) implanted previously deep frozen patellar tendon allografts in the knees of one group of dogs and autograft patellar tendons in the knees of a second group. Both the allografts and autografts exhibited the same maximum load relative to their contralateral ligaments 30 weeks after implantation (35%). This percentage of control did not change at 52 weeks postop. Subsequent evaluation of patients with frozen allografts showed that 31 of 50 had returned to full sporting activity (Shino et al, 1986). Webster and Werner (1983) examined the mechanical behavior of deep frozen flexor tendon allografts of the canine anterior cruciate ligament eight months after surgery. They too found that these grafts were about 30% of both control ACL and autograft strength. Curtis et al (1985) found that freeze-dried fascia lata replacements of the anterior cruciate ligament in dogs underwent large reductions in strength by 4 weeks postop. However they then observed that the graft strength returned to 64% of the ACL value. This is one of the largest percentages which authors have reported in the literature. However, since only one or two grafts were examined at each time period, these experiments need to be repeated in larger numbers of animals.

Even more impressive were the results of Nikolaou et al (1986) who replaced the canine ACL with autografts and cryopreserved ACL allografts. Their rationale for using an ACL graft was that parallel-fibered tendons could not provide the detailed fiber geometry that the natural ligament could. Their results showed that the allografts and autografts had achieved 90 percent of control ligament strength by 36 weeks with no abnormal vascularity, structural degradation or immunological reaction present. Jackson et al (1987a,b) also studied ACL allografts, but preserved them by freeze-drying. One year after implantation, the operated knees had almost four times the A/P laxity of the control knees, and 35% and 25% of ACL stiffness and maximum load, respectively (Jackson et al, 1987a). When a synthetic ligament augmentation device (LAD) was placed in parallel with the ACL allograft, knee laxity was reduced (3 times control) and graft/LAD stiffness and maximum load increased to 53% and 43% of control ACL values, respectively (Jackson et al,

1987b). These results, while not comparable to those of Nikolaou (1986), are similar to the autograft results of Butler et al (1989) one year after surgery.

Summary and Conclusions

Selected functions of the anterior cruciate ligament in the knee have been presented. The mechanical properties of the ACL have also been discussed as well as the properties of autograft and allograft replacements at "time-zero" and after implantation. The ACL functions to restrain not only anterior drawer but tibial rotation and varus-valgus as well. The many functions of the ligament are believed to result in its complicated structure. Despite this complexity, its subunits have more predictable material properties, like those of other ligaments in the knee. Replacement of the ACL depends upon many factors which were discussed. While selecting a strong and stiff replacement like the patellar tendon is advantageous, even its mechanical properties undergo significant reductions after implantation. Allografts undergo many of the same changes as autografts after implantation. Deleterious effects also occur at time zero when high levels of gamma irradiation sterilization are used.

Much more research is required to understand how the macrostructure and microstructure influence anterior cruciate mechanical properties. Further, much more needs to be learned about how mechanical factors affect the mechanical properties and biology of anterior cruciate ligament replacements. Only then can the anterior cruciate be reconstructed to provide both a strong and durable structure, enabling patients to resume preinjury activity levels.

ACKNOWLEDGMENTS:

The authors wish to acknowledge the support of the Musculoskeletal Diseases Program of the National Institute of Arthritis, Metabolic, Digestive, and Kidney Diseases (AR38719), and the National Science Foundation (EET 8910393). The authors also acknowledge the technical assistance of Ms Linda Moeller.

References

Abbott LC, Saunders JB deC M, Bost FC, Anderson CE: Injuries to the ligaments of the knee joint. J Bone and Joint Surg 1944;26:503-521.

Ahmed AM, Hyder A, Burke DL, Chan KH: In-vitro ligament tension pattern in the flexed knee in passive loading. J Orthop Res 1987;5:217-230.

Alm A, Ekstrom H, Stromberg B: Tensile strength of the anterior cruciate ligament in the dog. Acta Chir Scand 1974;44:15-23.

Alm A, Stromberg B: Transposed medial third of patellar ligament in reconstruction of the anterior cruciate ligament: Surgical and morphological study in dogs. Acta Chir. Scand. Suppl. 1974; 445:37.

Amiel D, Kleiner JB, Akeson W: The natural history of the anterior cruciate ligament autograft of patellar tendon origin. Am J Sports Med 1986;14(6):449-462.

Arms SW, Pope MH, Johnson RJ, Fischer RA, Arvidsson I, Eriksson E: The biomechanics of anterior cruciate ligament rehabilitation and reconstruction. Am J Sports Med 1984;12(1):8-18.

Arnoczky SP, Tarvin GB, Marshall JL: Anterior cruciate ligament replacement using patellar tendon: an evaluation of graft revascularization in the dog. J. Bone Joint Surg. 1982; 64(2):217-224.

Arnoczky SP, Warren RF, Ashlock MA: Replacement of the anterior cruciate ligament using a patellar tendon allograft. J Bone Joint Surg 1986;68A(3):376-385.

Bain JR: Body size and tensile strength of the mammalian anterior cruciate ligament. Trans Orthopaedic Research Society, 1989;14:325.

Ballock RT, Woo S-LY, Lyon RM, Hollis JM, Akeson WH: Use of patellar tendon autograft for anterior cruciate ligament reconstruction in the rabbit: A long-term histologic and biomechanical study. J Orthop Res 1989;7:474-485.

Barad S, Cabaud HE, Rodrigo JJ: Effects of storage at -80°C as compared to 4°C on the strength of rhesus monkey anterior cruciate ligaments,. Trans Orthop Res Soc 1982; 7:378.

Beynnon BD, Pope MH, Fleming JG, Howe RJ, Johnson AR, Erickson CM, Wertheimer C, Nichols: An in-vivo study of the ACL strain biomechanics in the normal knee. Trans Orthopaedic Research Society, 1989;14:324.

Beynnon B, Wertheimer C, Fleming B, Erickson A, Pope MH, Howe JG, Johnson RJ, Nichols CE: An in-vivo study of the anterior cruciate ligament strain biomechanics during functional knee bracing. Trans Orthopaedic Research Society 1990;15:223.

Bradley J, FitzPatrick D, Shercliff DD, O'Connor J: Orientation of the cruciate ligament in the sagittal plane and length change with flexion. J Bone Joint Surg 1988;70B:94-99.

Brand RA: Knee ligaments: A new view. J. Biomech Eng 1986; 108:106-110.

Brantigan OC, Voshell AF: The mechanics of the ligaments and menisci of the knee joint. J Bone Joint Surg 1941;23:44-66.

Bright AE, Burchardt H: The biomechanical properties of preserved bone grafts, In: Osteochondral Allografts. Biology, Banking, and Clinical Applications, ed by GE Friedlaender, HJ Mankin, and KW Sell, Boston/Toronto, Little, Brown and Company, First Edition, 1983, 241-247.

Bright RW, Burstein AH: Material properties of preserved cortical bone. Trans Orthop Res Soc 1978; 3:210.

Bridges AE, Olivo JP, Chandler VL: Relative resistance of microorganisms to cathode rays. II. Yeasts and molds. Appl Microbiol 1956; 4:147-149.

Butler DL, Grood ES, Noyes FR, Olmstead ML, Hohn RB, Arnoczky SP, Siegel MG: Mechanical properties of primate vascularized vs nonvascularized patellar tendon grafts; changes over time. J Orthopaedic Res 1989; 7:68-79.

Butler DL, Grood ES, Noyes FR, Sodd AN: On the interpretation of our anterior cruciate ligament data: Clin Orthop Rel Res 1985;196:26-34.

Butler DL, Grood ES, Noyes FR, Zernicke RF, Brackett K: Effects of structure and strain measurement technique on the material properties of young human tendons and fascia. J Biomechanics 1984;17(8):579-596.

Butler DL, Hulse DA, Kay MD, Grood ES, Shires PK, D'Ambrosia R, Shoji H: Biomechanics of cranial cruciate ligament reconstruction in the dog: II. Mechanical properties. Vet Surg 1983a;12:113-118.

Butler DL, Kay MD, Stouffer DC: Comparison of material properties of fascicle- bone units from patellar tendon and knee ligaments. J Biomechanics 1986;19:425-432.

Butler DL, Martin ET, Kaiser AD, Grood ES, Chun KJ, Stouffer DC: The effects of flexion and tibial rotation on the 3-D orientations and lengths of human anterior cruciate ligament bundles. Trans Orthop Res Soc 1988;13:59.

Butler DL, Noyes FR, Grood ES: Measurement of the biomechanical properties of ligaments. in CRC Handbook on Bioengineering and Biology, ed. Bahnik, G and Burstein A, 1978a;1:279-314.

Butler DL, Noyes FR, Grood ES: Ligamentous restraints to anterior-posterior drawer in the human knee. A biomechanical study. J Bone and Joint Surg 1980;62A:259-270.

Butler DL, Noyes FR, Grood ES, Miller EH, Malek M: Mechanical properties of transplants for the anterior cruciate ligament. Trans Orthop Res Soc 1979;4:81.

Butler DL, Noyes FR, Grood ES, Olmstead ML, Hohn RB: The effects of vascularity on the mechanical properties of primate anterior cruciate ligament replacements. Trans Orthop Res Soc 1983b;8:93.

Butler DL, Noyes FR, Walz KA, Gibbons MJ: Biomechanics of human knee ligament allograft treatment. Trans Orthop Res Soc 1987; 12:128.

Butler DL, Sheh MY, Stouffer DC, Samaranayake VA, Levy MS: Surface strain variation in human patellar tendon and knee cruciate ligaments. J Biomech. Engn. 1990;112:38-45.

Butler DL, Stouffer DC: Tension-torsion characteristics of the canine anterior cruciate ligament: II: Experimental observations. J Biomech Engr 1983;105:160-165.

Butler DL, Zernicke RF, Grood ES, Noyes FR: Biomechanics of ligaments and tendons. Exercise and Sports Science Review, Hutton R (ed), Franklin Insitute Press, 1978b;6:125-182.

Bylski-Austrow DI, Grood ES, Hefzy MS, Holden JP, Butler DL: Anterior cruciate ligament replacements: A mechanical study of femoral attachment location, flexion angle at tensioning, and initial tension. J Orthop Res (in press, 1990).

Cabaud HE, Feagin JA, Rodkey WG: Acute anterior cruciate ligament injury and augmented repair. Am J Sports Med 1980;8:395-401.

Cabaud HE, Rodkey WG, Feagin, JA: Experimental studies of acute anterior cruciate ligament injury and repair. Am J Sports Med 1979;7:18-22.

Campbell WC: Reconstruction of the ligament of the knee. Amer. J. of Surg. 1939;43:473-480.

Castaing J, Burdin PH, Mougin M: Les condition de la stabilite passive du genou . Revue de Chirurgie orthopedique. Supplement 1 tome. 1972;58:34-48.

CDC: Transmission of HIV through bone transplantation: case report and public health recommendations, MMWR 1988; 37(39):597-599.

Chen EH and Black J: Material Design Analysis of the Prosthetic Anterior Cruciate Ligament. Journal of Biomedical Materials Research 1980;14:567-586.

Christensen EA, Kristensen H, Sehestad K: Radiation sterilization, In: Principles and Practices of Disinfection, Preservation and Sterilization, ed by AD Russell, WB Huge, GA Ayliffe, Oxford, Blackwell Scientific Publications 1982; 513-533.

Clancy WG Jr, Narechania RG, Rosenberg TD, Gmeiner JG, Wisnefske DD, Lang TA: Anterior-posterior cruciate ligament reconstruction in rhesus monkeys. J Bone Joint Surg 1981;63A:1270-1284.

Curtis RJ, DeLee JC, Drez DJ, Jr: Reconstruction to the anterior cruciate ligament with freeze-dried fascia lata allografts in dogs. Am J Sports Med 1985;13(6):408-414.

Darmady EM, Hughes KEA, Burt MM, Freeman BM, Powell DS: Radiation sterilization. J Clin Path 1961; 14:55-58.

DeHaven K: Diagnosis of acute knee injuries with hemarthrosis. Am J Sports Med 1980;8(1):9-14.

Drouin G, Gely P, Dupont L: Biomechanics of the anterior cruciate ligament: A problem definition. Canadian Conference of Applied Mechanics, 1981, 179-180.

Edwards RG, Lafferty JF, Lange KO: Ligament strain in the human knee joint. Journal of Basic Engineering 1970; 131-136.

England R: Repair of the ligaments about the knee. Orthop Clin North Am 1976;7:195-204.

Eriksson E: Reconstruction of the anterior cruciate ligament. Orthop Clin of North Am 1976;7:165-179.

Feagin JA, Cabaud HE, Curl WW: The anterior cruciate ligament. Radiographic and clinical signs of successful and unsuccessful repairs. Clin Orthop Rel Res 1982;164:54-58.

Feagin JA, Curl WW: Isolated tear of the anterior cruciate ligament. Five- year follow-up study. Am J Sports Med 1976;4:95-100.

Fick R: Anatomie und mechanik der Gelenke (Gustav Fischer, Jena). Part 1: Anatomie der gelenke. 1904.

Figgie HE, Bahniuk EH, Heiple KG, Davy DT: The effects of tibial-femoral angle on the failure mechanics of the canine anterior cruciate ligament. J Biomechanics 1986;19(2):89-91.

Fleming BC, Beynnon BD, Erickson AR, Pope MH, Johnson RJ, Nichols CE, Howe JG: An in vivo study of the reconstructed anterior cruciate ligament at time of implantation. Trans Orthopaedic Research Society 1990;15:84.

Fukubayashi T, Torzilli PA, Sherman MF and Warren RF: An in Vitro Biomechanical Evaluation of Anterior - Posterior Motion of the Knee. J Bone and Joint Surg 1982;64A:258-264.

Furman W, Marshall JL, Girgis FG: The anterior cruciate ligament. A functional analysis based on postmortem studies. J Bone Joint Surg 1976;58A:179-185.

Fuss FK: Anatomy of the cruciate ligaments and their function in extension and flexion of the human knee joint. Am J Anatomy 1989;184:165-176.

Gibbons MJ, Butler DL, Grood ES, Chun KJ, Noyes FR, Bukovec DB: Dose-dependent effects of gamma irradiation on the material properties of frozen bone-patellar tendon-bone allografts. Trans. Orthopaedic Research Society, 1989; 14:513.

Girgis FG, Marshall JL, Al Monajem ARS: The cruciate ligaments of the knee joint. Anatomical, functional and experimental analysis. Clin Orthop Rel Res 1975;106:216-231.

Grood ES, Butler DL, Noyes FR: Models of ligament repairs and grafts. In: American Academy of Orthopaedic Surgeons Symposium on Sports Medicine: The Knee. C. V. Mosby Company 1985;169-184.

Grood ES, Hefzy MS, Butler DL, Noyes FR: Intra-articular vs over-the-top placement of anterior cruciate ligament substitutes. Trans Orthop Res Soc 1986;11:79.

Grood ES, Noyes FR: Diagnosis of Knee Ligament Injuries: Biomechanical Precepts. The Crucial Ligaments: Diagnosis and Treatment of Ligamentous Injuries About the Knee, Feagin, JA (ed) New York, Churchill Livingstone, 1988;245-260.

Grood ES, Noyes FR, Butler DL, Suntay WJ: Ligamentous capsular restraints preventing straight medial and lateral laxity in intact human cadaver knees. J Bone Joint Surg 1981;63A:1257-1269.

Grood ES, Suntay WJ, Noyes FR, Butler DL: Biomechanics of the knee - extension exercise. Effect of cutting the anterior ligament. J Bone Joint Surg 1984; 66-A:725-734.

Haut RC: Tensile failure properties of fresh frozen human tendon allografts: effects of irradiation. Report to the Michigan Tissue Bank, 1987.

Haut RC, Little RW: Rheological Properties of Canine Anterior Cruciate Ligaments. J. Biomech. 1969;2:289-298.

Haut RC, Powlison AC: Order of irradiation and lyophilization on the strength of patellar tendon allografts. Trans Orthop Res Soc 1989; 14:514.

Hefzy MS, Grood ES: Sensitivity of insertion locations on length patterns of anterior cruciate ligament fibers. J Biomech Engr 1986;108:73-82.

Henning CE, Lynch MA, Glick KR: An in vivo strain gage study of elongation of the anterior cruciate ligament. Am J Sports Med 1985;13(1):22-26.

Hey Groves, EW: Operation for the repair of the cruciate ligaments. Lancet 1917;2:674-675.

Hollis JM, Marcin JP, Horibe S, Woo SL-Y: Load determination in ACL fiber bundles under knee loading. Trans. Orthop Research Society, 1988;13:58.

Hollis JM, Horibe S, Adams DJ, Marcin JP, Woo SL-Y: Force distribution in the anterior cruciate ligament as a function of flexion angle. Torzilli PA, Friedman MH (eds): Biomechanics Symposium. New York, American Society of Mechanical Engineers, 1989:41-44.

Honigschmied J: Leichenexperimenten uber die Zerreissungen der Bander im Kniegelenk. Deutsch Zeitsch. f. Chri.1893;36:587-620.

Hughston, JC: The posterior cruciate ligament in the knee joint. J. Bone Joint Surg. 1969;51A:1045-1046.

Hughston, JC, Andrews, JR, Cross MJ, Moschi, A: Classification of knee ligament instabilities. I. The medial compartment and cruciate ligaments. J Bone Joint Surg 1976;58A:159-172.

Hulse DA, Butler DL, Kay MD, Noyes FR, Shires PK, D'Ambrosia R, Shoji H: Biomechanics of cranial cruciate ligament reconstruction in the dog. In vitro laxity testing. Vet Surg 1983;12(3):109-112.

Jackson DW, Grood ES, Arnoczky SP, Butler DL, Simon TM: Freeze dried anterior cruciate ligament allografts. Am J Sports Med 1987a;15(4):295-303.

Jackson DW, Grood ES, Arnoczky SP, Butler DL, Simon TM: Cruciate reconstruction using freeze dried anterior cruciate ligament allograft and a ligament augmentation device (LAD). Am J Sports Med 1987b; 15:528-538.

Johnson RJ: The anterior cruciate: A dilemma in sports medicine. Int J Sports Med 1982;3:71-79.

Johnson RJ, Eriksson E, Haggmark T, Pope MH: Five-to ten-year follow-up evaluation after reconstruction of the anterior cruciate ligament. CORR 1984;183:122-140.

Jones KG: Reconstruction of the anterior cruciate ligamnet. J Bone Joint Surg 1963; 45A:925-932.

Kennedy JC, Hawkins RJ, Willis RB, Danylchuk KD: Tension studies of human knee ligaments. J. Bone Joint Surg. 1976;58A:350-355.

Kennedy JC, Hawkins RJ, Willis RB: Strain gauge analysis of knee ligaments. Clin Orthop. 1977; 129:225-229.

Kennedy JC, Weinberg HW and Wilson AS: The Anatomy and Function of the Anterior Cruciate Ligament, As Determined by Clinical and Morphological Studies. J. Bone Joint Surg. 1974;56-A:223-235.

Komender A: Influence of preservation on some mechanical properties of human haversian bone. Mater Med Pol 1976; 8:13.

Kurosaka M, Yoshiya S, Andrish JT: A biomechanical comparison of different surgical techniques of graft fixation in anterior cruciate ligament reconstruction. Am J Sports Med 1987;15(3):225-229.

Lenggenhager, K: Ueber Genese, Symptomatogie und Therapie des Schubladen symptoms des Kniegelenkes. Zentrallblatt f. Chir. 1940; 67:1810-1825.

Lawrence WH, Turner JE, Autian J: Toxicity of ethylene chlorhydrin. I: Acute toxicity studies, J Pharm Sci 1971; 60:568-571.

Lewis JL, Lew WD, Schmid J: A note on the application and evaluation of the buckle transducer for knee ligament force measurement. J. Biomech. Eng. 1982; 104:125-128.

Lewis JL, Lew WD, Shybut GT, Jasty M, Hill JA: Biomechanical function of knee ligaments. In: American Academy of Orthopaedic Surgeons Symposium on Sports Medicine: The Knee. C. V. Mosby Company. 1985;152-168.

Liljedahl S, Lindvall N, Wattersfors J: Early diagnosis and treatment of acute ruptures of the anterior cruciate ligament. J Bone Joint Surg 1965;47A:1503-1513.

Markolf LK, Kochan A, Amstutz CH: Measurement of Knee Stiffness and Laxity in Patients with Documented Absence of the Anterior Cruciate Ligament. J Bone Joint Surg 1984;66A:242-253.

Markolf KL, Mensch JS, Amstutz HC: Stiffness and laxity of the knee - The contributions of the supporting structures. A quantitative in vitro study. J Bone Joint Surg 1976;58A:583-594.

Marshall JL, Rubin RM: Knee ligament injuries - A diagnostic and therapeutic approach. Orthop Clin North Am 1977;8:641-668.

Marshall JL, Warren RF, Wickiewicz TL: Primary surgical treatment of anterior cruciate ligament lesions. Am J Sports Med 1982;10:103-107.

Martin ET, Butler DL, Grood ES, Chun KJ, Sodd AN: Technique for measuring the 3-dimensional configuration of the human cruciate ligaments. ASME Advances in Bioengineering 1987;3-4.

McDaniel WJ, Dameron TB: Untreated ruptures of the anterior cruciate ligament: A follow-up. J Bone Joint Surg 1980;62A:696-705.

McDaniel WJ, Dameron TB: The untreated anterior cruciate ligament rupture. Clin Orthop Rel Res 1983;172:158-163.

Morrison JB: Bioengineering Analysis of Force Actions Transmitted by the Knee Joint. Biomech. Eng. 1968;3:164-170.

Morrison JB: Function of the Knee Joint in Various Activities. Biomech Eng. 4:573-580, 1969.

Morrison JB: The Mechanics of the Knee Joint In Relation to Normal Walking. J. Biomech. 1970;3:51-61.

Nikolaou PK, Seaber AV, Glisson RR, Ribbeck BM, Bassett FH: Anterior cruciate ligament allograft transplantation: Long-term function, histology, revascularization, and operative technique. Am J Sports Med 1986;14(5):348-360.

Noyes FR: Functional properties of knee ligaments and alterations induced by immobilization. A correlative biomechanics and histological study in primates. Clin Orthop Rel Res 1977;123-210.

Noyes FR, Bassett RW, Grood ES, Butler DL: Arthroscopy in acute traumatic hemarthrosis of the knee. Incidence of anterior cruciate tears and other injuries. J Bone Joint Surg 1980;62A:687-695.

Noyes FR, Butler DL, Grood ES, Zernicke RF, Hefzy MS: Biomechanical analysis of human ligament grafts used in knee ligament repairs and reconstructions. J Bone Joint Surg 1984;66A:344-352.

Noyes FR, Butler DL, Paulos LE, Grood ES: Intraarticular cruciate reconstruction. I. Perspectives on graft strength, vascularization, and immediate motion after replacement. Clin Orthop Rel Res 1983a;172:71-77.

Noyes FR, DeLucas JL, Torvik PJ: Biomechanics of anterior cruciate ligament failure: An analysis of strain-rate sensitivity and mechanisms of failure in primates. J Bone Joint Surg 1974a;56A:236-253.

Noyes FR, Grood ES: Diagnosis of Knee Ligament Injuries: Clinical Concepts. The Crucial Ligaments: Diagnosis and Treatment of Ligamentous Injuries About the Knee, Feagin, JA (ed) New York, Churchill Livingstone, 1988;261-285.

Noyes FR, Grood ES: The strength of the anterior cruciate ligament. Age and species-related changes. J Bone Joint Surg 1976;58A:1074-1082.

Noyes FR, Matthews DS, Mooar PA, Grood ES: The symptomatic anterior cruciate-deficient knee. II. The results of rehabilitation, activity modification and counseling on functional disability. J Bone Joint Surg 1983b;65A:163-174.

Noyes FR, Torvik PJ, Hyde WB, DeLucas JL: Biomechanics of ligament failure II. An analysis of immobilization, exercise and reconditioning effects in primates. J Bone Joint Surg 1974b;56A:1406-1418.

O'Donoghue DH, Frank GR, Jeta GL, Johnson W, Zeiders JW, Kenyon R: Repair and reconstruction of the anterior cruciate ligament in dogs. Factors influencing long-term results. J Bone Joint Surg 1971;53A:710-718.

O'Donoghue DH, Rockwood CA, Frank GR, Jack SC, Kenyon R: Repair of the anterior cruciate ligament in dogs. J Bone Joint Surg 1966;48A:503-519.

Pagenstecher:Die isolierte Zerreissung der Kreuzbander des Knies. Deutsche Med Wochenschr 1903;29:872-875.

Palmer I: On the injuries to the ligaments of the knee joint. A clinical study. Acta Chir Scandinavica, Supplementum 1938;53.

Paulos LE, France EP, Rosenberg TD, Jayaraman G, Abbott PJ, Jaen J: The biomechanics of lateral knee bracing. Part I: Response of the valgus restraints to loading. Am J Sports Med 1987;15(5):419-429.

Paulos LE, France EP, Rosenberg TD, Drez DJ, Abbott PJ, Straight CB, Hammon DJ, Oden RR: Comparative material properties of allograft tissues for ligament replacement. Effects of type, age, sterilization and preservation. Trans Orthop Res Soc 1987; 12:129.

Paulos LE, Noyes FR, Grood ES, Butler DL: Knee rehabilitation after anterior cruciate ligament reconstruction and repair. Am J Sports Med 1981;9(3):140-149.

Pelker RP, Friedlander GE, Markham TC: Biomechanical properties of bone allografts. Clin Orthop Rel Res 1983; 174:54-57.

Pelker RP, Friedlander GE, Markham TC, Panjabi MM, Moen CJ: Effects of freezing and freeze-drying on the biomechanical properties of rat bone, J Orthop Res 1984; 1:405-411.

Penner DA, Daniel DM, Wood P, Mishra D: An in vitro study of anterior cruciate ligament graft placement and isometry. Am J Sports Med 1988;16(3):238-243.

Piziali RL, Rastegar J, Nagel DA and Schurman DJ: The Contribution of the Cruciate Ligaments to the Load - Displacement Characteristics of the Human Knee Joint. J Biomech. Eng. 1980;102:277-283.

Renstrom P, Arms SW, Stanwyck TS, Johnson RJ, Pope MH: Strain within the anterior cruciate ligament during hamstring and quadriceps activity. Am J Sports Med 1986;14(1):83-87.

Rosenberg DT, Rasmussen LG: The Function of the Anterior Cruciate Ligament During Anterior Drawer and Lachman's Testing, An in Vivo Analysis in Normal Knees. Am J Sports Med 1984;12(4):318-322.

Roth JH, Kennedy JC: Intra-articular reconstruction of the anterior cruciate ligament in rabbits. Trans Orthop Res Soc 1980;5:109.

Ryan JR, Drompp BW: Evaluation of tensile strength of reconstructions of the anterior cruciate ligament using the patellar tendon in dogs. South Med J 1966;59:129.

Santora SD, Daniels AU, Dunn HK: The effect of an anterior cruciate reconstruction on knee ligament force distribution. Trans Orthopaedic Research Society 1984;9:111.

Schutte MJ, Dabezies EJ, Zimny ML, Happel LT: Neural anatomy of the human anterior cruciate ligament. J Bone Joint Surg 1987;69A:243-247.

Schultz RA, Miller DC, Kerr CS, Micheli L: Mechanoreceptors in human cruciate ligaments. J Bone Joint Surg 1984;66A:1072-1076.

Seedholm BB and Terayama K: Knee Forces During the Activity of Getting Out of a Chair With and Without the Aid of Arms. Biomed. Eng. 1976;11:278-282.

Seering WP, Piziali RL, Nagel DA, Schurman DJ: The Function of the Primary Ligaments of the Knee in Varus - Valgus and Axial Rotation. J. Biomech. 1980;13:785-794.

Selvik G: A roentgen stereophotogrammetric method for the study of the kinematics of the skeletal system. Thesis. Lund (1974).

Sheh MY, Butler DL, Stouffer DC, Kay MD: Correlation between structure and material properties in human ligaments and tendons. ASME Joint Biomech Symp 1985;17-20.

Shiavi R, Limbird T, Frazer M, Stivers K, Strauss A, Abramovitz J: Helical motion analysis of the knee-II. Kinematics of uninjured and injured knees during walking and pivoting. J Biomech 1987;20(7):653-665.

Shino K, Kawasaki T, Hirose H, Gotoh I, Inoue M, Ono K: Replacement of the anterior cruciate ligament by an allogenic tendon graft: An experimental study in the dog. J Bone Joint Surg 1984;66B:672-681.

Shino K, Kimura T, Hirose H, Inoue M, Ono K: Reconstruction of the anterior cruciate ligament by allogeneic tendon graft. J Bone Joint Surg 1986;68B:739-746.

Sidles JA, Larson RV, Garbini JL, Downey DJ, Matsen FA III: Ligament length relationships in the moving knee. J Orthop Res 1988;6:593-610.

Solomonow M, Baratta R, Zhou BH, Shoji H, Bose W, Beck C, D'Ambrosia R: The synergistic action of the anterior cruciate ligament and thigh muscles in maintaining joint stability. Am J Sports Med 1987;15(3):207-213.

Solonen KA, Hjelt L, Rinne T: Anterior cruciate ligament reconstruction by a vascularized and innervated graft. An experimental study on rabbits. Acta Orthop Scandinav 1968;39:82-90.

Sommer RE: The effects of ionizing radiation on fungi. In: Manual on Radiation Sterilization of Medical and Biological Materials, Tech Report Series No. 149, Vienna, International Atomic Energy Agency, 1973; 73-79.

Spire B, Barre-Sinoussi F, Dormant D, Montagnier L, Chermann JC: Inactivation of lymphadenopathy associated virus by heat, gamma ray, and ultraviolet light. Lancet 1985;26:188-189.

Stouffer DC, Butler DL, Hosny D: The relationship between crimp pattern and mechanical response of human patellar tendon-bone units. J Biomech Eng 1985;107:158-165.

Stouffer DC, Butler DL, Kim H: Tension-torsion characteristics of the canine anterior cruciate ligament:Part I: Theoretical framework. J Biomech Engr 1983;105:154-159.

Sullivan D, Levy M, Sheskier S, Torzilli PA, Warren FR: Medial Restraints to Anterior - Posterior Motion of the Knee, J Bone Joint Surg 1984;66A:930-936.

Tkaczuk H: Tensile properties of human lumbar longitudinal ligaments, Acta Orthop Scand (suppl) 1968; 115.

Torg JS, Conrad W, Kalen V: Clinical diagnosis of anterior cruciate ligament instability in the athlete. Am J Sports Med 1976;4:84-93.

Torzilli PA, Greenberg RL, Hood RW, Pavlov H, Insall JN: Measurement of anterior-posterior motion of the knee in injured patients using a biomechanical stress technique. J Bone Joint Surg 1984;66A(9):1438-1442.

Trent PS, Walker PS, Wolf B: Ligament length patterns, strength, and rotational axes of the knee joint. Clin Orthop. 1976; 117:263-270.

Triantafyllou N, Sotiropoulos E, Triantafyllou J: The mechanical properties of the lyophilized and irradiated bone grafts. Acta Orthop Belg 1975; 41:35.

Turner TC, Bassett AL, Pate JW, Sawyer PN, Trump JG, Wright K: Sterilization of preserved bone grafts by high-voltage cathode irradiation. J Bone Joint Surg 1956; 38(4):862-844.
Van Dijk R: The behavior of the cruciate ligaments in the human knee. Thesis, Univ. Nijmegan, 1983.
Viidik A, Lewin T: Changes in tensile strength characteristics and histology of rabbit ligament induced by different modes of postmortem storage. Acta Ortho Scand 1966; 37:141-155.
Viidik A, Sandqvist L, and Magi ML: Influence of postmortal storage on tensile characteristics and histology of rabbit ligaments. Acta Ortho Scand 1965;79, Supplementum.
Wang CJ and Walker JE: The effects of flexion and rotation on the length patterns of the ligaments on the knee. J. Biomech. 1973;6:587-596.
Weber W and Weber E: Mechanik der menschlichen gehwerkzeuge. Part II Ueber das Kniegelenk, Gottingen 1836:161-202.
Webster DA, Werner, FW: Freeze-dried flexor tendon in anterior cruciate ligament reconstruction. Clin Orthop Rel Res 1983;181:238-243.
Wheeler Haines R: A note on the actions of the cruciate ligaments of the knee joint. J Anatomy 1941;75:373-375.
Woo SL-Y: Mechanical properties of tendons and ligaments. I. Quasi-static and nonlinear viscoelastic properties. Biorheology 1982;19:385-396.
Woo SL-Y, Gomez MA, Seguchi Y, Endo CM, Akeson WH: Measurement of mechanical properties of ligament substance from a bone-ligament-bone preparation. J Ortho Res 1983;1:22-29.
Woo SL-Y, Hollis JM, Roux RD, Gomez MA, Inoue M, Kleiner JB and Akeson WH: Effect of knee flexion on the structural properties of the rabbit femur - anterior cruciate ligament - tibia complex (FATC). J Biomech 1987;20:557-563.
Woo SL-Y, Orlondo CA, Camp JF, Akeson WA: Effects of postmortem storage by freezing on ligamnet tensile behavior. J Biomech 1986; 19(5):399-404.
Wroble RR and Brand RA: Function of knee ligaments: An historical review of two perspectives. Iowa Orthop Journal 1988;8:62-67.
Yoshiya S, Andrish JT, Manley MT, Bauer TW: Graft tension in anterior cruciate ligament reconstruction: An in vivo study in dogs. Am J Sports Med 1987;15(5):464-470.
Zernicke RF, Butler DL, Grood ES, Hefzy MS: Strain topography during failure of young human fascia and tendons. J Biomech Engn 1984;106:177-180.
Zimny ML, Schutte M, Dabezies E: Mechanoreceptors in the human anterior cruciate ligament. Anat Record 1986;214:204-290.

Chapter 5

New Insights Into Load Bearing Functions of the Anterior Cruciate Ligament

K.L. Markolf, J.F. Gorek, J.M. Kabo, M.S. Shapiro, G.A.M. Finerman

Introduction

The anterior cruciate ligament (ACL) is well recognized as a key structure in providing stability to the knee. A detailed understanding of its biomechanical function is of particular interest to orthopaedic surgeons who elect to repair, augment or replace this structure. Although numerous ligament sectioning studies have defined the role of the ACL in limiting tibiofemoral motions (Butler 1980, Fukubayashi, 1982, Piziali, 1980, 1981), the forces developed in the ligament itself are not known. This is due to a lack of suitable experimental techniques for measuring total ligament force as external forces and moments are applied to the knee. Knowledge of forces developed in the ACL is important in understanding common injury mechanisms, and for formulating rehabilitation exercises which will limit forces in ligaments which have undergone surgical repair, or have been replaced with soft tissue or synthetic substitutes.

Direct measurement of ACL force has presented a formidable challenge to biomechanical investigators. We have successfully recorded forces in a Gore-Tex synthetic substitute ligament used as a replacement for the ACL (More, 1988), but it is fair to say that no satisfactory method presently exists to study the total force generated in the natural ligament itself. Nonetheless, various approaches to this problem have been presented.

Buckle transducers have been used to measure forces in selected fiber bundles of the ACL (Ahmed, 1986, Barry, 1986, Lewis, 1982, 1987, Pauolos, 1981). These miniature devices can measure force only in those fibers which pass directly through the buckle. When the entire ligament is instrumented, the recorded forces are frequently subject to errors due to impingement of the buckle frame within the joint. In either case, foreshortening of the tissue which passes through the buckle may alter the forces recorded in the structure.

Direct measurements of ligament strain have been reported using mercury filled strain gauges which were sutured to selected ligament fibers (Edwards, 1979, Kennedy, 1977). Fiber strain measurements also have been recorded by attaching miniature Hall effect transducers to the ACL with sharp barbs which penetrate into the ligament substance (Arms, 1984, 1986). Unfortunately, localized measurements of ligament strain cannot be correlated directly with total ligament force. A complicating factor with all of these techniques is the fact that specific bands of the ligament are tensioned at different portions of the loading cycle.

Strain gauges have been applied to the tibial plateau near the ACL insertion site to measure changes in bone strain due to ligament loading (France, 1983). Again, these measurements cannot be related directly to ligament force; the recorded bone strain is also sensitive to compressive forces applied across the joint.

In this study, we describe a completely new experimental approach to the direct measurement of ACL force, and present the results of a series of loading experiments during which ligament force levels were recorded in fresh cadaver specimens before and after section of the medial collateral ligament (MCL). The unique advantages of this method are: (1) the ligament fibers themselves are not altered in any way during the measurement, (2) the total resultant force within the ligament is recorded directly (as opposed to localized measurements in specific bands of the ligament).

Methods and Materials

Seventeen fresh frozen cadaveric knee specimens from individuals 56 to 68 years of age were used for this study. All knees were examined for instability, range of motion, and flexion contractures. The presence of normal joint space was verified by radiographs, and the articular cartilage was inspected at arthrotomy. Knees with findings of arthritis or instability were excluded from the study. The tibia and femur were sectioned in the midshaft area and scraped clean of soft tissue to within 10 cm of the joint line. The bone ends were potted in cylindrical molds of polymgwhylmethacrylatgwacrylic cement for gripping in the test fixtures.

The knee specimens were then mounted in special test fixtures on a model 812 Materials Test System (MTS) machine for a series of loading tests. Anterior-posterior force vs displacement response curves (at ± 200N of applied tibial force) and torque vs rotation response curves (at ± 10 N-m applied tibial torque) were recorded at full extension and 20 degrees of flexion without and with the presence of 925N (207 lbs) of tibiofemoral contact force. For these tests, full extension (0 degrees flexion) was defined as the tibiofemoral angle which resulted when 2.5 N-m of extension moment was applied to the specimen. Details of test fixture design, our techniques for balancing and applying joint load and the procedures for testing have been fully documented in a prior publication from this laboratory (Markolf, 1981).

Insertion of the Load Cell

After completion of the MTS tests on intact knees, the specimens were prepared for attachment of a special load transducer designed to measure force in the ACL. In this procedure, a guide hole is drilled in the tibia which exits at the center of the insertion of the ACL in the tibial plateau; this hole is approximately in line with the fibers of the ACL. Using a series of cannulated

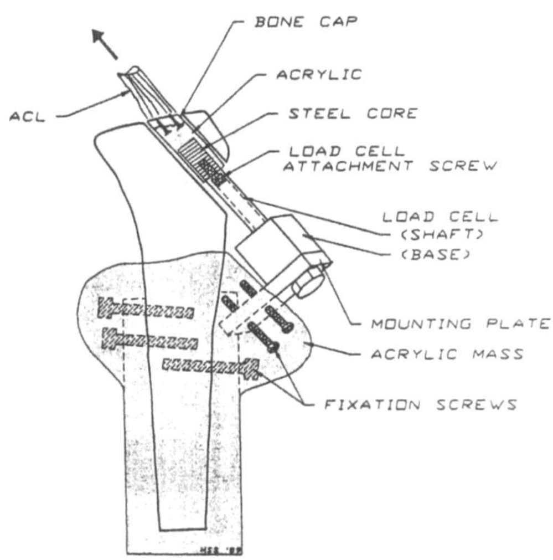

Figure 1. Schematic view of the load cell-bone plug construct. The shaft of the load cell is attached by an internal screw to a steel core imbedded within a cylinder of acrylic. The proximal end of this acrylic mass also incorporates small wood screws inserted into the undersurface of a mechanically isolated bone cap which contains the base of the tibial attachment of the ACL. The base of the load cell is secured by a hex head bolt to a metal mounting plate. A large acrylic mass incorporates the base of the mounting plate, the potted tibial shaft, and screws within the plate and potted tibiagwnto a solid structural base. All force generated by the ACL passes through the load cell to the tibia through this acrylic mass.

drills and a cylindrical reamer, a section of cancellous bone beneath the ACL is partially isolated. Prior to complete mechanical isolation of a bone cap containing the tibial insertion fibers of the ACL, six miniature wood screws are fixed to its undersurface. The porous cancellous bone and protruding screw heads are incorporated into an acrylic cylinder containing a steel core. This core is connected by an attachment screw to the shaft of a specially designed miniature load cell. The base of the load cell is attached by a hex head bolt to a mounting plate, which in turn is incorporated into a large acrylic mass surrounding screws fixed into the tibial shaft. After final mechanical isolation of the bone cap with a special coring cutter, all ligament force passes directly through the load cell. A schematic diagram of the load cell installed on a tibial specimen is shown in Figure 1. An important feature of this technique is the fact that the base of the ligament remains in its precise anatomical location with respect to the tibia.

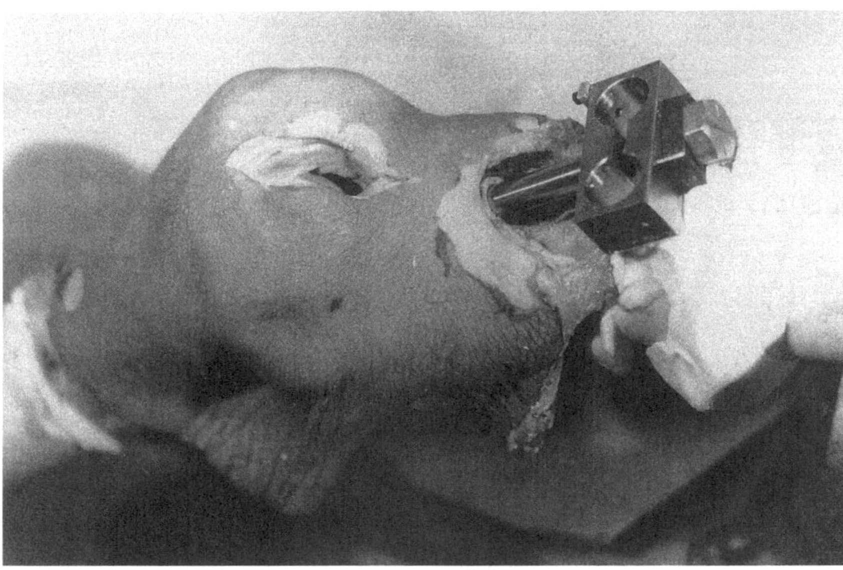

Figure 2. A mock load cell mounted in position on the knee specimen. The proximal load cell shaft is connected to the acrylic cylinder which is incorporated into the partially isolated bone cap. The hex head bolt connects the load cell base to a mounting plate which is incorporated with the tibial shaft by the large acrylic mass.

A load cell mounted on a knee specimen is shown in Figure 2; the wiring and strain gages have been removed for clarity. Two pairs of strain gauges bonded to the base of the load cell shaft in half bridge configurations measured the two orthogonal components of force acting perpendicular to the shaft axis. The component of force acting along the axis of the shaft was measured by four strain gauges bonded to the inner and outer surfaces of the circular cut-outs in the rectangular portion of the transducer.

Prior to each test session, the load cell was calibrated by hanging weights at its tip. These moment calibration factors were scaled for each specimen to reflect the actual distance from the ACL insertion to the tip of the load cell. The three components of force were referred to an origin located at the geometric center of the ACL attachment on the surface of the tibia. As the ligament was loaded during testing, the force components were recorded with directions corresponding to the orthogonal arrangement of the transducer gages. A computerized data acquisition system was used to record the force components, and to compute and display the resultant force in real time. The maximum error in the resultant force vector (principally due to slight errors in gage alignment and minor distortion strains in the axial gages generated by transverse force components) was 10 per cent for the extremes of the angles of ACL pull generated in these experiments. For angles of pull more closely aligned with the long axis of the load cell, the error in the resultant force was less than three per cent.

Tibial Loading Tests

With the load cell in place, the MTS tests described above were repeated. The ligament force was recorded simultaneously with force vs displacement or torque vs rotation measurements. Upon completion of the repeat MTS tests, a series of bench tests was performed with the load cell in place.

For the flexion-extension tests, the potted femoral shaft was clamped and a goniometer linkage was attached to the tibia to record knee flexion angle (Figure 3). The tibia was extended manually from 90 degrees of flexion to five degrees of hyperextension as ACL force vs flexion angle was recorded. The extension moment was applied in such a way as to allow the tibia unconstrained rotation throughout the range of flexion.

In a related test, a 200N weight was attached through a pulley system to a cord sutured in the quadriceps tendon with the knee at 90 degrees flexion. The knee extension moment produced by the quadriceps tendon force was resisted by manual pressure as the knee was allowed to extend slowly. This test simulated a knee extension exercise against light tibial resistance throughout a 90 degree range of motion.

For the tibial torque tests, an electronically instrumented handle was attached to the end of the potted distal tibia and a manual torque of ± 15 N-m

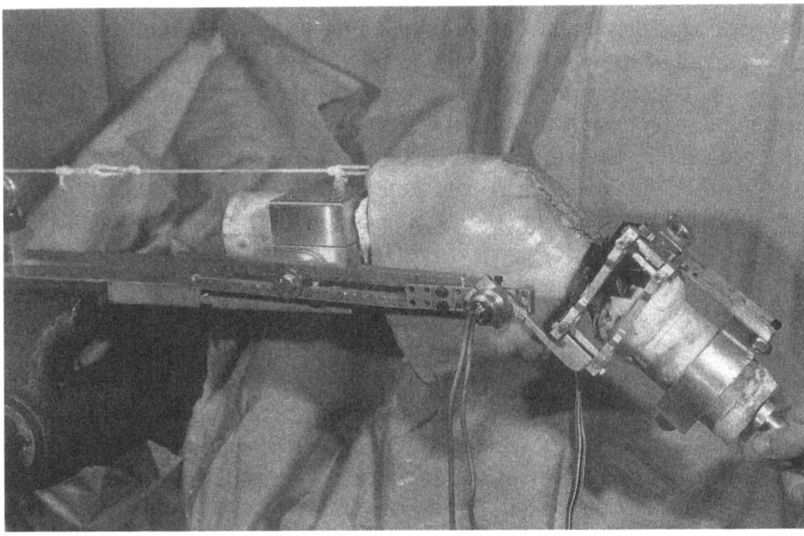

Figure 3. The flexion\extension bench test. A goniometer mounted on the linkage connected to the potted tibial shaft records flexion angle as the tibia is extended manually against gravity. The cord extending to the left is used to apply a constant 200N pull to the quadriceps tendon for selected tests.

was applied at flexion angles of 0, 10, 20, and 45 degrees (Figure 4). A goniometer attached to a four bar linkage recorded the tibial rotation as torque was applied. Ligament force and tibial rotation were recorded vs applied tibial torque without and with 200N quadriceps tendon pull. In a variation of this test, the knee was inverted and a low friction roller bearing was mounted co-axially on the potted tibial shaft. A weight was suspended from the bearing to produce a constant 10 N-m hyperextension moment while ligament force vs applied torque was recorded as described above (Figure 5).

For the varus-valgus tests, another electronically instrumented handle was used to apply and monitor bending moments of ± 15 N-m to the tibia at the same knee flexion angles used in the rotation tests (Figure 6). A fixed horizontal bar which contacted the potted tibia was used to maintain the desired flexion angle as bending moment was applied; the tibia was not allowed to rotate about its long axis during the test. Ligament force vs bending moment were recorded simultaneously at each flexion angle without and with 200N quadriceps tendon pull.

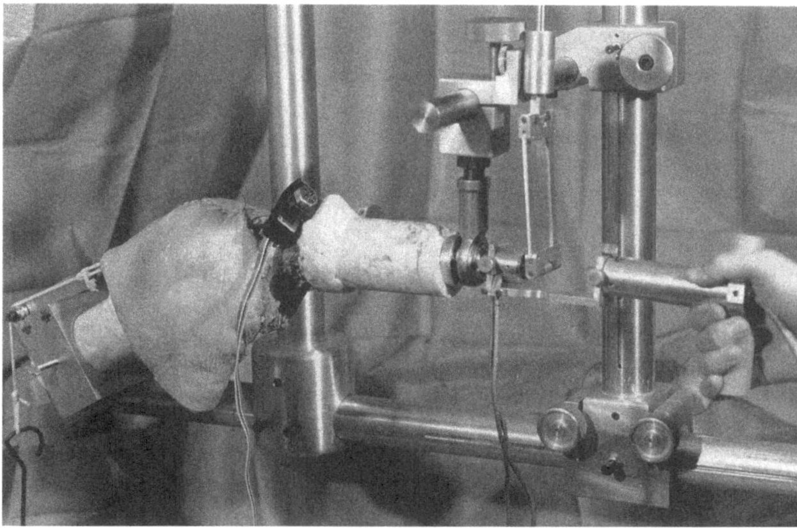

Figure 4. The tibial torque bench test. A goniometer mounted on the four bar linkage records tibial rotation. A spherical rod end bearing which supports the rod extending from the end of the tibial shaft permits the knee to seek its own axis for tibial rotation as internal or external torque is applied through an electronically instrumented handle.

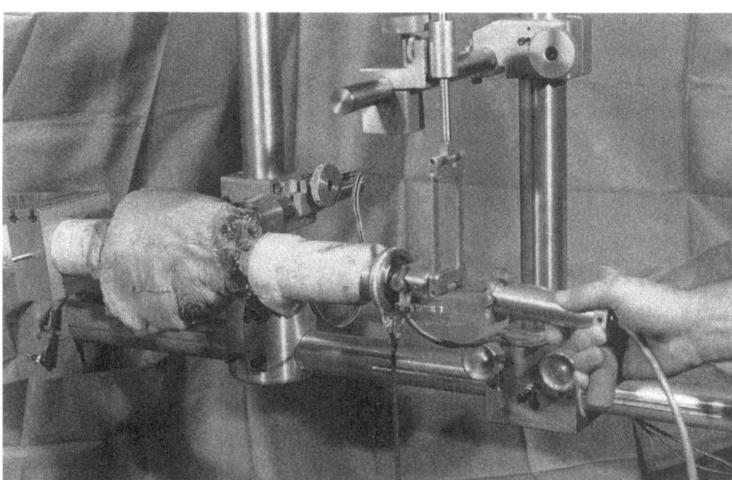

Figure 5. A variation of the tibial torque test with the knee inverted (patella facing down). A weight suspended from a low friction pulley bearing on the end of the tibia produces a constant 10 N-m hyperextension moment while tibial torque is applied with the instrumented handle.

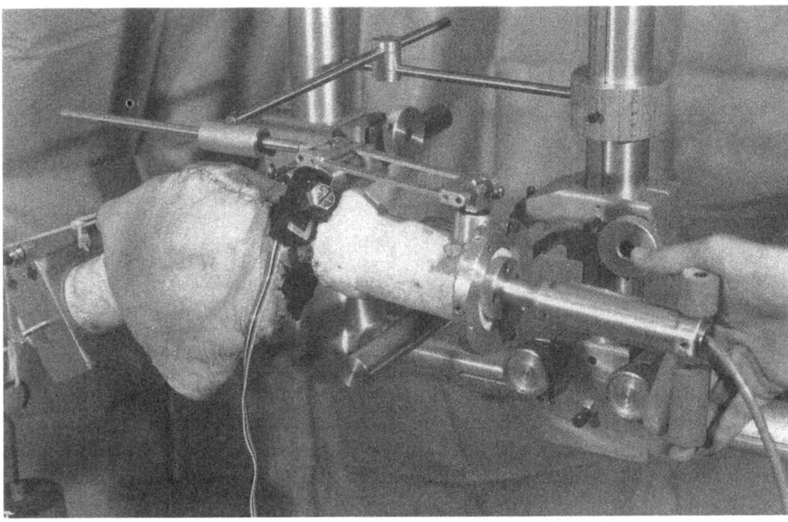

Figure 6: The varus-valgus bench test. Varus-valgus moment is applied to the end of the tibia by the instrumented handle shown. A horizontal bar which contacts the potted tibia is used to maintain a constant flexion angle during the test. No tibial rotation of the tibia is allowed as varus-valgus moment is applied.

Statistical Analysis

All test data consisted of ligament force values (the dependent variable) which were recorded continuously as functions of either applied tibial torque, applied tibial bending moment, applied anterior tibial force or manually generated knee extension angle (the independent variables). A first or second order regression curve was fit to data for each individual knee specimen for each specific test condition. An acceptable fit was defined by a correlation coefficient (r) of 0.9 or greater. A linear regression model was used to evaluate differences in regression curve coefficients and intercepts between knee flexion angles, quadriceps loading conditions, status of MCL section, and joint load conditions. A significance level of $p<.05$ was used to indicate differences in regression curve coefficients and intercepts.

Results

Intact Knees

Passive Knee Flexion/Extension

Although there was considerable variation in the magnitudes of ligament forces generated by passive extension of the knee without quadriceps tendon pull, the shapes of the response curves were quite similar (Figure 7). Ligament forces at

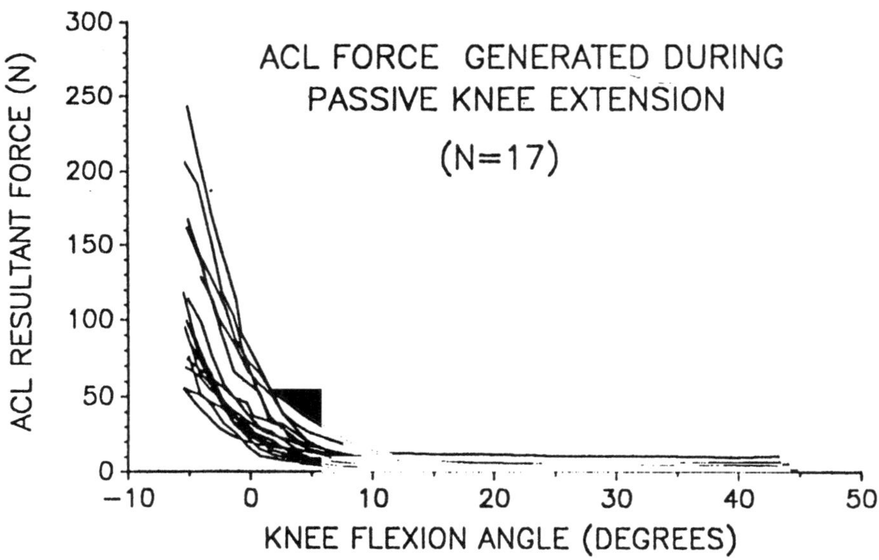

Figure 7. Force generated in the ACL during passive knee extension for all specimens in the study. There was considerable scatter in the force levels between 10 degrees of flexion and 5 degrees of hyperextension. Ligament force was minimal beyond 10 degrees of flexion.

full extension ranged from 16N to 87N, and from 50N to 241N at 5 degrees of hyperextension. Ligament forces beyond 10 degrees of flexion were negligible; ACL force increased rapidly as the knee was forced into hyperextension. When a 200N quadriceps tendon pull was applied and the knee was allowed to extended slowly against tibial resistance, ligament force was recorded throughout the flexion range (Figure 8). This force arose from the anteriorly directed

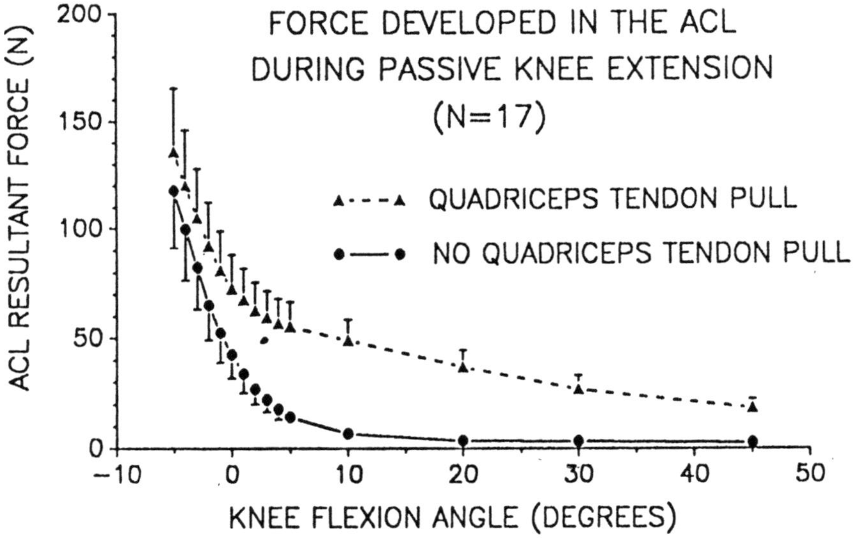

Figure 8. Mean curves of ACL force vs knee flexion angle for specimens during manual knee extension against gravity (solid curve) and for specimens extended slowly against tibial resistance by an applied 200N quadriceps tendon pull (dashed curve). Error bars indicate the 95 per cent confidence interval for the mean. The effects of quadriceps tendon pull are diminished as the knee is hyperextened.

component of the patellar tendon force which acted to sublux the tibia forward. The effect of quadriceps tendon force in increasing ACL force diminished as the knee was extended from 5 degrees of flexion to 5 degrees of hyperextension.

Tibial Torque Bench Tests

Internal tibial torque always generated greater ACL force than external torque. The ligament forces generated from application of both internal and external torque increased as the knee was extended; the highest ligament forces were recorded when tibial torque was applied to a knee which sustained a constant superimposed hyperextension moment of 10 N-m (Figure 9).

Quadriceps tendon pull had no significant effect on the ligament force generated when internal torque was applied to the tibia. Ligament force generated during application of 10 N-m of external tibial torque was greater when 200N of quadriceps tendon force was present; the increases averaged 26 per cent at full extension, 45 per cent at 10 and 20 degrees of knee flexion, and 90 per cent at 45 degrees of flexion.

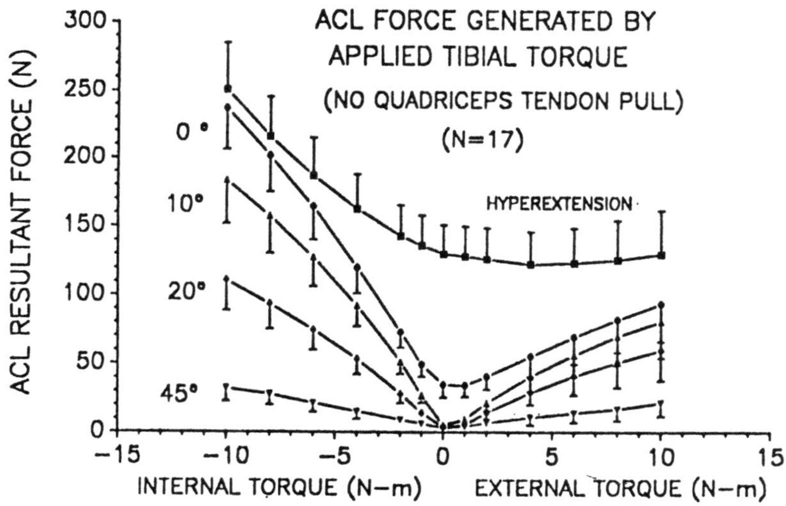

Figure 9. Mean curves of ACL force generated by application of internal and external tibial torque. Error bars indicate the 95 per cent confidence interval for the mean. The curve labeled "hyperextension" represents specimens with a constant applied extension moment of 10 N-m. All mean curves shown are significantly different from one another.

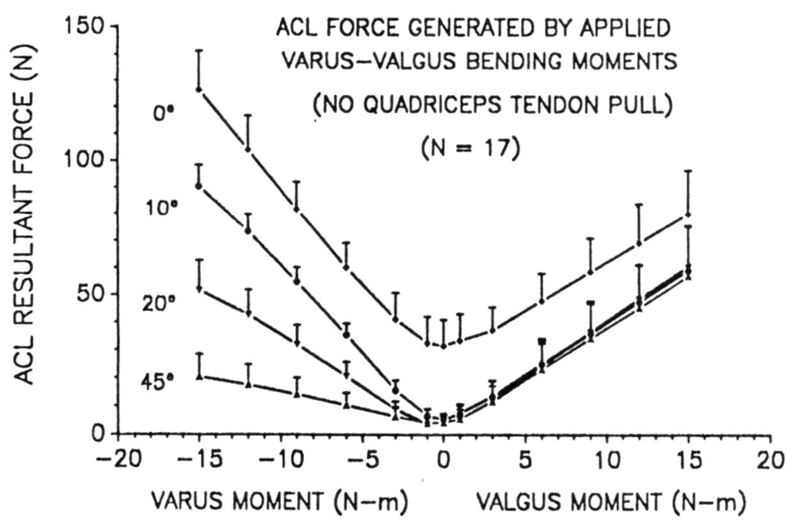

Figure 10. Mean curves of ACL force generated by application of varus and valgus bending moments to the tibia. Error bars indicate the 95 per cent confidence interval for the mean. For applied varus moment, ligament force levels are significantly different between flexion angles. Beyond 10 degrees of flexion, the ACL force generated by applied valgus moment is unchanged. The slopes of all mean valgus curves shown are equivalent.

Varus-Valgus Bench Tests

Ligament force was generated for both varus and valgus applied moments. For a given varus moment, ACL force declined steadily as the knee was flexed from 0 to 45 degrees (Figure 10). This was not the case for applied valgus moments, where ligament force was unchanged for flexed knee positions. Quadriceps tendon pull had no significant effect on the ACL force generated by 15 N-m of applied varus moment. In contrast, when 15 N-m valgus moment was applied to the knee, application of 200N quadriceps tendon pull increased ACL force by the following amounts: + 41 per cent (0 degrees of flexion), + 100 per cent (10 degrees and 20 degrees of flexion), ± 50 per cent (45 degrees flexion).

Anterior-Posterior Tests

Total anterior-posterior laxity of the seventeen intact knee specimens (defined as the tibiofemoral displacement between ± 200N of applied anterior tibial force) averaged 7.7 mm at full extension, and 11.3 mm at 20 degrees of flexion. There was a mean total laxity increase of 0.8 mm at both flexion positions after insertion of the load cell. When 925N of tibiofemoral contact force was applied to the knee specimens at full extension and 20 degrees flexion, a mean force of 52N was recorded. This force was directed medially, and represented an artifact since application of joint load to a balanced knee would not be expected to strain the ACL. This medial force was generated by the anterior ligamentous attachment of the medial meniscus which inserted on the isolated bone plug near the base of the ACL. As tibiofemoral contact force was applied, circumferential expansion of the medial meniscus tensioned this ligamentous attachment. This spurious force component was only observed in the loaded knee tests. The medial ACL force component values for the loaded anterior tibial force tests were adjusted to reflect the proportional changes in the other two force components (which were equivalent). This correction was based on the assumption that the angle of ACL pull did not change significantly between unloaded and loaded tests.

In the unloaded knee, application of 200N of anterior force to the tibia (at the joint line) generated a mean resultant ligament force of 207N at full extension and 201N at 20 degrees of flexion. The posteriorly directed horizontal component of the ligament force (which resisted the applied anterior force) averaged 135N, and the vertical force component averaged 136N. Under 925N of tibiofemoral contact force, the resultant ACL force was decreased an average of 36 per cent at 0 degrees flexion, and 46 per cent at 20 degrees of flexion.

Torque vs Rotation Tests

Total torsional laxity (defined as the tibiofemoral rotation at ± 10 N-m of tibial torque) averaged 23.6 degrees at full extension and 37.2 degrees at 20 degrees of flexion before installation of the load cell. Insertion of the load cell increased total torsional laxity an average of 2.4 degrees at full extension and 3.2 degrees at 20 degrees of knee flexion.

Ligament force values generated during the unloaded MTS torque vs rotation tests were not significantly different than those measured during the manual bench rotation tests. A medially directed force component generated by the anterior ligamentous attachment of the medial meniscus was also observed in the loaded torsional tests.

Wide variability in the patterns of ACL force change were observed when tibial torque was applied to knees with joint load. In some loaded specimens there was no increase in ACL force as torque was applied, while in others applied torque produced ACL force increases which were similar to those observed for unloaded specimens. Due to these inconsistencies between specimens, no definite conclusions could be drawn regarding the effects of joint load on ACL force generated from applied tibial torque.

MCL Deficient Knees

ACL Force Measurements After MCL Section

Section of the MCL did not significantly change the ACL force generated by applied varus moment. For valgus loading, ACL force increased after MCL section for all specimens at all flexion angles (Figure 11); the force increase ratio (mean force after MCL section / mean force prior to ACL section) varied significantly with knee flexion angle as follows: 1.7 (0 degrees), 2.5 (10 degrees), 3.3 (20 degrees) and 4.6 (45 degrees). When valgus moment was applied to an MCL deficient knee, the ACL force increased as the knee was placed in greater flexion. This is in marked contrast to an intact knee for which the ACL force did not change significantly with knee flexion (Figure 11).

For applied internal tibial torque, the results of MCL section were inconclusive. Some specimens registered force increases after MCL section, while others showed force decreases. This variability appeared to be related to a change in the axis of tibial rotation for some specimens; internal torque often produced a posterior subluxation of the medial tibial condyle. For applied

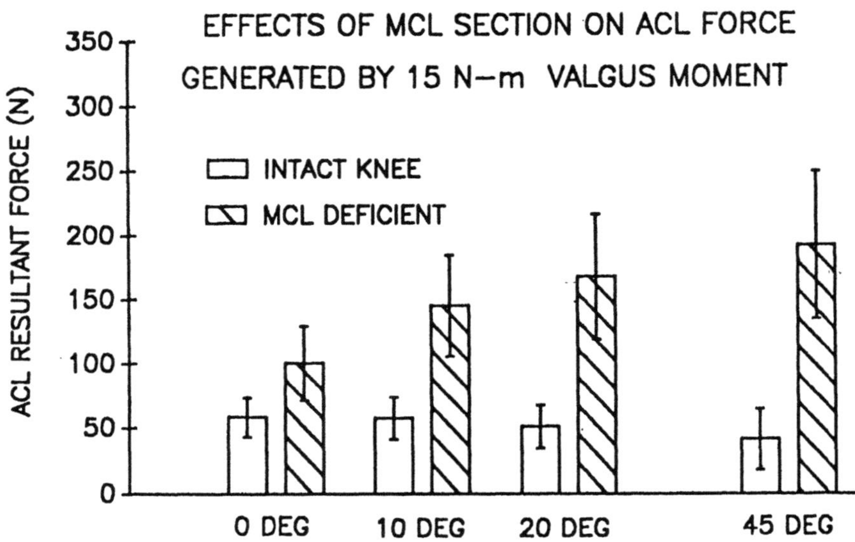

Figure 11. ACL force generated by 15 N-m of applied valgus tibial bending moment for ten specimens at four flexion angles. Mean force levels are shown before and after MCL section; error bars indicate the 95 per cent confidence interval for the mean.

external torque, marked increases in ACL force were recorded for all specimens at all flexion angles after MCL section (Figure 12). The force increase ratio varied significantly with knee flexion as follows: 1.6 (full extension), 2.5 (10 degrees flexion), 4.0 (20 degrees flexion), and 7.4 (45 degrees flexion). After MCL section, the ACL force generated by external torque <u>increased</u> as the knee was placed in greater flexion. This is in direct contrast to the intact specimens , for which the ACL force <u>decreased</u> with knee flexion.

Total laxity (as defined as the tibial rotation between ± 10 N-m of applied tibial torque) increased significantly after MCL section as follows: +12.6 degrees (full extension), +12.9 degrees (10 degrees flexion), +15.5 degrees (20 degrees flexion), and +19.6 degrees (45 degrees flexion). The increases for internal and external laxity were approximately equal.

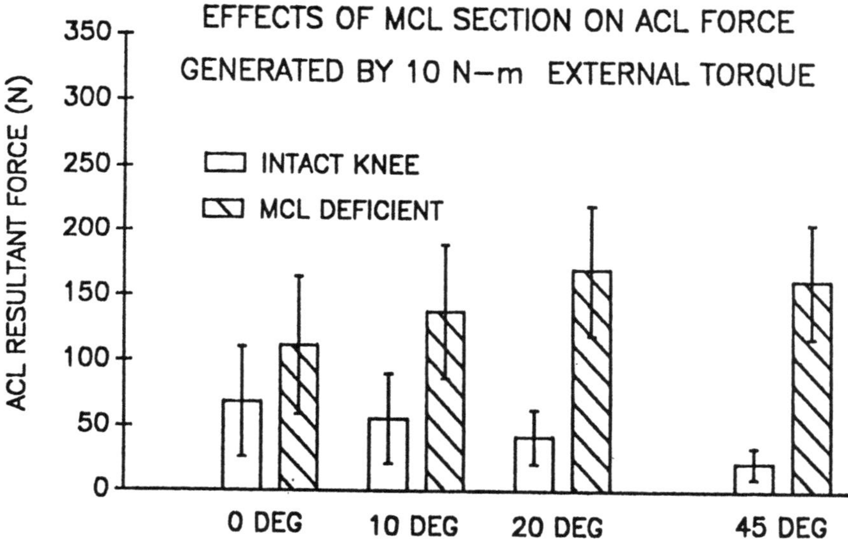

Figure 12. ACL force generated by 10 N-m of applied external tibial torque for ten specimens at four flexion angles. Mean force levels are shown before and after MCL section; error bars indicate the 95 per cent confidence interval for the mean.

Discussion

In the past, information on ACL loading has come indirectly from ligament sectioning studies, from direct measurements of select fiber strains, or from buckle transducers which produce significant foreshortening of the fiber bundles which are instrumented. This study presents a totally new technique for direct measurement of the resultant force generated in the ACL. The resultant force measurements reported in this study represent the contributions of numerous ligament fiber bundles of the ACL which become tensioned during defined external loading states at specific flexion angles. We have made no attempt to identify which bands of the ligament are responsible for the resultant force readings. The distribution of fiber bundle forces over the tibial insertion of the ACL is complex and beyond the scope of the present investigation. The force measurements reported here reflect the gross function of the ligament in resisting applied forces and moments. This load carrying function is particularly important when one considers replacing the ACL with a soft tissue reconstruction or synthetic prosthesis, structures which cannot replicate the complex loading patterns within the fiber bundles of the natural ACL. The ligament force data presented here are useful as a standard to which future loading studies with ligament substitutes can be compared.

Comparison of results from this study with other studies is difficult since our data represent the first direct measurement of resultant force in the natural ACL. In a prior study from our laboratory using fresh cadaver knees, the force generated in the Gore-Tex synthetic ligament was recorded by a force transducer attached to the distal tibial eyelet (More, 1988). In that study, the ligament was placed in an "over the top" femoral route and tensioned such that the knee laxity matched that of the intact knee (prior to ligament implantation) at 20 degrees of flexion. The mean Gore-Tex ligament force generated at full extension averaged 40N as compared to 42N mean force in the present study. A 200N quadriceps tendon pull increased the Gore-Tex force an average of 26N at 10 degrees of flexion, as compared to a mean increase of 43N in the present study. At full extension, the force in the natural ACL was 60 per cent greater than the Gore-Tex force for 7.5 N-m of applied internal and external torque. At 20 degrees flexion, ligament force generated by 7.5 N-m of internal tibial torque was the same for both studies; force in the natural ACL was twice that recorded in the Gore-Tex ligament for external applied torque. Resultant ligament force generated by an applied anterior tibial force of 200N in the unloaded knee averaged 206N at full extension in both studies. At 20 degrees of flexion, mean ligament force in the natural ACL was 201N as compared to 246N in the Gore-Tex ligament. Reductions in the above ligament forces due to 925N of tibial-femoral contact force were similar in both studies.

The similarities in ligament force magnitudes and patterns of force generation between the two studies is unexpected considering the marked differences between the Gore-Tex ligament and the natural ACL. The greater stiffness of the Gore-Tex ligament, its over the top placement, and the marked sensitivity of Gore-Tex ligament force to initial tension are all factors which could have produce marked deviations from normal ACL behavior.

There was considerable variation in the ACL force levels generated when the knee was passively extended against gravity. Similar scatter was observed in our prior Gore-Tex study, and represents specimen differences related to geometric variations, and possibly the "tightness or looseness" of the individual knees. This scatter could also be a consequence of our definition of full extension, which set 0 degrees as the tibiofemoral angle resulting from 2 N-m of applied knee extension moment. The tightness of the posterior capsule influenced the tibiofemoral angle attained by each specimen, thereby moderating the generated ligament force.

The high ligament forces recorded beyond full extension suggest that hyperextension can contribute to ACL rupture. The absence of ligament force beyond 10 degrees of flexion suggests that passive range of motion beyond this point would be safe for a knee undergoing rehabilitation after a ligament injury or reconstruction. The increases in ACL force observed during application of quadriceps tendon pull would suggest that active quadriceps extension against resistance in the flexion range 0 to 45 degrees would not be advisable if one desired to limit forces in the ACL or a ligament substitute. If a surgically implanted ligament substitute is overtensioned at 20 or 30 degrees of knee flexion, forcing the knee to full extension can generate high forces in the graft and possibly compromise graft fixation in the tunnel holes.

The change in ACL force due to an applied valgus moment was surprisingly constant between 0 and 45 degrees of knee flexion. This implies that the restraining moments generated by other medial structures (primarily the MCL) were also constant over this flexion range. In contrast, the ACL force generated from an applied varus moment decreased with increasing knee flexion, indicating possible recruitment of additional lateral structures. Thus for applied varus moment, the ACL is markedly more susceptible to high ligament forces when the knee is extended, an observation which is consistent with a mode of ACL injury which involves cutting maneuvers to the inside away from planted foot with the knee near extension.

The patterns of ACL force generation from tibial torsion also aids our understanding of commonly observed ACL injury mechanisms. The ACL force generated by both internal and external tibial torque decreases as the knee is flexed from 0 to 45 degrees, indicating that a flexed knee may be less vulnerable to ACL injury from twisting. Hyperextension of an externally rotated tibia markedly increased ACL force. This is consistent with a mechanism for ACL rupture during skiing whereby a skier "catches a tip" and applies high external tibial torque to a hyperextended knee (often with associated valgus stress). Near extension, the ACL force generated by internal torque is more than double that generated by external torque. Internal tibial torque near extension can be produced when a skier "crosses the tips" and the upper body is thrust forward over an extended knee.

The substantial increases in ACL force produced by quadriceps pull in combination with external tibial torque and valgus moment are unusual findings. Application of quadriceps pull acts to increase ACL force by increasing the anterior component of the patellar tendon force acting on the tibia. It is reasonable to assume that this mechanism is also acting during the varus-valgus and tibial torsion tests. However, one would expect increases in ACL force for torque and bending moments in both directions. We have no explanation as to why increases in ACL force due to quadriceps tendon pull were observed in one direction only during these tests.

Our results suggest an interesting mechanism by which the ACL resists an applied anterior tibial force. When 200N of anterior tibial force was applied to the tibia of an unloaded knee, the mean posteriorly directed horizontal component of the ACL force averaged only 135N. Therefore 65N of resistive force must be accounted for by other mechanisms. Force vs displacement tests in unloaded specimens with the bone plug disconnected from the load cell (simulating an

ACL deficient knee) showed that the remaining tissues were not capable of providing substantial resistive force at intact knee displacements corresponding to 200N of applied anterior force. The 65N of posterior force necessary to satisfy joint equilibrium could be explained by a net tangential force created by the 136N vertical component of the resultant force which acts to compress the menisci and congruent joint surfaces. This mechanism has also been proposed to explain observed decreases in knee laxity in the presence of joint load (Markolf, 1988).

The increases in ACL force after MCL section are especially interesting in light of the fact that many athletes with residual medial laxity from a prior MCL injury continue to participate in sports. External torque and valgus bending moment are loading modes which normally tension the MCL. It is not surprising to find that section of this important structure would alter ACL loading patterns. However, the magnitudes of the force increases after MCL section were unexpected. Also surprising was the finding that the MCL is clearly more active in limiting ACL force when the knee is in a flexed position; that is to say an intact MCL acts to protect a flexed knee from excessive ACL forces generated by these loading modes. We conclude that an MCL deficient knee is most vulnerable to ACL injury from applied external torque and valgus bending moment between 20 and 45 degrees of flexion. This emphasizes the importance of knee musculature as a first line of defense for protecting knees with residual medial laxity from high ACL forces; our findings indicate that such a knee is at increased risk for ACL injury.

Finally, the magnitudes of ACL forces recorded in this study merit consideration. The highest ligament force for an individual specimen (340N) was recorded when 10 N-m of internal tibial torque was applied to a hyperextended knee. The highest force recorded for a hyperextended knee in external rotation was 305N. The maximum load levels we were able to apply to the specimens were limited by fixation strength of the bone cap to the acrylic cylinder; bone cap failure did occur in some specimens and they were eliminated from the study.

In a prior study from our laboratory (Shoemaker, 1982), 31N-m to 55N-m of external tibial torque was required to produce ligamentous failure in knee specimens from elderly individuals at 20 degrees of knee flexion. A reasonable failure level to assume for younger individuals might be 60 N-m of external torque. It might also be reasonable to further assume that the failure torque for internal rotation is roughly the same magnitude. A linear extrapolation of the mean ACL force level for 10 N-m of applied internal torque (240N) would yield an ACL force level of 1500N for a hyperextended knee. The commonly quoted strengths for a young human ACL are 1735N, and for older humans 734N (14). Our data suggest that ACL rupture would be possible at reported gross structural failure levels for the knee.

Summary

We have developed an new and unique experimental technique for direct measurement of the resultant ACL force in cadaver specimens. In this study, we report the first direct measurements of resultant force generated in the natural ACL during a series of controlled loading experiments, and document changes in ACL force for selected tests after section of the medial collateral ligament (MCL). These measurements have identified loading modes which could produce ACL injury, and have provided a rational basis for formulating recommendations for post-operative rehabilitation exercises designed to limit forces generated in a ligament which has undergone repair, augmentation, or substitution. The changes in ACL force patterns observed after MCL section have direct clinical bearing for a knee which has sustained prior MCL injury and has healed with residual medial laxity. The risk factors for subsequent ACL injury of a knee in this condition are presently unknown.

Intact Knees

Passive extension of the knee generated ligament force only during the last 10 degrees of extension. This would suggest that passive flexion-extension motions in the range from 10 degrees to full flexion would be safe for a knee undergoing rehabilitation after repair or reconstruction of the ACL. When a 200N quadriceps tendon pull was applied to a knee which was extending slowly against tibial resistance, the ACL force increased at all knee flexion angles. This indicates that active quadriceps extension against resistance in the flexion range 0 to 45 degrees would not be advisable if one desired to limit forces in the ACL or a ligament substitute.

Internal tibial torque always generated greater ligament force than external tibial torque; ligament forces generated by tibial torque were greater as the knee was extended. We conclude that a flexed knee should be less vulnerable to ACL injury from applied tibial torque. The greatest ligament forces in this study (133N to 370N) were generated when 10 N-m of internal tibial torque was applied to a hyperextended knee. This is consistent with commonly observed ACL injury mechanisms during skiing; "catching a tip" and "crossing the tips" are both injury modes which involve application of tibial torque to a hyperextended knee.

For applied varus moment, the ACL is markedly more susceptible to elevated ligament forces when the knee is near full extension; this is consistent with a mode of injury which involves cutting maneuvers to the inside away from a planted foot with the knee near extension. For applied valgus moment, the ACL force remained unchanged with knee flexion.

The force in the ACL during straight anterior tibial translation was approximately equal to the applied anterior tibial force. Therefore, joint load acts to protect the knee from high ACL forces generated by applied straight anterior tibial force. No such protective mechanism was demonstrated for applied internal or external tibial torque.

MCL Deficient Knees

Section of the MCL did not change the ACL force generated by applied varus moment. For applied valgus moment, ACL force increased dramatically after MCL section; these changes were greatest at 45 degrees of flexion. When valgus moment was applied to an MCL deficient knee, the ACL force increased for greater angles of knee flexion.

For applied internal tibial torque, effects of MCL section were variable; posterior subluxation of the medial tibial condyle was often observed. For applied external torque, marked increases in ACL force were recorded after MCL section; as for applied valgus moment, these increases were most dramatic at 45 degrees of flexion. In an MCL deficient knee, the ACL force generated by external torque increased as the knee was placed in greater flexion.

For applied external torque and valgus bending moment, the MCL is clearly more active in limiting ACL force when the knee is in a flexed position; that is to say an intact MCL helps protect the ACL from excessive forces generated by these loading modes. Conversely, an MCL deficient knee is most vulnerable to ACL injury from these loading modes between 20 and 45 degrees of flexion.

References

Ahmed AM, Burke DL, Hyder A: Effect of tibial prerotation on the ligamentous response of the flexed knee to passive anterior shear. Trans Ortho Res Soc 1986; 1:127.

Arms SW, Pope MH, Johnson RJ, Fischer RA, Aruidsson I, Ericksson E: The biomechanics of anterior cruciate ligament rehabilitation and reconstruction. Am J Sports Med 1984:12:8-17.

Arms SW, Pope MH, Renstrom P, Johnson RJ: The determination of zero strain within the anteromedial fibers of the anterior cruciate ligament. Trans Ortho Res Soc 1984;11:239.

Barry D, Ahmed AM: Design and performance of a modified buckle transducer for the measurement of ligament tension. J Biomech Eng 1986;108:148-152.

Butler DL, Noyes FR, Grood ES: Ligamentous restraints to anterior-posterior drawer in the human knee. J Bone Joint Surg 1980;62-A:259-270.

Edwards RG, Lafferty JF, Lange KO: Ligament strain in the human knee. J Basic Eng, ASME Trans 1979;92:131-136.

France FP, Daniels AU, Goble EM, Dunn HK: Simultaneous quantification of knee ligament forces. J Biomech 1983;16:553-564.

Fukubayashi B, Torzilli PA, Sherman MF, Warren RF: An in vitro biomechanical evaluation of anterior-posterior motion of the Knee. J Bone Joint Surg 1982;64-A:258-264.

Kennedy JC, Hawkins RJ, Willis RB: Strain gauge analysis of knee ligaments. Clin Ortho Rel Res 1977;129:225-229.

Lewis JL, Hill JA, Ohland K, Lew WD: Knee joint laxity and ligament force changes with ACL repairs. Trans Ortho Res Soc 1987; 12:270.

Lewis JL, Lew WD, Schmidt J: A note on the application and evaluation of the buckle transducer for knee ligament force measurement. J Biomech Eng 1982;104:125-128.

Markolf KL, Bargar WL, Shoemaker SC, Amstutz HC: The role of joint load in knee stability. J Bone Joint Surg 1981;63-A:570-585.

More RC, Markolf KL: Measurement of stability of the knee and ligament force after implantation of a synthetic anterior cruciate ligament;in vitro measurement. J Bone Joint Surg 1988;70-A:1020-1031.

Noyes FR, Grood ES: The strength of the anterior cruciate ligament in humans and rhesus monkeys. J. Bone Joint Surg 1976;58-A:1074-1082.

Paulos LE, Noyes FR, Grood ES, Butler DL: Knee rehabilitation after anterior cruciate ligament reconstruction and repair. Am J Sports Med 1981;9:140-149.

Piziali RL, Seering WP, Nagel DA, Schurman DJ: The function of primary ligaments of the knee in anterior-posterior and medial-lateral motions. J Biomech 1980;13:777-784.

Shoemaker SC, Markolf KL: Effects of joint load on the stiffness and laxity of ligament deficient knees. J Bone Joint Surg 1985;67-A:136-146.

Shoemaker SC, Markolf KL: In vivo rotatory knee stability-ligamentous and muscular contributions. J Bone Joint Surg 1982;64-A:208-216.

Chapter 6

Structure and Biology of the Knee Meniscus

S.P. Arnoczky

Introduction

The menisci are C-shaped discs of fibrocartilage interposed between the condyles of the femur and tibia. Once described as the functionless remains of leg muscle (Sutton 1987) the menisci are now realized to be integral components in the complex biomechanics of the knee joint (Arnoczky et al 1988). This realization has resulted in an renewed interest in the basic science of the meniscus in terms of its structure, physiology, and function. This chapter will examine the structure and biology of the menisci of the knee joint.

Gross Anatomy

The menisci of the knee joints are actually extensions of the tibia which serve to deepen the articular surfaces of the tibial plateau to better accommodate the condyles of the femur. The peripheral border of each meniscus is thick, convex, and attached to the inside capsule of the joint; the opposite border tapers to a thin free edge (Warren et al 1986). The proximal surfaces of the menisci are concave and in contact with the condyles of the femur; their distal surfaces are flat and rest on the head of the tibia (Figure 1).

The medial meniscus is somewhat semicircular in form. It approximately 3.5 cm in length and considerably wider posteriorly than it is anteriorly (Warren et al 1986). The anterior horn of the medial meniscus is attached to the tibial plateau in the area of the anterior intercondylar fossa in front of the anterior cruciate ligament (Figure 2). The posterior fibers of the anterior horn attachment merge with the transverse ligament, which connects the anterior horns of the medial and lateral menisci. The posterior horn of the medial meniscus is firmly attached to the posterior intercondylar fossa of the tibia between the attachments of the lateral meniscus and the posterior cruciate ligament. The periphery of the medial meniscus is attached to the joint capsule throughout its length. The tibial portion of the capsular attachment is often referred to as the coronary ligament. At its midpoint, the medial meniscus is more firmly attached to the femur and tibia through a condensation in the joint capsule known as the deep medial collateral ligament.

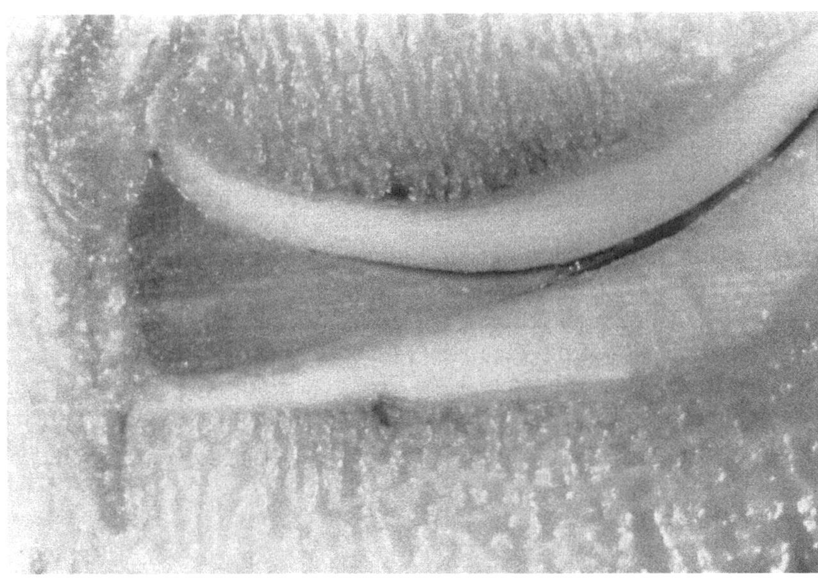

Figure 1. Frontal section of the medial compartment of a human knee illustrating the articulation of the menisci with the condyles of the femur and tibia. (From: Warren RF, Arnoczky SP, and Wickiewicz TL: Anatomy of the Knee, in Nicholas JA, and Hershman EB (eds): The Lower Extremity and Spine in Sports, CV Mosby Co. 1986, pp 657-694)

The lateral meniscus is almost circular and covers a larger portion of the tibial articular surface than the medial meniscus; it is approximately the same width from front to back (Figure 2). The anterior horn of the of the lateral meniscus is attached to the tibia in front of the intercondylar eminence and behind the attachment of the anterior cruciate ligament, with which it partially blends. The posterior horn of the lateral meniscus is attached behind the intercondylar eminence of the tibia in front of the posterior end of the medial meniscus. While there is no attachment of the lateral meniscus to the lateral collateral ligament, there is a loose peripheral attachment to the joint capsule (Warren et al 1986).

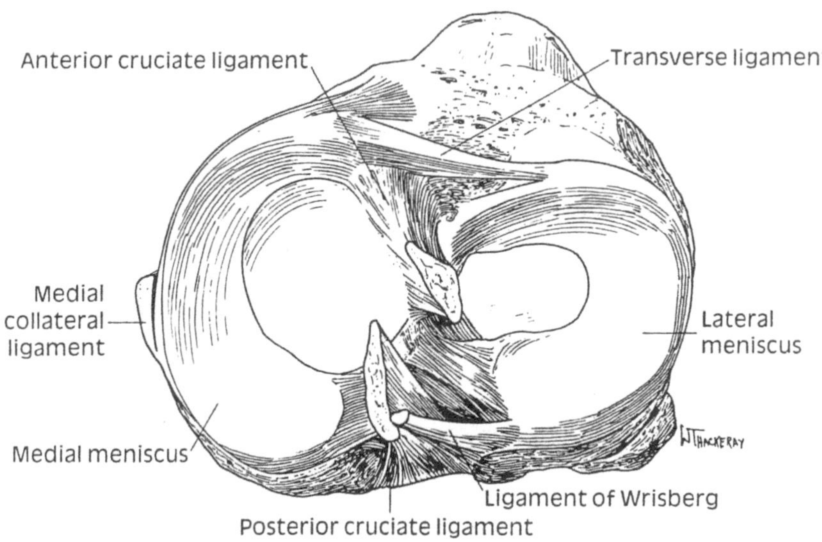

Figure 2. Drawing of a human tibial plateau showing the relative size and attachments of the medial and lateral menisci. (From: Warren RF, Arnoczky SP, and Wickiewicz TL: Anatomy of the Knee, in Nicholas JA, and Hershman EB (eds): The Lower Extremity and Spine in Sports, CV Mosby Co. 1986, pp 657-694)

Several ligaments run from the posterior horn of the lateral meniscus to the medial femoral condyle, either just in front of or behind the origin of the posterior cruciate ligament. These are known as the anterior meniscofemoral ligament (ligament of Humphrey) and the posterior meniscofemoral ligament (ligament of Wrisberg)(Warren et al 1986).

Ultrastructure and Biochemistry

Histologically, the meniscus is a fibrocartilaginous tissue composed, primarily, of an interlacing network of colgwgen fibers interposed with cells (Figure 3). In addition, the extracellular matrix consists of proteoglycan molecules and glycoproteins.

The cells of the meniscus are responsible for synthesizing and maintaining the extracellular matrix. There is still some debate as to whether the cells of the meniscus are fibroblasts, chondroctyes, or a mixture of both and whether the tissue should be classified as fibrous tissue or fibrocartilage (Ghadially 1983). The cells have been termed fibrochondrocytes because of their condrocytic

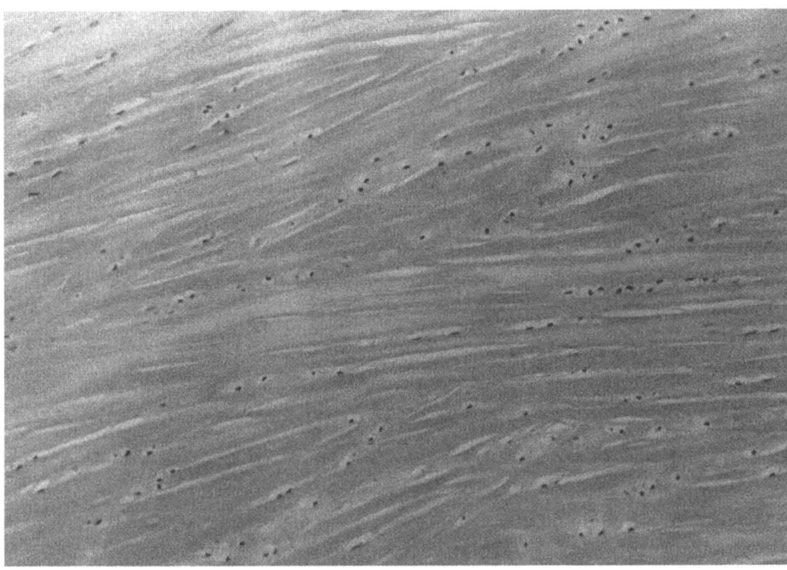

Figure 3. Photomicrograph of a longitudinal section of human meniscus showing the histologic appearance of meniscal fibrocartilage. (hematoxylin and eosin X 100).

appearance and their ability to synthesize a fibrocartilage matrix. Two basic types of fibrochondroctyes have been described within the meniscus: a fusiform cell found in the superficial zone of the meniscus and an ovoid or polygonal cell found throughout the remainder of the tissue (Ghadially 1978). Although the fusiform cells resemble fibroblasts, they are situated in well-formed lacunae and resemble the chondrocytes found in the superficial (tangential) zone of articular cartilage (Ghadially 1978, 1983). Both cell types contain abundant endoplasmic reticulum and Golgi complexes. Mitochondria are only occasionally visualized, suggesting that, as in articular chondroctyes, the major pathway for energy production for the fibrochondroctyes in their avascular surroundings is probably anaerobic glycolysis (McDevitt and Webber 1990).

The extracellular matrix of the meniscus is composed primarily of collagen (60-70% of the dry weight) (Eyre et al 1983). It is mainly Type I collagen (90%) although Type II, III, V, and VI have been identified within the meniscus (Eyre et al 1983). The circumferential orientation of these collagen fibers appears to be directly related to the function of the meniscus. In a classic study describing the orientation of the collagen fibers within the menisci it was noted that although the principal orientation of the collagen fibers is circumferential, a few small, radially disposed fibers appear on both the femoral and tibial surfaces of the menisci as well as within the substance of the tissue (Bullough et al 1970).

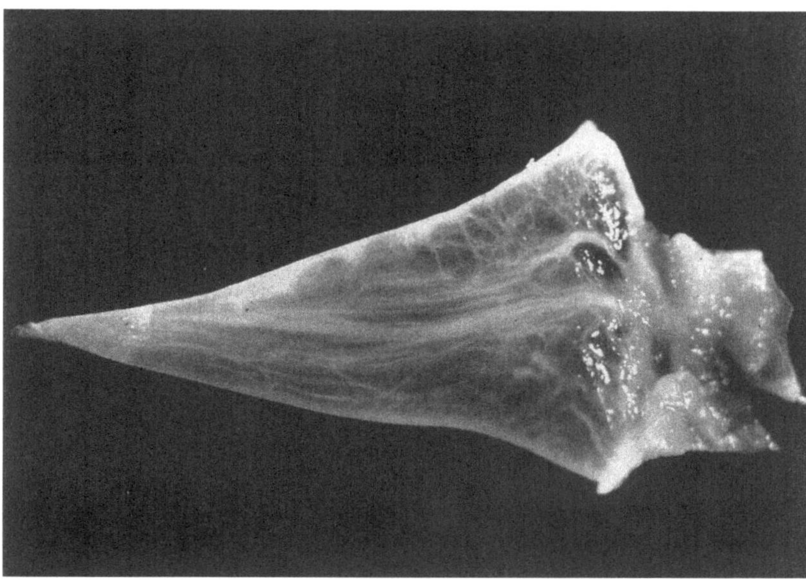

Figure 4. Cross section of a lateral meniscus showing the radial orientation of fibrous "ties" within the substance of the meniscus. (From: Arnoczky SP, and Torzilli PA: The Biology of Cartilage, in Hunter LY, and Funk FJ Jr.(eds): Rehabilitation of the Injured Knee, CV Mosby Co. 1984, pp 148-209)

It is theorized that these radial fibers act as "ties" to provide structural rigidity and help resist longitudinal splitting of the menisci resulting from undue compression (Figure 4). Subsequent light and electron microscopic examinations of the menisci revealed three different collagen framework layers: a superficial layer composed of a network of fine fibrils woven into a mesh-like matrix, a surface layer just beneath the superficial layer composed, in part, of irregularly aligned collagen bundles, and a middle layer in which the collagen fibers are larger and coarser and are oriented in a parallel, circumferential direction (Yasui 1978) (Aspden et al 1985) (Figure 5). It is this middle layer which allows the meniscus to resist tensile forces and function as a transmitter of load across the knee joint.

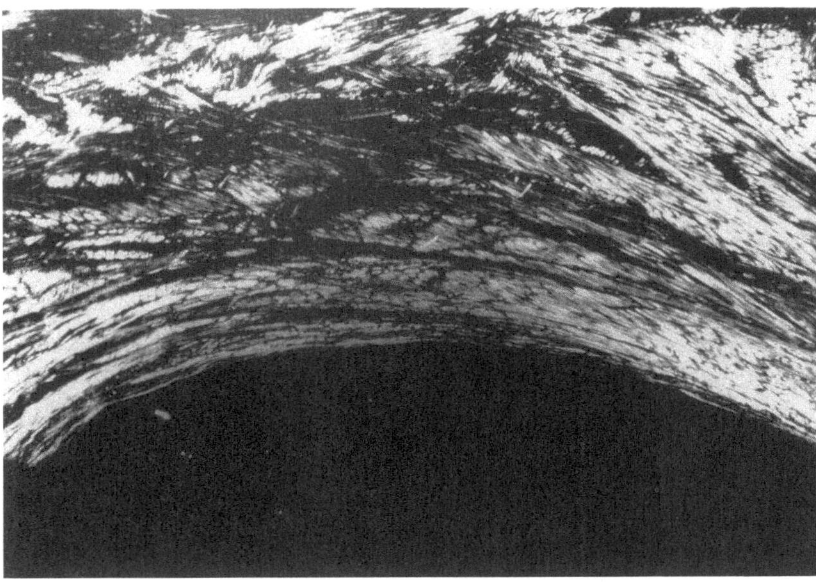

Figure 5. Photomicrograph of a longitudinal section of a meniscus under polarized light demonstrating the orientation of the coarse, deep, circumferentially oriented collagen fibers. (From: Arnoczky SP, Adams ME, DeHaven K, Eyre D, and Mow VC: Meniscus, in Woo S-LY, and Buckwalter J (eds): Injury and Repair of the Musculoskeletal Soft Tissues, American Academy of Orthopaedic Surgeons, 1988)

In addition to collagen, the extracellular matrix of the meniscus also consists of proteoglycans, matrix glycoproteins, and elastin (Adams et al 1983, Ingman et al 1974). The proteoglycan content of the adult meniscus is approximately 10% of that in hyaline cartilage although this has been shown to vary with age and location within the tissue. A study in the porcine meniscus has shown a higher (2 to 4 times) content of hexosamine and uronic acid in the inner third of the meniscus as compared to the outer two thirds (Nakano et al 1986). There was also a trend towards higher concentrations in the anterior horn as compared to the posterior horn in both the medial and lateral meniscus (Nakano et al 1986). The glycosaminoglycan profile of the adult human meniscus has been reported to consist of chondroitin 6-sulfate (40%), chondroitin 4- sulfate (10-20%), dermatan sulfate (20-30%), and keratan sulfate (15%) (Herwig et al 1984, McNicol and Roughley 1980, Roughley et al 1981).

Matrix glycoproteins, such as the link proteins which stabilize the proteoglycan- hyaluronic acid aggregates and a 116-k- Dalton protein of unknown consequence, have also been within the extracellular matrix (Fife 1985). In addition, adhesive glycoproteins such as Type VI collagen (McDevitt and Webber 1990), fibronectin (McDevitt and Webber 1990), and thrombospondin (Miller and McDevitt 1988) have also been isolated from the meniscus. These macromolecules have the property to bind to other matrix macromolecules and/or cell surfaces and may play a role in the supramolecular organization of the extracellular molecules of the meniscus (McDevitt and Webber 1990).

Vascular Anatomy of the Menisci

The menisci of the knee are relatively avascular structures whose limited peripheral blood supply originates predominantly from the lateral and medial geniculate arteries (both inferior and superior) (Arnoczky and Warren 1982). Branches from these vessels give rise to a perimeniscal capillary plexus within the synovial and capsular tissues of the knee joint. This plexus is an arborizing newtork of vessels that supplies the peripheral border of the meniscus throughout its attachment to the joint capsule (Arnoczky and Warren 1982) (Figure 6). These perimeniscal vessels are oriented in a predominantly circumferential pattern, with radial branches directed toward the center of the joint (Figure 7). Anatomic studies have shown that the degree of vascular penetration is 10% to 30% of the width of the medial meniscus and 10% to 25% of the width of the lateral meniscus (Arnoczky and Warren 1982).

The middle genicular artery, along with a few terminal branches of the medial and lateral genicular arteries, also supplies vessels to the meniscus through the vascular synovial covering of the anterior and posterior horn attachments. These synovial vessels penetrate the horn attachments and give rise to endoligamentous vessels that enter the meniscal horns for a short distance and end in terminal capillary loops. A small reflection of vascular synovial tissue is also present throughout the peripheral attachment of the medial and lateral menisci on both the femoral and tibial articular surfaces. (An exception is the posterolateral portion of the lateral meniscus adjacent to the area of the popliteal tendon.) This

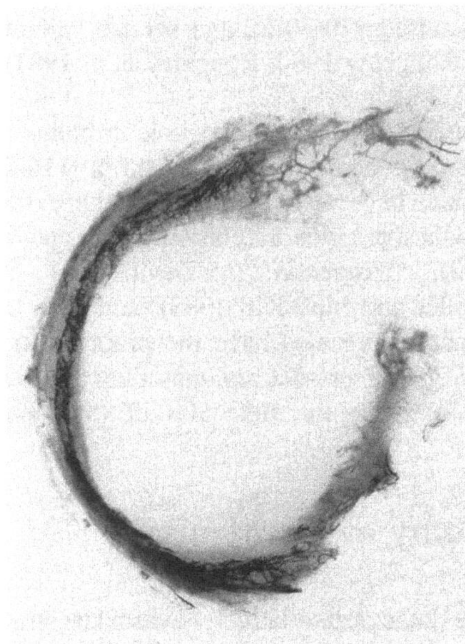

Figure 6. Superior aspect of a medial meniscus after vascular perfusion with India ink and tissue clearing with a modified Spalteholz technique. Note the vascularity at the periphery of the meniscus as well as at the anterior and posterior horn attachments. (From: Arnoczky SP, and Warren RF: Microvasculature of the human meniscus, Am. J. Sports Med. 1982;10:90-95)

"synovial fringe" extends for a short distance (1 to 3 mm) over the articular surfaces of the menisci and contains small, terminally looped vessels. While this vascular synovial tissue adheres intimately to the articular surfaces of the menisci, it does not contribute vessels into the meniscal tissue (Arnoczky and Warren 1982).

Meniscal Healing

The vascular response of the meniscus to injury has been studied experimentally and it has been demonstrated that the peripheral meniscal blood supply is capable of producing a reparative response similar to that observed in other connective tissues (i.e., exudation, organization, vascularization, cellular proliferation, and remodeling)(King 1936, Arnoczky and Warren 1983, Cabaud et al 1981, Heatley 1980).

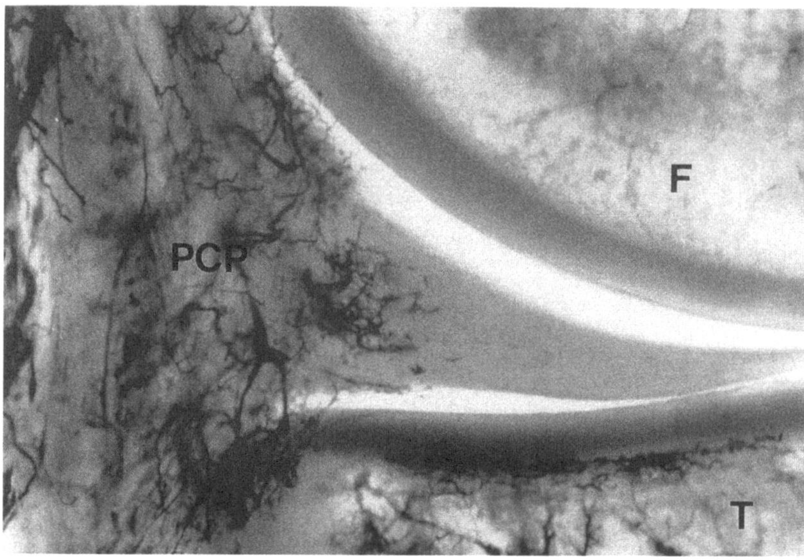

Figure 7. A 5 millimeter-thick frontal section of the medial compartment of a human knee (Spalteholz preparation). Branching radial vessels from the perimeniscal capillary plexus (PCP) penetrate the peripheral border of the medial meniscus. F=femur, T=tibia. (From: Arnoczky SP, and Warren RF: Microvasculature of the human meniscus, Am. J. Sports Med. 1982;10:90-95)

Following injury within the peripheral vascular zone of the meniscus, a fibrin clot forms that is rich in inflammatory cells. Vessels from the perimeniscal capillary plexus proliferate into this fibrin "scaffold" accompanied by the proliferation of undifferentiated mesenchymal cells. Eventually the lesion is filled with a cellular, fibrovascular scar tissue which "glues" the wound edges together and appears continuous with normal adjacent meniscal fibrocartilage (Figure 8)(Arnoczky and Warren 1983). Vessels from the perimeniscal capillary plexus as well as a proliferative vascular pannus from the "synovial fringe" penetrate the fibrous scar support this healing response (Figure 9). Experimental studies have shown that lesions within the vascular portion of the meniscus are completely healed by a fibrovascular scar by ten weeks (Arnoczky and Warren 1983, Cabaud et al 1981). Modulation of this scar tissue into "normal appearing" fibrocartilage, however, requires several months. The strength of this repair tissue as a function of time has not been delineated and further study is needed to document the material properties of this repair.

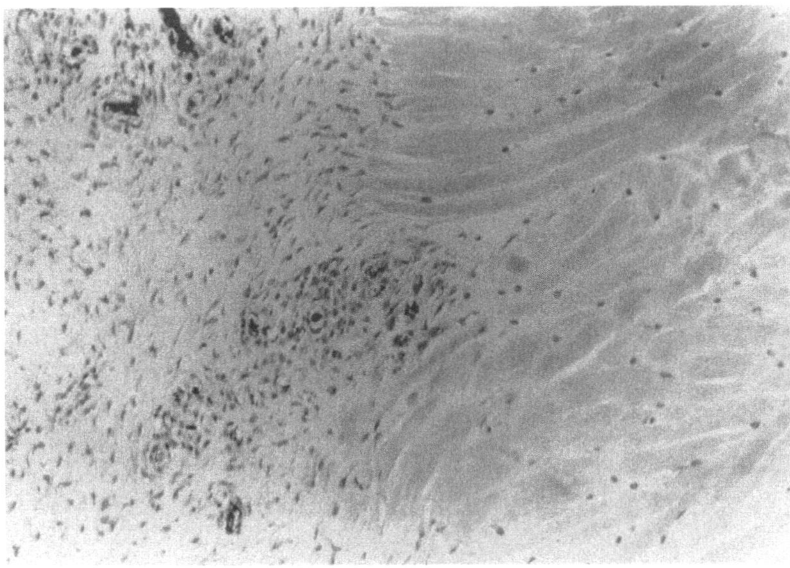

Figure 8. Photomicrograph of the junction of the meniscus and the fibrovascular repair tissue at six weeks. (hematoxylin and eosin X 100) (From: Arnoczky SP, and Warren RF: The Microvasculature of the Meniscus and Its Response to Injury. An Experimental Study in the Dog, Am. J. Sports Med. 1983;11:131-141)

Meniscal Regeneration

The ability of a meniscus or a meniscus-like structure to regenerate following total meniscectomy has been the subject of much controversy (Doyle et al 1966, Evans 1963, King 1936, Smillie 1944). This controversy may have arisen from confusion about the extent of meniscectomy (partial versus total) orthe fact that much of the data regarding meniscal regeneration is derived from investigations in animals.

Studies in dogs (DeYoung et al 1980)(Ghosh et al 1983) and rabbits (Kim and Moon 1979) have demonstrated that following total meniscectomy there is regrowth of a structure that is similar in shape and texture to the removed meniscus. Initially, this regenerated tissue has the histologic appearance of fibrous connective tissue. However, with time a fibrocartilagenous metaplasia occurs within the tissue and by 7 months it resembles fibrocartilage (DeYoung et al 1980).

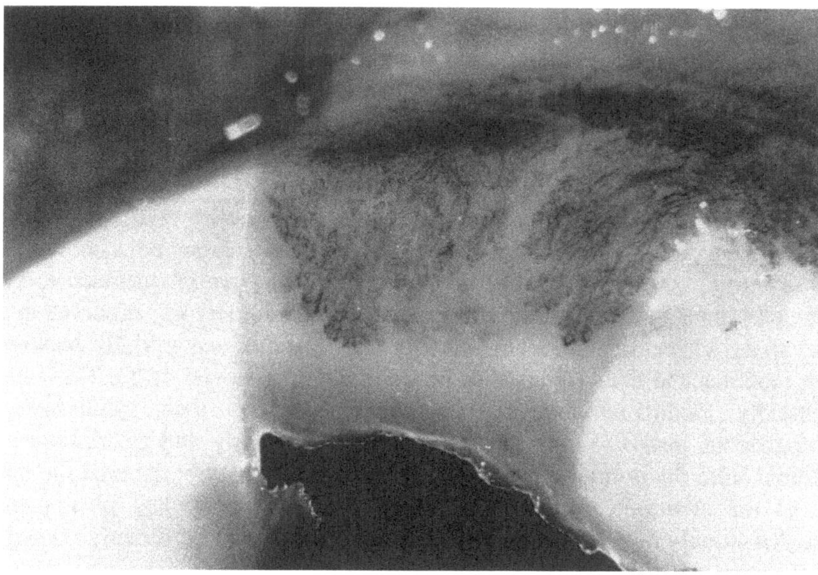

Figure 9. Photograph of a meniscus six weeks following the creation of a radial lesion. The fibrovascular scar tissue has filled the defect, and vascular proliferation from the synovial fringe can be seen. (From: Arnoczky SP, and Warren RF: The Microvasculature of the Meniscus and Its Response to Injury. An Experimental Study in the Dog, Am. J. Sports Med. 1983;11:131-141)

For a fibrocartilagenous tissue to regenerate following meniscectomy the entire meniscus must be resected to expose the peripheral vascular connective tissue. Experimental studies have shown the importance of this peripheral synovial tissue in meniscal regeneration (Kim and Moon 1979). In rabbits in which synovectomy accompanied total resection of the meniscus there was no evidence of tissue regrowth at twelve weeks. However, regrowth of a meniscus-like structure following total meniscectomy alone was observed in 83% (15 of 18) of the animals.

It appears, therefore, that the synovial and peripheral meniscal vasculature are capable of generating a connective tissue replacement for a resected meniscus. However, it should be noted that this regeneration is not always complete and does not occur in all cases. In addition, the material properties and functional adequacy of this regenerated tissue has yet to be determined.

Meniscal Remodeling

Although meniscal regeneration has been shown to occur only after total or subtotal (into the peripheral vascular zone) meniscectomy, a remodeling response has been observed in the avascular zone of the meniscus after partial meniscectomy (Arnoczky et al 1985). Because previous studies have shown the meniscus to be incapable of mounting a reparative response in the absence of a blood supply the origin of this remodeling response was unknown.

An experimental study demonstrated that this remodeling response probably results from an extrameniscal accretion of new tissue adjacent to the meniscectomy site (Arnoczky et al 1985). Following partial meniscectomy a fibrin clot (presumably resulting from residual hemarthrosis) was observed in the dead space adjacent to the meniscectomy site. The clot was initially populated with mononuclear cells (thought to be free-floating synovial cells). These cells eventually modulated into fibrochondroctyes which then synthesized a homogeneous matrix. While this new tissue was grossly and microscopically different from the normal meniscus it appeared to completely remodel the inner rim of the meniscus. It should be noted that this remodeling phenomenon occurred in only 67% of the cases studied and appears to be directly related to the presence of a hemarthrosis.

Experimental studies in tissue culture have demonstrated that when meniscofibrochondrocytes were exposed to chemotactic and mitogenic factors normally present in a wound hematoma the cells were capabale of proliferation and matrix synthesis (Webber et al 1985). The presence of hemarthrosis adjacent to the meniscectomy site therefore provides not only a potent mitogenic and chemotactic stimuli (platelet derived growth factor) but also a fibrin scaffold to support the proliferative and synthetic response.

Experimental and clinical studies have used an exogenous fibrin clot to support a reparative response in the avascular portion of the meniscus (Arnoczky et al 1988, Henning et al 1987, Webber et al 1987). While the biomechanical and biochemical character of this avascular repair tissue has yet to be determined this technique represents an intriguing concept in would repair.

The meniscus is a specialized tissue whose structure and biology reflect its functional role within the knee joint. While knowledge of the physiology of the meniscus has helped define the biologic capabilities and limitations of this tissue little is known about its material properties. Biomechanical characterization of the meniscus will be a critical contribution to the overall understanding and appreciation of this unique tissue.

References

Adams ME, Billingham MEJ, and Muir H: The glycosaminoglycans in menisci in experimental and natural osteoarthritis. Arthritis Rheum 1983;26:69-76.

Arnoczky SP, Adams ME, DeHaven K, Eyre D, and Mow VC: Meniscus in Woo S-LY, and Buckwalter J (eds): Injury and Repair of the Musculoskeletal Soft Tissues. Park Rodge, Illinois, American Academy of Orthopaedic Surgeons, 1988.

Arnoczky SP, and Warren RF: Microvasculature of the human meniscus. Am J Sports Med 1982;10:90-95.

Arnoczky SP, Warren RF: The microvascular of the meniscus and its response to injury: An experimental study in the dog. Am J Sports Med 1983;11:131-141.

Arnoczky SP, Warren RF, and Spivak J: Meniscal Repair Using an Exogenous Fibrin Clot: An experimental study in the dog. J Bone and Joint Surg.

Arnoczky SP, Warren RF, Kaplan N: Meniscal remodeling following partial meniscectomy: An experimental study in the dog. Arthroscopy 1985;1:247-252.

Aspden RM, Yarker YE, Hukins DWL: Collagen orientations in the meniscus of the knee. Joint J Anat 1985;140:371-380.

Bullough PG, Munuera L, Murphy J, and Weinstein AM: The strength of the menisci of the knee as it relates to their fine structure. J Bone and Joint Surg 1970;52B:564-570.

Cabaud HE, Rodkey WG, Fitzwater JE: Medial meniscus repairs: An experimental and morphologic study. Am J Sports Med 1981;9:129-134.

De Young DJ, Flo GL, Tvedten H: Experimental medial meniscectomy in dogs undergoing cranial cruciate ligament repair. J Am Anim Hosp Assoc 1980;1 639-645.

Doyle JR, Eisenberg JH, Orth MW: Regeneration of knee menisci: A preliminary report. J Trauma 1966;6:50-55.

Evans DK: Repeated regeneration of a meniscus in the knee. J Bone Joint Surg 1963;45B:748-749.

Eyre DR, Koob TJ, and Chun LE: Biochemistry of the meniscus:Unique profile of collagen types and site dependent variations in composition. Orthop Trans 1983;8:56.

Fife RS: Identification of link proteins and a 116,000-dalton matrix protein in canine meniscus. Arch Biochem Biophys 1985;240:682-688.

Ghadially FN: Fine Structure of Synovial Joints. London, Butterworths, 1983.

Ghadially FN, Thomas I, Yong N, et al: Ultrastructure of rabbit semilunar cartilages. J Anat 1978;125:499-517.

Ghosh P, Taylor TKF, Pettit GD, Horsburgh BA, and Bellenger CR: Effect of Postoperative Immobilization on the Regrowth of the Knee Joint Semilunar Cartilage:An Experimental Study. 1983;1:153-164.

Heatley FW: The meniscus-can it be repaired? An experimental study in the rabbits. J Bone Joint Surg 1980;62B:397-402

Henning CE, Lynch MA, Clark JR: Vascularity for healing of meniscus repair. Arthroscopy 1987;3:13-18.

Herwig J, Egner E, Buddecke E: Chemical changes of human knee joint menisci in various stages of degeneration. Ann Rheum Dis 1984;43:635-640.

Ingman AM, Ghosh P, Taylor TKF: Variation of collagenous and non-collagenousproteins of human knee joint menisci with age and degeneration. Gerontologia 1974;20:212-223.

Kim J-M, Moon MS: Effects of synovectomy upon regeneration of meniscus in rabbits. Clin Orthop 1979;141:287-294.

King D: Regeneration of the semilunar cartilage. Surg Gynecol Obstet 1936;62:167-170.

King D: The healing of semilunar cartilages. J Bone Joint Surg 1936;18:333-342.

McDevitt CA, and Webber RJ: The Ultrastructure and Biochemistry of Meniscal Cartilage. Clinical Orthop 1990;252:8-18.

Miller RR, and McDevitt CA: The presence of thrombospondin in ligament, meniscus, and intervertebral disc. Glycoconjugate J 1988;5:312.

McNicol D, Roughley PJ: Extraction and characterization of proteoglycan from human meniscus. Biochem J 1980;185:705-713.

Nakano T, Thompson JR, Aherne FX: Distribution of glycosamino-glycans and the non-reducible collagen crosslink, pyridinoline in porcine menisci. Can J Vet Res 1986;50:532-536.

Roughley PJ, McNicol D, Santer V, et al: The presence of a cartilage-like proteoglycan in the adult human meniscus. Biochem J 1981;197:77-83.

Smilie IS: Observations on the regeneration of the semilunar cartilages in man. Br J Surg 1944;31:398-401.

Sutton, JB: Ligaments: Their Nature and Morphology. London, MK Lewis & Co., 1897.

Warren R, Arnoczky SP, Wickiewicz TL: Anatomy of the knee, in Nicholas JA, Hershman EB (eds): The Lower Extremity and Spine in Sports Medicine. St. Louis, CV Mosby Co. 1986, pp 657-694.

Webber RJ, Harris MG, Hough AJ Jr: Cell culture of rabbit meniscal fibrochondrocytes: Proliferative and synthetic response to growth factors and ascorbate. J Orthop Res 1985;3:36-42.

Webber RJ, York L, Vander Schilden JL, et al: Fibrin clot invasion by rabbit meniscal fibrochondrocytes in organ culture. Trans Orthop Res Soc 1987;12:470.

Yasui K: The dimensional architecture of human normal menisci. J Jpn Orthop Assoc 1978;52:391-399.

Chapter 7

Structure and Function of the Meniscus: Basic and Clinical Implications

M.A. Kelly, D.C. Fithian, K.Y. Chern, V.C. Mow

Introduction

The menisci are fibrocartilaginous structures that are essential to normal function of the knee. Once thought to be functionless, investigations have demonstrated that the menisci serve a number of important functions in the knee (King 1936b; Fairbank 1948; MacConaill 1932; Seedholm and Hargreaves 1979; Voloshin and Wosk 1983; Fukubayashi et al., 1980; Kurosawa et al. 1980; Ahmed and Burke 1983). These functions include load bearing, shock absorption and joint lubrication. Although increased knee joint laxity after meniscectomy has been reported, a consensus of opinion regarding the stabilizing role of the meniscus in an otherwise intact knee has not been achieved. Shoemaker and Markolf and Levy and coworkers suggest that the menisci do provide increasing joint stability in the anterior cruciate ligament deficient knee (Shoemaker et al., 1986; Levy et al., 1982).

King first demonstrated the importance of the menisci in load bearing in 1936 (King 1936b). Using advanced experimental techniques, a number of investigators have determined that the menisci distribute large loads across the knee joint. Recent studies by Ahmed and Burke (1983) using a microindentation transducer demonstrated that the menisci bear at least 50 per cent of the compressive load of the knee in extension and that their contribution to load bearing increases to 85 percent at 90 degrees of flexion. Shrive and associates (1978) analyzed a section of the meniscus and proposed a model of load distribution within the tissue.

Clinicians commonly refer to the meniscus as the "shock absorber" of the knee. Investigations determining the compressive load-deformation response of the pre- and post-meniscectomy knee suggest that the meniscus may attenuate the intermittent shock waves that are generated in the normal gait cycle (Krause et al., 1976; Seedholm and Hargreaves 1979; Voloshin and Wosk 1981). The intrinsic material properties of the meniscus including its low compressive stiffness and low permeability are well suited for this function (Proctor et al., 1989).

The precise role of the meniscus in joint lubrication remains unclear and is worthy of further experimental evaluation. MacConaill suggested that the menisci play an important role in assisting fluid film lubrication of the knee joint (1932). Although the role of fluid transport through articular cartilage under load for lubrication has been documented, this information is not known for the meniscus.

Profound alterations in load transmission across the knee joint occur following total meniscectomy. These changes include increased peak stress, reduced contact areas and greater stress concentration (Ahmed and Burke 1983) and decreased shock absorption (Seedholm and Hargreaves 1979; Voloshin and Wosk 1983). Ahmed and Burke determined that medial meniscectomy reduces contact area by 50-70 percent, with greater reductions at increased loads. Partial as well as total meniscectomy significantly alters the strain distribution in the proximal tibia (Bourne et al., 1984). Odgaard et al. (1989) reported increased subchondral bone density in the medial tibial plateau five to ten years following partial and medial total meniscectomy. Presumably, this remodelling will lead to further alteration in contact pressures and strain distribution with the passage of time. The long term effects of bone remodelling following meniscectomy are being investigated (Bylski-Austrow et al., 1990). The disappointing long term clinical results following meniscectomy reflect these basic changes in knee joint mechanics.

It is likely that loss of meniscus due to either partial or total meniscectomy allows overloading of the involved articular cartilage with subsequent joint degeneration. In 1948, Fairbank described the early radiographic degenerative changes following meniscectomy which include joint space narrowing, flattening of the marginal aspect of the condylar articular surface and the formation of an osteophytic ridge on the involved femoral condyle. A number of investigators have confirmed these observations (Dandy and Jackson 1975; Gear 1967; Huckell 1965; Jackson 1967; Tapper and Hoover 1969). The severity of the degenerative joint changes appears proportional to the amount of meniscus removed (Cox et al., 1975). A number of experimental models have been developed utilizing removal of the meniscus to initiate early osteoarthritic changes in the articular cartilage (Moskowitz et al., 1979; Shapiro and Glimcher 1980; Hoch et al., 1983).

Due to the disappointing clinical results following total meniscectomy, partial meniscectomy has become increasingly common. This has been enhanced by the diagnostic and surgical techniques provided by arthroscopy of the knee. However, there is experimental evidence that partial meniscectomy also can contribute to knee joint degeneration (Cox et al., 1975). A growing body of clinical evidence also suggests that partial meniscectomy may have deleterious long-term effects (Jackson and Dandy 1976; Lynch et al., 1983; McGinty et al., 1977; Gillquist 1990). These results have further accelerated interest in meniscal preservation.

Historically, indications for meniscal repair have been limited to tears in the narrow peripheral margin of the meniscus, due to the limited capacity of central lesions to heal (King 1936a; Cabaud et al., 1981; Heatley 1980; Pontarelli et al., 1983; Redman and Haynes 1983). Investigations by Arnoczky and Warren and others have improved our understanding of meniscal microvasculature and the importance of the perimeniscal synovium (Arnoczky and Warren 1982; Limbird et al., 1987). This has allowed further refinement in patient selection and motivated the search for newer techniques of repair (Gershuni et al., 1985; Veth et al., 1983; Ghadially et al., 1986). Early experience with meniscal repair using an open surgical technique was reported by DeHaven and Hales (1983). Scott et al. (1986) reported promising results in a review of 178 meniscal repairs using an arthroscopically assisted intra-articular technique combined with a posterior incision. Similar encouraging results have been reported by Hamberg et al. (1983) and DeHaven et al. (1990) who have a 4.6 year average follow-up of meniscal repair in an athletic population. Meniscal cells are capable of proliferation and matrix production *in vitro* when they are exposed to certain trophic and mitogenic factors (Webber et al., 1985; Webber 1990). Experimental work by Arnoczky et al. (1986) suggested the use of exogenous fibrin clot to further improve meniscal healing rates. This technique has accounted for significant improvement in healing rates of isolated meniscal repairs (Henning et al., 1990).

Severely damaged menisci may not be amenable to surgical repair. One alternative to removal currently under investigation is replacement of the meniscus with a meniscal allograft. The hope is that successful transplantation of such an allograft could serve to eliminate the degenerative changes associated with meniscectomy. Recent experimental and clinical work lends promise to the applicability of meniscal allografting in the future (Arnoczky et al., 1990a,b; Zukor et al., 1990; Jackson et al., 1990; Garrett 1990).

Experimental and clinical investigations have established the important role the menisci play in normal knee function. Understanding meniscal function requires knowledge of their intrinsic material properties and local variations of these properties as well as their gross and microscopic anatomy. Tissue composition and ultrastructural organization have a significant influence on tissue material properties. A firm understanding of these meniscal features is essential. Considerable experimental investigation of meniscal material properties has been performed in the authors' laboratory. These properties may be determined from load deformation studies using precisely prepared specimens and loading conditions. We will review our current understanding of

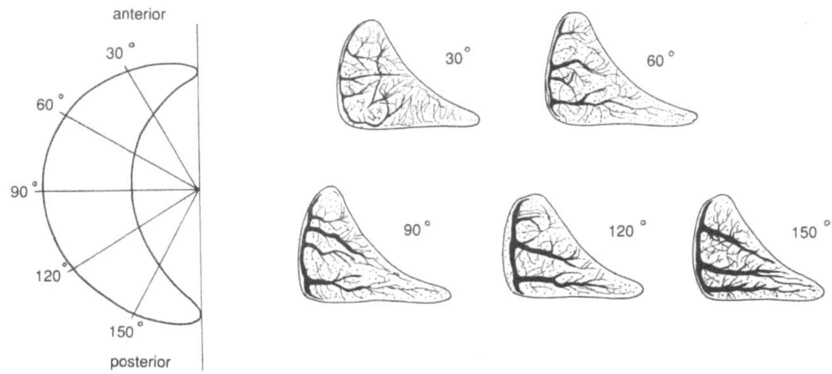

Figure 1. The distribution of radial fibers in bovine medial meniscus is inhomogeneous.

the meniscus structure-function relationships in the context of those previously established for normal articular cartilage.

Composition and Matrix Organization

Collagen

The meniscus contains coarse fibers of Type I collagen (Aspden et al., 1985; Bullough et al., 1970; Yasui 1978). These fibers dominate the gross and microscopic appearance of the tissue. On the surfaces, the collagen fibers are primarily random with some preference toward radial orientation (Aspden et al., 1985; Proctor et al., 1989; Yasui 1978). In the interior, or deep zone, which comprises the bulk of the meniscal substance, the fibers are grouped together into large fascicles which run predominantly in the circumferential direction, along the capsule parallel to the periphery of the meniscus. These fascicles, or bundles of 50-150 micron diameter, appear to be continuous with those of the anterior and posterior ligamentous horns which anchor the menisci firmly to bone.

The deep zone also contains radially oriented fibers which emanate from the periphery, weaving among the circumferential fiber bundles (Bullough et al., 1970). The functional significance of these fibers is not known. Bullough believed them to serve as tie fibers, capable of restraining the relative motion among the circumferential collagen bundles. Mow and Whipple suggested that they may serve as a mechanism of fiber bundle recruitment under conditions of circumferential tensile loading, and to control shearing along the interfaces as the bundles move over one another (Mow and Whipple 1984). Until recently, little was known about the properties of the radial fibers. Thus, their role remained largely a matter of conjecture.

Architectural studies suggest that the distribution and organization of collagen fibers in the meniscus is inhomogeneous (Figure 1). Radial fibers are larger, more numerous, and have a higher degree of horizontal orientation in the posterior medial meniscus than in the remainder of the tissue (Warden and Mow 1990). On the other hand, circumferential fiber bundles in this region appear less highly oriented with respect to the peripheral attachments than in other regions. Whereas in the anterior region of the medial meniscus and in the lateral meniscus the bundles run nearly parallel to one another, those in the posterior medial meniscus display a herring-bone pattern under polarized light (Figure 2) (Fithian et al., 1989b). While these differences in degree of orientation are difficult to quantify, the distribution and orientation of collagen fibers within meniscal tissue appears to correlate with tensile stiffness and strength for the regions studied (Skaggs and Mow 1990; Fithian et al., 1989b).

The most important mechanical properties of collagen fibers are their tensile stiffness and strength. They make their greatest contribution to tissue material properties when they are aligned along the direction of the load, as they are in tendons and ligaments. Although the nature of loading and stress in articular cartilage and meniscus is more complex, the basic assumption that collagen fibers tend to align with the principal tensile stress seems to be valid (Hukins et al., 1984; Mow et al., 1989; Mow and Rosenwasser 1988; Poole et al., 1984; Shrive et al., 1978). For articular cartilage, compressive loading develops: 1) large tensile stress parallel to the surface at the surface, 2) tensile stresses at various angles in the middle zone, and 3) tensile stresses at 45 degrees relative to the tidemark at the calcified-uncalcified tissue junction (Mow and Lai 1980). The actual collagen ultrastructure of articular cartilage and meniscus thus tends to reflect the local functional requirements within the tissue.

Proteoglycans

Proteoglycans are large (10^6 daltons) negatively charged hydrophyllic molecules which can entrain water fifty times their weight in free solution. The meniscus contains considerably less proteoglycan (<1% wet weight) than articular cartilage (7% wet weight) (Adams and Ho 1987; Adams and Muir 1981). Some data indicate that the distribution of proteoglycan within the meniscus matrix is inhomogeneous (Adams and Ho 1987; Eyre and Wu 1983; Nakano et al., 1986). For human menisci, differences between proteoglycan content of medial and lateral menisci have been reported (Adams and Ho 1987). However, we found little evidence of inhomogeneity in the total sulfated glycosaminoglycan content or water content of normal human medial and lateral menisci (Fithian et al., 1989a).

High fixed charge density and charge-charge repulsion forces cause proteoglycans to be stiffly extended in the matrix, providing the tissue with a high capacity to resist large compressive loads (Mow et al., 1984; Rosenberg et

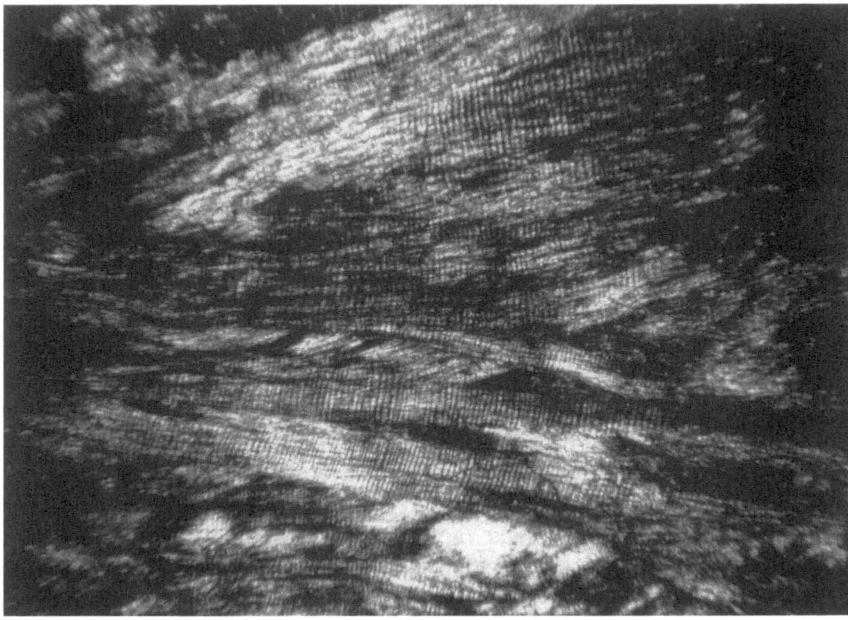

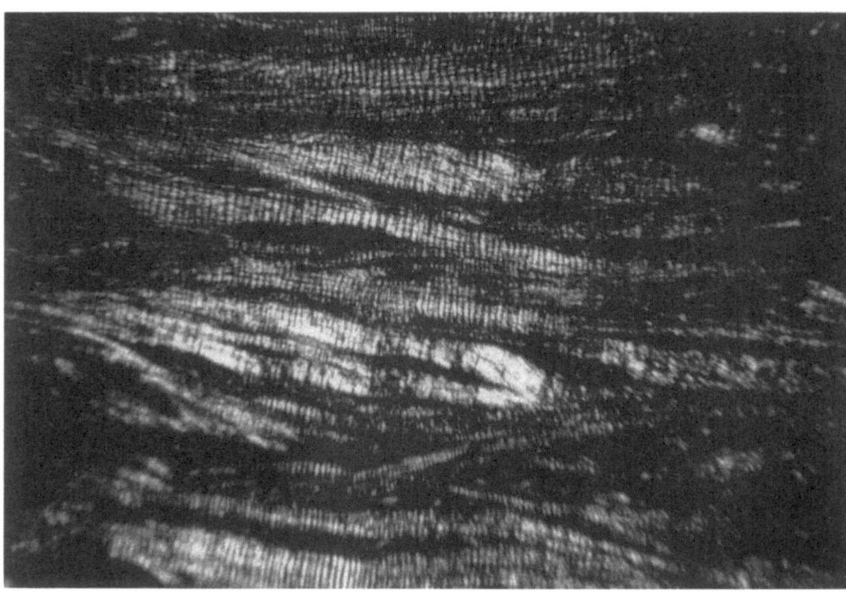

Figure 2. (*top*) Circumferential fiber bundles in the posterior region of medial human meniscus reveal a herring-bone pattern when viewed under polarized light. (*bottom*) Bundles in the anterior region of lateral human meniscus are more uniformly oriented.

al., 1988). In addition, these negatively charged molecules attract many positive counterions in the aqueous bath, creating a Donnan osmotic pressure which further resists compressive load. Proteoglycans are immobilized in the matrix by their entanglement in the meshwork of collagen fibers. The ability of proteoglycans to form aggregates *in situ* further helps to immobilize them within the collagen fibrillar meshwork (Buckwalter and Rosenberg 1982; Hardingham 1979; Hardingham and Muir 1974; Muir 1983). These aggregates are made up of 100-200 proteoglycan monomers attached to a single backbone of hyaluronic acid. The binding of the monomers to the hyaluronate is stabilized by link protein (Hardingham and Muir 1974; Hascall and Hascall 1981; Tang et al., 1979), which has been identified in the meniscus (Fife 1985). These interactions cause the proteoglycan-collagen matrix to behave as a fiber-reinforced solid material capable of resisting compressive, tensile, and shear stress.

Material Properties, Structure and Function in the Meniscus

Mechanically, the matrix may be considered to be composed of two phases, a solid phase (26% wet weight) and a fluid phase (74% wet weight). The solid matrix consists mostly of collagen, proteoglycans and other non-collagenous proteins, and its load-deformational behavior is that of a fiber-reinforced composite material which is also porous and permeable (Armstrong and Mow 1982; Mow et al., 1984; Mow and Lai 1980; Read and Dean 1978; Proctor et al., 1989). The fluid phase consists of water and interstitial electrolytes, and most of it may be forced to flow through the porous-permeable matrix by a hydraulic pressure gradient and matrix compaction (Linn and Sokoloff 1965; Maroudas 1979; Torzilli 1985). The flow of water through the porous-permeable matrix also plays an important mechanical role in governing deformational behavior of the tissue (Kwan et al., 1984; Mow et al., 1984; Proctor et al., 1989). In the following sections, the intrinsic mechanical behavior of the meniscus is discussed in light of its composition and structural organization.

In recent years, a biphasic theory has been used to determine the contributions each phase makes to the overall mechanical properties of hydrated soft tissues such as articular cartilage and meniscus (Mow et al., 1980; Mow et al., 1984; Mow and Lai 1980). In this theory, the intrinsic properties of the collagen-proteoglycan solid matrix, along with interstitial fluid flow, govern the deformability of the tissue. When such a material is acted upon by a constant tensile or compressive load, or deformation, the kinetics of the time-dependent creep and stress-relaxation viscoelastic responses are determined by the frictional drag of fluid flow through the porous matrix. In addition, the intrinsic viscoelastic or "flow-independent" response in shear of the solid matrix may be attributed to molecular relaxation effects from motion of long chain polymers such as collagen and proteoglycans (Hayes and Bodine 1978; Mow et al., 1982). The component of viscoelasticity due to interstitial fluid flow is known as the biphasic viscoelastic behavior of the tissue, and the component of viscoelasticity due to molecular motion is known as the flow-independent or intrinsic viscoelastic behavior of the collagen-proteoglycan solid matrix. (See chapter by Mow et al., in these volumes for a detailed discussion of cartilage and meniscus properties.)

The phenomena of creep and stress-relaxation are of the utmost importance in understanding the functional characteristics of articular cartilage and meniscus. The significance of the creep response is that when the joint is loaded over a long period of time, the contact area will gradually increase, spreading the compressive load over an ever increasing area. During this transient phase, which may last for several hours in the major load-bearing joints, interstitial fluid is exuded from the tissue into the joint space. The fluid is imbibed again when the load is released and the tissue regains its original dimensions. This creates a natural circulation pattern important for cell nourishment. It also provides a source of lubricant for fluid film lubrication. This fluid film lubrication process minimizes surface friction (Mow et al., 1982). (See chapter by Hou et al., in these volumes for a detailed discussion of fluid film lubrication.) The phenomenon of stress-relaxation is equally important in that it is exceedingly difficult to maintain high stresses in the collagen-proteoglycan solid matrix for extended periods of time. Stresses may reach high levels momentarily, but interstitial fluid redistribution will always occur to allow relaxation of the porous-permeable solid matrix with time. These two biphasic creep and stress-relaxation effects may be understood more easily if one models the response of the tissue as the summation of two separate responses linked in parallel: 1) the viscous response due to transient fluid flow through the porous-permeable solid matrix, and 2) the elastic response due to deformation of the solid matrix.

Behavior in Compression

Compression studies of bovine meniscal tissue of specimens taken perpendicular to the tibial plateau surface have indicated that these tissues are roughly one-half as stiff and one-sixth as permeable in confined compression as bovine articular cartilage (Proctor et al., 1989). These studies also confirm the biphasic nature of meniscus tissue predicted by Mow and coworkers (1984). The combination of low compressive stiffness and low permeability suggests that the menisci, as structures, should function as highly efficient shock absorbers per unit mass. Since the combined mass of the menisci is much greater than that of the articular cartilage bearing load across the tibiofemoral joint, it is likely that most of the shocks generated by knee joint loading are absorbed by the menisci. The menisci with their low stiffness distribute load well by virtue of being more deformable. More recent studies also indicate that meniscal tissue is anisotropic in compression, i.e. the material properties vary with the direction of loading (Chern et al., manuscript in preparation). These observations provide further insight into how the meniscus may carry load in compression.

Behavior in Shear

The meniscus is believed to sustain significant shear stress under normal loading conditions (Arnoczky et al., 1988a). Its response to shear, particularly in the two planes parallel to the axis of its large fiber bundles, may be important in the development of vertical and horizontal tears (Smillie 1978). Bovine meniscus has been studied under dynamic (oscillating) pure (torsional) shear conditions in order to eliminate the effects of fluid flow on tissue behavior (Chern et al., 1990). On average, the meniscus is one-sixth to one-tenth as stiff in dynamic shear as bovine articular cartilage (Chern et al., 1990, Roth et al., 1982). Bovine meniscus is anisotropic under dynamic shear. The anisotropy reflects the organization of the collagen fibers in the matrix. The tissue is 20-33% stiffer when the plane of shear is perpendicular to the coarse fiber bundles than when it is parallel to them (Chern et al., 1990). Increasing the torsional frequency has a stiffening effect on the matrix which has been observed for cartilage (Chern et al., 1989; Hayes and Bodine 1978; Roth et al., 1982). At the same time, the energy dissipation remains relatively constant, suggesting that elastic stiffening of the collagen-proteoglycan matrix is responsible for this effect. Elastic stiffening of bovine meniscus under dynamic shear is also observed when compressive clamping strain is increased (Figure 3a) (Roth et al., 1982, Chern et al., 1990).

To our surprise, increasing shear strain causes the opposite effect: the shear stiffness decreases (figure 3a) while the relative energy dissipation increases (figure 3b). Since this effect is seen at the low shear strains tested, 0.5-5% strain, it is likely to occur under physiologic loading conditions. It appears to be due to the highly oriented ultrastructure of the matrix collagen and the tenuous interactions between these fibers and the proteoglycans, which allows the molecules to slide over one another as the opposing articular surfaces are sheared. This "conformability" of the meniscal matrix as evidenced by its very low shear modulus maximizes joint congruity in all joint positions without constraining joint motion. Since two of the major functions of the menisci are to bear and distribute load, it would seem that the ability to change shape offers maximimum load-carrying efficiency at all joint angles.

Behavior in Tension

Typical tensile stress-strain curves of meniscal tissue resemble those of other collagenous tissues (Woo et al., 1981, 1982; Roth and Mow 1980). Studies of bovine meniscus by Proctor and coworkers (1989) have shown that the tissue is roughly ten times stiffer in the direction of the collagen fiber bundles than at right angles to them. These investigators have also compared the tensile properties of circumferentially oriented specimens from the surface to those of the deep layers of bovine menisci. Specimens from the surface were neither as stiff nor as strong as those from the deep layers of the same region.

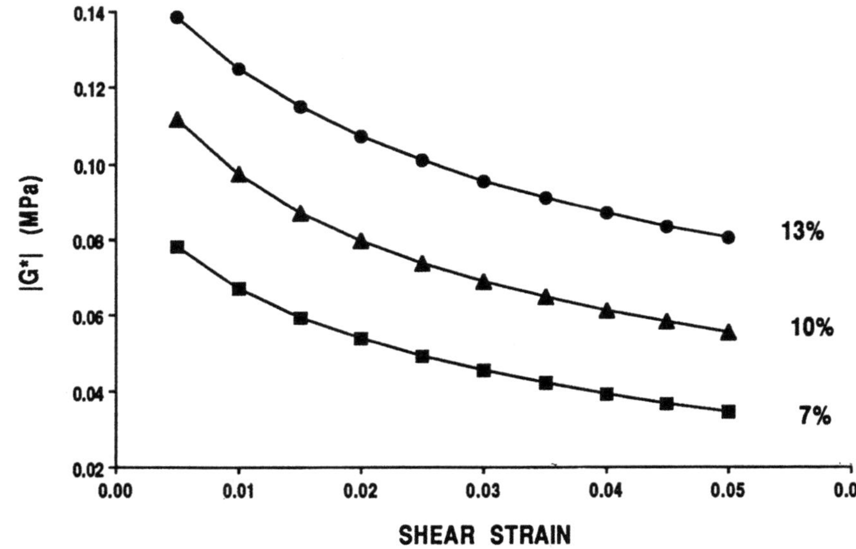

Figure 3a. Amplitude of dynamic shear modulus of bovine meniscus at 7%, 10%, and 13% clamping strain, plotted as a function of shear strain (mean of n=8 specimens in a plane parallel to circumferential collagen bundles)

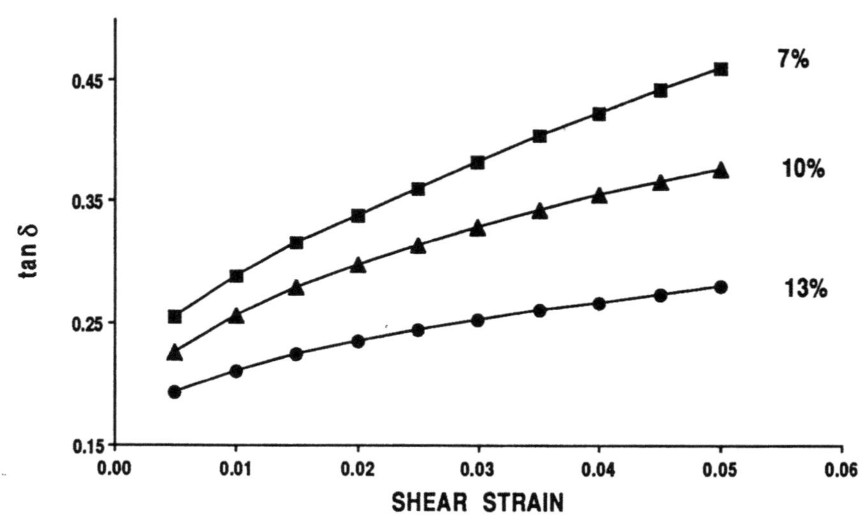

Figure 3b. Relative dissipation (tan δ) of bovine meniscus at 7%, 10%, and 13% clamping strain, plotted as a function of shear strain (mean of n=8 specimens).

Table 1. Composition of Meniscus by Region

Region*	n	S-GAG•	Water	H-Pro•
LA	18	1.80±0.50	75.02±2.14	14.3±3.7
LC	18	1.68±0.56	72.99±2.40	13.2±2.0
LP	18	1.75±0.45	73.39±2.44	15.2±3.1
MA	12	2.20±1.01	72.12±9.73	13.2±3.6
MC	14	2.06±0.68	76.77±2.68	13.9±3.4
MP	18	1.94±0.83	74.88±7.32	13.9±3.6

* LA=lat.ant.; LC=lat.central; LP=lat.post.
MA=med.ant.; MC=med.central; MP=med.post.
• % dry weight

More recently, we found that specimens from the inner one-third of the medial meniscus of skeletally mature steers are significantly less stiff in circumferential tension than specimens from the peripheral two-thirds of the tissue. This is consistent with differences in composition and collagen fiber architecture that have been noted previously (Ghosh et al., 1983; Nakano et al., 1986; Wagner 1976; Yasui 1978).

Although the menisci function under compression in the knee, the circumferential hoop and radial tensile stresses which develop in the tissue under load probably dominate both their normal function and their failure. In a recent study, we undertook to study the tensile behavior of normal human meniscus under uniaxial tension in the circumferential direction (Fithian et al., 1989a). Tensile stiffness was compared for the medial and lateral meniscus in the anterior, central and posterior regions. In order to evaluate the effects of tissue composition and structure on the these properties, correlative biochemical and polarized light microscopic studies were also performed.

We observed significant regional variation in the stiffness and strength of normal human meniscus tested in circumferential tension (Figure 4). This variation was not explained by differences in biochemical composition of the matrix, which showed little variation among the regions studied (Table 1). Rather, patterns of tensile stiffness did appear to follow fiber bundle architecture (Ghosh et al., 1983; Wagner 1976; Yasui 1978). Under polarized light, there appeared to be a greater degree of fiber bundle orientation in areas which demonstrated superior tensile stiffness and strength. This suggests that collagen ultrastructure and perhaps intermolecular interactions (such as collagen cross-linking) are the predominant factors influencing the tensile response of the meniscus in the circumferential direction.

Recent work by Skaggs and Mow (1990) has shown that radial fibers strongly influence the behavior of meniscus under radially applied tension. In the posterior horn of bovine medial meniscus, radial fibers are present in greater numbers and have a more horizontal orientation than in the anterior horn (Figure 1). This regional variation in radial fiber structure is reflected in the greater

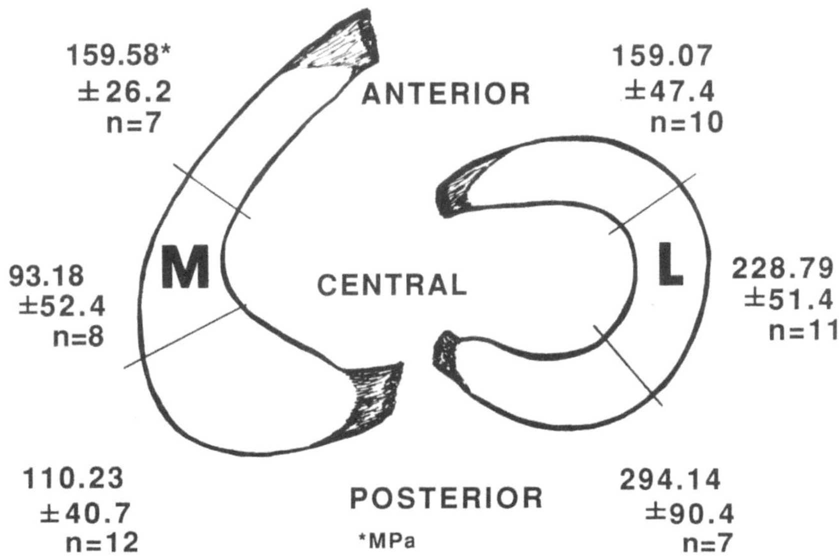

Figure 4. Mean Young's modulus in tension by region for normal adult human meniscus (MPa±SD).

mean tensile stiffness and strength of samples from the posterior region. When bundles of radial fibers were included in radially oriented specimens undergoing uniaxial tensile testing, tensile stiffness and strength increased ten-fold to values close to those observed for circumferential specimens (Proctor et al., 1989; Fithian et al., 1989a). Thus it would appear that radial fibers, although far fewer in number and less regular in distribution and orientation, possess tensile properties similar to those of circumferential fibers. We have observed that when the tissue fails in circumferential tension, the plane of failure is frequently the interface between two adjacent circumferential fiber bundles, and the failure proceeds in shear along this weak plane (Proctor et al., 1989; Fithian et al., 1989a). Similarly for radial samples, failure does not generally initiate with breakage of individual fibers, but with separation at the interface between the radial fibers and the surrounding matrix. The disposition of fibers, both radial and circumferential, within the matrix may thus be an important factor in the development and morphology of meniscal tears.

Modeling of Meniscal Function

The mechanical functions of the menisci are determined not only by their material properties but also by their shape, the shapes of the femoral and tibial condyles, their position in the joint, anatomical attachments (constraints), and the magnitude and direction of the load applied to the knee. An accurate model of the meniscus must include an accurate representation of the material properties of the tissue, anatomically appropriate attachments and constraints, and appropriate loading conditions (Huiskes and Chao 1983).

Early attempts at modeling have demonstrated the need for a more accurate representation of the material properties of the meniscus than that of a linear elastic model (Aspden 1985; Hefzy and Zoghi 1988; Sauren et al., 1984). Material nonlinearities displayed by meniscal tissue (Fithian et al., 1989b; Chern et al., 1989), anisotropies and biphasic flow effects (Proctor et al., 1989; Chern et al., 1990) all must be taken into account for a realistic structural model of the meniscus to be constructed.

In addition, constraints on meniscal displacement along the periphery must be considered (Fithian et al., 1989b; Tissakht et al., 1989; Wagner 1976). Because the menisci are wedge-shaped and occupy the periphery of the joint, axial loading of the knee creates extrusive forces which tend to displace the meniscus from the joint (Fairbank 1948; Shrive et al., 1978). The strong insertions at the anterior and posterior horns prevent this displacement. Thus, although the primary function of the meniscus may be to bear compressive loads, in doing so it must support enormous hoop tensile forces directed along the circumferential direction. Recent evidence suggests that the insertions at the anterior and posterior horns are not the only important constraints to meniscal displacement. Tissakht and coworkers recently have shown evidence that the attachments between the medial meniscus and MCL are also important in constraining the motion of the medial meniscus (Tissakht et al., 1989). Our own data support this finding (Fithian et al., 1989a). These considerations make simple stress analysis of the meniscus as a structure a very challenging task indeed for future research.

An accurate model for the meniscus should allow predictions of its response under various loading conditions in the intact joint. Since it is apparent that tissue composition and architecture, as well as loading conditions, affect the morphology of meniscal tears, it is interesting to speculate on how the combination of these factors affects strain within the meniscus. Spilker et al. (1990) used an axisymmetric biphasic finite element model and experimentally derived material coefficients for normal human and bovine meniscus to predict strain distributions within the meniscus at time $t=1$ second under physiologic loading conditions. They found that: 1) predicted axial strain was compressive, 2) radial and circumferential strain were tensile, and 3) radial strain in some instances reached as high as 25% (Figure 5). Their predictions were generally within an order of magnitude of known failure strains (Proctor et al., 1989; Skaggs and Mow 1990). Once a tear is initiated, its propagation may depend on the architecture of the matrix at the apex of the tear. Meniscal modeling could be used to predict the local stress and strain at the leading edge of a meniscus tear.

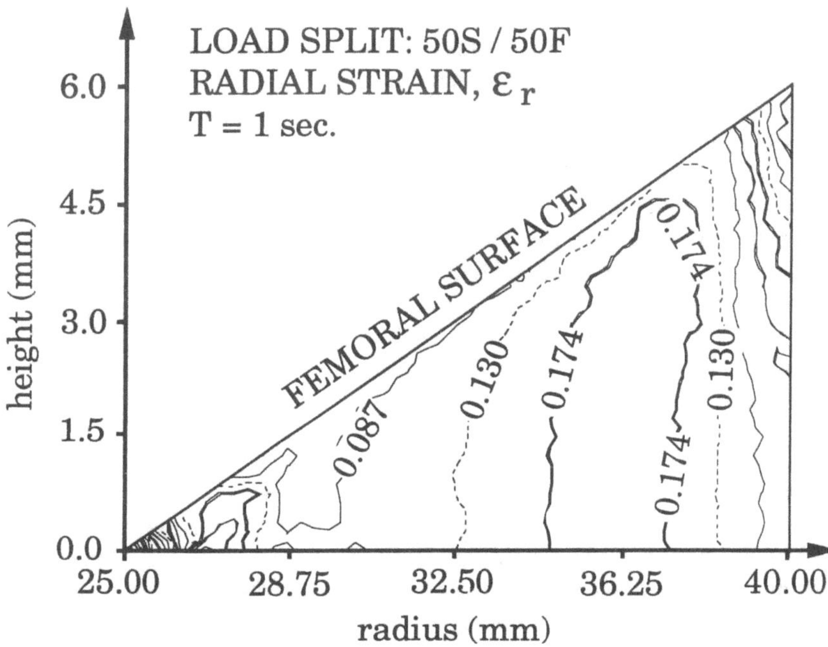

Figure 5. Predicted radial strain distribution for a cross section of an axisymmetric biphasic meniscus model under compressive load.

Perhaps a more important application of meniscal modelling would be to assess the effects of treatment, such as partial meniscectomy and repair. Each of these modalities is likely to alter the pattern of strain distribution in the remaining meniscal matrix. The function of the meniscus after partial resection or following repair is a matter of great clinical concern. Biologic healing of meniscal tears following repair has been demonstrated, and the rate of healing has improved with the appropriate use of fibrin clot (Arnoczky et al., 1986; Henning 1990). However, the mechanical effects of these techniques have not been evaluated.

Another useful application for such a model of the meniscus is in establishing the design characteristics of any material that would enable it to survive and function within the knee as a meniscal substitute or prosthesis. The ability of the menisci to dissipate energy, conform to constantly changing loading conditions, and distribute loads rapidly over a large area are important not only to lasting function of the joint as a whole, but probably to the survival of the meniscus itself. Under such harsh conditions, many materials will fail in time. It is thus desirable that some effort be made to predict the stresses and strains allografts, collagen scaffolds, and other meniscal replacements must face within the knee joint.

Summary

1. The meniscus behaves in load-deformation as a fiber-reinforced porous- permeable composite material in which frictional drag caused by fluid flow governs its creep and stress-relaxation behavior.
2. The meniscus is a functionally distinct load-bearing structure in the knee. Because of its intrinsic material properties, it is ideally suited for load distribution and shock absorption.
3. The ultrastructural organization of collagen fibers appears to dominate over tissue composition in determining the material properties of meniscal tissue.
4. Local variations in the geometry of femur, tibia and meniscus; mobility caused by capsular constraints (attachments); and loading may be expected to alter the local mechanical environment in different areas of the joint. These factors probably play a role in determining the tissue ultrastructure and intrinsic properties in different regions of the menisci.

Future Directions

Statistics indicate that over 1,500,000 knee injuries occur each year, of which a significant number involve damage to the meniscus (Grazier et al., 1984). Of acute knee injuries requiring surgery, meniscal tears are among the most frequent findings. The introduction of arthroscopic surgery has improved the diagnosis and treatment of meniscal tears. Despite these advances, little basic information is available on the mechanical function of these repaired menisci. The current level of research interest, both clinical and basic, in the meniscus reflects the importance of these structures in normal knee function. Promising research has begun to define the mechanical properties of normal human meniscus and develop accurate models for its behavior. This knowledge is essential to further our clinical understanding of meniscal tear patterns and their surgical treatment. Further, the future of successful meniscal allografting or prosthetic replacement will have its roots in such research. This will certainly have a significant clinical impact in the treatment of both acute and chronic knee injuries.

Acknowledgements

This work was supported by NIH grant AR-38728.

References

Adams ME, Muir H: The glycosaminoglycans of canine menisci. Biochem J 1981; 197:385.

Adams ME, Ho YA: Localization of glycosaminoglycans in human and canine menisci and their attachments. Conn Tiss Res 1987;16:269.

Ahmed AM, Burke DL: *In vitro* measurement of static pressure distribution in synovial joints, part 1: Tibial surface of the knee. J Biomech Eng 1983; 105:216.

Armstrong CG, Mow VC: Biomechanics of normal and osteoarthrotic articular cartilage. *In* Wilson, P.D., and Straub, L.R. (eds): Clinical Trends in Orthopaedics. New York: Thiem-Stratton, 1982, p. 189.

Arnoczky SP, Warren RF: Microvasculature of the human meniscus. Am J Sports Med 1982;10:90.

Arnoczky SP, McDevitt CA, Warren RF, Spivak J, Allen A: Meniscal repair using an exogenous fibrin clot: An experimental study in the dog. Trans Orthop Res Soc 1986;10:327.

Arnoczky SP, Adams ME, DeHaven KE, Eyre DR, Mow VC: Meniscus. *In* Woo, S.L-Y., and Buckwalter, J.A. (eds): Injury and repair of the musculoskeletal soft tissues. Park Ridge, Ill: American Academy of Orthopaedic Surgeons, 1988a, p. 427.

Arnoczky SP, McDevitt CA, Schmidt MB, Mow VC, Warren RF: The effect of cryopreservation on canine menisci: A biochemical, morphological, and biomechanical evaluation. J Orthop Res 1988b;6:1.

Arnoczky SP, Milachowski KA: Meniscal Allografts: Where Do We Stand? *In* Ewing JW (ed): Articular Cartilage and Knee Joint Function: Basic Science and Arthroscopy. New York: Raven Press, 1990a, p 129.

Arnoczky SP, Warren RF, McDevitt CA: Meniscal replacement using a cryopreserved allograft: An experimental study in the dog. Clin Orthop Rel Res 1990b;252:121.

Aspden RM, Yarker YE, Hukins DWL: Collagen orientations in the meniscus of the knee joint. J Anat 1985;140:371.

Aspden RM: A Model for the function and failure of the meniscus. Engin Med 1985;14:119.

Bourne RB, Finlay JB, Papadopoulos P, Andreae P.: The effect of medial meniscectomy on strain distribution in the proximal part of the tibia. J Bone Jt Surg 1984;66A:1431.

Buckwalter JA, Rosenberg LC: Electron microscopic studies of cartilage proteoglycans: Direct evidence for the variable length of the chondroitin sulfate-rich region of proteoglycan subunit core protein. J Biol Chem 1982; 257:9830.

Bullough PG, Munuera L, Murphy J, Weinstein A M: The strength of the menisci of the knee as it relates to their fine structure. J Bone Jt Surg 1970;52B:564.

Bylski-Austrow DI, Meade TI, Malumed J, Noyes FR, Grood ES, Arnoczky SP: Medial Meniscectomy and Irradiated Meniscal Allografts: Preliminary Mechanical and Vascular Studies in the Goat. Presented at the Meniscal Transplantation Study Group, American Academy of Orthopaedic Surgeons, New Orleans, 1990.

Cabaud HE, Rodkey WG, Fitzwater JE: Medial meniscus repairs: An experimental and morphologic study. Am J Sports Med 1981;9:129.

Chern KY, Zhu WB, Mow VC: Anisotropic viscoelastic shear properties of meniscus. Adv Bioeng WAM ASME 1989;15:105.
Chern KY, Zhu WB, Kelly MA, Mow VC: Anisotropic shear properties of bovine meniscus. Trans Orthop Res Soc 1990;5:246.
Cox JS, Nye CE, Schaefer WW, Woodstein IJ: The degenerative effects of partial and total resection of the medial meniscus in dog knees. Clin Orthop Rel Res 1975;109:178.
Cox JS, Cordell LD: The degenerative effects of medial meniscus tears in dog knees. Clin Orthop Rel Res 1977;126:236.
Dandy DJ, Jackson RW: The diagnosis of problems after meniscectomy. J Bone Jt Surg 1975;57B:349.
DeHaven KE, Hales W: Peripheral meniscus repair in a young athlete. Orthop Consultant 1983;4:7.
DeHaven KE: Decision-making factors in the treatment of meniscus lesions. Clin Orthop Rel Res 1990;252:49.
Eyre DR, Wu JJ: Collagen of fibrocartilage: a distinctive molecular phenotype in bovine meniscus. FEBS Letters 1983:158(2):265.
Fairbank TJ: Knee joint changes after meniscectomy. J Bone Jt Surg 1948;30B:664.
Fife RS: Identification of link proteins and a 116,000-dalton matrix protein in canine meniscus. Arch Biochem Biophys 1985;240:682.
Fithian DC, Schmidt MB, Ratcliffe A, Mow VC: Human meniscus tensile properties: Regional variation and biochemical correlation. Trans Orthop Res Soc 1989a;14:205.
Fithian DC, Zhu WB, Kelly MA, Ratcliffe A, Mow VC: Exponential law representation of tensile properties of human meniscus. Proc Inst Mech Engin, London, 1989b;5:85.
Fukubayashi T, Kurosawa H: The contact area and pressure distribution pattern of the knee. Acta Orthop Scand 1980;51:871.
Garrett J: Personal communication 1990.
Gear MW: The late results of meniscectomy. Br J Surg 1967;54:270.
Gershuni DH, Skyhar MJ, Danzig LA, et al: Healing of tears in the avascular segment of the canine lateral meniscus. Trans Orthop Res Soc 1985;10:294.
Ghadially FN: Fine structure of joints. *In* Sokoloff L (ed): The Joints and Synovial Fluid. New York, Academic Press, 1978, p 105.
Ghadially FN, Wedge JH, Lalonde JMA: Experimental methods of repairing injured menisci. J Bone Jt Surg 1986;68B:106.
Ghosh P, Ingman AM, Taylor TKF. Variations in collagen, non-collagenous proteins, and hexosamine in menisci derived from osteoarthritic and rheumatoid arthritic knee joints. J Rheum 1975;2(1):100.
Ghosh P, Taylor TKF, Pettit GD, Horsburgh BA, Bellenger CR: Effect of postoperative immobilization on the regrowth of knee joint semilunar cartilage: An experimental study. J Orthop Res 1983;1:153.
Gillquist J: Knee stability: Its effect on articular cartilage. *In* Ewing JW (ed): Articular Cartilage and Knee Joint Function: Basic Science and Arthroscopy. New York: Raven Press, 1990, p 267.
Grazier KL, Holbrook TL, Kelsey JL, Stauffer RN: The frequency of occurence, impact and cost of musculoskeletal conditions in the United States. AAOS, 1984.

Hamberg P, Gillquist J, Lysholm J: Suture of new and old peripheral meniscus tears. J Bone Jt Surg 1983;65A:193.

Hardingham TE, Muir H: Hyaluronic acid in cartilage and proteoglycan aggregation. Biochem J 1974;139:565.

Hardingham TE: The role of link-protein in the structure of cartilage proteoglycan aggregates. Biochem J 1979;177:237.

Hardingham TE, Muir H, Kwan MK, et al: Viscoelastic properties of proteoglycan solutions with varying proportions present as aggregates. J Orthop Res 1987;5:36.

Hascall VC, Sajdera SW: Proteinpolysaccharide complex from bovine nasal cartilage: The function of glycoprotein in the formation of aggregates. J Biol Chem 1969;244(9):2384.

Hascall VC, Hascall GK: Proteoglycans. *In* Hay ED (ed): Cell Biology of Extracellular Matrix. New York, Plenum Press, 1981, p. 39.

Hayes WC, Bodine AJ: Flow-independent viscoelastic properties of articular cartilage matrix. J Biomech 1978;11:407.

Heatley FW: The menisacus - can it be repaired?: An experimental investigation in rabbits. J Bone Jt Surg 1980;62B:397.

Hefzy MS, Zoghi M: The menisci: A finite element model. Trans Orthop Res Soc 1988;13:149.

Henning CE, Lynch MA, Yearout KM, et al: Arthroscopic meniscal repair using an exogenous fibrin clot. Clin Orthop Rel Res 1990;25:264-72.

Hoch DH, Grodzinsky AJ, Koob TJ, Albert ML, Eyre DR: Early changes in material properties of rabbit articular cartilage after meniscectomy. J Orthop Res 1983;1:4.

Huckell, JR: Is meniscectomy a benign procedure?-- A long-term follow-up study. Can J Surg 1965;8:254.

Huiskes R, and Chao EYS: A survey of finite element analysis in orthopedic biomechanics: The first decade. J Biomech 1983;16:385.

Hukins DWL, Aspden RM, Yarker YE: Fibre reinforcement and mechanical stability in articular cartilage. Engin Med 1984;13:153.

Hunziker EB, Schenk RK: Cartilage ultrastructure after high pressure freezing, freeze substitution, and low temperature embedding. J Cell Biol 1984;98:277.

Hunziker EB, Herrmann W: *In situ* localization of cartilage extracellular matrix components by immunoelectron microscopy after cryotechnical tissue processing. J Histochem Cytochem 1987;35:647.

Jackson DW, McDevitt CA, Atwell AT, Arnoczky SP, Simon TM: Meniscal transplantation using fresh and cryopreserved allografts: An experimental study in goats. Trans Orthop Res Soc 1990;15:221.

Jackson JP: Degenerative changes in the knee after meniscectomy. J Bone Jt Surg 1967;49B:584.

Jackson RW, Dandy DJ: Partial meniscectomy (abs). J Bone Jt Surg 1976;58B;142.

King D: The function of semilunar cartilages. J Bone Jt Surg 1936a;18:1069.

King D: The healing of semilunar cartilages. J Bone Joint Surg 1936b;18:333.

Krause WR, Pope MH, Johnson RJ, et al.: Mechanical changes in the knee after meniscectomy. J Bone Joint Surg, 1976; 58A:599.

Kurosawa H, Fukubayashi T, Nakajima H: Load-bearing mode of the knee joint: Physical behavior of the knee joint with or without menisci. Clin Orthop Rel Res 1980;149:283.

Kwan MK, Lai WM, Mow VC: Fundamentals of fluid transport through cartilage in compression. Ann Biomed Eng 1984;12:537.

Levy IM, Torzilli IM, Warren RF: The effect of medial meniscectomy on anterior-posterior motion of the knee. J Bone Jt Surg 1982;64A:883.

Limbird T, Swiontkowski MF, Schler F, et al: Direct, *in vivo* measurement of meniscal blood flow. Presented at the interim meeting of the American Orthopaedic Society for Sport Medicine, San Francisco,California, Jan 21, 1987.

Linn FC, Sokoloff L: Movement and composition of interstitial fluid of cartilage. Arthritis Rheum 1965;8:481.

Lynch MA, Henning CE, Glick KR Jr: Knee joint surface changes: Long-term follow-up meniscus tear treatment in stable anterior cruciate ligament reconstruction. Clin Orthop Rel Res 1983;172:148.

McDevitt CA, Webber RJ: The ultrastructure and biochemistry of meniscal cartilage. Clin Orthop 1990;252:8.

McGinty JB, Geuss FL, Marvin RA: Partial or total meniscectomy. J Bone Jt Surg 1977;57A:763.

MacConaill, MA: The functions of intra-articular fibro-cartilages with special reference to the knee and inferior radio-ulnar joints. J Anatomy 1932;66:210.

Maroudas, A: Physicochemical properties of articular cartilage. *In* Freeman MAR (ed): Adult Articular Cartilage. Tunbridge Wells, England, Pitman Medical, 1979, p 215.

Moskowitz RW, Davis W, Sammarco J, Martens M, Baker J, Mayor M, Burstein AH, Frankel VH: Experimentally induced degenerative joint lesions following partial meniscectomy in the rabbit. Arth Rheum 1973;16:397.

Moskowitz RW, Howell DS, Goldberg VM, Muniz O, Pita JC: Cartilage proteoglycan alterations in an experimentally induced model of rabbit osteoarthritis. Arth Rheum 1979;22:155.

Mow VC, Lai WM: Recent developments in synovial joint biomechanics. SIAM Rev 1980; 22:275.

Mow VC, Kuei SC, Lai WM, Armstrong CG: Biphasic creep and stress relaxation of articular cartilage in compression: Theory and experiments. J Biomech Eng 1980;102:73.

Mow VC, Lai WM, Holmes MH: Advanced theoretical and experimental techniques in cartilage research. *In* Huiskes R, van Campen D, de Wijn J. (eds): Biomechanics: Principles and Applications. The Hague, Martinus Nijhoff, 1982, p. 42.

Mow VC, Holmes MH, Lai WM: Fluid transport and mechanical properties of articular cartilage: A review. J Biomech 1984;17:377.

Mow VC, Mak AF: Lubrication of diartrodial joints. *In* Skalak R, Chien S (eds): Handbook of Bioengineering. New York, McGraw-Hill, 1986, p 5.1.

Mow VC, Rosenwasser MP: Articular cartilage biomechanics. *In* Woo SLY, Buckwalter JA (eds): Injury and Repair of the Musculoskeletal Soft Tissues. Park Ridge, Ill, American Academy of Orthopaedic Surgeons, 1988, p 427.

Mow VC, Fithian DC, Kelly MA: Fundamentals of articular cartilage and meniscus function. *In* Ewing JW (ed): Articular Cartilage and Knee Joint Function: Basic Science and Arthroscopy, New York, Raven Press, 1989, p 1.

Mow VC, Whipple RR: The biology and mechanical properties of cartilage and menisci. *In* Resources for Basic Sciences Educators VI. Williamsburg, Va, AAOS, 1984, p 165.

Muir H: Proteoglycans as organizers of the extracellular matrix. Biochem Soc Trans 1983;11:613.

Nakano T, Thompson JR, Aherne FX: Distribution of glycosaminoglycans and the nonreducible collagen crosslink pyridinoline in porcine menisci. Can J Vet Res 1986;50:532.

Odgaard A, Pedersen CM, Bentzen SM, Jorgensen J, Hvid I: Density changes at the proximal tibia after medial meniscectomy. Trans Orthop Res Soc 1989;14,51.

Pontarelli WR, Albright JP, Martin RK, et al: Meniscus suture repair. Trans Orthop Res Soc 1983;8:58.

Poole CA, Flint MH, Beaumont BW: Morphological and functional interrelationships of articular cartilage matrices. J Anat 1984;138:113.

Proctor CS, Schmidt MB, Whipple RR, Kelly MA, Mow VC: Material properties of the normal medial bovine meniscus. J Orthop Res 1989;7(6):771-782.

Read BE, Dean GD: The determination of dynamic properties of polymers and composites. John Wiley and Sons, 1978, p 21.

Redman DS, Haynes DW: Meniscal repair: An experimental study in the rabbit. Trans Orthop Res Soc 1983;8:59.

Rosenberg LC, Buckwalter JA, Coutts R, Hunziker E, Mow VC: Articular cartilage *In* Woo SLY, Buckwalter JA, (eds): Injury and Repair of the Musculoskeletal Soft Tissues. Park Ridge, Ill, American Academy of Orthopaedic Surgeons, 1988, p 401

Roth V, Mow VC: The intrinsic tensile behavior of the matrix of bovine articular cartilage and its variation with age. J Bone Jt Surg 1980;62A:1102.

Roth V, Schoonbeck JM, Mow VC: Low frequency dynamic behavior of articular cartilage under torsional shear. Trans Orthop Res Soc 1982;7:150.

Sauren AAHJ, Huson A, Schouten RY: An axisymmetric finite element analysis of the mechanical function of the meniscus. Int J Sports Med 1984;5:93.

Scott GA, Jolly BL, Henning CE: Combined posterior incision and arthroscopic intra-articular repair of the meniscus. J Bone Jt Surg 1986;68A:847.

Seedholm BB, Hargreaves DJ: Transmission of the load in the knee joint with special reference to the role of the menisci. Eng Med 1979;8:220.

Shapiro F, Glimcher M: Induction of osteoarthrosis in the rabbit knee joint: Histological changes following meniscectomy and meniscal lesions. Clin Orthop Rel Res 1980;147:287.

Shoemaker SC, Markolf KL: The role of the meniscus in the anterior-posterior stability of the loaded anterior cruciate-deficient knee. J Bone Jt Surg 1986;68A:71.

Shrive NG, O'Connor JJ, Goodfellow JW: Load bearing in the knee joint. Clin Orthop Rel Res 1978;131:279.

Smillie IS: Injuries of the Knee Joint (5th ed), London, Churchill-Livingstone, 1978.

Skaggs DL, Mow VC: Function of radial tie fibers in the meniscus. Trans Orthop Res Soc 1990;15;248.

Spilker RL, Maxian TA, Mow VC: A fibrous biphasic finite element model of the meniscus. Trans Orthop Res Soc 1990;15,244.

Tang LH, Rosenberg L, Reiner A, Poole AR: Proteoglycans from bovine nasal cartilage--properties of a soluble form of link protein. J Biol Chem 1979;254:10523.

Tapper EM, Hoover NW: Late results after meniscectomy. J Bone Jt Surg 1969; 51A:517.

Tissakht M, Farinaccio R, Ahmed AM: Effect of ligament attachments on the response of the knee menisci in compression and torsion: A finite element study. Trans Orthop Res Soc 1989;14:203.

Torzilli P: Influence of cartilage conformation on its equilibrium water partition. J Orthop Res 1985;3:473.

Veth RPH, den Heeten GJ, Jensen HWB, et al: Repair of the meniscus: An experimental investigation in rabbits. Clin Orthop ReL Res 1983;175:258.

Voloshin AS, Wosk J: Shock absorption of meniscectomized and painful knees: A comparative *in vivo* study. J Biomed Eng 1983;5:157.

Wagner HJ: Die kollagenfaserarchitektur der menisken des menschlichen kniegelenkes. Z Mikrosk Anat Forsch 1976;90(2):302.

Warden WH, Mow VC: Unpublished data 1990.

Webber RJ, Harris MG, Hough AJ Jr: Cell culture of rabbit meniscal fibrochondrocytes: Proliferative and synthetic response to growth factors and ascorbate. J Orthop Res 1985;36.

Webber, RJ: Biological response of lateral and medial menisci in culture. Trans Orthop Res Soc 1990;15:217.

Woo SLY, Gomez MA, Akeson WH. The time and history-dependent viscoelastic properties of the canine medial collateral ligament. J Biomech Eng 1981;103:293.

Woo SLY, Gomez MA, Woo YK, et al: Mechanical properties of tendons and ligaments II: The relationships of immobilization and exercise on tissue remodeling. Biorheology 1982;19:397.

Yasui K: Three dimensional architecture of normal human menisci. J Jpn Orthop Assoc 1978;52:391.

Zhu WB, Lai WM, Mow VC: Intrinsic quasi-linear viscoelastic behavior of the extracellular matrix of cartilage. Trans Orthop Res Soc 1986;11:407.

Zukor DJ, Rubins IM, Daigle MR, et al: Allotransplantation of frozen irradiated menisci in rabbits. Trans Orthop Res Soc 1990;15:219.

Zukor DJ, Oakeshott RD, Brooks PJ, McAuley JP, Langer F, and Gross AE: Fresh, Small Fragment Osteochondral Allografts for Post-traumatic Defects of the Knee.*In* Ewing JW (ed): Articular Cartilage and Knee Joint Function: Basic Science and Arthroscopy. New York: Raven Press, 1990, p 153.

Part II
Cartilage Biomechanics

Chapter 8

Biphasic and Quasilinear Viscoelastic Theories for Hydrated Soft Tissues

V.C. Mow, J.S. Hou, J.M. Owens, A. Ratcliffe

Introduction

The major connective tissues of the musculoskeletal system include tendons, ligaments, articular cartilage, meniscus and intervertebral disc. Their main purpose is to connect the muscles and bones of the body together forming joints of various shapes and sizes (the anatomy of joint surfaces and its influence on joint motion are covered by other chapters in these volumes), thereby enabling the wide ranges of motion required by the body during daily activities. These connective tissues are strong enough to transmit large loads from one bone to another or from muscles to bones. In addition, they provide structural stability for the musculoskeletal system and constrain the motion of joints when required. Under normal conditions they are able to maintain these properties with little or no damage or change. In this chapter, we present a brief account of three of these tissues: articular cartilage, meniscus and intervertebral disc. Descriptions of joint motion and other tissues, such as bone, tendons and ligaments, may be found in other chapters of these volumes.

Although each of the three tissues is compositionally and structurally unique, the macromolecules that provide the mechanical properties of the tissues, collagen and proteoglycans, are similar (Muir, 1980). In mechanical terms, these tissues are also similar in that they can be considered as composed of two immiscible phases: a solid phase and a fluid phase (Mow et al 1980, 1984a). The solid phase represents 20-30% of the tissue by wet weight (Maroudas 1979; Muir 1980, 1983). However, in the solid phase, the collagen type and fibrillar network are quite different, and the distribution of the proteoglycan component is distinct for these three tissues (Adams and Ho 1987; Aspden and Yarker 1985; Buckwalter et al 1987; Clark 1985; Clarke 1971; Poole et al 1984). The fluid phase, chiefly water and dissolved inorganic salts, saturates this solid matrix (Linn and Sokoloff, 1963). The inorganic salts dissolved in the interstitial fluid yield ions which are required to balance the electric charges along the proteoglycans (Eisenberg and Grodzinsky 1985; Maroudas 1975; Lai et al 1989, 1990). Most of the fluid component may be moved by an application of a pressure gradient or by compression (Edwards 1967; Mansour and Mow 1976; Maroudas 1975). The movement of this fluid dominates the material properties of these tissues and is essential for their function (Mow et al 1980, 1984a).

Each phase and each distinct constituent of both the solid and fluid phases (including the ion phase; please refer to the chapter on the triphasic theory for cartilage for a detailed treatment of the ion phase) contributes to the material properties of these tissues. The intent of this chapter is to provide: 1) a succinct summary of the these tissues, their composition, molecular and ultrastructural organization; and 2) a precis of the biphasic theories and problems commonly used to obtain the permeability and intrinsic elastic properties of the solid matrix.

Composition and Structure of Articular Cartilage, Meniscus, and Intervertebral Disc

The components of articular cartilage, meniscus, and intervertebral disc are mainly collagen, proteoglycans, and water. These and other quantitatively minor constituents form the highly ordered structures which determine their individual mechanical behaviors. In brief, the relative amounts of the various biochemical components of these tissues are presented in Table I.

Tissue	Collagen (% dry wt.)	Proteoglycan (% dry wt.)	H_2O (% wet wt.)
Articular cartilage	50-73	15-30	58-78
Meniscus	75-80	2-6	~70
Intervertebral disc - nucleus pulposus	15-25	~50	70-90
- annulus fibrosus	50-70	10-20	60-70

Table I. Composition of articular cartilage, meniscus, and intervertebral disc.

Articular Cartilage

Early studies of the fine structure in cartilage showed elongated split-line patterns produced on the articular surface when round holes were punched into the cartilage. These patterns were believed to reflect the preferred collagen fiber directions at the surface (Figure 1) (Benninghoff, 1925; Hultkrantz, 1898). These observations were later supported by polarized light microscopy and India ink staining studies of Bullough and Goodfellow (1968).

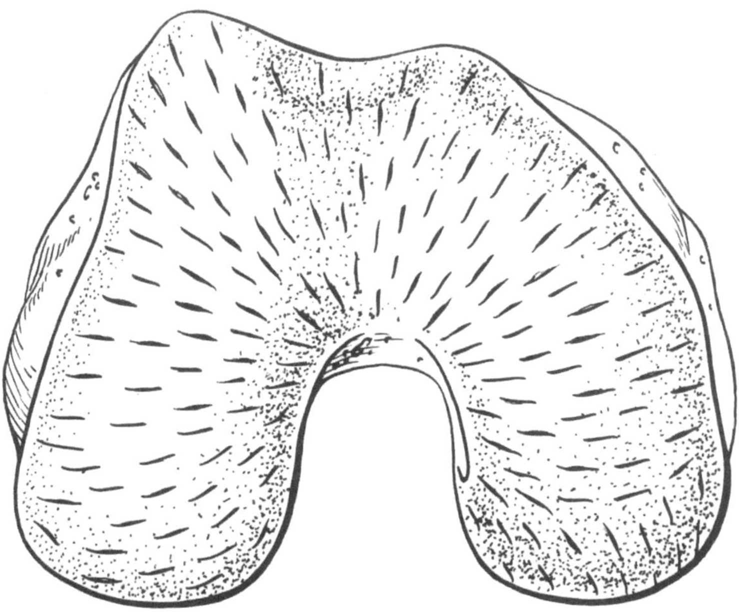

Figure 1. Split-lines on the surface of the femoral condyles showing distinct and consistent patterns.

The composition and structure of articular cartilage changes with depth from the joint surface (Buckwalter et al 1987; Clarke 1973; Lane and Weiss 1975; Lipshitz et al 1976; Muir et al 1970; Ratcliffe et al 1984). Although these variations are continuous, articular cartilage has been classified into four distinct zones or layers referred to as the superficial zone, the middle or transitional zone, the deep or radial zone, and the zone of calcified cartilage (Figure 2). Proteoglycan occupies the interfibrillar space and its concentration increases from the surface to a maximum in the middle zone, then diminishes toward the deep zone (Muir 1980; Poole et al 1982; Ratcliffe et al 1984). Within each zone, regions of specific cellular organization exist (Stockwell 1971, 1987). These regions include the pericellular and territorial matrices, which provide the cells with their immediate biochemical and mechanical environment. For articular cartilage, a vast interterritorial matrix exists with chondrocytes accounting for only approximately 5% of the tissue volume (Buckwalter et al 1987).

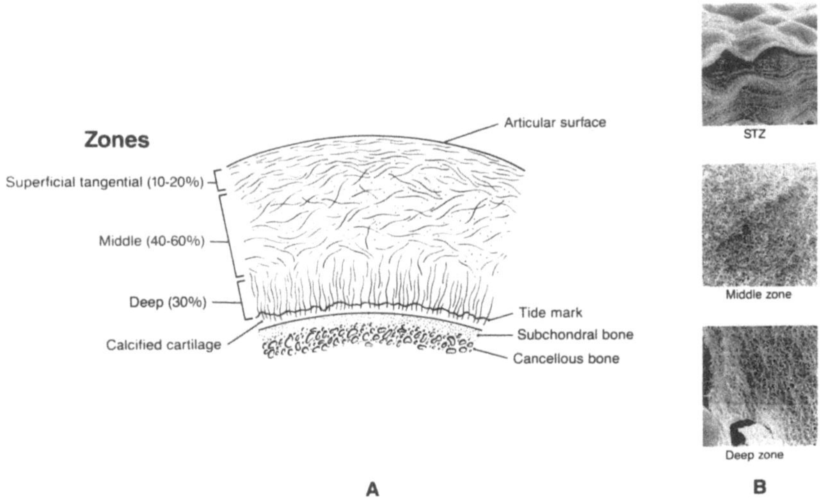

Figure 2. Schematic diagram of articular cartilage depicting the collagen fibril ultrastructure, along with scanning electron micrographs (×3000), throughout the depth of the tissue.

The layered inhomogeneity and orientation of the collagen fibrils have significant effects on the material properties of the tissue. It has been shown that the tensile properties of articular cartilage demonstrate marked inhomogeneity and anisotropy strongly reflecting the biochemical character of the tissue (Kempson et al 1973; Roth and Mow 1980; Woo et al 1976). The tensile properties also vary significantly with distribution of collagen cross-link density (Schmidt et al 1987), age (Roth and Mow 1980) and pathologic changes (Kempson 1979; Akizuki et al 1986, 1987).

The superficial zone, the thinnest of the four zones of articular cartilage, forms the articulating surface for the tissue. This layer of matrix consists primarily of fine densely packed collagen fibrils organized parallel to the articular surface, and a relatively low concentration of proteoglycan (Clarke 1971; Lane and Weiss 1975; Redler and Zimny 1970). A high density of oblong chondrocytes, with their long axis parallel to the surface, reside in this region (Figure 3) (Stockwell, 1971). Within each of the matrix zones the chondrocytes are surrounded by their own pericellular and territorial matrices, providing the cells with their immediate metabolic and mechanical environment. In the transitional or middle zone, the collagen fibrils have much larger diameters and appear to be more randomly arranged. The cells are round in shape and are separated by the interterritorial matrix. In the deep zone, the cells tend to form columns parallel to the radially oriented collagen fiber bundles. The large fiber bundles insert across the tidemark, the boundary between the uncalcified cartilage and the calcified cartilage, to securely anchor articular cartilage to the bone (Redler et al., 1975). The zone of calcified cartilage separates uncalcified or hyaline cartilage from the subchondral bone, and contains a low density of relatively small cells.

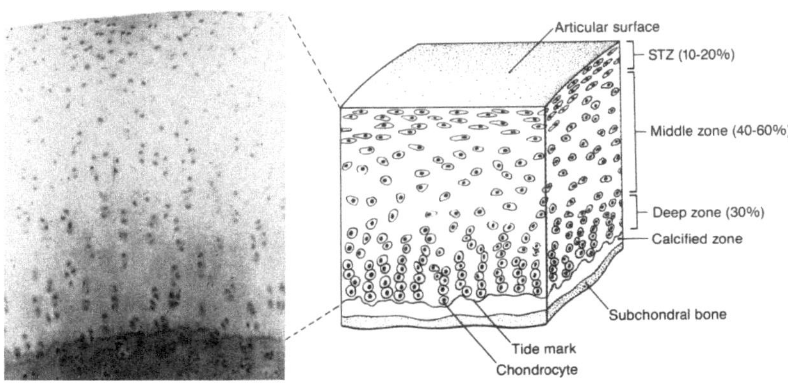

Figure 3. A schematic depiction of the distribution of the chondrocytes throughout the depth of the articular cartilage.

Meniscus

The meniscus is a semi-lunar shaped fibrocartilaginous tissue (Figure 4), and resides in the knee at the tibial-femoral articulation. It is composed mainly of a dense network of type I collagen fibers. The interfibrillar space contains proteoglycans, other glycoproteins, cells and water (see Table I). Little is known of the cellular distribution within the meniscus, however, the collagen ultrastructure has been extensively studied (Aspden et al., 1985; Bullough et al 1970; Proctor et al 1989). The reader is referred to chapters by Arnoczky and co-workers and Kelly and co-workers in volume I for a detailed discussion of the meniscus. The surface layer, approximately 200 μm thick, contains fine fibers which are randomly distributed in the plane of the surface. In the deep layers the collagen fibers are circumferential, with a few, usually small fibers running in the radial direction (Figure 4). Organized as such, the radial fibers act to 'tie' the large circumferential fiber bundles together, providing cohesion and strength to the meniscus. The structural inhomogeneity and anisotropy of meniscus have also been shown to dominate the tensile behavior of the tissue (Proctor et al 1989; Fithian et al 1990).

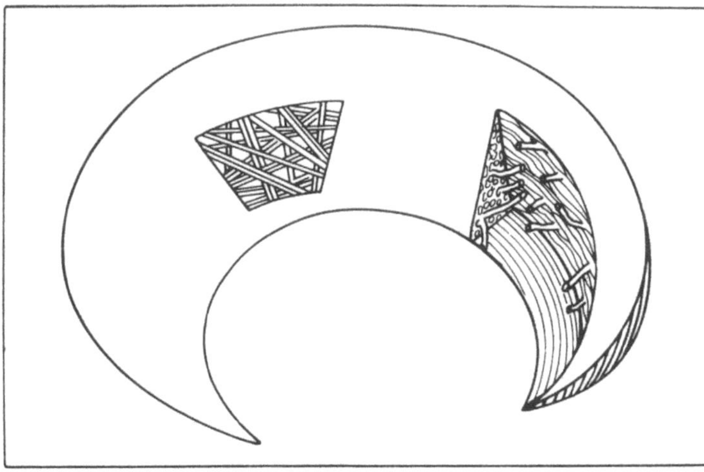

Figure 4. Collagen ultrastructure of the meniscus, showing the surface (S) and the deep zone (D). Radial fibers (r) are also shown.

Intervertebral Disc

The intervertebral disc is structurally organized into the outer annulus fibrosus, the inner nucleus pulposus, and the cartilaginous end-plates. The annulus fibrosus consists of an outer rim of circumferential type I collagen fibers (Eyre 1979), surrounding a less dense fibrocartilage, and the transitional zone (Buckwalter, 1982). The collagen fibers are arranged in cylindrical lamellae. They are parallel within each lamella, but have a changed orientation between the adjacent lamellae. The complex organization of the collagen fibers in the annulus fibrosus enables them to provide tensile stress reinforcement during torsional, bending or compressive loading (Hickey and Hukins 1980). The densely packed collagen fibers of the outer annulus gradually decrease in concentration and become more randomly distributed throughout the fibrocartilaginous and transitional zones before they merge with the nucleus pulposus. The centrally located nucleus pulposus consists of a soft matrix of proteoglycan and randomly oriented type II collagen network (Eyre 1979). The end-plates are located on the upper and lower surfaces of the disc, and together with the annulus fibrosus confine the nucleus pulposus within the intervertebral disc. The reader is referred to: "The Biology of the Intervertebral Disc. Vols. I-II." edited by Peter Ghosh which provides an up to date summary of intervertebral disc composition and structure.

The large regional variations in tissue consistency are due to changes in the biochemical constituents and their relative contents. As mentioned above, the collagen fibrils in the outer annulus fibrosus are mainly type I, while those in the nucleus pulposus are almost exclusively type II. The collagen cross-link density of intervertebral disc has been shown to be one of the highest of any vertebrate connective tissue (Eyre 1984). Though mechanical testing of this tissue is difficult due to its propensity to swell, Galante (1967) has demonstrated the strongly anisotropic tensile character of the annulus fibrosus.

Proteoglycan and water contents are greatest in the center of the disc and lowest at its periphery (Urban and Maroudas 1981). In young tissue the proteoglycans of the intervertebral disc closely resemble those found in hyaline cartilage. However, maturation (Buckwalter 1985) and age-related changes (Adams et al 1977) have been shown to result in a reduction of the proportion of proteoglycan able to aggregate. Furthermore, mature disc proteoglycans have been noted to be smaller than and are compositionally different from those generally found in hyaline cartilages (Berthet et al 1978). Such biochemical variations might be expected to manifest themselves in the mechanical properties of these tissues. Indeed, the compressive stiffness of the annulus fibrosus has been shown to decrease with increasing glycosaminoglycan content (Best et al 1989), the opposite relationship of that found for articular cartilage (Kempson 1971; Armstrong and Mow 1982a). The high water content of the nucleus pulposus reflects the tendency of proteoglycan to swell (Urban and Maroudas 1981; Panagiotacopulos et al 1979) and plays a significant role in the viscoelastic behavior of the disc under loading (Anderson and Schultz 1979).

Major Components of the Extracellular Matrix

Collagens

There are several genetically distinct types of collagen in these connective tissues. Type I collagen is the major collagen of meniscus, and type II is the primary collagen of articular cartilage. Intervertebral disc contains significant amounts of both type I and type II collagen, their relative concentrations depending upon the location within the tissue. The collagens form the typical cross-banded fibrillar structure noted by electron microscopy (Buckwalter et al 1987; Eyre 1980; Muir 1980; Nimni 1983; Nimni and Harkness 1988). A major extracellular modification of the collagen molecules, which occurs after fibril formation, is the development of covalent interfibrillar cross-links (Eyre et al 1981, 1987a, 1988). These collagen-collagen interactions are very important in determining the tensile stiffness and strength of the collagen network (Schmidt 1987).

The quantitatively minor collagens may also make important contributions to the structure of the matrix. For example, type IX collagen, a short non-fibrillar collagen (which contains a glycosaminoglycan chain and is therefore also considered a proteoglycan), binds covalently to type II collagen fibrils and may help link fibrils together or bind fibrils to other matrix molecules (Bruckner et al 1985; Eyre and Wu 1987; Van der Rest and Mayne 1988). Type XI collagen, a minor fibrillar collagen, may be involved in controlling the diameter of the type II fibrils (Eyre and Wu 1987; Van der Rest and Mayne 1988; Mayne and Irwin 1986). Other collagens, including type V and type VI, may also form part of the matrix, but their function and location in the matrix molecular framework is as yet undetermined.

The most important mechanical properties of collagen fibers are their tensile stiffness and strength (Akizuki et al 1986; Kempson et al 1973; Kempson 1979; Roth and Mow 1980; Woo et al 1976). The density of the fibers, the fiber diameter and orientation, and the amount of cross-links contribute to the overall mechanical stability and high tensile strength of the collagen network (Nimni and Harkness 1988; Kempson et al 1973; Schmidt et al 1986, 1987). In this chapter, we shall present an analysis of a constant strain-rate experiment commonly used to determine the tensile properties of cartilage modeled as a biphasic medium.

Proteoglycans

In articular cartilage proteoglycans constitute the second largest portion of the solid phase, accounting for 5-10% of the wet weight (Maroudas and Venn 1977; Maroudas et al 1980; Muir 1980, 1983). The proteoglycans of the cartilage matrix consist mainly of the large aggregating type (Figure 5) and large non-aggregating proteoglycans, with distinct small proteoglycans also being present (Heinegard et al 1981; Sampaio et al 1988).

Proteoglycans of cartilage contribute significantly to the compressive and swelling properties of these tissues (Akizuki et al 1987; Armstrong and Mow 1982a, 1982b; Eisenberg and Grodzinsky 1985; Lai et al 1989, 1990; Maroudas 1975, 1979; Myers et al 1984a, 1984b, 1988). It is believed that the large, high molecular weight proteoglycan monomers (M_r 1×10^6 - 4×10^6) contribute most significantly to these properties (Hardingham, 1981). These large proteoglycan monomers (Figure 5) consist of an extended protein core with several distinct regions: an N-terminal region with two globular domains, G1 and G2 (Weidemann et al 1984), a keratan sulfate-rich domain, a longer chondroitin sulfate rich domain which may also contain some interspersed keratan sulfate and neutral oligosaccharide chains, and a C-terminal globular domain G3. Aggregates are formed by many proteoglycan monomers binding to a chain of hyaluronate (Hardingham and Muir 1972, 1974; Hascall and Heinegard 1974a, 1974b) at the G1 globular domain (Hardingham 1979). Each proteoglycan-hyaluronate bond is stabilized by a separate globular link protein (M_r 41,000-48,000) (Hardingham 1979; Choi et al 1985).

The structure of proteoglycan in cartilage is not uniform. Differences in amount and chain length of keratan sulfate and chondroitin sulfate, length of the protein core, and the degree of aggregation all contribute to the structural and compositional variations of proteoglycans within the tissue. As already mentioned above, proteoglycans are also inhomogeneously distributed throughout the cartilage matrix. In normal cartilage their concentration is highest in the

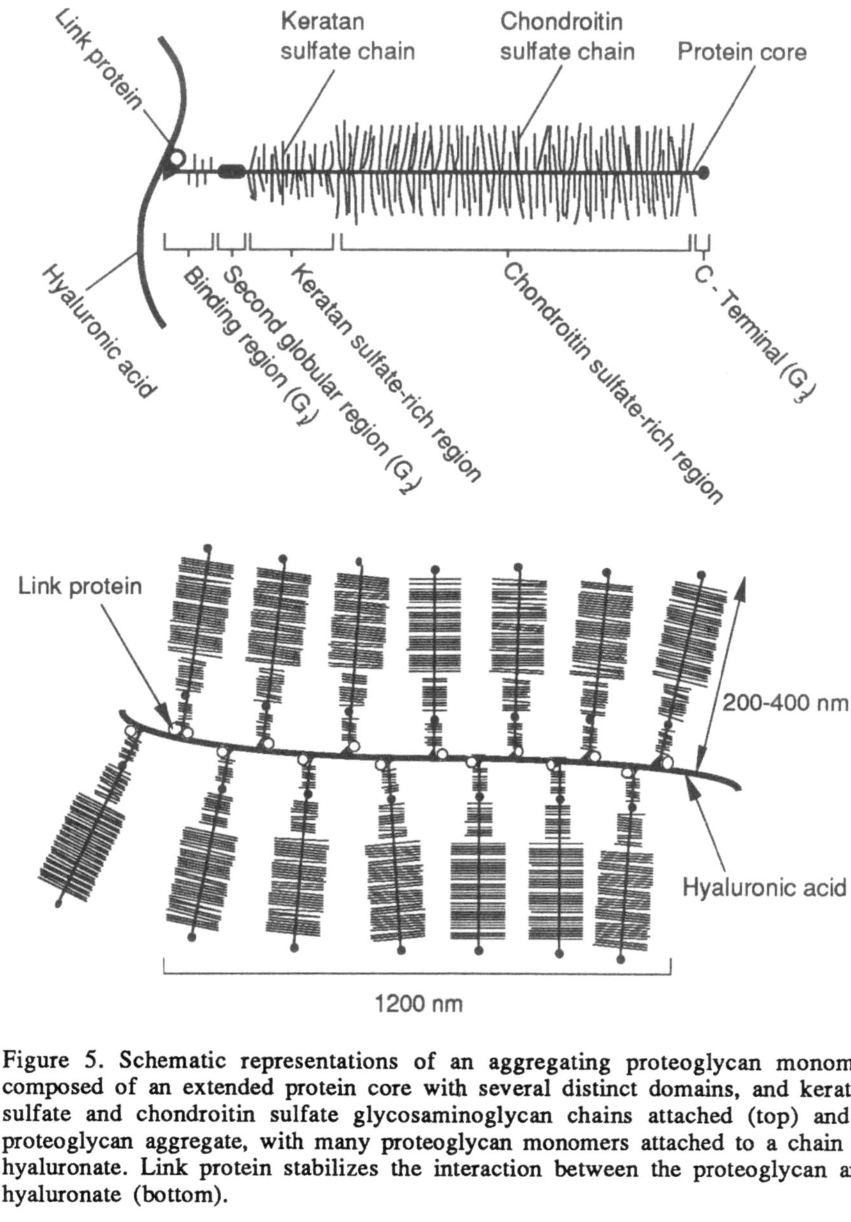

Figure 5. Schematic representations of an aggregating proteoglycan monomer composed of an extended protein core with several distinct domains, and keratan sulfate and chondroitin sulfate glycosaminoglycan chains attached (top) and a proteoglycan aggregate, with many proteoglycan monomers attached to a chain of hyaluronate. Link protein stabilizes the interaction between the proteoglycan and hyaluronate (bottom).

mid-zone and lowest in the superficial zone (Maroudas et al 1980; Muir 1980; Ratcliffe et al 1984). Furthermore, the composition, structure and distribution of proteoglycans varies with both age and disease (Buckwalter and Rosenberg 1982; Carney et al 1985; Manicourt et al 1988; McDevitt and Muir, 1976).

The size, structural rigidity and complex molecular conformations of normal proteoglycan aggregates make important contributions to the behavior of articular cartilage. Undoubtedly, the sheer size of proteoglycan will arrest or minimize diffusion or hydrodynamic convective transport of the molecules through the extracellular matrix due to steric exclusion or intermolecular frictional effects (Hascall and Hascall 1981; Pottenger et al 1982). The size and complex organization are also known to promote proteoglycan-proteoglycan networking and proteoglycan-collagen interactions (Hunziker and Schenk 1987; Muir 1983). Recent studies of pure proteoglycan solutions have confirmed that proteoglycans do form strong networks at concentrations similar to those found *in situ*, which are capable of storing energy elastically (Hardingham et al 1987; Mow et al 1984b, 1989; Zhu, 1989). See the chapter on viscometric flow of proteoglycans in these volumes for more details on this subject. This networking capacity of proteoglycans undoubtedly will contribute to their functional role in cartilage by maintaining and adding to the stiffness and strength of the extracellular matrix. However, little is currently known of proteoglycan-collagen interactions and their specific contribution to articular cartilage behavior.

Non-collagenous Proteins and Glycoproteins

Several specific non-collagenous proteins have been identified, including anchorin and chondronectin. However, their compositions and functions remain poorly understood (Hewitt et al 1982; Von der Mark et al 1986). The most well characterized of these proteins is link protein, which functions as a stabilizer of proteoglycan aggregation, influences proteoglycan aggregate size and provides structural strength to proteoglycan networks formed in concentrated solutions (Hardingham 1979; Mow et al 1989).

Water

Water is the most abundant component of articular cartilage, meniscus and intervertebral disc, comprising from 65-85% of the weight of the tissue (Armstrong and Mow 1982b; Fithian et al 1990; Linn and Sokoloff 1965; Lipshitz et al 1976; Mankin and Thrasher 1975; Maroudas 1979; Proctor et al 1989). In the tissues, it occupies two distinct compartments: 1) the proteoglycan solution domain which contains approximately 70% of the water (Hascall and Hascall, 1981; Muir, 1983), and 2) the collagen intrafibrillar space which contains the remaining 30% of the water (Maroudas and Schneidermann 1987; Torzilli 1985, 1988). Although water makes up 65-80% of these tissues, the "pore" size within these tissues has been estimated from hydraulic permeation experiments to range from 30 Å to 65 Å (Maroudas 1979; Mow et al 1984a). Inorganic ions such as sodium, calcium, chloride and potassium are dissolved in the tissue water (Linn and Sokoloff 1965; Maroudas 1979). These ions balance the fixed charges on the proteoglycans and generate significant swelling pressure

(Donnan 1924; Eisenberg and Grodzinsky 1985; Lai et al 1989, 1990; Maroudas 1975, 1976; 1979; Myers et al 1984a, 1984b).

The water content in cartilage is inhomogeneously distributed throughout the depth, decreasing in concentration from 80% at the surface to 65% in the deep zone (Lipshitz et al 1976). Most of the interstitial water may be extruded from the tissue by applying a pressure gradient across the tissue or compressing the solid matrix (Edwards 1967; Linn and Sokoloff 1965; Maroudas 1975; Mansour and Mow 1976; Mow et al 1980). The permeability of these tissues is extremely low because the frictional resistance to interstitial fluid flow through the porous-permeable solid matrix is very high (Best et al 1989; Mow et al 1980; 1984a; Proctor et al 1989). We shall see later how this high frictional force dominates the compressive viscoelastic behavior of articular cartilage, meniscus and the intervertebral disc.

Interactions Among Connective Tissue Components

The material properties of connective tissues are dependent upon the complex chemical, physical, electrochemical and mechanical interactions of the organic components. The solid phase consists of collagen, proteoglycans, minor collagen types and other non-collagenous proteins and glycoproteins. The interactions between these components produce a strong, cohesive, porous and permeable solid matrix capable of sustaining large loads for long periods. These interactions have been intensively studied over the past decades and are summarized below.

Proteoglycan-proteoglycan Interactions

Proteoglycans possess unique chemical and structural features which enable them to make important contributions to the mechanical properties of these connective tissues. Proteoglycan-proteoglycan interactions have been shown to include proteoglycan-hyaluronate-link protein interactions to form proteoglycan aggregates (Hardingham and Muir, 1972, 1974; Hascall and Heinegard, 1974a, 1974b; Muir 1983; Ratcliffe et al 1986), and proteoglycan network formation (Hardingham et al 1987, Mow et al 1984b, 1989). Further, by virtue of their abundant charge and hydroxyl groups they are soluble in solution and are able to entrain up to 50 times their weight in water (Hascall 1977; Muir 1983). This expanded conformational state results mainly from three factors: 1) to maintain electroneutrality, osmotically active counter-ions (e.g., Na^+) enter the molecular domain resulting in an osmotic swelling pressure; 2) the negative charges on the glycosaminoglycan chains exert electrostatic repulsive forces on one another; and 3) a highly solvated, extended molecule is entropically favored since it maximizes the number of possible conformational states of the molecule (Rees, 1975).

Studies on pure proteoglycan solutions at concentrations similar to those found in articular cartilage have shown that proteoglycans are capable of interacting with one another to form strong networks (Hardingham et al 1987; Mow et al 1984b, 1989; Zhu 1989). However, this network is less permanent, being subject to turnover from normal metabolic activities. This topic is also treated extensively in another chapter of these volumes. In summary, the viscometric studies on concentrated proteoglycan solutions indicate that the strength of the interaction sites and the energy storage capacity of the proteoglycan networks were noted to increase with the degree of proteoglycan aggregation and with link protein stabilization.

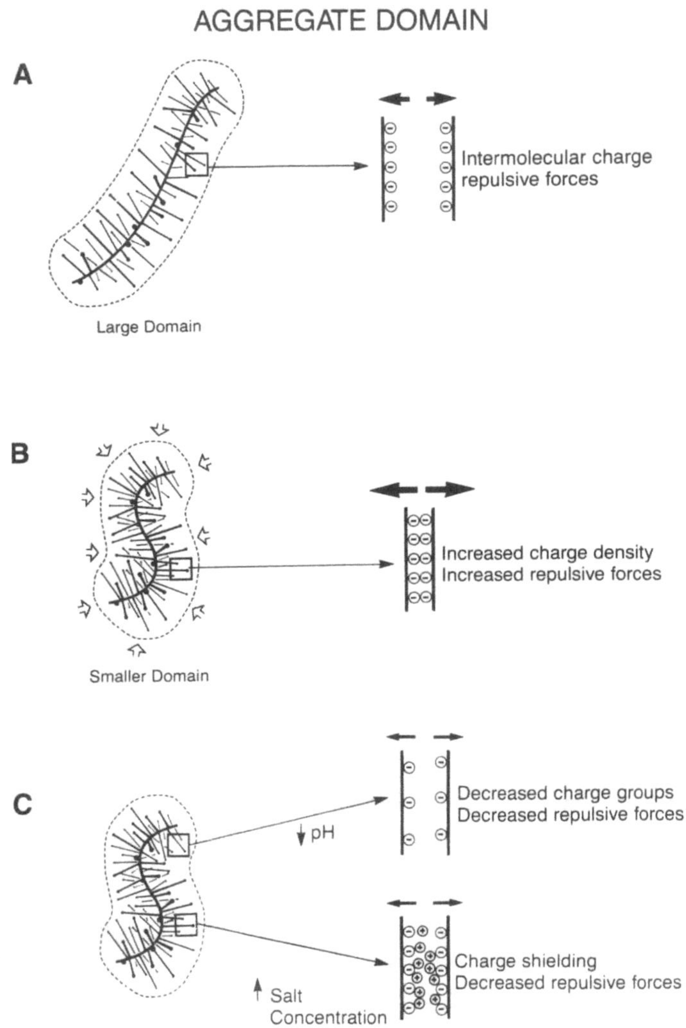

Figure 6. Proteoglycans carry a high density of charge groups (SO_4^-, COO^-) which are firmly attached to the glycosaminoglycan chains. Compression of the tissue would bring these charge groups closer together thereby increasing the Donnan osmotic pressure and charge-to-charge repulsive forces.

Within the tissue matrix the conformation and interactions of the proteoglycan molecules are dramatically altered. In articular cartilage, for example, the normally water soluble proteoglycan molecules are prevented by the collagen mesh from passing into solution. They are restrained to less than 20% of their free solution volume (Hascall 1977; Muir 1983). Such conformational changes
concentrate the neutralizing cations (Figure 6) which gives rise to a significant increase of the osmotic swelling effect (Donnan 1924) and bring the fixed negative charges into closer proximity thereby increasing the electrostatic repulsive forces (Lai et al 1989, 1990). The magnitude of the osmotic pressure in articular cartilage has been measured to approach 0.35 MPa and is dependent upon the negative charge density of the proteoglycans (Maroudas 1975, 1979). These internal swelling forces are balanced by tension in the surrounding collagenous network (Maroudas 1976). As a result, connective tissues rich in proteoglycan possess high water content, but low hydraulic permeabilities and high compressive stiffness (Armstrong and Mow 1982a, 1982b).

Collagen-collagen Interactions

The principal structural protein of all mammalian tissues is collagen. As mentioned earlier, it confers tensile strength and stiffness on connective tissues. However, if the collagen molecules were lying side by side with no molecular interactions they would slide relative to one another under loading. To prevent such an occurrence, both inter- and intra-molecular crosslinks exist between collagen molecules (Eyre et al 1981; Nimni and Harkness 1988; Yamaguchi and Mechanic 1988). These cross-links interlock the molecules and their presence has been experimentally shown to further increase the tensile strength and stiffness of articular cartilage (Schmidt et al 1987).

Collagen-proteoglycan Interactions

The interactions between collagens and proteoglycans are poorly understood. This comes as no surprise given the very complex nature of the constituents. Proteoglycans are highly polydisperse and both proteoglycans and collagen types vary not only between connective tissues but in their distributions within a given connective tissue. Such structural diversity leads to a great variety of possible chemical and physical interactions (figure 7).

Experimental observations suggest that the interactions between the two macromolecules generally involve mechanical entanglement, electrostatic bonds and excluded volume effects. Physical entanglement is felt to be assisted by the complexing of proteoglycan monomers to form large multimolecular aggregates (Pottenger et al 1982). Proteoglycan networking also helps to immobilize the proteoglycans in the collagen meshwork (Muir 1983; Hardingham et al 1987; Mow et al 1989; Nimni and Harkness 1988). From tensile creep and enzymatic proteoglycan extraction studies, Schmidt et al (1990) showed that frictional forces

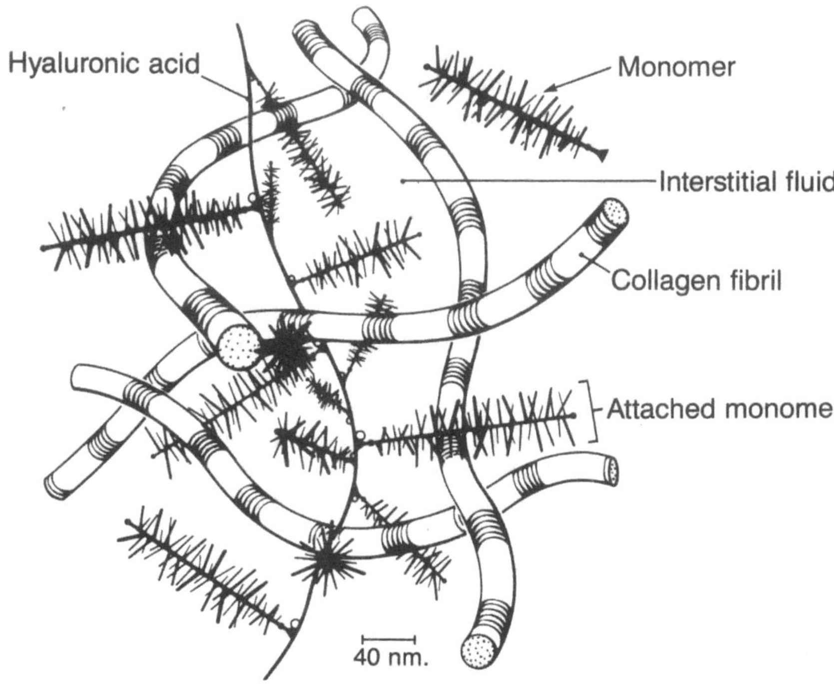

Figure 7. Schematic representation of the molecular organization of cartilage. Collagen and proteoglycan interact to form a porous solid matrix which is swollen with water.

between the collagen network and the proteoglycan network retard fibril movement in the extracellular matrix. Electrostatic interactions have been implicated in making strong contributions to the cohesive nature of the solid matrix (Scott 1988). Both the negative charges of the polysaccharide subunits that make up the glycosaminoglycan chains and those of the protein core have been shown to be important in collagen binding (Toole 1976). In addition, molecular charge density and the spatial distribution of charged groups are important characteristics in establishing binding affinity (Obrink 1973).

Excluded volume effects arise when a given molecule sterically inhibits neighboring molecules from interacting with the water in its hydrodynamic domain. As a result, more compact configurations of the molecular species are favored. This also tends to alter the swelling behavior of the molecules by increasing their osmotic activities (Edmond and Ogston 1968). Proteoglycan-collagen interactions may also play significant roles in regulating collagen fibril formation (Muthiah 1973; Wood 1960), size (Scott 1988) and spacing (Ruggeri and Benazzo 1984). Consequently, structural interactions not only have strong influences on the mechanical properties of a given tissue but also have important implications in terms of its assembly and organization.

Constitutive Modeling of Hydrated Soft Tissues

In order to understand the function of any material, constitutive laws must be developed to describe its stress-strain relationship (Truesdell and and Toupin 1960; Truesdell and Noll 1965). All constitutive laws must satisfy certain axioms, the most important of which is the Principle of Material Objectivity. This principle asserts that no properly formulated constitutive law may depend on the observer, i.e., these constitutive laws must be objective. In practical terms, this principle asserts that all stress-strain relationships must use only objective measures of deformation (strain, rate of deformation, Cauchy-Green tensor, Rivlin-Erickson tensors). These tensors are all invariant under an arbitrary transformation of the observer's reference frame, i.e., rotation, translation and time shift.

Many constitutive laws exist. The most commonly used stress-strain laws are: 1) the generalized Hooke's law for the theory describing idealized linear elastic solids; and 2) the Newtonian fluid for the Navier-Stokes theory of idealized linearly viscous fluids. For materials which are not ideally elastic nor ideally viscous, viscoelastic constitutive laws have been developed (Truesdell and Noll 1965; Ferry 1970; Fung 1965, 1972, 1981). The most commonly used linear viscoelastic stress-strain laws are: 1) the Maxwell model for a viscoelastic fluid; 2) the Kelvin-Voigt model for a viscoelastic solid; 3) the three element standard viscoelastic body; and 4) the Boltzmann superposition principle for a general viscoelastic material (Fung 1965). The latter two could be used to describe either a solid or a fluid. More recently, Fung (1972, 1981) developed a quasi-linear viscoelastic theory specifically for soft tissues whose stress-strain behavior are not too strain-rate sensitive. Historically, all these single phase constitutive laws have been used to describe articular cartilage, meniscus and intervertebral disc (Colleti et al 1970; Hirsch 1944; Hayes 1971, 1972; Kempson 1979; Sokoloff 1963; Spilker et al 1986; Spirt et al 1988).

Linear elasticity theory (single phase) has been used for stress-strain analysis of articular cartilage and intervertebral disc (Askew and Mow 1978; Brown et al 1985; Hayes et al 1972; Hirsch 1944; Hock et al 1983; Jurvelin et al 1987; Kempson 1971, 1979; Sokoloff 1963; Spilker et al 1986; Shirazi-Adl et al 1986). However, linearly elastic materials do not exhibit viscoelastic creep nor stress-relaxation behaviors as do these tissues. Therefore, in practical terms, it is impossible to choose the appropriate material properties (for example, the Young's modulus and Poisson's ratio) to use for any desired stress-strain analysis. Consequently, the results from the stress-strain analysis using linearly elastic models are of limited value. In addition, material coefficients for a constitutive model may not be determined in an arbitrary manner. For example, the method of Kempson et al (1971) to determine a "2-second" modulus for cartilage compressive stiffness (using linear elasticity theory) is subjective since it depends on the observer's choice of time in taking the data. The arbitrary imposition of this "2-second" requirement violates the time-shift transformation invariance condition for constitutive laws. Therefore, this method to determine the modulus of elasticity for cartilage can not be theoretically justified.

Single phase viscoelastic models have also been employed to describe the creep and stress-relaxation behaviors of these tissues (Colleti et al 1972; Hayes and Mockros 1971: Parsons and Black 1977, 1979; Sprit et al 1988; Woo et al 1976, 1981). However, to date, no attempt has been made to perform stress-strain analysis for these tissues using single phase viscoelastic models.

The constitutive models most commonly used for stress-strain analyses to describe the viscoelastic creep and stress-relaxation behaviors of hydrated soft tissues are the general theoretical formulations for mixture by Truesdell and Toupin (1960), Mow et al (1980) and Bowen (1980) (Kwan et al 1990; Lai et al 1989, 1990; Mak 1986; Holmes 1986; Mow et al 1984a, 1986; Spilker et al 1988) or formulations similar to those commonly used in soil mechanics (Biot 1941, 1955; Kenyon 1976, 1980; Simon and Gaballa 1988).

In this chapter, we shall use only the mixture theory approach developed by Mow and co-workers (1980) pertinent to the measurement of the material properties of these tissues. This biphasic theory assumes the solid matrix and the interstitial fluid of the tissue to be immiscible, and each phase to be, by itself, intrinsically incompressible. The interstitial fluid may be moved through the tissue by a pressure gradient or the "apparent" compression of the solid matrix. Viscous dissipation in the tissue is dominated by the frictional drag of interstitial fluid flow through the porous-permeable collagen-proteoglycan solid matrix. In this chapter, we present a summary of this theory, and the mathematical analyses of the most often used experimental configurations to determine the intrinsic material properties of these hydrated soft tissues. A summary of relevant material coefficients is also presented, see Table II. We shall restrict ourselves in this chapter to the infinitesimal strain theory, i.e., the linear KLM biphasic theory (constant permeability) and the nonlinear KLM biphasic theory (strain-dependent permeability). The reader is referred to references by Mow et al (1986), Holmes (1986) and Kwan et al (1990) for complete descriptions of finite deformation biphasic theories for cartilage, and the reference by Spilker and co-workers in these volumes for a detailed discussion of the finite element formulation of the biphasic theories for soft hydrated tissues.

The KLM Biphasic Theory

The KLM biphasic constitutive equations for hydrated soft tissues assume each phase to be intrinsically incompressible. For these assumptions, the balance of mass for the tissue is expressed by the following continuity equation:

$$\operatorname{div}(\phi^s \boldsymbol{v}^s + \phi^f \boldsymbol{v}^f) = 0\,, \tag{1}$$

where ϕ^s and ϕ^f are the volume fractions of the solid phase and the fluid phase, and $\boldsymbol{v}^s$ and $\boldsymbol{v}^f$ are their velocities respectively. These volume fractions must also

	Human[1]	Bovine[2]	Dog[3]	Monkey[4]	Rabbit[5]
LFC	0.70	0.89	0.60	0.78	0.54
PFG	0.53	0.47	0.55	0.52	0.51
Patella	0.78	—	—	—	—
Meniscus	—	0.41*	—	—	—
IVD	0.34	—	—	—	—

Table IIA. Equilibrium aggregate modulus (MPa)

	Human[1]	Bovine[2]	Dog[3]	Monkey[4]	Rabbit[5]
LFC	1.18	0.43	0.77	4.19	1.81
PFG	2.17	1.42	0.93	4.74	3.84
Patella	0.47	—	—	—	—
Meniscus	—	0.81	—	—	—
IVD	0.28	—	—	—	—

Table IIB. Permeability coefficient (10^{-15} m^4/Ns)

	Human[1]	Bovine[2]	Dog[3]	Monkey[4]	Rabbit[5]
LFC	0.10	0.40	0.30	0.24	0.34
PFG	0.00	0.25	0.09	0.20	0.21
Patella	0.00	—	—	—	—

Table IIC. Poisson's ratio of cartilage

1. Young normal; 2. 18 mos. to 2 yrs old; 3. Mature beagles;
4. Mature cynomologous monkey; 5. Mature New Zealand white rabbits;

Key: LFC=Lateral Femoral Condyle; PFG=Patellar Femoral Groove;
IVD=Intervertebral Disc.

Data from: 1) Armstrong and Mow, 1982b. 2) Athanasiou KA et al, Interspecies comparison of in situ biomechanical properties of knee joint cartilage. Trans Orthop Res Soc 1989;14:149. 3) Froimson MI et al, Patellar cartilage mechanical properties vary with site and biochemical composition. Trans Orthop Res Soc 1989;14:150.

satisfy the constraint equation given by: $\phi^s + \phi^f = 1$. For quasi-static situations, the equations of motion for the solid phase and the fluid phase are:

$$\text{div}\sigma^s + \pi = \mathbf{0}\ , \tag{2}$$

$$\text{div}\sigma^f - \pi = \mathbf{0}\ , \tag{3}$$

where σ^s and σ^f are the stress tensors acting on the solid phase and fluid phase, respectively, and π is the action-and-reaction interaction force between the two phases which is often called the momentum supply from one phase to the other. For infinitesimal strains, the KLM theory assumes the solid phase is a linearly elastic solid and the fluid phase is a Newtonian viscous fluid. Under these conditions, the constitutive relations for the stresses and the momentum supply are given by:

$$\sigma^s = -\phi^s p\mathbf{I} + \lambda_s \text{tr}(\mathbf{E})\mathbf{I} + 2\mu_s\mathbf{E}\ , \tag{4}$$

$$\sigma^f = -\phi^f p\mathbf{I} - \frac{2}{3}\mu_a(\text{div}\nu^f)\mathbf{I} + 2\mu_a\mathbf{D}\ , \tag{5}$$

$$\pi = p\nabla\phi^f + K(\nu^f - \nu^s)\ , \tag{6}$$

where λ_s and μ_s are Lamè constants for the solid phase, μ_a is the apparent viscosity of the fluid phase in cartilage, $\mathbf{E}$ is the infinitesimal strain tensor for the solid matrix, $\mathbf{D}$ is the rate of the deformation tensor for the interstitial fluid, and K is the coefficient of the diffusive drag caused by the relative motion between the two phases (Mow et al 1980). These equations may be written in a more compact form by deriving the Navier's equations of motion for the biphasic material. To do this, we insert constitutive equations (4)-(6) into the equations of motion (2) and (3). This yields the Navier's equations for the solid phase and the fluid phase:

$$-\phi^s\nabla p + (\lambda_s+\mu_s)\nabla(\text{div}\boldsymbol{u}) + \mu_s\nabla^2\boldsymbol{u} + K(\nu^f - \nu^s) = \mathbf{0}\ , \tag{7}$$

$$-\phi^f\nabla p + \frac{1}{3}\mu_a\nabla(\text{div}\nu^f) + \mu_a\nabla^2\nu^f + K(\nu^s - \nu^f) = \mathbf{0}\ , \tag{8}$$

where $\boldsymbol{u}$ is the displacement vector of the solid matrix. For infinitesimal deformation the velocity of the solid matrix is given by:

$$\nu^s = \frac{\partial \boldsymbol{u}}{\partial t}\ . \tag{9}$$

Equations (1) through (9) form the complete biphasic theory for hydrated soft tissues with constant permeability. Lai and Mow (1980) showed that the coefficient of the diffusive drag K is related to the permeability coefficient k by the equation:

$$k = \frac{\phi^{f2}}{K}. \tag{10}$$

For the strain-dependent permeability case, it was shown experimentally that the permeability function (figure 8) is given by:

$$k = k_o e^{Mtr(\mathbf{E})}, \tag{11}$$

where M is a material constant, and tr(**E**) is the dilatation of the solid matrix.

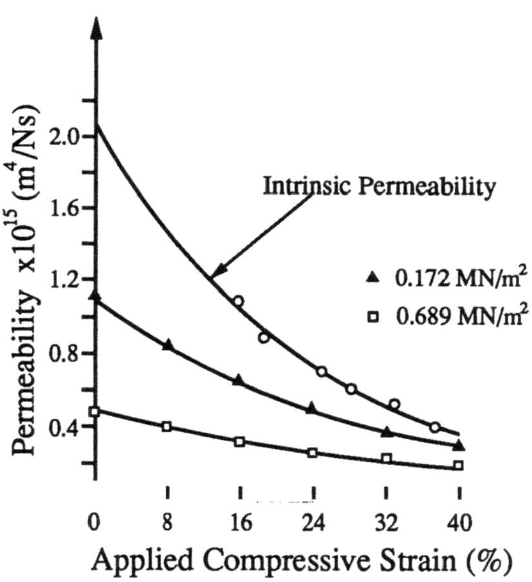

Figure 8. Permeability of articular cartilage, at two levels of pressure P_A, as a function of the applied clamping strain. The intrinsic permeability is obtained from the limited case of $P_A \rightarrow 0$ from six levels of P_A.

In this chapter, we shall present the mathematical solutions to the following commonly used experiments: 1) steady state uniaxial filtration with constant permeability and the strain-dependent permeability; 2) confined compression creep and stress-relaxation; 3) unconfined compression creep and stress-relaxation; 4) indentation creep; 5) the steady-state sinusoidal confined compression; and 6) uniaxial tension. These mathematical solutions provide the simplest equations for determination of the material properties of hydrated soft tissues in some commonly used experimental configurations.

Steady State Uniaxial Filtration Problem

The complete mathematical solution of this problem is described by Lai and Mow (1980). Here we provide a summary of the results only. In this problem, we define z as the axis in the thickness direction of a cylindrical tissue specimen of thickness h (figure 9). The specimen is confined in the radial (lateral) r-direction and is supported at its surface z=h by a free-draining rigid-porous block. Thus, at z=h, the solid matrix displacement $u_z=0$. For the filtration problem, at the upstream surface, the hydrostatic pressure is P_A, and at the downstream surface, it is zero:

$$p(0) = P_A \quad \text{and} \quad p(h) = 0. \tag{12}$$

A clamping strain of the tissue (ε_c) may be achieved by a surface displacement $u_z(0)=\varepsilon_c h$ imposed to the upstream rigid-porous block. If no compression is imposed, then the total-stress boundary condition is given by its continuity with the hydrostatic pressure, i.e., $\sigma_{zz}(0) = -P_A$.

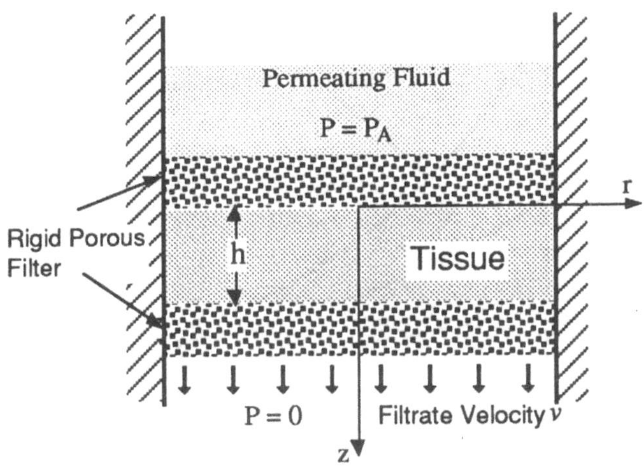

Figure 9. Schematic representation of one-dimentional permeation of cartilage.

Let Q be the volume flux of fluid per unit total cross-section area for the pressure drop P_A. For the steady state condition, $v_z^s=0$ and $\phi^f v_z^f=Q$. By the continuity condition, equation (1), Q must be constant throughout the specimen thickness. From the momentum equation for the fluid phase and the definition of the permeability, one obtains:[1]

[1] For all the problems presented in this chapter, the effect of interstitial fluid viscosity is negligible, i.e., $\mu_a=0$, (see Mow et al 1980 for theoretical justification). In other words, energy dissipation associated with the interstitial fluid viscosity, equation (8), in these problems manifests itself in the diffusive drag coefficient.

$$-k\frac{\partial p}{dz} = Q\,. \tag{13}$$

If k is constant, then this simple differential equation, along with the boundary conditions given above, define Darcy's laws for the hydraulic permeability k, and the experimental conditions by which k may be determined. These equations show that k is simply given by the measured pressure drop P_A, the fluid volume flux Q and specimen thickness h:

$$k = Q\frac{h}{P_A}\,. \tag{14}$$

If the specimen is maintained under a clamping strain ε_c, the compressive strain ε_{zz} in the solid matrix can be obtained from equation (7):

$$\varepsilon_{zz}(z) = -\frac{\partial u_z}{\partial z} = \varepsilon_c + \frac{P_A}{H_A}\left(\frac{z}{h} - \frac{1}{2}\right). \tag{15}$$

If no compression is applied, then the tissue surface at z=0 is free to move and the compressive strain in the tissue is given by:

$$\varepsilon_{zz}(z) = \frac{P_A}{H_A h}\,z. \tag{16}$$

For the strain-dependent permeability case, equation (11), the compressive strain throughout the tissue is more complex and can be obtained from the integration of equation (7). For the case where ε_c=0, the apparent permeability is given by

$$k_{app} = k_o\frac{1-\exp(-MP_A/H_A)}{MP_A/H_A}\exp\left[-M\varepsilon_c + \left(M\frac{P_A}{H_A} + 1 - M\frac{MP_A/H_A}{1-\exp(-MP_A/H_A)}\right)\right]. \tag{17}$$

The compressive strain for this case can be shown to be

$$\varepsilon_{zz}(z) = \frac{1}{M}\ln\left[\frac{MhQ}{H_A k_o}\left(\frac{1}{1-\exp(-MP_A/H_A)} - \frac{z}{h}\right)\right], \tag{18}$$

where the fluid flux Q is given by

$$Q = -k_{app}\frac{P_A}{h}. \tag{19}$$

We also provide the relationship between the apparent permeability k_{app} of the test specimen and the applied P_A for the case $\varepsilon_c=0$,

$$k_{app} = \frac{k_o H_A}{M P_A}\left[1-\exp\left(-M\frac{P_A}{H_A}\right)\right], \tag{20}$$

as well as a correlation between the predicted strain-dependent permeability and experimental data. The accuracy of these strain-dependent permeability coefficients (k_o,M) has been verified by calculations based upon data obtained from independent confined compression stress-relaxation experiments (Holmes et al 1985).

Confined Compression Creep and Stress-relaxation Problems

In a confined compression experiment, a thin cylindrical plug of tissue is confined laterally by an impermeable-frictionless ring so that there is no radial displacement nor fluid flow. The tissue surface at z=h is supported by a rigid-impermeable plate and the other surface is in contact with a rigid-porous loading platen. In a creep experiment, a step load $F_oH(t)$ is applied in the axial direction, where H(t) is the Heaviside function. The governing equation for the matrix displacement is a diffusion-type equation given by:

$$H_A k \frac{\partial^2 u_z}{\partial z^2} = \frac{\partial u_z}{\partial t}. \tag{21}$$

The boundary conditions for this creep problem are:

$$u_z(h,t)=0 \quad \text{and} \quad \frac{\partial u_z(0,t)}{\partial z} = -\frac{F_o}{H_A}H(t). \tag{22}$$

If the permeability k is constant, the solution for the creep displacement u_z has been obtained (Mow et al 1980):

$$\frac{u_z(0,t)}{h} = \frac{F_o}{H_A}\left[1 - \frac{2}{\pi^2}\sum_{n=1}^{\infty}\frac{1}{(n+\frac{1}{2})^2}\exp\left(-\frac{H_A k(n-\frac{1}{2})^2\pi^2}{h^2}t\right)\right]. \tag{23}$$

For the initial time period ($t \ll h^2/(kH_A)$), this creep may be simplified to the asymptotic expression:

$$u_z(0,t) = 2F_o\sqrt{\frac{kt}{\pi H_A}} + \cdots. \tag{24}$$

For the strain-dependent permeability k given by equation (11), and for short creep time, the asymptotic expression for the creep displacement is given by

$$u_z(0,t) = 2F_o\left(1 - \frac{MF_o}{\pi H_A}\right)\sqrt{\frac{kt}{\pi H_A}} + \cdots. \tag{25}$$

These asymptotic results offer very simple analytical expressions relating the tissue creep response and the material properties. A creep curve for a typical set of cartilage material properties (H_A,k) calculated from equation (23) is shown in Figure 10a. This creep solution has been used to determine the aggregate modulus H_A and permeability k of articular cartilage, meniscus and the intervertebral disc (Armstrong and Mow 1982b; Kwan et al 1989; Proctor et al 1989, Best et al 1989). Typical numerical values of these material coefficients are given in Tables II.

In a stress-relaxation experiment, the displacement of the specimen surface at z = 0 is given by a prescribed motion of the rigid-porous loading platen. Since the stress-relaxation problem remains unidirectional, equation (21) remains the governing differential equation. We now consider the following stress-relaxation experimental procedure: 1) during the compression phase, the specimen is subjected to a constant ramp compression rate (constant speed V at the surface); and 2) during the stress-relaxation phase, i.e., when a predetermined strain ε_o is attained at time $t=t_o$ ($t_o=\varepsilon_o h/V$), the specimen is then kept at this level of compression for $t>t_o$ until the stress-relaxation process has been completed. This prescribed boundary condition is given by the following mathematical expression:

$$u_z(h,t)=0 \quad \text{and} \quad u_z(h,t) = \begin{cases} \varepsilon_o h\dfrac{t}{t_o}, & \text{for } t<t_o, \\ \varepsilon_o h, & \text{for } t\geq t_o, \end{cases} \tag{26}$$

For the constant permeability case, the mathematical solution can be obtained by using an elementary separation of variable technique (see Mow et al 1980). In order to analyze the experimental data in a simpler manner, we provide an asymptotic solution for slow rate of compression experiments. For the initial time period ($t<<t_o$), the compressive stress response is given by the asymptotic expression (Holmes 1983):

$$\sigma_{zz} = H_A\varepsilon_o\frac{2}{\sqrt{\pi}}\sqrt{\frac{h^2}{H_A k t_o}\frac{t}{t_o}} + \cdots. \tag{27}$$

For high compression rates, the stress response during the compression phase is given by the asymptotic formula:

$$\sigma_{zz} = H_A \varepsilon_o \frac{2}{\sqrt{\pi}} \sqrt{\frac{h^2}{H_A k t_o}} \frac{t}{t_o} + \cdots. \tag{28}$$

However, for high compression rates, very large local strains may be produced near the surface z=0. Thus, care must be exercised in an experiment so that the compression rate $V=\varepsilon_o h/t_o$ is not chosen to produce internal strains beyond the infinitesimal strain assumption of the linear KLM biphasic theory. These simple formulas can be used to determine the average permeability of the tissue from the ramp phase of the stress-relaxation experiment if H_A is known. This can be measured by the linear equilibrium stress-strain relationship (Mow et al 1980). We note that similar expressions may also be obtained to describe the stress-relaxation phase of the experiment (Mow et al 1980; Holmes 1983). For the slow-rate compression experiment, an asymptotic expression for the stress relaxation is given by:[2]

$$\sigma_{zz} = \sigma\Big|_{t=t_o} - H_A \varepsilon_o \frac{2}{\sqrt{\pi}} \sqrt{\frac{h^2}{H_A k t_o}\left(\frac{t}{t_o} - 1\right)} + \cdots. \tag{29}$$

With this expression, we may calculate the permeability of the tissue from the experimental stress-relaxation data. This determination of permeability may be used as an independent verification of the permeability determined during the compression phase of the experiment.

For the strain-dependent permeability case, equation (11), the governing equation (21) becomes nonlinear. In this case the elementary separation of variable technique can no longer be used to solve the problem. No exact solution exists and asymptotic perturbation methods must be used to obtain an approximate solution (Holmes, 1983; Holmes et al., 1985). For the slow compression rate problem, defined parametrically by the inequality $t_o=h\varepsilon_o/V>>h^2/(H_A k)$, the compressive stress is given by the expression:

$$\sigma_c = H_A \varepsilon_o \left(\frac{t}{t_o} + \frac{1}{3} \frac{h^2}{H_A k_o t_o} e^{-M\varepsilon_o t/t_o} + \cdots\right) \tag{30}$$

while the stress response during the initial period of relaxation is given by

$$\sigma_c = \sigma_c\Big|_{t=t_o} - H_A \varepsilon_o \frac{2}{\sqrt{\pi}} \sqrt{\frac{h^2}{H_A k_o t_o \exp(M\varepsilon_o)}\left(\frac{t}{t_o} - 1\right)} + \cdots. \tag{31}$$

---

[2]Only the slow rate of compression stress-relaxation result is provided here since, as discussed above, the high-rate result has limited applicability.

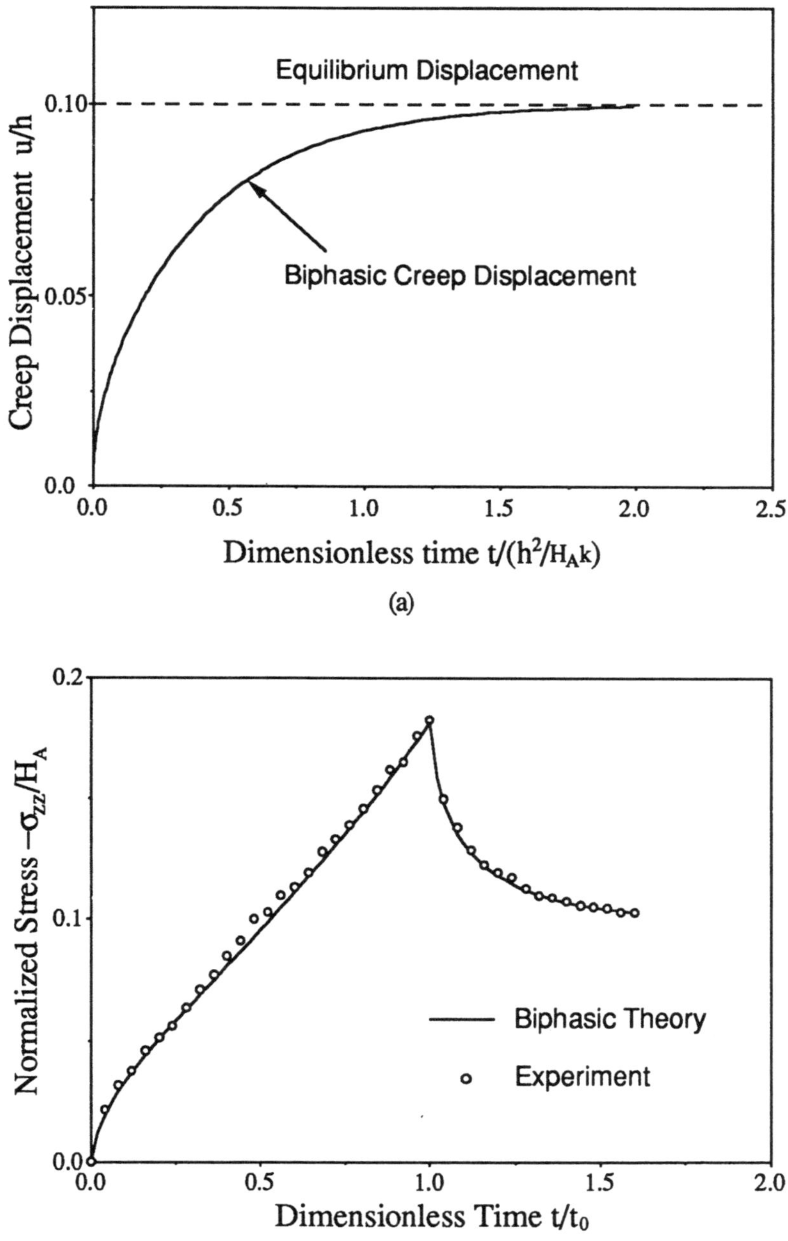

(b)

Figure 10. (a) Biphasic creep behaviour of articular cartilageb. (b) Biphasic stress-relaxation of cartilage under controlled displacement. Comparison between the theoretical prediction of the biphasic model and the experimental results shows excellent agreement.

These two equations have been used in curve-fitting procedures with experimental data to obtain the permeability parameters ko and M of equation (11). Figure 10b provides an example of the excellent curve-fit from the calculations with experimental stress response data. Similar mathematical expressions for the stress response in a high rate of compression stress-relaxation experiment may be found in Holmes et al (1985). The utilities of these high rate compression results are limited because these rates may produce very large local strains near the loaded surface at z=0, beyond the range of validity for the infinitesimal strain theory used.

Unconfined Compression Stress-Relaxation and Creep Problems

Armstrong and co-workers (1984) provided an analysis of the unconfined compression experiment where thin, circular disks of the tissue were squeezed between two perfectly smooth (frictionless) impermeable plates. This problem was solved for both creep, with an imposed load F(t), and stress-relaxation, with an imposed strain $\varepsilon(t)$ in the axial z direction. Unlike the confined compression problem, here a radial expansion is caused by the applied axial compression. At the cylindrical surface of the specimen, r=R, the solid matrix and the interstitial fluid may move in an unconstrained manner. Since contact with the plates is assumed to be frictionless, then, by symmetry, the deformation would be independent of z. Thus, this axisymmetric problem becomes a one-dimensional problem in r with the loading applied in the z direction. The governing equation, from equation (7), for the radial displacement u_r is given by

$$H_A k\left(\frac{\partial^2 u_r}{\partial r^2} + \frac{1}{r}\frac{\partial u_r}{\partial r} - \frac{u_r}{r^2}\right) = \frac{\partial u_r}{\partial t} + \frac{r}{2}\dot{\varepsilon}(t). \tag{32}$$

The boundary condition for the displacement u_r is obtained from the stress-free condition $\sigma_{rr}=0$ on the surface r=R, and it is given by

$$\lambda_s\left(\frac{\partial u_r}{\partial r} + \frac{u_r}{r} + \varepsilon(t)\right) + 2\mu_s\frac{\partial u_r}{\partial r} = 0. \tag{33}$$

In equations (32) and (33), e(t) is the overall surface-to-surface axial compression. For the creep problem with loading F(t) in the z-direction, $\varepsilon(t)$ is unknown and is part of the solution. In this case, the equation for the total stress σ_{zz} at the loading platen:

$$\int_0^R 2\pi\sigma_{zz} r\,dr = F(t), \tag{34}$$

provides the condition used for calculating the creep response $\varepsilon(t)$.

For constant permeability k, equation (32), with initial and boundary conditions, can be solved by using the Laplace transform technique. For the stress-relaxation spectrum where a step axial strain $\varepsilon(t) = -\varepsilon_c H(t)$ is imposed, the average compressive stress $\bar{\sigma}_c$ (total compressive force divided by area) response is given by

$$\bar{\sigma}_c = E_s\varepsilon_c\left[1 + \frac{(1-\nu_s)(1-2\nu_s)}{(1+\nu_s)}\sum_{n=1}^{\infty}\frac{1}{(1-\nu_s)^2\alpha_n^2-(1-2\nu_s)}\exp\left(-\frac{\alpha_n^2 H_A k}{R^2}\,t\right)\right]. \quad (35)$$

where E_s and ν_s are the Young's modulus and Poisson's ratio of the solid matrix, α_n are the roots of the characteristic equation $J_1(x) - (1-\nu_s)xJ_0(x)/(1-2\nu_s) = 0$, and J_0 and J_1 are Bessel functions. The lateral expansion of the specimen at all times is given by

$$\frac{u_r(R,t)}{R} = \varepsilon_c\left[\nu_s + (1-\nu_s)(1-2\nu_s)\sum_{n=1}^{\infty}\frac{1}{(1-\nu_s)^2\alpha_n^2-(1-2\nu_s)}\exp\left(-\frac{\alpha_n^2 H_A k}{R^2}\,t\right)\right]. \quad (36)$$

For short time intervals after the application of $\varepsilon(t)$, one obtains the asymptotic expressions for the average compressive stress and the lateral expansion:

$$\bar{\sigma}_c = 3\mu_s\varepsilon_c\left(1 - \frac{4\mu_s}{3H_A}\sqrt{\frac{H_A k}{\pi R^2}\,t} + \cdots\right). \quad (37)$$

and

$$\frac{u_r(R,t)}{R} = \frac{1}{2}\varepsilon_c\left(1 - \frac{4\mu_s}{H_A}\sqrt{\frac{H_A k}{\pi R^2}\,t} + \cdots\right). \quad (38)$$

These simple mathematical solutions may be readily used for determining tissue compressive properties if the frictionless platen condition is a good approximation for the experimental configuration (Brown and Singerman 1986).

For the case of unconfined-compression creep under a step loading, i.e., $F(t) = -F_o H(t)$, where $H(t)$ is the Heaviside function, the axial creep (compressive) strain ε_c is given by

$$\varepsilon_c = \frac{F_o}{\pi R^2 E_s}\left[1 - \sum_{n=1}^{\infty}\frac{(1-\nu_s^2)(1-2\nu_s)}{9(1-\nu_s)^2\beta_n^2-8(1+\nu_s)(1-2\nu_s)}\exp\left(-\frac{\beta_n^2 H_A k}{R^2}\,t\right)\right]. \quad (39)$$

where β_n are the roots of the characteristics equation

$$J_0(x) - \frac{4(1-2\nu_s)}{3(1-\nu_s)}\frac{J_1(x)}{x} = 0. \quad (40)$$

For this problem, the lateral expansion is

$$\frac{u_r(R,t)}{R} = \frac{F_o}{\pi R^2 E_s}\left[\nu_s + \sum_{n=1}^{\infty} \frac{4(1-\nu_s^2)(1-2\nu_s)}{9(1-\nu_s)^2\beta_n^2 - 8(1+\nu_s)(1-2\nu_s)} \exp\left(-\frac{\beta_n^2 H_A k}{R^2}t\right)\right]. \quad (41)$$

For short time, one obtains the following asymptotic expansions for these expressions yield

$$\varepsilon_{zz} = \frac{F_o}{\pi R^2}\left[\frac{1}{3\mu_s} + \frac{2}{3H_A}\sqrt{\frac{H_A k}{\pi R^2}t} + \cdots\right]. \quad (42)$$

and the radial displacement:

$$\frac{u_r(R,t)}{R} = \frac{F_o}{\pi R^2}\left[\frac{1}{6\mu_s} - \frac{4}{9H_A}\sqrt{\frac{H_A k}{\pi R^2}t} + \cdots\right]. \quad (43)$$

As above, these solutions could provide ways to determine intrinsic tissue material properties if the frictionless assumption is a good one for the experiment at hand (Brown and Singerman 1986). For unconfined compression, no solution exists for the strain-dependent permeability nonlinear biphasic theory. However, this problem has been solved numerically using the finite element method (see chapter by Spilker et al in these volumes).

Biphasic Indentation Creep Problem

The indentation creep experiment has been used extensively in the literature to determine articular cartilage compressive behavior (Bar, 1926; Elmore et al 1963; Gocke 1927; Hirsch 1944; Kempson et al 1971; Colleti et al 1972; Hock et al 1983; Hori and Mockros 1976; Jurvelin et al 1987). The analysis of this indentation problem using the linear KLM biphasic theory was derived by Mak et al (1987), and later used by Mow et al (1989b) to determine the intrinsic properties of this tissue. Mak and co-workers modeled the cartilage on the joint surface as a layer of linear KLM biphasic material of thickness h bonded to an impervious, rigid bony substrate. The creep indentation is performed by applying a constant step load $F_oH(t)$ to a circular, flat-ended, rigid-porous indenter of radius R. The contact surface (z=0) between the tissue and the indenter tip is assumed to be frictionless. Under these assumptions, the boundary conditions are

$$p(r,0,t) = 0, \quad (44a)$$

$$(r,0,t) = 0, \quad (44b)$$

$$u_z(r,0,t) = u(t), \quad \text{for } r < R, \tag{44c}$$

$$\sigma_{zz}(r,0,t) = 0, \quad \text{for } r > R. \tag{44d}$$

For creep problems, the indenter displacement u(t) is unknown. However, similar to the creep problem for unconfined-compression configuration, the additional equation for obtaining u(t) is derived from the loading condition:

$$\int_0^R 2\pi\sigma_{zz} r\,dr = -F_o. \tag{44e}$$

Using a double Laplace and Hankel transform technique, an integral equation of the Fredholm type for the indentation creep was derived derived by Mak and co-workers. The creep solutions can be obtained by inversion of the Laplace transform integral equation (Mak et al 1987). Figure 11 shows a family of normalized creep curves (indenter displacement) for changing Poisson's ratio ν_s. Because these curves depend parametrically on ν_s, they may be used to calculate all three intrinsic biphasic coefficients for articular cartilage: H_A from the equilibrium displacement, ν_s from the shape of the creep displacement curve, and k from the rate of creep (Mow et al 1989b).

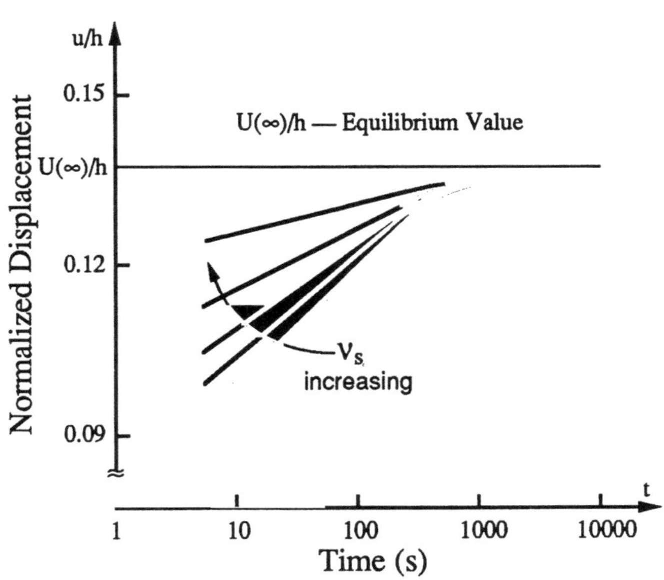

Figure 11. Biphasic indentation creep curves of articular cartilage when normalized to the equilibrium value.

Mak et al (1987) also derived the asymptotic expressions for the indentation creep for $t \to 0$ and $t \to \infty$. For $t \to 0$, the instantaneous behavior of the layer of biphasic tissue under a Heaviside load is the same as that of an equivalent incompressible (ν_s=0.5) elastic layer. This instantaneous response is given by

$$\nu_s = \frac{F_o}{8Ru_o\kappa(R/h,0.5)}, \tag{45}$$

where u_o is the instantaneous displacement of the indenter and κ is a scale factor which is numerically determined from an integral equation derived by Hayes et al (1972). As $t \to \infty$, interstitial fluid flow will cease and indentation will reach an equilibrium value. Here, the response of the linear KLM biphasic layer also agrees with the elastic layer indentation solution derived by Hayes and associates (1972). This expression can be used to determine the elastic constants of the solid matrix λs and μs. Details on the numerical algorithm required to use this mathematical solution for calculating of H_A, ν_s and k are provided in Mow et al (1989b).

Sinusoidal Confined Compression Problem

Oscillation-compression experiments are often used to determine the properties and energy dissipation mechanism of soft tissues (Higginson and Snaith 1976; Lee et al 1978; Mow et al 1986; Sah et al 1989). In this section we shall restrict our attention to the confined compression experiment. First, an offset compressive strain ε_o is applied to the tissue specimen by a slow ramp and held, then stress-relaxation is allowed to take place until equilibrium. A sinusoidal displacement is then imposed at t=0 on the specimen surface (z=0) through the rigid-porous loading platen. The boundary conditions for this oscillation problem are

$$u_z(0,t) = h[\varepsilon_o + \varepsilon_1 \sin(2\pi\omega t)], \quad \text{and} \quad u_z(h,t) = 0, \tag{46}$$

where ε_1 is the amplitude of the oscillating strain and ω is the frequency (Hz) of oscillation. The initial condition is given by the equilibrium strain solution provided by $u_z(z,t) = \varepsilon_o(h-z)$.

In this problem, the total energy dissipation per unit area during each oscillation cycle is calculated from the integral:

$$\Phi_{tot} = \varepsilon_1 h \int_0^{1/\omega} \sigma_c d[\sin(2\pi\omega t)]. \tag{47}$$

where σ_c is the compressive stress measured in the experiment (Mow et al 1987). For the case with a constant permeability k, this problem can be solved by using Fourier's series. The compressive stress response to the oscillating surface displacement is found to be

$$\sigma_c = H_A\Bigg\{\varepsilon_o + \varepsilon_1\Bigg[\sin(2\pi\omega t) -$$

$$\sum_{n=1}^{\infty}\frac{4\pi(n\pi R)^2}{(n\pi R)^4+4\pi^2}\Bigg(\cos(2\pi\omega t) + \frac{2\pi}{(n\pi R)^2}\sin(2\pi\omega t) - e^{(n\pi R)^2\omega t}\Bigg)\Bigg]\Bigg\}. \tag{48a}$$

where the dimensionless characteristic parameter is $R^2=H_Ak/(\omega h^2)$. Of interest is the steady state harmonic response as $t\rightarrow\infty$. This is given by the following equation:

$$\frac{\sigma_c}{H_A} = \varepsilon_o + \varepsilon_1\Bigg[\sin(2\pi\omega t)-\sum_{n=1}^{\infty}\frac{4\pi(n\pi R)^2}{(n\pi R)^4+4\pi^2}\Bigg(\cos(2\pi\omega t)+\frac{2\pi}{(n\pi R)^2}\sin(2\pi\omega t)\Bigg)\Bigg]. \tag{48b}$$

The low frequency response of the tissue is often studied in experiments. The asymptotic approximation of this equation for low frequencies (defined by the condition $\omega<<H_Ak/h^2$) is given by the following simple expression

$$\frac{\sigma_c}{H_A} = \varepsilon_o + \varepsilon_1\Bigg[\sin(2\pi\omega t) + \frac{2\pi}{3R^2}\cos(2\pi\omega t)\Bigg] + \cdots. \tag{49}$$

For the strain-dependent permeability k case, equation (11), an asymptotic approximation for the compressive stress for slow frequencies is also available. This is given by:

$$\frac{\sigma_c}{H_A} = \varepsilon_o + \varepsilon_1\Bigg[\sin(2\pi\omega t) + \frac{2\pi}{3R^2}\cos(2\pi\omega t)e^{M[\varepsilon_o+\varepsilon_1\sin(2\pi\omega t)]}\Bigg] + \cdots. \tag{50}$$

As with the stress-relaxation problem, fast compression rates can cause very large stresses and strains to be developed on or near the surface, thus invalidating the use of this theory. In general, a slow compression rate (i.e., $R^2\sim1$) is desired experimentally and theoretically. For all biphasic materials, there exists a natural recovery speed when the load is removed from the surface. This recovery speed is dictated by the elasticity of the solid matrix, and the frictional resistance it offers against interstitial fluid flow. For example, a stiff porous-permeable elastic solid matrix (H_A is large) with high permeability (k is large) will have a very fast recovery speed, and vice versa. Therefore, for each specimen, a critical frequency exists beyond which the loading platen will move faster than the recovery speed and "lift-off" from the tissue surface. We define the lift-off frequency to be that frequency when the surface stress $\sigma_c=0$, i.e., the frequency at which the terms in the brackets of equations (49) and (50) cancel the compressive stress caused by the imposed ε_o. When this happens, there is a separation between the cartilage surface and the loading platen, and no force will be measured through the transducer.

In our experiments on cartilage, this lift-off phenomenon has been observed repeatedly at frequencies around 0.1 Hz. Using the linear biphasic theory, we can determine the lift-off frequency and its dependence on the stiffness H_A, permeability k, thickness h, off-set strain ε_o and the amplitude of the oscillation strain ε_1. The theory predicts that lift-off happens when the parameter $R^2<0.05$, with $\varepsilon_o = 0.1$ and $\varepsilon_1 = 0.01$. For example, if $H_A = 0.5$ MPa, $k = 4\times10^{-15}$ m^4/Ns and h = 2 mm, with an off-set strain $\varepsilon_o = 0.1$ and oscillation strain $\varepsilon_1 = 0.01$, the "cut-off" frequency ω at which lift-off occurs may be as low as 0.025 Hz; for these values $R^2 = 0.02$, Figure 12. The figure also shows the calculated surface speed when compared with the sinusoidal loading platen speed. At point L, lift-off will occur. This effect may explain the discrepancy between the predictions of the linear KLM biphasic theory and experimental data in their sinusoidal confined compression study where frequencies as high as 20 Hz were used (Lee et al 1981).

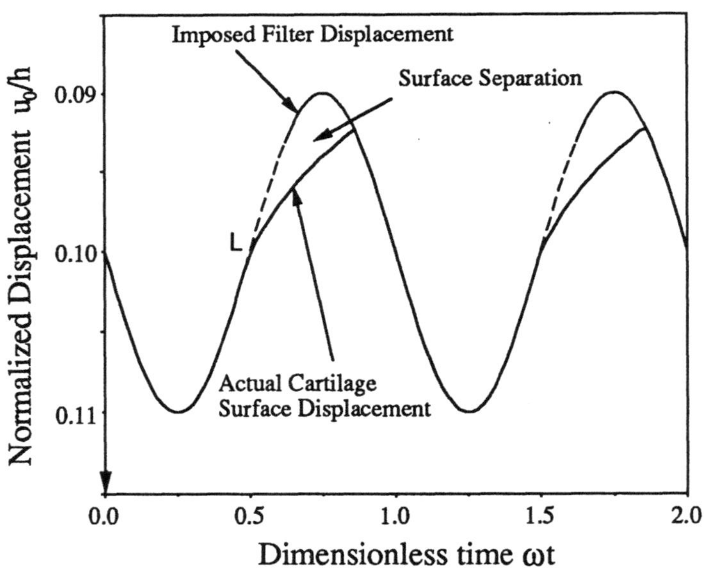

Figure 12. Normalized displacement of the articular surface relative to that of an oscillating loading platen. For example, at frequencies $\omega>50H_Ak/h^2$ — lift-off of the platen from the cartilage surface occurs at point L.

Uniaxial Tension Problem

The tensile characteristics of articular cartilage are indicative of the tensile behavior of the native collagen network within the tissue (Kempson 1979; Woo et al 1976; Roth and Mow 1980) and have been used as a method of quantifying the structural disorganization of the solid matrix found in degenerate and aging articular cartilage (Kempson 1979). Tensile properties of tendons, ligaments and meniscus have also been extensively studied (see for example chapters by Kelly et al, Viidik et al, and Woo et al, in these volumes). Most of the early tensile studies of collagenous tissues used spring, dashpot and friction element viscoelastic models to describe their stress-strain behaviors (Frisen et al 1969, Haut and Little 1972). Woo and co-workers (1981) used the quasi-linear viscoelastic (QLV) theory proposed by Fung to describe the constant strain-rate and cyclic experimental results of cartilage and the medial collateral ligament.

In this section, the linear KLM biphasic theory is used to describe the unidirectional constant-strain rate tensile experiment for articular cartilage. The typical dimensions of the gauge section of a tensile specimen are (l × w × t) = (10mm×1.5mm×300μm). Here, tensile strain rate is used as the experimental parameter of study. In our theoretical formulation, the x-axis is along the length, y is along the width and z is along the thickness directions, respectively. Since the length of the specimen is much greater than both the width and thickness, the theoretical problem can be shown to be approximated by a one dimensional problem, where the pressure, stresses and strains are functions of z and t only. In this case, the governing equation for the pressure is given by:

$$H_A k \frac{\partial^2 p}{\partial z^2} = \frac{\partial p}{\partial t} + \frac{\mu_s}{\lambda_s+\mu_s} \frac{\partial}{\partial t}\left(\frac{2}{h} \int_0^{h/2} p\,dz \right) + \frac{\mu_s H_A}{\lambda_s+\mu_s} \dot{\varepsilon}. \tag{51}$$

This equation is solved with the boundary condition p = 0 at z = ±h/2. Once the pressure distribution p is obtained from this equation, the total tensile force per unit cross-section area can then be calculated from the following formula:

$$\bar{\sigma}_{xx} = E_s \dot{\varepsilon} t - \frac{\mu_s}{\lambda_s+\mu_s}\left(\frac{2}{h} \int_0^{h/2} p\,dz \right). \tag{52}$$

The contractions in the z- and y- directions, $-\bar{\varepsilon}_z$ and $-\bar{\varepsilon}_y$, are given by the formulas:

$$-\bar{\varepsilon}_z = \frac{1}{4}\left(\dot{\varepsilon} t - \frac{1}{\lambda_s+\mu_s} \frac{2}{h} \int_0^{h/2} p\,dz \right), \tag{53}$$

$$-\bar{\varepsilon}_y = \frac{1}{4}\left(\dot{\varepsilon} t - \frac{1}{\lambda_s} \frac{2}{h} \int_0^{h/2} p\,dz \right). \tag{54}$$

For initial short time, an asymptotic approximation for the average tensile stress is given by a very simple formula in terms of the material coefficients, specimen thickness and time:

$$\bar{\sigma}_{xx} = 3\mu_s\dot{\varepsilon}t\left(1 - \frac{8\mu_s}{9h}\sqrt{\frac{kt}{\pi H_A}} - \frac{2k\mu_s^2 t}{3H_A h^2} + \cdots\right). \tag{55}$$

The ratios of the lateral strains, in the y and z directions respectively, versus the longitudinal strain (x) for initial short time are given by:

$$-\frac{\bar{\varepsilon}_y}{\dot{\varepsilon}t} = \frac{1}{2} - \frac{2(1-2\nu_s)}{3(1-\nu_s)}\sqrt{\frac{H_A k}{\pi h^2}t} + \cdots, \tag{56}$$

$$-\frac{\bar{\varepsilon}_z}{\dot{\varepsilon}t} = \frac{1}{4(1-\nu_s)} - \frac{(1-2\nu_s)^2}{3(1-\nu_s)^2}\sqrt{\frac{H_A k}{\pi h^2}t} + \cdots. \tag{57}$$

Equations (55)-(57) are three very simple equations for the three unknown intrinsic material coefficients of the linear KLM biphasic material (H_A,μ_s,k).[3]

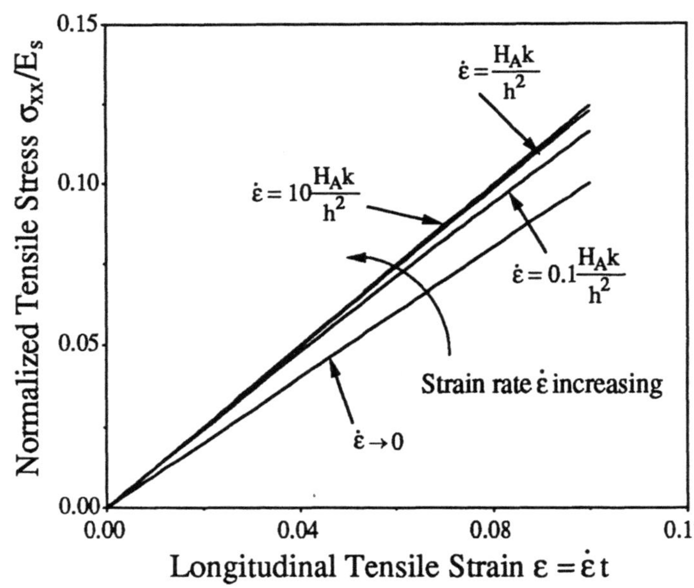

Figure 13. Average tensile stress of the uniaxial tension of articular cartilage as predicted by the biphasic theory. Higher strain rate produces higher tensile stress.

[3]By virtue of the assumed isotropy of the solid matrix, only two independent constants exist, i.e., if we know H_A and μ_s, then we may calculate ν_s.

Figure 13 shows the average tensile stress for different values of parameter $R^2=H_A k/(\dot{\varepsilon}h^2)$ with an assumed value of Poisson's ratio $\nu_s = 0.2$. When $R\rightarrow\infty$, it represents either an extremely slow strain rate ($\dot{\varepsilon}\rightarrow 0$) or a very high permeability ($k\rightarrow\infty$). In either case, the diffusive drag caused by the relative motion between the solid and fluid phases offers no contribution to the tissue behavior, and therefore the strain-stress response is the same as the equilibrium elastic curve. Experimentally, the Poisson's ratio effect in the lateral contraction in the width direction (y) can be measured (e.g., see Woo et al 1986). It would indeed be very difficult to determine the lateral contraction in the thickness direction (z). Thus, in practical terms, it would be very difficult to determine all three intrinsic material coefficients of a biological material from these constant strain-rate tensile experiments (Li et al 1983).

Flow Independent Viscoelastic Behavior of the Solid Matrix — QLV Theory

The previous discussions on hydrated soft tissues have focused on how interstitial fluid flow influences the viscoelastic creep and stress-relaxation behavior of cartilage, meniscus and intervertebral disc materials. Interstitial fluid flow always occurs when these tissues are compressed or stretched since a volume change always occurs, or when a pressure gradient is applied. However, when these tissues are subjected to the action of pure shear, no volume change occurs and no pressure gradients exist; thus no interstitial fluid flow occurs. When tissue specimens are subjected to pure shear, the response is that offered by the intrinsic viscoelasticity of the collagen-proteoglycan solid matrix. This is sometimes known as the "flow-independent" viscoelastic behavior of the solid matrix (Hayes and Bodine 1978; Mow et al 1982; Myers et al 1988; Sprit et al 1987). For pure shear experiments on cartilage, we have found that the quasi-linear viscoelastic (QLV) model proposed by Fung (1972, 1981) provides an excellent theory to describe the response of the collagen-proteoglycan solid matrix (Zhu et al 1986; Myers et al 1988).

The essentials of the QLV theory are similar to the linear superposition theory of Boltzmann. The history of the stress response $K(\lambda,t)$ due to a step increase in elongation (λ) is assumed to be of the form:

$$K(\lambda,t) = G(t)T^e(\lambda), \quad \text{with} \quad G(0) = 1, \tag{58}$$

where $G(t)$ is the (normalized) reduced relaxation function, and $T^e(\lambda)$ is known as the elastic response. Using the superposition principle, the response of the total stress due to a continuous stretch $T^e[\lambda(t)]$, history can be written in the form

$$T(t) = \int_{-\infty}^{t} G(t-\tau)\dot{T}^e(\tau)d\tau. \tag{59}$$

We note that equation (59) uses an elastic stress $T^e(\lambda)$, which in general need not be a linear function, together with a linear superposition integral. This provides the quasi-linear name for this viscoelasticity theory. The inverse of equation (59) defines the reduced creep function J(t) which yields the stretch, $\lambda(t)$, due to a continuous loading history T(t):

$$T^e[\lambda(t)] = \int_{-\infty}^{t} J(t-\tau)\dot{T}(\tau)d\tau. \tag{60}$$

If the motion starts at time t = 0 rather than $-\infty$, then equation (60) reduces to

$$T(t) = T^e(0+)G(t) + \int_{0}^{t} G(t-\tau)\frac{\partial T^e[\lambda(t-\tau)]}{\partial \tau}\,d\tau. \tag{61}$$

It can be easily shown that this equation may also be written in the following experimentally more convenient form given by:

$$T(t) = T^e[\lambda(\tau)] + \int_{0}^{t} T^e[\lambda(\tau)]\frac{\partial G(\tau)}{\partial \tau}\,d\tau, \tag{61}$$

where $T^e(\lambda)$ is directly measured (Woo et al 1981). In using the QVL theory, a reduced relaxation function G(t) must be chosen. This is usually taken to be a sum of exponential functions as:

$$G(t) = \frac{\sum C_i e^{-\nu_i t}}{\sum C_i} . \tag{63}$$

For biological materials which are relatively strain-rate insensitive, Fung (1981) proposed a continuous distribution of the exponents ν_i for the reduced relaxation function given by:

$$G(t) = \frac{1 + \int_{0}^{\infty} S(\tau)e^{-t/\tau}d\tau}{1 + \int_{0}^{\infty} S(\tau)d\tau} , \tag{64}$$

with a specific spectrum function S(t):

$$S(\tau) = \begin{cases} \frac{c}{\tau}, & \text{for } \tau_1 \le \tau \le \tau_2 , \\ 0, & \text{for } \tau < \tau_1 , \tau > \tau_2, \end{cases} \tag{65}$$

where c is a constant. A number of authors have used this quasi-linear model to study the intrinsic viscoelastic behavior of the solid matrix of biological soft tissue, such as ligament and cartilage in tension (Woo et al 1981, 1986) cartilage in shear (Mak 1986; Spirt et al 1989; Zhu et al 1986).

Discussions and Conclusions

In this chapter, we have provided detailed discussions on some major connective tissues, i.e., articular cartilage, meniscus and intervertebral disc. Because these connective tissues play essential roles in the function of the musculoskeletal system, and because their pathologies lead to severe disabilities, much research has been devoted to them in order to understand their composition, molecular and ultrastructural organization, material properties and function. Although each of the three tissues discussed in this chapter is compositional and structurally unique, the macromolecules that provide the mechanical properties of the tissues are similar — collagen and proteoglycans. The viscoelastic behavior of these tissues have been modeled by either the biphasic theories (or triphasic theory — see chapter by Lai et al in these volumes) proposed by Mow and co-workers (1980, 1984a, 1986) or the quasi-linear viscoelastic theory proposed by Fung (1972, 1981).

The collagen-proteoglycan solid phase represents 20-30% of the tissue by wet weight, and the fluid phase, chiefly water and dissolved inorganic salts, saturates this solid matrix and comprises the remainder of the tissue. The inorganic salts dissolved in the interstitial fluid yield ions at high concentration which contribute to the large osmotic swelling pressure exhibited by cartilage and intervertebral disc. Each phase and each distinct constituent of both the solid and fluid phases contribute to the material properties of these tissues enabling them to ultimately fulfill the functional demands required by the body.

Often, for biologists and biomedical researchers, the notion of theoretical modeling of material behavior seems confusing. We have provided some simple discussions on how theoretical modeling of material behaviors should be done in general, and how the behavior of hydrated soft tissues should be modeled specifically. The reader is referred to the extensive treatise by Truesdell and Noll (1965) for a complete and thorough discussion on constitutive modeling of material properties. The most commonly used constitutive models to describe the viscoelastic creep and stress-relaxation behaviors of hydrated soft tissues and for stress-strain analyses are the general theoretical formulations for binary mixture theory by Mow et al (1980) and Bowen (1980). This biphasic theory can describe the viscoelastic creep and stress-relaxation behaviors of articular cartilage, meniscus and intervertebral disc. A summary of important mathematical solutions for the biphasic theory has been presented. These mathematical solutions correspond to the following experiments: 1) steady state uniaxial filtration with constant permeability and the strain-dependent permeability; 2) confined compression creep and stress-relaxation; 3) unconfined compression creep and stress-relaxation; 4) indentation creep; 5) the steady-state sinusoidal confined compression; and 6) uniaxial tension. These are very useful mathematical solutions. They provided the simplest equations for the analyses of common experimental configurations used to determine the material properties of hydrated soft tissues such as articular cartilage, meniscus and intervertebral disc. These simple solutions also provide insights into the mechanisms giving rise to hydrated soft tissue viscoelasticity. Finally, we provide some cautionary advice for investigators attempting to use these theories. Every theory and every mathematical solution has it limitations. When used inappropriately, the theory can not be expected to provide good results. We believe, nevertheless, the current biphasic and quasi-linear viscoelastic theories provide sufficient flexibility and power to describe the deformational behaviors of most hydrated soft tissues.

The ability of articular cartilage, meniscus and intervertebral disc to function is dependent on their unique material properties which are in turn dependent on their composition, microstructural organization and anatomical form. Pathologic situations (such as osteoarthritis and intervertebral disc degeneration) alter the composition of articular cartilage and their microstructural organization. These changes can alter the material properties of cartilage; in general, there is a decrease of stiffness in tension and compression, and an increase of permeability. These changes impair the ability of these tissues to bear load in joints, thus making it more vulnerable to further injuries and degeneration. When an imbalance occurs between rates of maintenance or repair and degradation of the collagen-proteoglycan network, tissue failure occurs with the likely development of osteoarthritis or low back pain. During the next decade, we expect that biomechanics will play a major role in determining the pathophysiology of these diseases.

References

Adams ME, Muir H: The glycosaminoglycans of canine meniscus. Biochem J 1981;197:385-389.

Adams P, Eyre DR, Muir H: Biochemical aspects of development and aging of human intervertebral discs. Rheum Rehab 1977;16:22-29.

Akizuki S, Mow VC, Müller F, Pita JC, Howell DS, Manicourt DH: Tensile properties of knee joint cartilage: I. Influence of ionic conditions, weight bearing, and fibrillation on the tensile modulus. J Orthop Res 1986;4:379-392.

Akizuki S, Mow VC, Müller F, Pita JC, Howell DS: Tensile properties of knee joint cartilage: II. Correlations between weight bearing and tissue pathology and the kinetics of swelling. J Orthop Res 1987;5:173-186.

Anderson G, Schultz A: Effects of fluid injection on mechanical properties of intervertebral discs. J Biomech 1979;12:453-458.

Armstrong CG, Mow VC: Biomechanics of normal and osteoarthrotic articular cartilage. In Wilson PD Jr, Straub LR (eds): Cilinical Trends in Orthopaedics. Thiem-Stratton Inc, 1982a, pp 189-197.

Armstrong CG, Mow VC: Variations in the intrinsic mechanical properties of human articular cartilage with age, degeneration, and water content. J Bone Joint Surg 1982b;64A:88-94.

Armstrong CG, Mow VC, Lai WM: An analysis of unconfined compression of articular cartilage. J Biomech Engng 1984;106:165-173.

Askew MJ, Mow VC: The biomechanical function of the collagen ultrastructure of articular cartilage. J Biomech Eng 1978;100:105-115.

Aspden RM, Yarker YE, Hukins DWL: Collagen orientations in the meniscus of the knee joint. J Anat 1985;140:371-381.

Bar E: Elasticiatssprufunger der gelenkknorpel. Arch Entwickklungsmech Organ 1926;108:739-760.

Benninghoff A. Form und Bau der Gelenkknorpel in ihren Beziehungen zur Funktion: Zweiter Teil. Der Aufbau des Gelenkknorpels in Seinen Bezienhungen zur Funktion. Z Zellforsch Mikrosk Anat 1925;2:783-862.

Berthet C, Hulmes DJS, Miller A, Timmins PA: Structure of collagen in cartilage of IVD. Science 1978;199(4328):547-549.

Best BA, Setton LA, Guilak F, Ratcliffe A, Weidenbaurm M, Mow VC: Permeability and compressive stiffness of annulus fibrosus: variation with site and composition. Tran Orthop Res Soc 1989;14:354.

Biot MA: General theory of three-dimensional consolidation. J App Phys 1941; 12:155-164.

Biot MA: Theory of elasticity and consolidation for a porous anisotropic solid. J App Phys 1955;26:182-185.

Bowen RM: Incompressible porous media models by use of the theory of mixtures. Int J Eng Sci 1980;18:1129-1148.

Brown TD, Radin EL, Martin RB, Burr DB: Finite element studies of some juxtarticular stress changes due to localized subchondral stiffening. J Biomech 1984;17:11-24.

Brown TD, Singerman RJ: Experimental determination of the linear biphasic constitutive coefficients of human fetal proximal femoral chondroepiphysis. J Biomech 1986;19:597-605.

Bruckner P, Vaughan L, Winthalter KH: Type IX collagen from sternal cartilage of chicken embryo contains covalently bound glycosaminoglycans. Proc Natl Acad Sci USA, 1985;82:2608-2615.

Buckwalter JA, Pedrini-Mille A, Pedrini V, Tudisco C: Proteoglycans of human infant intervertebral disc: Electron microscopic and biochemical studies. J Bone Joint Surg 1985;67A:284-294.

Buckwalter JA, Rosenberg LC: Electron microscopic studies of cartilage proteoglycans: Direct evidence for the variable length of the chondroitin sulfate rich region of the proteoglycan subunit core protein. J Biol Chem 1982; 257:9830-9839.

Buckwalter JA: The fine structure of human intervertebral disc, in White III, AA, Gordon, SL (eds): Symposium on Idiopathic Low Back Pain. Am Acad Orthop Surg 1982, pp 108-143.

Buckwalter JA, Hunziker E, Rosenberg LC, Coutts R, Adams M, Eyre D: Articular Cartilage: Composition and Structure. In Woo SLY, Buckwalter JA (eds): Injury and Repair of the Musculoskeletal Soft Tissues. Am Acad Orthop Surg 1987, pp 405-425.

Bullough P, Goodfellow J: The significance of the fine structure of articular cartilage. J. Bone Joint Surg, 1968;50B:852-857.

Bullough PG, Munuera L, Murphy J, Weinstein AM: The strength of the menisci of

the knee as it relates to their fine structure. J Bone Joint Surg 1970;52B:564-570.
Carney SL, Billingham MEJ, Muir H, Sandy JD: Structure of newly synthesized 35S-proteoglycans and 35S-proteoglycan turnover products of cartilage explant cultures from dogs with experimental osteoarthritis. J Orthop Res 1985;3:140-147.
Choi HU, Tang L-H, Johnson TL, Rosenberg L: Proteoglycans from bovine nasal and articular cartilages. Fractionation of the link proteins by wheat germ agglutinin affinity chromatography. J Biol Chem 1985;260:13370-13376.
Clark JM: The organization of collagen in cryofractured rabbit articular cartilage: A scanning electron microscopic study. J Orthop Res 1985;3:17-29.
Clarke IC: Articular cartilage: a review and electron microsope study. J Bone Joint Surg 1971;53B:732-750.
Colleti JM, Akeson WH, Woo SLY: A comparison of the physical behavior of normal articular cartilage and the arthroplasty surface. J Bone Joint Surg 1972; 54A:147-160.
Donnan FG: The theory of membrane equilibria. Chem Rev 1924;1:73-90.
Edmond E, Ogston AG: An approach to the study of phase separation in ternary aqueous systems. Biochem J 1968;109:569-576.
Edwards J: Physical characteristics of articular cartilage. Proc Inst Mech Engng, London 1967;181:16-24.
Eisenberg SR, Grodzinsky AJ: Swelling of articular cartilage and other connective tissues: electromechanochemical forces. J Orthop Res 1985;3:148-159.
Elmore SM, Sokoloff L, Norris G, Carmeci P: Nature of "imperfect" elasticity of articular cartilage. J App Physiol 1963;18:393-396.
Eyre DR: Biochemistry of the intervertebral disc. Int Rev Connect Tiss Res 1979;8:227-291.
Eyre DR: Collagen: Molecular diversity in the body's protein scaffold. Science, 207:1315-1322,1980.
Eyre DR, Grynpas MD, Shapiro FD, Creasman CM: Crosslink formation and molecular packing in articular cartilage collagen. Semin Arth Rheum 1981;11 Supp:46-48.
Eyre DR, Koob TJ, Van Ness KP: Quantitation of hydroxypyridinium cross-links in collagen by high-performance liquid chromatography. Anal Biochem 1984;137:380-388.
Eyre D, Apon S, Wu J-J, Ericsson LH, Walsh KA: Collagen Type IX: Evidence for covalent linkages to Type II Collagen in Cartilage. FEBS Letters, 1987a;320:337-341.
Eyre D, and Wu, J-J: Type IX of 1a2a3a Collagen. In Maine R, Burgeson RE (eds): Structure and Function of Collagen Types. Academic Press, 1987b.
Ferry JD: Viscoelastic Properties of Polymers. 2nd ed. New York, John Wiley & Sons Inc, 1970.
Frisen M, Magi M, Sonnerup L, Viidik A: Rheological analysis of soft collagenous tissue. Part II. J Biomech 1969;2:13-20.
Fung, YC: Foundations of Solid Mechanics. Englewood Cliff, NJ, Prentice-Hall, 1965.
Fung YC: Biomechanics: Its Foundation and Objectives. In Fung YC, Perrone N, M Anliker (eds): Englewood Cliff, NJ, Prentice-Hall, 1972.
Fung YC: Quasi-linear viscoelasticity of soft tissues. In Mechanical Properties of Living Tissues. New York, Springer-Verlag, 1981, pp 226-238.
Fithian DC, Kelly MA, Mow VC: Material properties and structure-function relationships in the menisci. Clin Orthop Rel Res 1990;252:19-31.
Galante J: Tensile properties of the human lumbar annulus fibrosus. Acta Orthop Scand 1967;100:7-91.

Ghosh P: The Biology of the Intervertebral Disc. Vols. I-II. Boca Raton, CRC Press Inc.,1988.
Gocke E: Elastizitats studien am junger und alten gelenkknorpel. Verh Deutsch Orthop Ges 1927;22:130-147.
Hardingham TE, Muir H.: The specific interaction of hyaluronic acid with cartilage proteoglycans. Biochim Biophys Acta, 1972;279:401-405.
Hardingham TE, Muir H: Hyaluronic acid in cartilage and proteoglycan aggregation. Biochem J 1974;139:565-581.
Hardingham TE: The role of link protein in the structure of cartilage proteoglycan aggregates. Biochem J 1979;177:237-247.
Hardingham TE. Proteoglycans: Their structure, interactions and molecular organization in cartilage. Biochem Soc Trans 1981;489-497.
Hardingham TE, Muir H, Kwan MK, Lai WM, Mow VC: Viscoelastic properties of proteoglycan solutions with varying proportions present as aggregates. J Orthop Res 1987;5:36-46.
Hascall VC, Heinegard D: Aggregation of cartilage proteoglycans I. The role of hyaluronic acid. J Biol Chem 1974a;249:4232-4241.
Hascall VC, Heinegard D: Aggregation of cartilage proteoglycans II. Oligosaccharide competitors of the proteoglycan-hyaluronic acid interaction. J Biol Chem 1974b;249:4242-4249.
Hascall VC: Interactions of cartilage proteoglycans with hyaluronic acid. J Supramol Struct 1977;7:101-120.
Hascall VC, Hascall GK: Proteoglycans. In Hay ED (ed): Cell Biology of Extracellular Matrix. Plenum Press, New York, 1981, pp 39-63.
Haut RC, Little RW: A constitutive equation for collagen fibers. J Biomech 1972;5:423-430.
Hayes WC, Mockros LF: Viscoelastic properties of human articular cartilage. J Appl Physiol 1971;31:562-568.
Hayes WC, Keer LM, Herrmann G, Mockros LF: A mathematical analysis for the indentation tests of articular cartilage. J Biomech 1972;11:407-419.
Hayes WC, Bodine AJ: Flow-independent viscoelastic properties of articular cartilage matrix. J Biomech 1978;11:407-419.
Heinegard D, Paulsson M, Inerot S, Carlstrom C: A novel, low molecular weight chondroitin sulfate proteoglycan isolated from cartilage. J BiochemJ 1981;197:355-366.
Hewitt AT, Varner HH, Silver MH: The role of chondronectin and cartilage proteoglycan in the attachment of chondrocytes to collagen. In Kelly RO, Goetinck PF, MacCabe JA (eds): Limb Development and Regeneration, Part B. Raven Press, 1982, pp 25-33.
Hickey DS, Hukins DWL: Relation between the structure of the annulus fibrosus and the function and failure of the intervertebral disc. Spine 1980;5:106-116.
Higginson GR, Snaith JE: The mechanical stiffness of articular cartilage in confined oscillating compression. I Mech E 1979;8:11-14.
Hirsch C: The pathogenesis of chondromalacia of the patella. Acta Chir Scand 1944;83Supp:1-106.
Hock DH, Grodzinsky AJ, Koob TJ, Albert ML, Eyre DR: Early changes in material properties of rabbit articular cartilage after meniscectomy. J Orthop Res 1983;1:4-12.
Holmes MH: A nonlinear diffusion equation arising in the study of soft tissue. Quart Appl Math 1983;61:209-220.
Holmes MH, Lai WM, Mow VC: Singular perturbation analysis of the nonlinear flow dependent compressive stress relaxation behavior of articular cartilage. J Biomech Eng 1985;107:206-218.
Holmes MH: Finite deformation of soft tissue: analysis of a mixture model in uni-

axial compression. J Biomech Eng 1986;108:372-381.
Hori RY, Mockros LF: Indentation tests of human articular cartilage. J Biomech 1976;9:259-268.
Hultkrantz W: Ueber die spaltrichtungen der gelenknorpel. Verh Dsch Anat Ges 1898;12:248.
Hunziker EB, Schenk RK: Structural organization of proteoglycans in cartilage. In Wight TW, Mecham RP (eds): Biology of Proteoglycans, Academic Press, 1987, pp 155-183.
Jurvelin J, Kiviranta I, Aronkoski J, Tammi M, Helminen HJ: Indentation study of the biomechanical properties of articular cartilage in canine knee. Engng Med 1987;16:16-22.
Kempson GE, Muir H, Swanson SAV, Freeman MAR: Correlations between stiffness and chemical constituents of cartilage on the human femoral head. Biochim Biophys Acta 1970;215:70-77.
Kempson GE, Muir H, Pollard C, Tuke M: The tensile properties of the cartilage of human femoral condyles related to the content of collagen and glycosaminoglycans. Biochim Biophys Acta 1973;297:456-472.
Kempson GE, Spivey CJ, Swanson SAV, Freeman MAR: Patterns of cartilage stiffness on normal and degenerate femoral heads. J Biomech 1971;4:597-609.
Kempson GE: Mechanical properties of articular cartilage, in Freeman MAR (ed): Adult Articular Cartilage, 2nd ed. Pitman Medical, 1979, pp 333-414.
Kenyon DE: The theory of an incompressible solid-fluid mixture. Arch Rat Mech Anal 1976;62:131-147.
Kenyon DE: A model for surface flow in cartilage. J Biomech 1980;13:129-134.
Kwan MK, Woo SLY, Amiel D, Kleiner JB, Field FP, Coutts RD: Neocartilage generated from rib perchondrium: A long term multi-disciplinary evaluation. Tran Orthop Res Soc 1987;12:277.
Kwan MK, Wayne JS, Woo SLY, Field FP, Hoover J, Meyers M: Histological and biomechanical assessment of articular cartilage from stored osteochondral shell allografts. J Orthop Res 1989;7:637-644.
Kwan MK, Lai WM, Mow VC: A finite deformation theory for cartilage and other soft hydrated connective tissues — I. Equilibrium results, J Biomech 1990;23:145-156.
Lai WM, Mow VC: Drag-induced compression of articular cartilage during a permeation experiment. Biorheol 1980;17:111-123.
Lai WM, Hou JS, Mow VC: A triphasic theory for articular cartilage swelling, Proc Biomech Symp ASME, 1989;AMD98:33-36.
Lai WM, Hou JS, Mow VC: A triphasic theory for the swelling and deformational behavior of cartilage, J Biomech Eng In Press, 1990.
Lane JM, Weiss C: Review of articular cartilage collagen research, Arth Rheum 1975;18:553-562.
Lee RC, Frank EH, Grodzinsky AJ, Roylance DK: Oscillatory compressional behavior of articular cartilage and its electromechanical properties. J Biomech Eng 1981;103:280-292.
Li JT, Armstrong CG, Mow VC: The effect of strain rate on mechanical properties of articular cartilage in tension. Biomech Symp ASME, 1983; AMD56:117-120.
Linn FC, Sokoloff L: Movement and composition of interstitial fluid of cartilage. Arth Rheum 1965;8:481-494.
Lipshitz H, Etheredge R, Glimcher MJ: Changes in the Hexosamine Content and Swelling Ratio of Articular Cartilage as Functions of Depth from the Surface. J Bone Joint Surg 1976;58A:1149-1153.
Mak AF: The apparent viscoelastic behavior of articular cartilage—the contributions from the intrinsic matrix viscoelasticity and interstitital fluid flow. J Biomech Eng 1986;108:123-130.

Mak AF, Lai WM, Mow VC: Biphasic Indentation of Articular Cartilage: I. Theoretical Analysis. J Biomech 1987;20:703-714.

Mankin HJ, Thrasher AZ: Water content and binding in normal and osteoarthritic cartilage, J Bone Joint Surg 1975;57A:76-80.

Manicourt DH, Pita JC, McDevitt CA, Howell DS: Superficial and deeper layers of dog normal articular cartilage: Role of hyaluronate and link protein in determining the sedimentation coefficients distribution of the non-dissociately extracted proteoglycans. J Biol Chem 1988;263:13121-13129.

Mansour JM, Mow VC: The permeability of articular cartilage under compressive strain and at high pressures. J Bone Joint Surg 1976;58A:509-516.

Maroudas A: Biophysical chemistry of cartilaginous tissues with special reference to solute and fluid transport. Biorheol 1975;12:233-248.

Maroudas A: Balance between swelling pressure and collagen tension in normal and degenerate cartilage. Nature 1976;260:808-809.

Maroudas A: Physicochemical properties of articular cartilage, in Freeman AR (ed): Adult Articular Cartilage. Turnbridge Wells, England, Pitman Medical, 1979, pp 215-290.

Maroudas A, Venn M: Chemical composition and swelling of normal and osteoarthritic femoral head cartilage. II: Swelling. Ann Rheum Dis 1977;36:399-406.

Maroudas A, Bayliss MT, Venn MF. Further studies on the composition of human femoral head cartilage. Ann Rheum Dis 1980;39:514-523.

Maroudas A, Schneidermann R: "Free" and "exchangeable" or "trapped" and "non-exchangeable" water in cartilage. J Orthop Res 1987;5:133-138.

Mayne R, Irwin MH: Collagen types in cartilage, in Kuettner, KE, Schleyerbachand R, Hascall VC (eds): Articular Cartilage Biochemistry. Raven Press, New York, 1986, pp 23-38.

McDevitt CA, Muir H: Biochemical changes in the cartilage of the knee in experimental and natural osteoarthritis in the dog. J Bone Joint Surg 1976; 58B:94-101.

Mow VC, Kuei SC, Lai WM, Armstrong CG: Biphasic creep and stress relaxation of articular cartilage in compression: Theory and experiments. J Biomech Eng 1980;102:73-84.

Mow VC, Lai WM, Holmes MH: Advanced theoretical and experimental techniques in cartilage research, in Huiskes R, van Campen DH, de Wijn JR (eds): Biomechanics: Principals and Applications. The Hague, Martinus Nijhoff Publishers, 1982, pp 47-74.

Mow VC, Holmes MH, Lai WM: Fluid transport and mechanical properties of articular cartilage. J Biomech 1984a;17:377-394.

Mow VC, Mak AF, Lai WM, Rosenberg LC, Tang LH: Viscoelastic properties of proteoglycan subunits and aggregates in varying solution concentrations. J Biomech 1984b;17:325-338.

Mow VC, Kwan MK, Lai WM, Holmes MH: A finite deformation theory for nonlinearly permeable soft hydrated biological tissues, in Schmid-Schonbein GW, Woo SLY, Zweifach BW (eds): Frontiers in Biomechanics, New York, Springer Verlag, 1986, pp 153-179.

Mow VC, Zhu WB, Lai WM, Hardingham TE, Hughes C, Muir H: Link protein effects on proteoglycan viscometric flow properties. Biochem Biophys Acta 1989a;112:201-208.

Mow VC, Gibbs MC, Lai WM, Zhu WB, Athanasiou KA: Biphasic indentation of articular cartilage — Part II. A numerical algorithm and an experimental study. J Biomech 1989b;22:853-861.

Muir H, Bullough P, Maroudas A: The distribution of collagen in human articular cartilage with some of its physiologic implications. J Bone Joint Surg

1970;52B:554-563.

Muir H: The chemistry of the ground substance of joint cartilage, in Sokolff, L (ed): The Joints and Synovial Fluid. Vol. II. Academic Press, 1980, pp 27-94.

Muir H: Proteoglycans as organizers of the extracellular matrix. Biochem Soc Trans 1983;11:613-622.

Muthiah P, Kuhn K: Studies on proteoglycans obtained from bovine knee joint and ear cartilages: sequential extraction, fractionation, characterization and their effect on fibril formation. Biochim Biophys Acta 1973;304:12-19.

Myers ER, Armstrong CG, Mow VC: Swelling pressure and collagen tension, in Hukins DWL (ed): Connective Tissue Matrix. MacMillan Press Ltd, 1984, pp 161-168.

Myers ER, Lai WM, Mow VC: A continuum theory and an experiment for the ion-induced swelling behavior of articular cartilage. J Biomech Eng 1984b; 106:151-158.

Myers ER, Zhu W, Mow VC: Viscoelastic properties of articular cartilage and meniscus, in Nimni ME (ed): Collagen, Vol II. CRC Press, 1988, pp 267-288.

Nimni ME: Collagen: Structure, Function, and Metabolism in Normal and Fibrotic Tissues. Sem Arth Rheum 1983;13:1-86.

Nimni ME, Harkness RD: Molecular structure and functions of collagen, in Nimni ME (ed): Collagen, Vol I. CRC Press, 1988, pp 1-78.

Obrink B: A study of the interactions between monomeric tropocollagen and glycosaminoglycans. Eur J Biochem 1973;33:387-400.

Panagiotacopulos N, Krauss H, Bloch R: On the mechanical properties of human intervertebral disc material. Biorheol 1979;16:317-330.

Parsons JR, Black JD: The viscoelastic shear behavior of normal rabbit articular cartilage. J Biomech 1977;10:21-29.

Parsons JR, Black JD: Mechanical behavior of articular cartilage: quantitative changes with alteration of ionic environment. J Biomech 1979;12:765-773.

Poole AR, Pidous I, Reiner A, Rosenberg LC: An immunoelectron microscope study of the organization of proteoglycan monomer link protein and collagen in the matrix of articular cartilage. J Cell Biol 1982;93:921-937.

Poole CA, Flint MH, Beaumont BW: Morphological and functional interrelationships of articular cartilage matrices. J Anat 1984;138:113-138.

Pottenger LA, Lyon NB, Hecht JD, Neustadt PM, Robinson RA: Influence of cartilage particle size and proteoglycan aggregation on immobilization of proteoglycans. J Biol Chem 1982;257:11479-11485.

Proctor CS, Schmidt MB, Whipple RR, Kelly MA, Mow VC: Material properties of normal bovine meniscus. J Orthop Res 1989;7:771-782.

Ratcliffe A, Fryer PR, Hardingham TE: The distribution of aggregating proteoglycans in articular cartilage: Comparison of quantitative immunoelectron microscopy with radioimmunoassay and biochemical analysis. J Histochem Cytochem 1984;32:193-201.

Ratcliffe A, Tyler JA, Hardingham TE: Articular cartilage cultured with interleukin 1: increased release of link protein, hyaluronate-binding region, and other proteoglycan fragments. Biochem J 1986;238:571-580.

Rees DA: Sterochemistry and binding behaviour of carbohydrate chains, in Whelan WJ (ed): MTP International Rerview of Science. Biochemistry, Series I, ed. Butterworth & Co Ltd, London, 1975, 5:1-42.

Redler I, Zimny ML: Scanning electron microscopy of normal and abnormal articular cartilage. J Bone Joint Surg 1970;52A:1395-1404.

Redler I, Zimny ML, Mansell J, Mow VC: The Ultrastructure and Biomechanical Significance of the Tidemark of Articular Cartilage. Clin Orthop Rel Res 1975;112:357-362.

Roth V, Mow VC, Lai WM, Eyre DR: Correlation of intrinsic compressive properties

of bovine articular cartilage with its uronic acid and water contents. Trans Orthop Res Soc 1981;6:49.
Roth V, Mow VC: The intrinsic tensile behavior of the matrix of bovine articular cartilage and its variation with age. J Bone Joint Surg 1980;62A:1102-1117.
Ruggeri A, Benazzo F: Collagen-proteoglycan interaction, in Ruggeri A, Motta PM (eds): Ultrastructure of Connective Tissue Matrix. Boston, Martinus Nijhoff Publishers, 1984, pp 113-125.
Sah RLY, Kim Y, Doong JY, Grodzinsky AJ, Plass AHK, Sandy JD: Biosyn-thetic response of cartilage explants to dynamic compression. J Orthop Res 1989;7:619-636.
Sampaio L de O, Bayliss MT, Hardingham TE, Muir H: Dermatan sulfate proteoglycan from human articular cartilage. Variation in its content with age and its structural comparison with a small chondroitin sulfate proteoglycan from pig laryngeal cartilage. Biochem J 1988;254:757-764.
Schmidt MB, Schoonbeck JM, Mow VC, Eyre DR, Chun LE: Effects of enzymatic extraction of proteoglycans on the tensile properties of articular cartilage. Trans Orthop Res Soc 1986;11:450.
Schmidt MB, Schoonbeck JM, Mow VC, Eyre DR, Chun, LE: The relationship between collagen cross-linking and the tensile properties of articular cartilage. Trans Orthop Res Soc 1987;12:134.
Schmidt MB, Mow VC, Chun LE, Eyre DR: Effects of enzymatic extraction of proteoglycans on the tensile properties of articular cartilage. J Orthop Res 1990;8:353-363.
Scott JE: Proteoglycan-fibrillar collagen interactions. Biochem J 1988;252:313-323.
Shirazi-Adl A, Ahmed AM, Shrivastava SC: A finite element study of a lumbar motion segment subjected to pure sagittal plane moments. J Biomech 1986; 19:331-350.
Simon BR, Gaballa MA: Poroelastic finite element models for the spinal motion segment including ionic swelling. In Spilker RL, Simon BR (eds): Computational Methods in Bioengineering, New York, ASME Publishers, 1988;93-99.
Sokoloff L: Elasticity of articular cartilage: effect of ions and viscous solutions. Science 1963;141:1055-1056.
Spilker RL, Jakobs DM, Schultz AB: Material constants for a finite element model ofthe intervertebral disc with a fiber composite annulus, J Biomech Engng, 1986;108:1-11.
Spilker RL, Suh JK, Mow VC: A finite element formulation of the nonlinear biphasic model for articular cartilage and hydrated soft tissues including strain-dependent permeability. In RL Spilker, BR Simon (eds). Computational Methods in Bioengineering, New York, ASME Publishers, 1988, pp 81-92.
Sprit AA, Mak AF, Wassell RP: Nonlinear viscoelastic properties of articular cartilage in shear. J Orthop Res 1989;7:43-49.
Stockwell RA: The interrelationship of cell density and cartilage thickness in mammalian articular cartilage, J Anat 1971;109:411-421.
Stockwell RA: Structure and function of the chondrocyte under mechanical stress. In Helminen HJ et al (eds): Loading, Biology and Health of Articular Structures. Bristol:Wright Publishers, 1987, Chapter 6.
Toole B: Binding and precipitation of soluble collagens by chick embryo cartilage proteoglycans. J Biol Chem 1976;251:895-897.
Torzilli PA: Influence of cartilage conformation on its equilibrium water partition. J Orthop Res 1985;3:473-483.
Torzilli PA: Water content and equilibrium partition in immature cartilage, J Orthop Res 1988;6:766-769.

Truesdell C, Toupin R: The Classical Field Theories, Handbuck der Physik, Berlin, Springer-Verlag, 1960, III/1.
Truesdell C, Noll W: The Nonlinear Field Theories of Mechanics, Handbuck der Physik, Berlin, Springer-Verlag, 1965,III/3.
Urban JPG, Maroudas A: Swelling of the intervertebral disc in vitro. Connect Tiss Res 1981;9:1-10.
Van der Rest M, Mayne R: Type IX Collagen Proteoglycan from Cartilage is Covalently Cross-linked to Type II Collagen. J Biol Chem 1988;263:1615-161.
von der Mark K, Mollenhauer J, Pfaffle M, van Menxel M, Müller, PK: Role of anchorin CII in the interaction of chondrocytes with extracellular collagen, in Kuettner KE, Schleyerbach R, Hascall VC (eds): Articular Cartilage Biochemistry. Raven Press, 1986, pp 125-141.
Weidemann H, Paulsonn M, Timpl R, Engel J, Heinegard D: Domain structure of cartilage proteoglycans revealed by rotary shadowing of intact and fragmented molecules. Biochem J 1984;224:331-333.
Woo SLY, Akeson WH, Jemmott GF: Measurements of nonhomogeneous directional mechanical properties of articular cartilage in tension. J Biomech 1976;9:785-791.
Woo SLY, Lai WM, Mow VC: Biomechanical Properties of Articular Cartilage, in Skalak R, Chien S (eds): Handbook of Bioengineering. New York, McGraw Hill Publishers, 1986, Chapter 4.
Woo SLY, Gomez MA, Akeson WH: The time and history-dependent viscoelastic properties of the canine medial collateral ligament. J Biomech Eng 1981;103:293.
Wood GC, Keech MK: The formation of fibrils from collagen solution. 1. The effect of experimental conditions: kinetic and electron-microscope studies. Biochem J 1960;75:588-598.
Yamauchi M, Mechanic G: Cross-linking of collagen, in Nimni ME (ed): Collagen: Biochemistry. CRC Press, Boca Raton, FL, 1988, pp 157-172.
Zhu WB, Lai WM, Mow VC: Intrinsic quasi-linear viscoelastic behavior of the extracellular matrix of cartilage. Trans Orthop Res Soc 1986;11:407.
Zhu WB: Nonlinear viscoelastic behavior of concentrated proteoglycan solutions, and articular cartilage in shear, PhD Thesis, Rensselaer Polytechnic Institute, 1989.

Chapter 9

Physicochemical and Bioelectrical Determinants of Cartilage Material Properties

E.H. Frank, A.J. Grodzinsky, S.L. Phillips,
P.E. Grimshaw

Introduction

Articular cartilage is the dense connective tissue that functions as a bearing material in synovial joints. Cartilage is composed of cells (less than 10% by volume) and an osmotically swollen extracellular matrix (ECM) (Schenk *et al.*, 1986; Buckwalter *et al.*, 1988). The high water content of the tissue (60–80% tissue wet weight (Mankin, 1978; Maroudas, 1979; Muir, 1980)) and its high resistance to fluid flow (low hydraulic permeability) are responsible in part for the complex biomechanical and electromechanical behavior of cartilage that characterizes its response to transient and cyclic loads (Kempson, 1979; Mow *et al.*, 1980; Lee *et al.*, 1981; Torzilli, 1984; Holmes *et al.*, 1985; Mak, 1986; Frank and Grodzinsky, 1987b).

The extracellular matrix is composed principally of hydrated collagen fibrils (50–60% of tissue dry weight), large proteoglycans (30–35% dry weight) and non-collagenous proteins and glycoproteins (10–20% dry weight) (Maroudas, 1979; Muir, 1980; Buckwalter *et al.*, 1988). While the biomechanical properties of articular cartilage have been related primarily to the structure and composition of the large aggregating proteoglycans and the collagen type II fibrils, significant attention has also been focused on the role of other smaller protein and polysaccharide constituents in the overall structure and assembly of the ECM (Heinegard and Oldberg, 1989).

Studies have shown that the chemical environment of cartilage has a profound effect on the mechanical and electromechanical properties of the tissue (Elmore *et al.*, 1963; Sokoloff, 1963; Maroudas, 1980; Grodzinsky *et al.*, 1981; Myers *et al.*, 1984; Eisenberg and Grodzinsky, 1985; Eisenberg and Grodzinsky, 1987; Frank and Grodzinsky, 1987a; Frank and Grodzinsky, 1987b). Further, during an electrolyte- or enzymatically-induced alteration of the tissue, the intrinsic material properties will evolve in space and time. The chemical environment within the extracellular matrix is determined by the electrolyte bath ion concentrations, the charge density of the matrix, and the titration isotherms of individual charge groups within the tissue. The chemical environment of soft tissues is also affected by the mechanical state of the tissue: compression increases the density of charge groups and thereby alters intratissue ion concentrations (Gray *et al.*, 1988).

The objectives of this study are to describe the effect of bath chemical environment (e.g., pH and salt concentration) on the mechanical, electrical, and electromechanical properties of cartilage. A theoretical model for the effect of pH and ionic strength on the titration of cartilage fixed charge groups is first presented, along with a model for the dependence of basic material properties on tissue fixed charge density and bath ion concentrations. Predictions of the models are compared to data primarily from experiments using adult bovine articular cartilage.

Previously we have described the experimentally observed frequency dependence of the mechanical-to-electrical and electrical-to-mechanical transduction response of cartilage in compression (Frank and Grodzinsky, 1987a). We have also presented a nonequilibrium electrokinetic theory coupled to a linear, poroelastic theory to describe the observed electromechanical behavior of the tissue (Frank and Grodzinsky, 1987b). In the absence of macroscopic concentration gradients, soft tissue electrokinetics can be modeled by the phenomenological equations of nonequilibrium thermodynamics (DeGroot and Mazur, 1969),

$$\begin{bmatrix} \vec{U} \\ \vec{J} \end{bmatrix} = \begin{bmatrix} -k_{11} & k_{12} \\ k_{21} & -k_{22} \end{bmatrix} \begin{bmatrix} \nabla P_f \\ \nabla V \end{bmatrix} \tag{1}$$

where $\vec{U}$ is the average fluid velocity with respect to the solid, $\vec{J}$ is the electric current density, P_f is fluid pressure, V is the macroscopic averaged electric potential, and the k_{ij} are the phenomenological coupling coefficients. In particular, we identify the (Darcy) hydraulic permeability of the tissue at zero current density as $k = k_{11} - k_{12}k_{21}/k_{22}$. We also identify the streaming potential coefficient as $k_e \equiv k_{21}/k_{22}$ (the ratio of electric potential to fluid pressure at zero current density), the coefficient of electroosmosis, $k_i \equiv k_{12}/k_{22}$ (ratio of fluid velocity to imposed current density at zero pressure drop), and the tissue electrical conductivity, k_{22}, which includes bulk ionic migration as well as convective (streaming) ion flow through the tissue. In general, all of these material parameters are not only functions of bath pH and ionic strength, but will vary with tissue composition and compression.

A constitutive law for the total stress, T_{ij}, that reflects the importance of the chemical environment for a homogeneous, isotropic, linear tissue sample and valid for small strain, ε_{ij}, is given by (Eisenberg and Grodzinsky, 1987),

$$T_{ij} = 2G(c)\varepsilon_{ij} + \{\lambda(c)\varepsilon_{kk} - \beta(c) - P_f\}\delta_{ij} \tag{2}$$

where the fluid pressure $P_f = (P - \Delta\Pi)$ includes both hydrostatic (P) and osmotic (Π) pressure (Eisenberg and Grodzinsky, 1987), the Lamé constants $G(c)$ and $\lambda(c)$ are functions of local chemical concentrations, c, and the chemical stress, $\beta(c)$, is the chemically dependent part of the equilibrium stress that would be felt at zero strain. In uniaxial confined compression, the compressive stress, $\sigma = -T_{zz}$, is related to the compressive strain, $\varepsilon = -\varepsilon_{zz}$, by,

$$\sigma = H_A\varepsilon + \beta(c) + P_f \tag{3}$$

where $H_A = 2G+\lambda$ is the equilibrium confined compression modulus (Mow *et al.*, 1984). Equation (2) is analogous to the general relations given by Biot (1962) and Rice and Cleary (1976) in the limit of incompressible fluid and solid constituents, although the chemical stress β and the chemical and osmotic dependence of G, λ, and P_f were not included in those developments.

Frank and Grodzinsky (1987b) combined Equations (1) and (2) with conservation of current and with laws (Biot, 1962; Mow *et al.*, 1980) for conservation of momentum and mass continuity to predict the self-consistent mechanical, electrical, and electromechanical transduction behavior of cartilage in confined compression within the linear regime. The basic material parameters necessary to characterize this behavior are the modulus, H_A, the hydraulic permeability, k, the electrical conductance, k_{22}, and the electrokinetic coefficients, $k_{12} = k_{21}$. The following developments are aimed at characterizing the dependence of these parameters on tissue fixed charge density and chemical environment such as bath pH and salt concentration.

Theoretical Titration of Cartilage

In this section, a model is derived for the dependence of cartilage fixed charge density on bath pH, salt concentration, and hydration. This titration model is then compared to data on the titration of intact cartilage tissue.

The ionization state (titration) of acidic and basic charge groups in a polyelectrolyte network (e.g., extracellular matrix) depends on the local pH at the molecular site of the charge group. The local pH, in turn, is affected by the presence of neighboring, ionized charge groups through electrostatic interactions. It is these electrostatic interactions that complicate the theory of titration of intact tissues, as compared to dilute, noninteracting molecules in solution. In general, the local concentration of hydrogen ions, $\bar{c}_H$, at position $\vec{r}$, depends on the local electrical potential, $\Phi(\vec{r})$, according to the Boltzmann relation (Glasstone, 1940),

$$\bar{c}_H = c_{\text{bath}} \exp(zF\Phi(\vec{r})/RT) \tag{4}$$

where z is the valence (+1), F is the Faraday constant (96,500 Coulombs/mole), R is the gas constant, and T is the temperature; RT/F is the "thermal voltage", $\simeq$ 25 mV at 25°C.

There are two distinct approaches by which $\Phi(\vec{r})$ in Equation (4) can be estimated. Microcontinuum theories solve the laws of electrostatics, e.g., the Poisson-Boltzmann equation, for the local, space-varying $\Phi(\vec{r})$ surrounding individual rod-like polyelectrolyte molecules in equilibrium with known bath constituents (Alexandrowicz and Katchalsky, 1963; Nagasawa *et al.*, 1965; Oosawa, 1971). The resulting potential is then used to compute an electrostatic interaction term accounting for the presence of charges along the macromolecule and on adjacent macromolecules of the polyelectrolyte matrix. This electrostatic term is added as a correction to the Henderson-Hasselbalch equation for the titration of an otherwise noninteracting charge group (Tanford, 1961), formulated in terms of the intrinsic dissociation constant at zero polyelectrolyte charge.

In contrast, macrocontinuum models represent the tissue as having a smoothed volume fixed charge density with an associated, smoothed intratissue electrical potential and mobile ion concentrations (Grodzinsky, 1983). Characteristic dimensions in this continuum contain many macromolecules, and are so large compared to an electrical Debye length that quasielectroneutrality is assumed valid everywhere within the tissue phase. (The Debye length $(1/\kappa)$ is related to bath salt concentration, c_o, by $(1/\kappa) = \sqrt{(\epsilon RT)/(2z^2F^2c_o)}$.) Mobile ions are thus assumed to be distributed within the tissue according to a smoothed Donnan equilibrium, which satisfies both electroneutrality and a macroscopically smoothed version of the Boltzmann law (4) which defines the Donnan potential difference between the intratissue space and the external bath. In this approach, the effect of electrostatic interactions on titration is represented by the difference between intratissue pH and bath pH induced by the presence of tissue fixed charge groups and the concomitant Donnan potential. Dissociation of charge groups is then represented by a constitutive law (e.g., Langmuir isotherm) that relates the concentration of ionized charge groups to the intrinsic dissociation constant and the computed intratissue pH.

In this study, we use the macrocontinuum approach to derive a theory for titration of intact tissue specimens (Phillips, 1984). This is consistent with our present objective of predicting the pH and ionic strength dependence of macroscopic, intrinsic material properties. These tissue properties are macroscopically smooth, but can be space varying. The following model is derived for the case of a bath containing NaCl, HCl, and NaOH. A significant body of data is available corresponding to these bath conditions; extension of the theory to include additional salt ions (Frank, 1987) and buffers (Gray *et al.*, 1988) adds complexity but is straight-forward.

The major charge groups in cartilage are amino (NH_3^+, on collagen and non-collagenous proteins), carboxyl (COO^-, on chondroitin sulfate, hyaluronate, and proteins), and sulfate (SO_3^-, on chondroitin and keratan sulfate) (Maroudas, 1979; Urban and Maroudas, 1979; Muir, 1980; Grodzinsky, 1983). The concentration of these charge groups determines the charge density, ρ_m (coul per liter tissue water),

$$\rho_m/F = [NH_3^+] - [SO_3^-] - [COO^-]\,. \tag{5}$$

Electroneutrality requires that the concentration of charge groups, (ρ_m/F), be balanced by the internal ion concentrations, $\bar{c}_{\mathrm{Na}}$, $\bar{c}_{\mathrm{Cl}}$, $\bar{c}_{\mathrm{H}}$, and $\bar{c}_{\mathrm{OH}}$,

$$(\rho_m/F) + \bar{c}_{\mathrm{Na}} - \bar{c}_{\mathrm{Cl}} + \bar{c}_{\mathrm{H}} - \bar{c}_{\mathrm{OH}} = 0. \tag{6}$$

The internal ion concentrations are related to the external bath ion concentrations via Donnan equilibrium,

$$\frac{c_{\mathrm{Na}}}{\bar{c}_{\mathrm{Na}}} = \frac{c_{\mathrm{H}}}{\bar{c}_{\mathrm{H}}} = \frac{\bar{c}_{\mathrm{Cl}}}{c_{\mathrm{Cl}}} = \frac{\bar{c}_{\mathrm{OH}}}{c_{\mathrm{OH}}}\,; \quad \frac{c_{\mathrm{NaCl}} + c_{\mathrm{NaOH}}}{\bar{c}_{\mathrm{Na}}} = \frac{\bar{c}_{\mathrm{Cl}}}{c_{\mathrm{NaCl}} + c_{\mathrm{HCl}}}\,. \tag{7}$$

where the ratio of intratissue to bath mean ion activity coefficients (MacInnes, 1961) is approximated as unity. The second set of equalities is written in terms of bath acid, base, and salt concentrations for the 4-ion system. The internal ion concentrations are of primary importance in determining the internal fluid conductivity as well as the ionic strength and pH dependence of other material properties.

The concentrations of ionized charge groups and neutralized charge groups are assumed to be related in equilibrium to the internal H^+ ion concentration and the intrinsic equilibrium dissociation reaction constants by the Langmuir isotherms (Tanford, 1961),

$$K_C = \frac{\bar{c}_{\mathrm{H}}[\mathrm{COO^-}]}{[\mathrm{COOH}]} = \frac{\bar{c}_{\mathrm{H}}[\mathrm{COO^-}]}{N_C - [\mathrm{COO^-}]} \tag{8}$$

$$K_S = \frac{\bar{c}_{\mathrm{H}}[\mathrm{SO_3^-}]}{[SO_3H]} = \frac{\bar{c}_{\mathrm{H}}[\mathrm{SO_3^-}]}{N_S - [\mathrm{SO_3^-}]} \tag{9}$$

$$K_A = \frac{[\mathrm{NH_2}]\bar{c}_{\mathrm{H}}}{[\mathrm{NH_3^+}]} = \frac{(N_A - [\mathrm{NH_3^+}])\bar{c}_{\mathrm{H}}}{[\mathrm{NH_3^+}]} \tag{10}$$

where K_C, K_S, and K_A are the intrinsic dissociation constants and N_C, N_S, and N_A are the site densities of the carboxyl, sulfate, and amino groups, respectively.

In general, the different carboxylate species on chondroitin sulfate and hyaluronate, and on collagen and other noncollagenous proteins can have distinct titration behavior resulting from their distinct spatial distribution, molecular structure, and local interactions. Each species could therefore be characterized by a given intrinsic dissociation constant, K_C^j, and site density, N_C^j (Tanford, 1961). Similarly the sulfate groups of CS and KS, and the amino groups of collagen and other noncollagenous proteins, would be characterized by distinct dissociation constants and site densities. However, many of these titration constants are yet unknown; thus, a general theory that distinguishes between all such groups is of limited value. Therefore, for simplicity in the present model, but without loss of generality, we have chosen to represent the carboxyl, sulfate, and amino groups each with an overall site density, N_i, and an average dissociation constant, K_i, in Equations (8)–(10).

The system of equations (5)–(10) yields a single master equation for the internal hydrogen concentration, $\bar{c}_{\mathrm{H}}$, in terms of the known bath concentrations and experimentally measurable site densities and dissociation constants,

$$\frac{N_A\bar{c}_{\mathrm{H}}}{\bar{c}_{\mathrm{H}} + K_A} - \frac{K_S N_S}{\bar{c}_{\mathrm{H}} + K_S} - \frac{K_C N_C}{\bar{c}_{\mathrm{H}} + K_C} + \frac{c_{\mathrm{Na}}\bar{c}_{\mathrm{H}}}{c_{\mathrm{H}}} - \frac{c_{\mathrm{Cl}}c_{\mathrm{H}}}{\bar{c}_{\mathrm{H}}} + \bar{c}_{\mathrm{H}} - \frac{c_{\mathrm{H}}c_{\mathrm{OH}}}{\bar{c}_{\mathrm{H}}} = 0\,. \tag{11}$$

The other intratissue ion concentrations and the tissue fixed charge density can then be obtained from Equations (7) and (6), respectively.

Charge Site Concentrations and Dissociation Constants

Collagen has approximately 230 carboxyl and 250 amino groups per molecule (Li and Katz, 1979), and is nearly charge neutral at neutral pH. Based on a water content of ~ 80% ($H_O \simeq 4$) and a collagen content of ~ 55% of tissue dry weight for adult bovine femoropatellar groove cartilage (Koob, 1982), and a tissue density of 1.08 kg/liter, the amino and carboxyl site concentrations for collagen, $N_A^{\rm col}$ and $N_C^{\rm col}$, are estimated to be

$$N_A^{\rm col} = \frac{250\text{ mole NH}_2}{\text{mole col}} \times \frac{\text{mole col}}{300\text{ kg col}} \times \frac{0.55\text{ kg col (dry)}}{\text{kg tissue (dry)}} \times \frac{1.08\text{ kg tissue}}{\text{liter tissue}} \times \frac{1}{H_O} = 0.13\text{ M}$$

$$N_C^{\rm col} = \frac{230\text{ mole COOH}}{\text{mole col}} \times \frac{\text{mole col}}{300\text{ kg col}} \times \frac{0.55\text{ kg col (dry)}}{\text{kg tissue (dry)}} \times \frac{1.08\text{ kg tissue}}{\text{liter tissue}} \times \frac{1}{H_O} = 0.12\text{ M}$$

We are not aware of titration data for the ~10–15% noncollagenous proteins in adult bovine femoropatellar groove cartilage. For the purpose of estimating the site densities and titration behavior of this constituent, we will assume that amino and carboxyl groups are present in roughly the same proportion and with similar dissociation constants as that of collagen.

Chondroitin sulfate (CS) and keratan sulfate (KS) are the major charge contributing glycosaminoglycans (GAGs) of cartilage. On the average, each CS disaccharide unit contains one ionizable carboxyl and sulfate group, while KS contains a single sulfate group. (While hyaluronic acid (HA) is very important to the formation of proteoglycan aggregates in cartilage, the concentration of ionized charge groups associated with HA is much less than that of CS and KS.) In adult bovine femoropatellar groove articular cartilage, glucuronic acid (the CS and HA disaccharide constituent containing the carboxyl site) comprises 5.4% of cartilage dry weight. HA comprises 0.2% of dry weight, and the ratio of CS to KS was measured to be approximately 3.3:1 (Koob, 1982). Based on these numbers, the GAG carboxyl site density is estimated to be,

$$N_C^{\rm gag} = \frac{0.054\text{ kg glu}}{\text{kg tissue}} \times \frac{\text{mole glu}}{179\text{ kg glu}} \times \frac{1.08\text{ kg}}{\text{liter}} \times \frac{1}{H_O} = 0.08\text{ M}$$

The sulfate site concentration is estimated to be 30% higher, due to the contribution of keratan sulfate, so that N_S=0.11 M.

The dissociation constants for the carboxyl and sulfate groups in intact tissue are difficult to estimate, compared to those of dilute molecular solutions. Data from Bowes and Kenten (1948) suggest that the pK of carboxyl groups in collagen is in the range 3.5. Reported values for the $\mathrm{p}K_C$ for carboxyl groups of CS are in the range 3.35–3.6 (Mathews, 1961; Park and Chakrabarti, 1978) and for HA in the range 3–3.4 (Cleland *et al.*, 1982; Park and Chakrabarti, 1978) We do not know of specific pK values reported for the $\mathrm{p}K_S$ of sulfate groups on CS and KS, though values in the range 1.5–2 are suggested (Kuettner and Lindenbaum, 1965; Comper, 1990). Based on the above data, we use the following "average" values to estimate the titration behavior of bovine femoropatellar groove cartilage: $\mathrm{p}K_C \simeq 3.4$, $\mathrm{p}K_S \simeq 1.5$–2, $N_S \simeq 0.11$ M, total $N_C \simeq 0.22$ M, and $N_A \simeq 0.15$ M. We will present theoretical and experimental results in the acid range pH 2–7; in this range, essentially all of the amino groups are assumed to be ionized, given their known dissociation constants $\mathrm{p}K_A \simeq 10.5$–12.5 (Bowes and Kenten, 1948).

Table 1: Titration and material parameters for adult bovine articular cartilage.

Titration Parameters		Value	Reference
amino groups (collagen)	N_A pK_A	0.15 M 11	Li and Katz (1979) Bowes and Kenten (1948)
carboxyl groups (collagen)	N_C pK_C	0.12 M 3.5	Li and Katz (1979) Bowes and Kenten (1948)
carboxyl groups (GAGs)	N_C pK_C	0.08 M 3.4	Koob (1982) Mathews (1961)
sulfate groups (GAGs)	N_S pK_S	0.11 M 1.5–2	Koob (1982)
charge density (0.15 M NaCl, pH 7)	ρ_m/F	0.18 M	Equation (5)
isoelectric point	pI	2.75	Frank and Grodzinsky (1987a) Grodzinsky *et al.* (1981)

Material Parameters		Value at 0.15 M NaCl, pH 7	Reference
hydraulic permeability ($\varepsilon = 0.15$)	k_{11}	$1 \times 10^{-15}\ m^2/Pa \cdot s$	Mow *et al.* (1984)
electrokinetic coefficient	k_e, k_i	13×10^{-9} V/Pa	Frank and Grodzinsky (1987b)
fluid conductivity	σ_o	0.5–1 S/m	Chammas (1989) Hasegawa *et al.* (1983)
bulk conductivity	k_{22}	1–1.5 S/m	Equation (29)
compressive modulus	H_A	0.55 MPa	Eisenberg and Grodzinsky (1985)

A summary of the charge site concentrations and dissociation constants, as well as the mechanical and electrical parameters used in this paper is given in Table 1.

Equation (11) was solved via Newton's method for the pH range 2–7 and NaCl concentration 0.001–1 M. From the resulting internal H^+ ion concentration, $\bar{c}_H$, the ion concentrations $\bar{c}_{Na}$ and $\bar{c}_{Cl}$ and charge density, ρ_m, were calculated using Equations (7) and (6). The predicted charge density versus bath pH at 0.15 M NaCl is shown in Figure 1. Intratissue pH, $\bar{c}_{Na}$, and $\bar{c}_{Cl}$ at 0.15 and 0.01 M NaCl are shown in Figure 2.

Two-Compartment Titration Model

Equations (5)–(11) above correspond to a model in which all charge groups are distributed uniformly within the tissue phase. Maroudas (1979) and Grushko *et al.* (1989) have distinguished between the collagen intrafibrillar space and the proteoglycan (extrafibrillar) space with regard to their respective water content, charge density, and osmotic swelling pressure. A titration theory can be derived for the individual collagen and proteoglycan compartments given estimates of their individual charge site densities and hydrations. (This approach can be extended to apply equally to any number of compartments.) Here, the collagen and proteoglycan compartments have water volume fractions, V_W^c and V_W^p, and

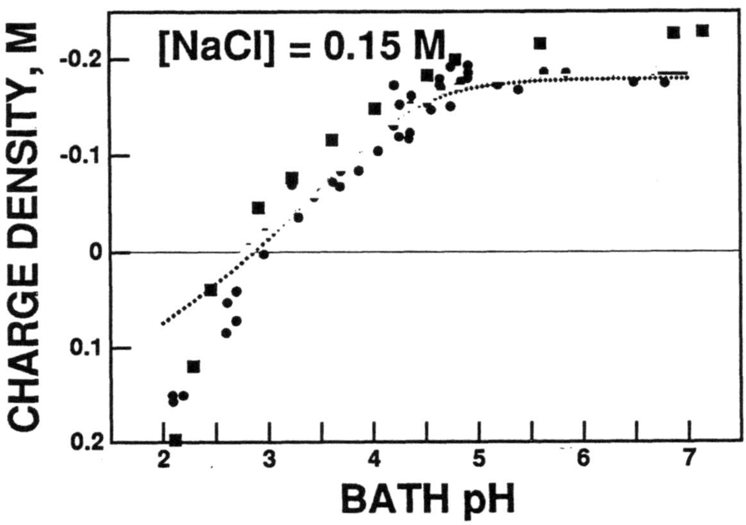

Figure 1: Cartilage fixed charge density versus bath pH computed from the theoretical titration model of Equation (11), using the parameter values N_A=0.15M, N_S=0.11M, N_C=0.22M, and pK_A = 11, pK_C = 3.4, pK_S = 1.5 (solid line) and pK_S = 2 (dotted line). The data (■) are measured fixed charge densities for adult bovine femoropatellar groove cartilage (Phillips, 1984), obtained by equilibrating 500–700 mg of 200 μm thick cartilage slices at neutral pH, 0.15 M NaCl, and sequentially reequilibrating the tissue at different pH values in the range 2–7. Also shown for comparison are data from adult human femoral head cartilage (●) (adapted from Maroudas (1979)).

solid volume fractions, V_S^c and V_S^p, respectively, such that,

$$V_W = V_W^c + V_W^p \tag{12}$$

$$V_S = V_S^c + V_S^p \tag{13}$$

where V_W and V_S are the total water and solid volume fractions, respectively, and, by definition, $V_W + V_S = 1$. Then in each compartment, the effective charge site densities, N_i, are given by

$$N_i^c = N_{io}^{\text{col}} \frac{V_W}{V_W^c} \; ; \; N_i^p = N_{io}^{\text{gag}} \frac{V_W}{V_W^p} \tag{14}$$

where N_{io}^{col} and N_{io}^{gag} are the contributions to the site densities based on total tissue water volume (as was done in the one-compartment model).

Given the effective site densities in each compartment, and assuming each compartment is in equilibrium with each other and the external bath, we can apply Equation (11) in each compartment and solve for $\bar{c}_H$ and the other intratissue ion concentrations. To compare the predictions of the two compartment model to those of the single compartment model, we calculate the average ion concentrations for the tissue as a whole,

$$\bar{c}_i = \bar{c}_i^p \frac{V_W^p}{V_W} + \bar{c}_i^c \frac{V_W^c}{V_W} \tag{15}$$

and the average charge density for the tissue as a whole,

$$\rho_m = \rho_m^p \frac{V_W^p}{V_W} + \rho_m^c \frac{V_W^c}{V_W} \tag{16}$$

where $\bar{c}_i^p$ and $\bar{c}_i^c$ are the ion concentrations for the ith species in the proteoglycan and collagen compartments, respectively, as obtained from Equations (11) and (7), and ρ_m^p and ρ_m^c are the corresponding charge densities each compartment as obtained from Equation (6). Figure 2 compares the pH dependence of ρ_m, intratissue pH, $\bar{c}_{\text{Na}}$, and $\bar{c}_{\text{Cl}}$ predicted by the 1- and 2-compartment models.

Effect of Hydration on Charge Density

Charge density is also a function of hydration and compressive strain. As the tissue is compressed, the site density necessarily increases. The dissociated ions in the fluid can not occupy the solid space. Thus, in Equations (5)–(11), all concentrations are in terms of fluid volume and not total volume. With hydration, H, defined as the ratio of fluid to solid volume, the charge site concentrations are related to hydration by

$$N_i = N_{io} \frac{H_O}{H} \tag{17}$$

where N_i is the site concentration of the ith species and N_{io} is the concentration at the initial equilibrium hydration, H_O. If the solid and fluid phases are assumed to be incompressible, tissue hydration, H, is related to the one-dimensional strain, ε, by

$$H = H_O - (H_O + 1)\varepsilon\ . \tag{18}$$

Macro-Continuum Charge Model of Cartilage Electrokinetic Parameters

In this section, we relate the electromechanical parameters, k_{ij}, of Equation (1) to tissue fixed charge density and ion concentrations described by the above titration theory. Once again, both microcontinuum and macrocontinuum approaches are available. Microcontinuum models for fluid flow and electrical double-layer interactions have been used to describe electrokinetics in simple pore structures (Matijevic, 1974) and more complicated assemblies of charged cylindrical molecules (Eisenberg and Grodzinsky, 1988; Kozak and Davis, 1989a; Kozak and Davis, 1989b). Micromodels are fundamentally based on the electroquasistatic limit of Faraday's Law and Gauss' Law, respectively, for the local electric field, $\vec{E}$,

$$\nabla \times \vec{E} = 0 \tag{19}$$

$$\nabla \cdot \epsilon \vec{E} = \rho_u \tag{20}$$

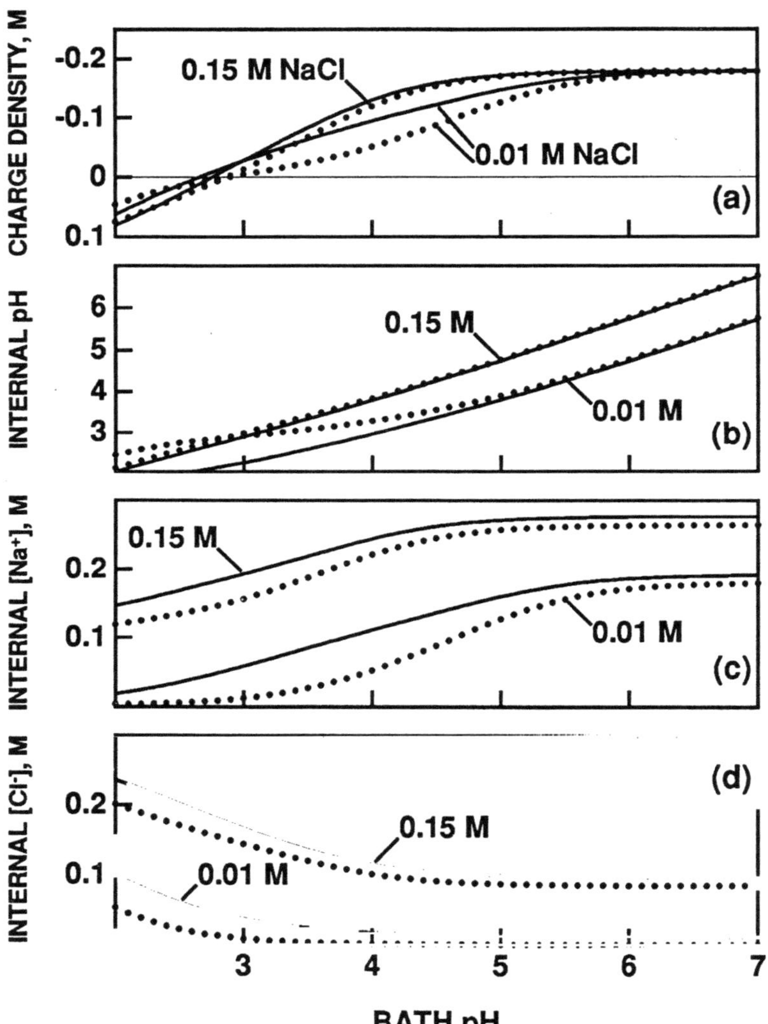

Figure 2: Intratissue pH, $\bar{c}_{Na}$, $\bar{c}_{Cl}$, and charge density from Equations (6), (7), and (11) (the 1-compartment (· · ·)) compared to the predictions of Equations (15) and (16) (2-compartment model (—)) using the parameters of Figure 1 with $pK_S = 1.5$.

conservation of current,

$$\nabla \cdot \vec{J} = -\frac{\partial \rho_u}{\partial t} \simeq 0 \tag{21}$$

and a constitutive law for current including ohmic conduction and convection,

$$\vec{J} = \sigma_o \vec{E} + \rho_u \vec{U} \tag{22}$$

where ϵ is the fluid dielectric constant, σ_o is the bulk fluid conductivity, and ρ_u is the net space charge in the fluid phase. In Equation (21), the charge relaxation time ϵ/σ_o for physiological conductivity is so short ($\sim 10^{-9}$ sec) that $(\partial \rho_u/\partial t \to 0)$ for frequencies less than $\sim$100 MHz. Equations (19)–(22) are combined with the Navier-Stokes equation in the limit of viscous dominated low Reynold's number flow, and the local fluid continuity equation, respectively,

$$\eta \nabla^2 \vec{v}_f - \nabla P + \rho_u \vec{E} = 0 \tag{23}$$

$$\nabla \cdot \vec{v}_f = 0 \tag{24}$$

where $\rho_u \vec{E}$ is the force density of electrical origin exerted by the electric field $\vec{E}$ on the fluid, and $\vec{v}_f$ is the local fluid velocity.

In the macromodel, equivalent macroscopic versions of these laws are used to describe electrokinetics. Taking the macroscopic view that individual ion concentrations are uniform throughout the fluid volume (or smoothly varying on a length scale much greater than a Debye length), Faraday's and Gauss' Laws are replaced by a statement of electroneutrality (Equation (6)),

$$\rho_m = -\rho_u = -F \sum_i z_i \bar{c}_i \, . \tag{25}$$

Assuming that fluid/solid drag forces are much more important than viscous forces within the fluid itself, the Navier-Stokes equation in the direction of transport is replaced by a macrocontinuum force balance including terms for the fluid/solid drag, pressure gradient, and electrical force density, respectively,

$$-\frac{\vec{U}}{k_{11}} - \nabla P_f + \rho_u \vec{E} = 0 \tag{26}$$

where the viscous drag of the fluid on the solid matrix is described by the Darcy permeability at zero field (potential gradient), k_{11}, as was the case in Frank and Grodzinsky (1987a), and $\vec{U}$ is the total area-averaged relative velocity of the fluid with respect to the solid matrix. Conservation of current in the form of Equation (21) is satisfied as before, and the continuity law (24) is replaced by an expression for the biphasic porous medium, written for the case of incompressible fluid and solid constituents (Armstrong *et al.*, 1984; Holmes, 1986) as,

$$\nabla \cdot \left(\phi \vec{v}_f + (1-\phi)\vec{v}_s\right) = 0\,; \quad \vec{U} \equiv \phi(\vec{v}_f - \vec{v}_s) \tag{27}$$

where the porosity, ϕ, is related to hydration by $\phi = H/(1+H)$, and $\vec{v}_s$ is the local solid velocity. The continuity law (27) can then be written in the form

$$(1+H)\nabla \cdot \vec{U} + \left(\vec{v}_s \cdot \nabla + \frac{\partial}{\partial t}\right) H = 0\, . \tag{28}$$

From Equations (22), (25), and (26), $\vec{U}$ and $\vec{J}$ can be written as,

$$\begin{bmatrix} \vec{U} \\ \vec{J} \end{bmatrix} = \begin{bmatrix} -k_{11} & \rho_m k_{11} \\ \rho_m k_{11} & -(\sigma_o + \rho_m^2 k_{11}) \end{bmatrix} \begin{bmatrix} \nabla P_f \\ \nabla V \end{bmatrix} \tag{29}$$

where we have substituted $\vec{E} = -\nabla V$. By comparing Equations (29) and (1), we see that $k_{12} = k_{21} = (\rho_m k_{11})$, consistent with Onsager reciprocity, and $k_{22} = (\sigma_o + \rho_m^2 k_{11})$ contains both ohmic conduction and convection components. The form of these relations for the k_{ij} were given previously by Helfferich (1962) for the case of electrokinetic interactions in ion-exchange membranes.

Fluid conductivity, σ_o, is given by the internal concentrations and diffusivities,

$$\sigma_o = \frac{F}{V_T} \sum_i \bar{D}_i \bar{c}_i \tag{30}$$

where $\bar{D}_i$ is the intratissue diffusivity of the ith species and $V_T = RT/F$ is the thermal voltage. The intratissue diffusivity has often been approximated (Maroudas, 1979; Grimshaw *et al.*, 1989) by using the Mackie and Meares (1955) tortuosity factor in terms of the hydration, H, and the ionic diffusivity at infinite dilution, D_i^∞,

$$\bar{D}_i = D_i^\infty \left(\frac{H}{2+H}\right)^2 . \tag{31}$$

In the macro-charge model the "open-circuit" hydraulic permeability, k, is given by

$$k = \left(k_{11} - \frac{k_{12}k_{21}}{k_{22}}\right) = k_{11}\left(1 - \frac{\rho_m^2 k_{11}}{\sigma_o + \rho_m^2 k_{11}}\right) . \tag{32}$$

This permeability can be profoundly influenced by the charge density; for values of $\rho_m^2 k_{11} \gtrsim \sigma_o$ the effective k will be a fraction of k_{11}. The electrokinetic coefficient k_e is given by

$$k_e = \frac{k_{21}}{k_{22}} = \frac{\rho_m k_{11}}{\sigma_o + \rho_m^2 k_{11}} . \tag{33}$$

Thus, for k_{22} dominated by conduction ($\rho_m^2 k_{11} < \sigma_o$), k_e is proportional to fixed charge density; in the opposite limit, k_e can decrease with increasing ρ_m.

Empirical Model of Equilibrium Swelling Stress

In equilibrium in the absence of fluid flow, an applied compressive stress, σ (Equation (3)), is balanced by an equilibrium swelling pressure, p, (Eisenberg and Grodzinsky, 1985),

$$p = H_A \varepsilon + \beta . \tag{34}$$

As described below, Eisenberg and Grodzinsky (1985) found that H_A and β decreased with increasing bath NaCl concentration in a manner that was well described by a simple exponential fit. Grimshaw (1982) and Grimshaw *et al.* (1983) measured the swelling stress of cartilage as a function of bath pH. After calculating the tissue fixed charge density, ρ_m, from bath pH using Equations (6)–(11), we found that the pH-dependence of the measured swelling stress (Grimshaw, 1982) could be well fit by a quadratic function in charge density. This suggested that the combined dependence of the equilibrium compressive modulus and chemical stress on bath pH and salt concentration could be described by the analytical expressions,

$$H_A(\rho_m, c_o) = H_A^{\infty} + (H_A^o - H_A^{\infty})\left(\frac{\rho_m}{\rho_{\text{ref}}}\right)^2 \exp\left(-\frac{c_o}{c_{\text{ref}}^H}\right) \quad (35)$$

$$\beta(\rho_m, c_o) = \beta_o\left(\frac{\rho_m}{\rho_{\text{ref}}}\right)^2 \exp\left(-\frac{c_o}{c_{\text{ref}}^{\beta}}\right) \quad (36)$$

where c_o is the external ionic strength, H_A^o and H_A^{∞} are the values of confined compression modulus in the limits of low and high ionic strength, respectively, β_o is the value of swelling stress in the limit of low ionic strength, and ρ_{ref}, c_{ref}^H, and c_{ref}^{β} are measured constants. The quadratic dependence of H_A and β on ρ_m is consistent with the form of previous theoretical models of the Donnan osmotic and electrostatic component of swelling and swelling pressure of polyelectrolyte materials, based on double layer repulsion stresses (Lazare *et al.*, 1956; Nussbaum, 1986). The analytical expressions (35) and (36), are convenient for including the chemical dependence of the equilibrium H_A and β in predictions of the chemical dependence of nonequilibrium stiffness and streaming potential, as shown below.

Chemical Dependence of Material Parameters: Comparison of Theory and Experiment

Titration of Articular Cartilage

To determine the titration behavior of bovine articular cartilage, specimens were harvested from the femoropatellar groove of 2-year old cattle as previously described (Eisenberg and Grodzinsky, 1985), and equilibrated in 0.15 M NaCl under a nitrogen atmosphere to eliminate the presence of CO_2. The cartilage was titrated by adding known amounts of HCl or NaOH to the solution and monitoring the resulting change in bath pH. The difference between measured bath H^+ concentration and the amount of H^+ added was assumed to represent the change in charge density (i.e., H^+ bound). The data of Figure 1 show the charge density computed from titration measurements on bovine cartilage in the range pH 2–7 and the known isoelectric pH (=2.75) of this same intact tissue (measured independently from streaming potential (Frank and Grodzinsky, 1987b) and isometric stress (Grodzinsky *et al.*, 1981) experiments). Also shown in Figure 1 for comparison is the fixed charge density of human femoral head cartilage as determined from radioisotope partitioning (Maroudas, 1979).

The reasonable correspondence between the data and theoretical curves of Figure 1 in the region pH>2.75 suggests that Equation (11) is useful in predicting tissue charge density in this region. We note that Equation (11) was *not* curve-fit to the data; there was no attempt to adjust the parameters of (11) to optimize the match between theory and experiment. Rather, estimates were obtained for all parameters from independent measurements in the literature. For pH>3, the shapes of the curves are dominated by titration of the carboxyl groups, which appears to be similar for human and bovine cartilage. For pH<3, theory and experiment diverge. This may be due to inaccuracies in the estimate of sulfate group pK, site densities, or both.

The 1- and 2-compartment titration models (Figure 2) predict similar ρ_m and $\bar{c}_i$ near pH 7 for all bath NaCl concentrations; similar ρ_m and $\bar{c}_H$ are predicted over the entire pH range at 0.15 M NaCl. The 2-compartment model predicts higher ρ_m and $\bar{c}_i$, especially apparent at low salt concentration in the acid pH range. Such predictions may be tested by radioisotope (Grushko *et al.*, 1989) or NMR (Lesperance *et al.*, 1990) measurement of intratissue ion concentrations.

Determination of k_{ij}

The above models for titration, electrokinetics, and the empirical expression for equilibrium swelling stress can now be combined and used to predict the pH and ionic strength dependence of the parameters k, $k_e = k_i$, k_{22}, σ_o, H_A, and β. The one-compartment titration model was first used to find tissue charge density and internal ion concentrations; the macro-continuum electrokinetic model was then used to predict values of k, k_e, k_{22}, and σ_o while the empirical swelling model was used to predict H_A and β. These values were then used in the electromechanical model of Frank and Grodzinsky (1987b) to predict the dynamic stiffness and streaming potential of cartilage in confined compression as a function of bath NaCl concentration and pH, and compared to experimental results. All theoretical predictions were based on the assumption of constant hydration over the pH and ionic strength range of interest. In adult bovine femoropatellar groove cartilage, water content was observed to change by only a few percent (Phillips, 1984; Eisenberg and Grodzinsky, 1985), and could not alone account for the significant changes in material properties with pH and NaCl.

We first recall from Equations (1) and (29) that $k_{21} = (k_e k_{22}) = \rho_m k_{11}$. This relation was used to compute the "short circuit" hydraulic permeability, k_{11}, at 0.15 M NaCl, pH 7, from: the value $\rho_m = -0.18$M predicted from Equation (11) for these bath conditions (Figure 1); the k_{22} calculated from the internal ion concentrations of Equation (7); and the experimental value $k_e \simeq 13$mV/MPa at 0.15 M NaCl, pH 7, based on the oscillatory stiffness and streaming potential measurements of Frank and Grodzinsky (1987b) at a static offset strain of 15%. The computed value of $k_{11} \simeq 10^{-15}\text{m}^2/(\text{Pa}\cdot\text{s})$ agrees well with the value of $0.9 \times 10^{-15}\text{m}^2/(\text{Pa}\cdot\text{s})$ reported by Mow *et al.* (1984) for adult bovine femoropatellar groove cartilage at 15% compression. Using the titration charge model to find the charge density and internal ion concentrations for bath pH 2–7 and 0.001 to 1 M NaCl, the open-circuit permeability, k (Figure 3), was computed using Equation (32) as a function of bath pH and NaCl concentration. In

Figure 3, the variation in the hydraulic permeability, k, is due to the electrokinetic backflow term in the expression $k = k_{11} - k_{12}k_{12}/k_{22}$. Physically, the flow-induced streaming potential gradient exerts an electrical force on the net counterion space charge in the fluid phase. This force acts to oppose fluid flow, effectively decreasing the hydraulic permeability. Maximum values of k in Figure 3 occur when electrokinetic interactions are minimal, i.e., at the isoelectric point or at high ionic strength. While there is some experimental evidence (Grodzinsky, 1983) that k increases with NaCl concentration for tissue maintained at constant volume, as suggested in Figure 3, these predictions remain to be extensively tested.

Figure 4 shows the streaming potential coefficient, k_e, versus pH and ionic strength as calculated using Equation (29). Experimental values of k_e, calculated from data on stiffness and streaming potential versus pH and NaCl concentration (Frank and Grodzinsky, 1987a) are shown for comparison. Taken together, the theory and data of Figure 4 show the effect of charge group titration and ionic shielding on k_e. For pH below the isoelectric point the sign of k_e is positive, corresponding to a positive fixed charge density. At high ionic strength, k_e tends toward zero. (Again, there was no attempt to fit the theory to the the data; the theory represents the use of the minimal number of independently determined parameters needed to describe trends with pH and salt concentration.)

Tissue conductivity, k_{22}, and fluid conductivity, σ_o, were calculated using Equations (30), (31), (18), and (17). Figure 5a shows that at zero strain, k_{22} is minimal near the isoelectric pH and increases with increasing ρ_m. Using human knee joint cartilage in a four-electrode measurement system, Hasegawa *et al.* (1983) found a linear correlation between σ_o and tissue fixed charge density at low ionic strength; charge density was measured independently using the radiotracer technique of Maroudas (1979). In Ringer's solution, values of σ_o were reported to be in the range 0.6–1 S/m. The measured conductivity, σ_o, versus compressive strain for disks of bovine articular cartilage (Chammas, 1989) is shown in Figure 5b. Although close in magnitude to the measured conductivity, the theoretical conductivity (Figure 5b) declines with strain, primarily due to the Mackie and Meares (1955) tortuosity factor. The measured conductivity increases with strain up to 30% compression before declining slightly (Chammas, 1989). Thus, the macromodel does not adequately predict the variation of σ_o with applied strain. Micromodels do predict increasing conductivity with strain, but tend to overpredict the conductivity magnitude (Chammas, 1989; Eisenberg and Grodzinsky, 1988).

Empirical model of Equilibrium Swelling Stress

Figure 6 shows the measured variation of equilibrium modulus, H_A, with bath pH and NaCl concentration, and the variation of the chemical stress, β, with NaCl, for adult bovine articular cartilage (Eisenberg and Grodzinsky, 1985; Grimshaw, 1982). Analytical expressions were fit to these data using Equations (35) and (36) (Figure 6). To implement this analytical model, the ionic strength, c_o, was computed as,

$$c_o = c_{\mathrm{NaCl}} + c_{\mathrm{HCl}} \qquad (37)$$

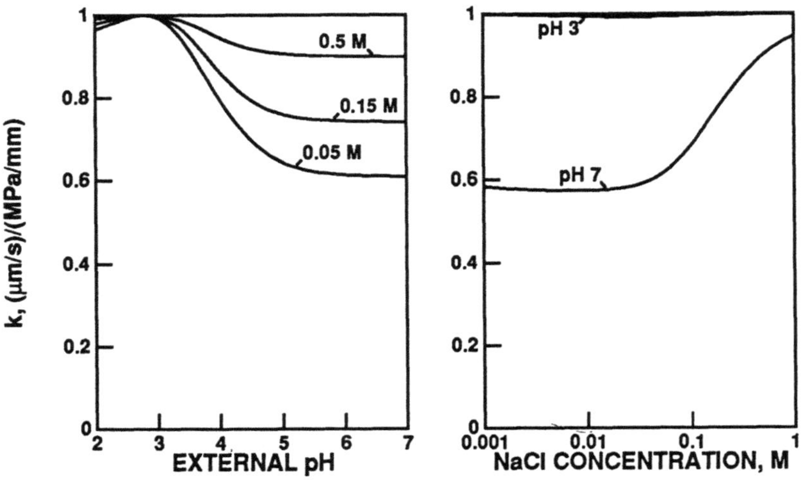

Figure 3: Hydraulic permeability, $k = k_{11} - (k_{12}k_{21}/k_{22})$, versus bath pH and NaCl concentration, predicted for tissue held at constant volume using Equation (32) with a value of $k_{11} \simeq 1 \times 10^{-15} \mathrm{m}^2/\mathrm{Pa} \cdot \mathrm{s}$.

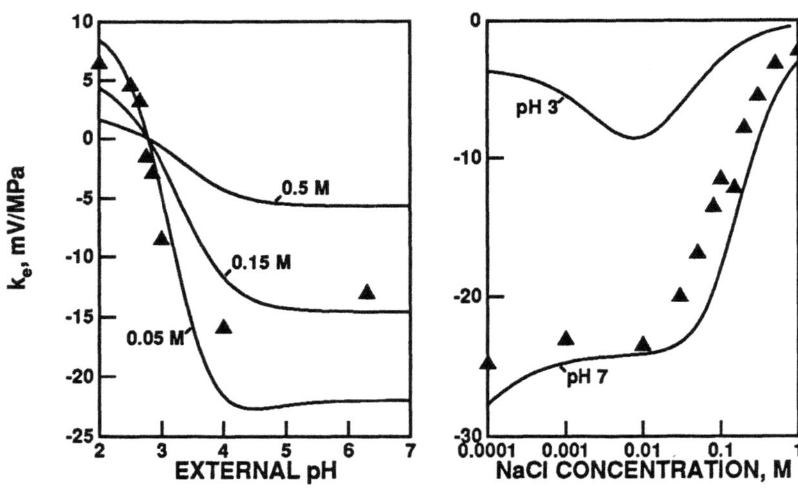

Figure 4: Streaming potential coefficient, k_e, versus bath pH and NaCl concentration. Experimental values of k_e (▲) are calculated from the stiffness and streaming potential data of Frank and Grodzinsky (1987a) using adult bovine articular cartilage. The experimental data shown in the left panel are from a cartilage specimen pre-equilibrated in 0.05 M NaCl, neutral pH, and reequilibrated at sequentially lower pH values. The data in the right panel are from a specimen pre-equilibrated at 0.0001 M NaCl, neutral pH, and reequilibrated at sequentially increasing bath NaCl concentrations.

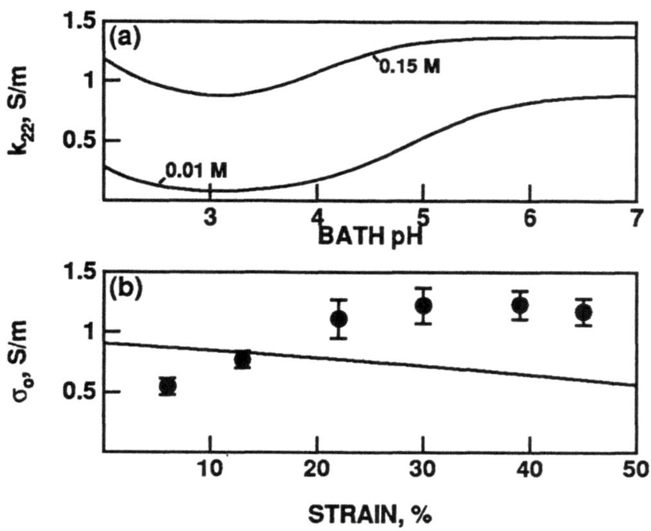

Figure 5: (a) Tissue conductivity, k_{22}, versus bath pH and NaCl concentration, calculated from Equations (29)–(31). (b) Tissue fluid conductivity, σ_o, versus applied static compressive strain, calculated from Equations (17), (18), (29), (30). The data are from disks of adult bovine femoropatellar groove cartilage (Chammas (1989); mean±SD, $n = 4$), with each specimen subjected to sequentially increasing uniaxial compressive strain in a 0.15 M NaCl at neutral pH.

and the charge density was computed from the titration model. The charge density was then incorporated self-consistently into Equations (35) and (36) to compute equilibrium H_A and β. With ρ_{ref} taken to be 0.18 M, the values of H_A^{∞}, H_A^o, β_o, c_{ref}^H, and c_{ref}^{β} that give reasonable fits to H_A and β are shown in Figure 6.

Comparison of Poroelastic Theory with Measured Stiffness and Streaming Potential

The analytical expressions for the *equilibrium* H_A and β (Equations (35), (36), and Figure 6) as a function of charge density and ionic strength provided a convenient means for incorporating the data of Figure 6 into predictions of the variation of *dynamic* stiffness and streaming potential on bath pH and NaCl concentration. These predictions were compared with stiffness and streaming potential data measured as a function of ionic strength (Figure 7) and pH (Figure 8).

Figure 7 shows the stiffness and streaming potential amplitude versus bath NaCl concentration (Frank and Grodzinsky, 1987a) at 0.1 Hz using 1% amplitude applied sinusoidal strain (displacement control) superimposed on a 15% offset strain for NaCl concentration between 0.0001 M and 1 M (neutral pH). The theoretical curves of Figure 7 were computed by incorporating the above model

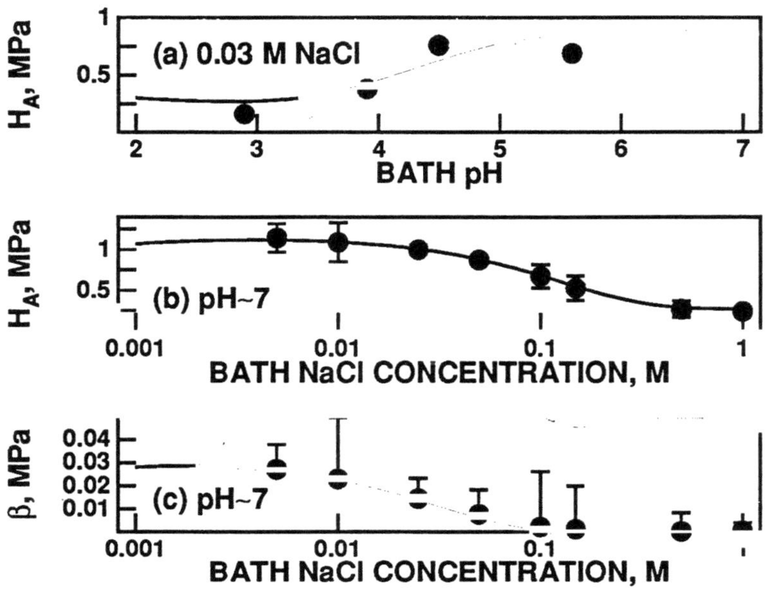

Figure 6: Empirical swelling model: compressive modulus, H_A, versus (a) ionic strength and (b) pH, and (c) chemical stress, β, versus NaCl concentration. Fitted parameters for the empirical model (Eisenberg, 1983) are H_A^o=1.17MPa, H_A^∞=0.27MPa, c_{ref}^H=0.13M, β_o=0.03MPa, c_{ref}^β=0.03M, and ρ_{ref}=0.18M.

for the NaCl concentration-dependence of k_e and k, and the empirical expressions for the NaCl-dependence of H_A into the equations for the dynamic stiffness and streaming potential given by Frank and Grodzinsky (1987b). Figure 8 shows the measured stiffness and streaming potential versus bath pH (Frank and Grodzinsky, 1987a) at 0.5 Hz for a constant offset stress of 130 kPa and 65 kPa dynamic stress (load control). The theoretical curves of Figure 8 were computed by incorporating the titration theory for the pH-dependence of k_e and k, and the empirical expressions for the pH-dependence of H_A into the equations for the stiffness and streaming potential. (For chemically homogeneous tissue, β does not enter into the expressions for sinusoidal stiffness and streaming potential.)

The trends predicted by the model were in good agreement with the experimental data of Figures 7 and 8 for reasonable values of model parameters. The streaming potential phase angle in Figure 8 shows a 180 degree shift near the isoelectric point, indicating a change in the sign of the fixed charge. Curve-fitting of theory to data in Figures 7 and 8 would give optimum parameter values perhaps more descriptive of the specimens used in these experiments. However, in the spirit of the approach used here, Figures 7 and 8 incorporate the "average" parameter values listed in Table 1.

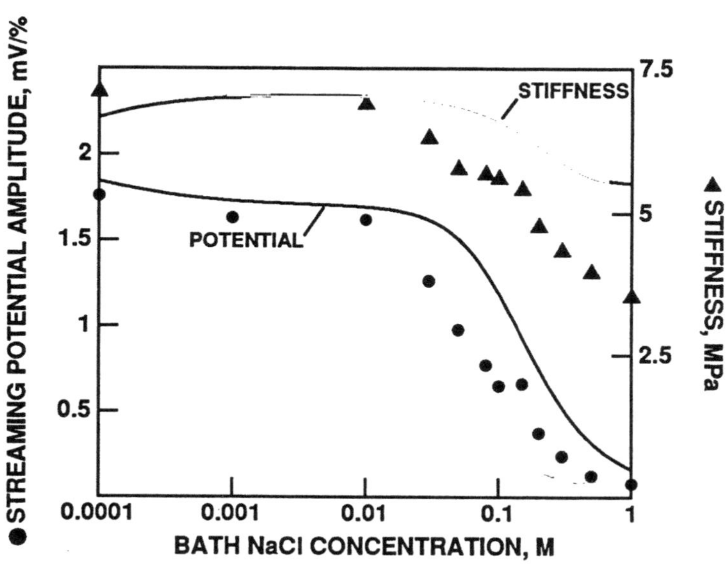

Figure 7: Comparison of the experimental and theoretical stiffness and streaming potential amplitude versus bath NaCl concentration. Experimental data (Frank and Grodzinsky, 1987a) are for a specimen of bovine articular cartilage equilibrated at neutral pH and at 15% static compression and subjected to sequentially increasing NaCl concentrations, while tested at 0.1 Hz, 1% dynamic amplitude. Solid lines are predictions of the macromodel for electrokinetics.

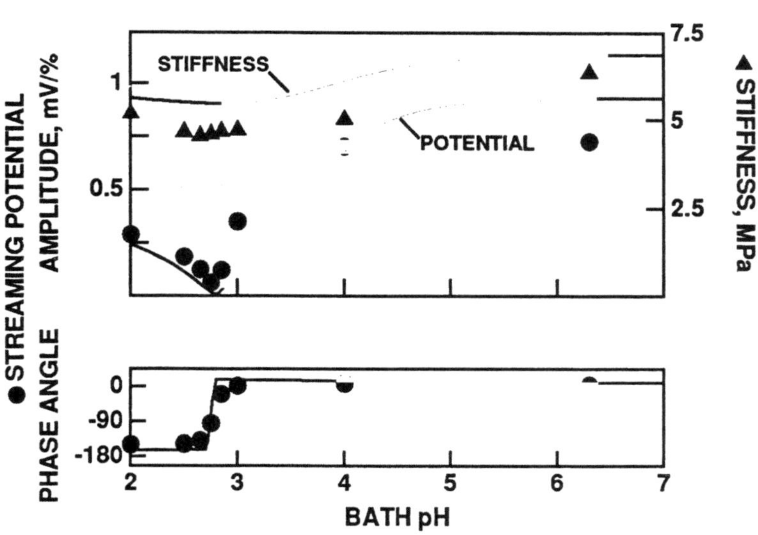

Figure 8: Comparison of the experimental and theoretical streaming potential amplitude versus pH for cartilage. Experimental data (Frank and Grodzinsky, 1987a) are for a specimen of bovine articular cartilage equilibrated at 0.05 M NaCl, neutral pH, and 130 kPa static stress, and subjected to sequentially decreasing bath pH while tested at 0.5 Hz. Solid lines are predictions of the macromodel for electrokinetics.

Summary

A theoretical model for titration has been used to self-consistently predict the internal ion concentrations and charge density of cartilage over a wide range of bath pH and ionic strength. The titration model can be coupled to an ion exchange macromodel to predict the electrokinetic transduction coefficients as functions of pH and ionic strength. By combining the titration model, electrokinetic model, and data on the chemical dependence of the equilibrium modulus, we can relate electromechanical properties directly to specific tissue constituents. The next goal is to apply these methodologies to model inhomogeneities in cartilage, such as the known variation in the fixed charge density of cartilage with depth, and as cartilage tissue undergoes changes from a normal to a degenerated state, either by chemically or enzymatically induced changes in the fixed charge density.

ACKNOWLEDGMENTS: This work was supported by NIH Grant AR33236 and NSF Grant BCS-8811371. The authors would like to thank Prof. Sol Eisenberg for his contributions to macro and micro models, and Paula Chammas for data on cartilage conductivity. We are also grateful to Dr. Alice Maroudas for data on titration and charge density of cartilage.

References

Alexandrowicz Z, Katchalsky A: Colligative properties of polyelectrolyte solutions in excess of salt. J Polymer Science 1963; 1:3231–3260

Armstrong CG, Lai WM, Mow VC: An analysis of the unconfined compression of articular cartilage. J Biomechanical Engineering 1984; 106:165–173

Biot MA: Generalized theory of acoustic propagation in porous dissipative media. J Accoust Soc Am 1962; 34:1254–64

Bowes JH, Kenten RH: The amino-acid composition and titration curve of collagen. Biochemical J 1948; 43:358–365

Buckwalter J, Hunziker E, Rosenberg L, Coutts R, Adams M, Eyre D: Articular Cartilage: Composition and Structure. American Academy of Orthopaedic Surgeons, Park Ridge, IL. pp. 405–425. 1988

Chammas P: Electromechanical Coupling in Articular Cartilage: An Electorkinetic Micromodel and Experimental Results. Master's thesis, Boston University. 1989

Cleland RL, Wang JL, Detweiler DM: Polyelectrolyte properties of sodium hyaluronate. 2. Potentiometric titration of hyaluronic acid. Macromolecules 1982; 15:386–395

Comper WD: Personal communication. 1990

DeGroot SR, Mazur P: Nonequilibrium Thermodynamics. North Holland, Amsterdam. 1969

Eisenberg SR: Nonequilibrium Electromechanical Interactions in Cartilage: Swelling and Electrokinetics. PhD thesis, MIT. 1983

Eisenberg SR, Grodzinsky AJ: Swelling of articular cartilage and other connective tissues: Electromechanochemical forces. J Orthopaedic Research 1985; 3:148–159

Eisenberg SR, Grodzinsky AJ: The kinetics of chemically induced nonequilibrium swelling of articular cartilage and corneal stroma. J Biomechanical Engineering 1987; 109:79–89

Eisenberg SR, Grodzinsky AJ: Electrokinetic micromodel of extracellular matrix and other polyelectrolyte networks. PhysicoChemical Hydrodynamics 1988; 10:517–539

Elmore SM, Sokoloff L, Norris G, Carmeci P: Nature of "imperfect" elasticity of articular cartilage. J Appl Physiol 1963; 18:393–396

Frank EH: Electromechanics of Normal and Degenerated Cartilage: Poroelastic Behavior and Electrokinetic Mechanisms. PhD thesis, MIT. 1987

Frank EH, Grodzinsky AJ: Cartilage electromechanics I: Electrokinetic transduction and the effects of electrolyte pH and ionic strength. J Biomechanics 1987; 20:615–627

Frank EH, Grodzinsky AJ: Cartilage electromechanics II: A continuum model of cartilage electrokinetics. J Biomechanics 1987; 20:629–639

Glasstone S: Text Book of Physical Chemistry. D Van Nostrand, New York. 1940

Gray ML, Pizzanelli AM, Grodzinsky AJ, Lee RC: Mechanical and physicochemical determinants of the chondrocyte biosynthetic response. J Orthopaedic Research 1988; 6:777–792

Grimshaw PE: The Response of Cartilage in Compression as it Undergoes Diffusion Limited Chemical Changes. Master's thesis, MIT. 1982

Grimshaw PE, Eisenberg SR, Grodzinsky AJ, Koob TJ, Eyre DR: The kinetics of in vitro neutralization and enzymatic extraction of cartilage charge groups: Characterization by isometric compressive stress. Trans 29th ORS 1983; 8:122

Grimshaw PE, Grodzinsky AJ, Yarmush ML, Yarmush DM: Dynamic membranes for protein transport: Chemical and electrical control. Chem Eng Sci 1989; 44:827–840

Grodzinsky AJ: Electromechanical and physicochemical properties of connective tissues. CRC Crit Rev Biomed Eng 1983; 9:133–199

Grodzinsky AJ, Roth V, Myers E, Grossman WD, Mow VC: The significance of electromechanical and osmotic forces in the nonequilibrium swelling behavior of articular cartilage in tension. J Biomechanical Engineering 1981; 103:221–231

Grushko G, Schneiderman R, Maroudas A: Some biochemical and biophysical parameters for the study of the pathogenesis of osteoarthritis: A comparison between the processes of ageing and degeneration in human hip cartilage. Connective Tissue Research 1989; 19:149–176

Hasegawa I, Kuriki S, Matsuno S, Matsumoto G: Dependence of electrical conductivity on fixed charge density in articular cartilage. Clinical Orthopaedics 1983; 177:283–288

Heinegard D, Oldberg A: Structure and biology of cartilage and bone matrix noncollagenous macromolecules. FASEB J 1989; 3:2042–2051

Helfferich F: Ion Exchange. McGraw-Hill, New York. 1962

Holmes MH: Finite deformation of soft tissue: Analysis of a mixture model in uni-axial compression. J Biomechanical Engineering 1986; 108:372–381

Holmes MH, Lai WM, Mow VC: Singular perturbation analysis for stress relaxation test of articular cartilage. J Biomechanical Engineering 1985; 107:206–218

Kempson GE: Mechanical Properties of Articular Cartilage. Pitman Medical, Kent, England. pp. 333–414. 1979

Koob TJ: Personal communication. 1982

Kozak MW, Davis EJ: Electrokinetics of concentrated suspensions and porous media: I. Thin electrical double layers. J Colloid and Interface Science 1989; 127:497–510

Kozak MW, Davis EJ: Electrokinetics of concentrated suspensions and porous media: II. Moderately thick electrical double layers. J Colloid and Interface Science 1989; 129:166–174

Kuettner KE, Lindenbaum A: Analysis of mucopolysaccharides in partially aqueous media. Biochim Biophys Acta 1965; 101:223–225

Lazare L, Sundheim BR, Gregor HP: A model for cross-linked polyelectrolytes. J Phys Chem 1956; 60:641–648

Lee RC, Frank EH, Grodzinsky AJ, Roylance DK: Oscillatory compressional behavior of articular cartilage and its associated electromechanical properties. J Biomechanical Engineering 1981; 103:280–292

Lesperance LM, Gray ML, Burstein D: Measurement of fixed charge density in intact

cartilage using NMR spectroscopy. Trans 36th ORS 1990; 15:342
Li S, Katz EP: Electrostatic Properies of Reconstituted Collagen Fibrils. Grune and Stratton, New York. p. 119. 1979
MacInnes DA: The Principles of Electrochemistry. Dover, New York. 1961
Mackie JS, Meares P: The diffusion of electrolytes in a cation-exchange resin. I. Theoretical. Proc Roy Soc A 1955; 232:498–509
Mak AF: The apparent viscoelastic behavior articular cartilage — The contributions from the intrinsic matrix viscoelasticity and interstitial fluid flows. J Biomechanical Engineering 1986; 108:123–130
Mankin HJ: The water of articular cartilage. University of Pennsylvania Press, Philadelphia. pp. 37–42. 1978
Maroudas A: Physicochemical Properties of Articular Cartilage. Pitman Medical, Kent, England. pp. 215–290. 1979
Maroudas A: Physical Chemistry of Articular Cartilage and the Intervertebral Disc. Academic Press, London. pp. 240–293. 1980
Mathews MB: Acid strength of carboxyl groups in isomeric chondrotin sulfates. Biochim Biophys Acta 1961; 48:402–403
Matijevic E: Surface and Colloid Science. Wiley-Interscience, New York. pp. 49–272. 1974
Mow VC, Kuei SC, Lai WM, Armstrong CG: Biphasic creep and stress relaxation of articular cartilage in compression: Theory and experiments. J Biomechanical Engineering 1980; 102:73–84
Mow VC, Holmes MH, Lai WM: Fluid transport and mechanical properties of articular cartilage: A review. J Biomechanics 1984; 17:377–394
Muir IHM: The Chemistry of the Ground Substance of Joint Cartilage. Academic Press, New York. pp. 28–94. 1980
Myers ER, Lai WM, Mow VC: A continuum theory and an experiment for the ion-induced swelling behavior of articular cartilage. J Biomechanical Engineering 1984; 106:151–158
Nagasawa M, Murase T, Kondo K: Potentiometric titration of stereoregular polyelectrolytes. J Phys Chem 1965; 69:4005–4012
Nussbaum JH: Electric field control of mechanical and electromechanical properties of polyelectrolyte gel membranes. PhD thesis, MIT: EECS. 1986
Oosawa F: Polyelectrolytes. Marcel Dekker, New York. 1971
Park JW, Chakrabarti B: Optical characteristics of carboxyl group in relation to the circular dichroic properties and dissociation constants of glycosaminoglycans. Biochim Biophys Acta 1978; 544:667–675
Phillips SL: The determination of charge density in articular cartilage via chemical titration. Master's thesis, MIT. 1984
Rice JR, Cleary MP: Some basic stress diffusion solutions for fluid saturated elastic porous media with compressible constituents. Rev Geophys Space Phys 1976; 14:227–241
Schenk RK, Eggli PS, Hunziker EB: Articular Cartilage Morphology. Raven Press, New York. pp. 3–22. 1986
Sokoloff L: Elasticity of articular cartilage: Effect of ions and viscous solutions. Science 1963; 141:1055–1057
Tanford C: Physical Chemistry of Macromolecules. John Wiley and Sons, New York. 1961
Torzilli PA: Mechanical response of articular cartilage to an oscillating load. Mechanics Research Communications 1984; 11:75–82
Urban JPG, Maroudas A: The measurement of fixed charge density in the intervertebral disk. Biochim Biophys Acta 1979; 586:166

Chapter 10

A Triphasic Theory for the Swelling Properties of Hydrated Charged Soft Biological Tissues

W.M. Lai, J.S. Hou, V.C. Mow

Introduction

Many hydrated soft tissues, such as articular cartilage, meniscus and intervertebral disc, change their dimensions, volume and weight when the ion concentration in the external bathing solution is changed (Parsons and Black 1979; Maroudas 1975, 1979; Maroudas and Bannon 1981; Myers et al 1984; Mow and Schoonbeck 1984; Eisenberg and Grodzinsky 1985, 1987). For example, for an unloaded specimen of cartilage soaked in NaCl solutions at constant temperature, the tissue dimensions decrease nonlinearly in an exponential manner with increasing NaCl concentration; this decrease approaches an asymptote at a high concentration, e.g., 2.5M NaCl (Mow and Schoonbeck 1984). Therefore, at the physiological state of 0.15M NaCl, cartilage is in a swollen state, with a swelling pressure resisted by the elastic stress developed in the collagen-proteoglycan solid matrix. This is often referred to as the collagen pre-stress or elastic stress in the solid matrix (Maroudas 1975, 1976, 1979; Maroudas and Bannon 1981; Grodzinsky et al 1981). For a normal cartilage bathed in 0.15M NaCl solution, the swelling pressure has been measured to be around 0.17 MPa (Maroudas 1975, 1979; Maroudas and Bannon 1981).

In cartilage, proteoglycan aggregates (PGA) are immobilized and restrained in the collagen meshwork. The PGA molecules, ranging from 100×10^6 to 200×10^6 daltons (Maroudas 1979; Muir 1983), contain a large number of fixed negative charge groups (SO_3^- and COO^-) along their glycosaminoglycan (GAG) chains. The density of these charges is called the fixed charge density (FCD). For example, for normal and degenerate femoral head cartilage, the FCD ranges from

0.04 to 0.18 mEq/(g wet tissue) (Maroudas 1975, 1979). Those negative charges require counter-ions to be nearby to maintain electro-neutrality. In a pure water environment, the concentration (c^F) of a univalent counter-ion (e.g., Na^+) is exactly equal to the FCD. The total ion concentration inside the tissue thus is larger than the ion concentration in the external bathing solution. This is true in a NaCl environment also. This imbalance of ions gives rise to a pressure in the interstitial fluid which is higher than the ambient pressure in the external bath. This pressure difference is known as the Donnan osmotic pressure. This osmotic pressure is one of the causes of cartilage swelling.

In the extracellular matrix (ECM), it is estimated that the PGA's may be restrained to 1/10th of their volume in free solution (Muir 1983; Hascall and Hascall 1983). Thus, the fixed charge groups along the GAG chains of the PG molecules are very close to each other, causing charge-to-charge repulsive forces to be exerted against each other. These forces may also cause the ECM to swell. The charge-to-charge electrostatic forces are modulated by the counter- and co-ions swarming around the PG molecules in solution. With increasing ion concentrations, the equivalent Debye length between the ion cloud and the fixed charges is decreased. This results in charge shielding which decreases the net charge-to-charge repulsive force (Gabler 1978), which is referred to as the chemical-expansion force.

In this chapter we shall describe how the above two effects, the Donnan osmotic pressure effect (excess ions) and the chemical-expansion effect (electrostatic repulsive forces) contribute to the total swelling behavior of cartilage and other hydrated soft tissues.

There exist two different views of cartilage, a fiber-reinforced charged fluid-solid gel as illustrated in Figure 1. The physicochemical view (Maroudas 1975, 1979; Urban and Maroudas 1979, 1981) of cartilage is based on the classical Donnan theory for aqueous polyelectrolyte solutions (Donnan 1924), with no field equations for stresses in the solid matrix and ions; while the biphasic view (Mow et al 1980, 1984, 1986) treats the collagen-proteoglycan matrix as a solid with the elastic properties depending on all the underlying physicochemical effects. Some attempts have been made to bridge this gap (Myers et al 1984; Mow and Schoonbeck 1984; Eisenberg and Grodzinsky 1985, 1987; Lanir 1987). However, these theories take the ionic effect into consideration in varying but incomplete ways.

In the present study, we propose a triphasic theory for cartilage which incorporates the Donnan ion distribution and osmotic pressure theory for polyelectrolytic solutions. This three phase model for cartilage is composed of two immiscible phases: 1) the interstitial fluid phase and 2) the collagen-proteoglycan solid phase; and a miscible fluid phase: 3) the ionic phase. In this triphasic theory, the stresses in the solid matrix and the chemical potentials for the interstitial fluid and ions are related to the Helmholtz energy functions in accordance with the laws of energy balance and entropy. The general theory for a mixture of one incompressible solid phase and N-1 incompressible fluid phases has been developed by Bowen (1980), in which the Helmholtz energy functions

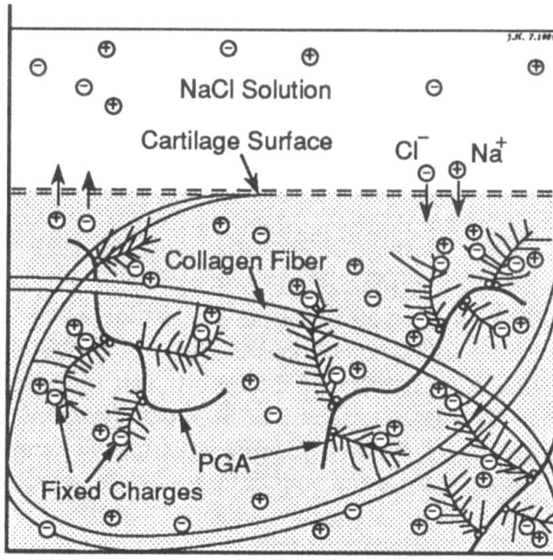

Figure 1. Schematic diagram of articular cartilage equilibrated with NaCl solution.

for the phases depend on temperature, the deformation of the solid matrix and the densities of the N−1 fluid phases. To include the fixed charge groups (c^F) of the solid matrix of cartilage, we assume specifically that the Helmholtz energy functions also depend on c^F. In addition, for the ion phase and the fluid phase, we incorporate the traditional chemical potentials for electrolyte and polyelectrolyte solutions into the theory, thus providing a theoretical bridge between the continuum mixture theory (Mow et al 1980, 1986; Bowen 1980) and physicochemical theory (Maroudas 1975, 1979; Urban and Maroudas 1979, 1981; Donnan 1924; Katchalsky 1965; Tomgs 1974). This triphasic theory will also subsume the biphasic theory for the deformational and flow behaviors of the tissue. Through applications to both equilibrium and transient problems, we will show how this theory can predict the experimentally observed swelling behaviors of cartilage.

A Triphasic Model

General Triphasic Mixture Formulations

Consider a mixture of three phases: an incompressible solid phase (the collagen-proteoglycan ECM), an incompressible fluid phase (interstitial water) and an ion phase (e.g., NaCl). Since the ions occupy only negligible volume (i.e., $dV^i/dV \approx 0$), the total mixture volume dV may be considered to be the sum of the solid dV^s and fluid (water) volume dV^w:

$$\phi^s + \phi^w = 1\,, \tag{1}$$

where $\phi^s = dV^s/dV$ is the solidity and $\phi^w = dV^w/dV$ the porosity of the material.

When no chemical reaction takes place, the mass balance for each phase is

$$\frac{\partial \rho^\alpha}{\partial t} + \operatorname{div}(\rho^\alpha \boldsymbol{v}^\alpha) = 0\,, \tag{2}$$

where α=s,w,i, denote the solid matrix, interstitial water and mobile salt respectively, and ρ^α is the apparent density (mass of α-phase per unit dV). In particular, ρ^i denotes the density of the mobile salt (not including c^F). The apparent densities are related to their true densities (mass of α-phase per unit volume of the α-phase) by $\rho^\alpha = \phi^\alpha \rho^\alpha_T$. From equations (1) and (2), one obtains the equation of continuity for an incompressible mixture in the following form:

$$\operatorname{div}(\phi^s \boldsymbol{v}^s + \phi^w \boldsymbol{v}^w) = 0\,. \tag{3}$$

The balance of linear momentum for each phase leads to the following equations of motion:

$$\rho^\alpha \frac{\partial \boldsymbol{v}^\alpha}{\partial t} + \rho^\alpha \boldsymbol{v}^\alpha \cdot \nabla \boldsymbol{v}^\alpha = \operatorname{div} \sigma^\alpha + \rho^\alpha \boldsymbol{b}^\alpha + \boldsymbol{\pi}^\alpha\,. \tag{4}$$

where σ^α is the apparent stress tensor, $\boldsymbol{b}^\alpha$ is the external body force per unit mass, and $\boldsymbol{\pi}^\alpha$ is the momentum supply to the α-phase from the other two phases. By the laws of balance of linear momentum for the mixture, the momentum supplies must satisfy

$$\boldsymbol{\pi}^s + \boldsymbol{\pi}^w + \boldsymbol{\pi}^i = \boldsymbol{0}\,. \tag{5}$$

Assuming no local supply of moment of momentum, then, from the balance of moment of momentum, we can conclude that the stress tensors are symmetric.

The balance of energy for each phase yields the following equations for the internal energy density e^α:

$$\rho^\alpha \frac{\partial e^\alpha}{\partial t} + \rho^\alpha \boldsymbol{v}^\alpha \cdot \nabla e^\alpha = \operatorname{tr}(\sigma^\alpha \mathbf{L}^\alpha) - \operatorname{div} \boldsymbol{q}^\alpha + \rho^\alpha r^\alpha + \varepsilon^\alpha\,. \tag{6}$$

where $\mathbf{L}^\alpha$ is the velocity gradient, $\boldsymbol{q}^\alpha$ is the heat flux vector, r^α is the internal heat supply and ε^α is the part of the energy supply to the α-phase from the other two phases which contributes to the increase of the internal energy. The total energy supply to each of the α-phase is $\delta^\alpha = \varepsilon^\alpha + \boldsymbol{\pi}^\alpha \cdot \boldsymbol{v}^\alpha$, and to be consistent with the balance of energy for the total mixture, we must have:

$$\delta^s + \delta^w + \delta^i = 0 . \tag{7}$$

The second thermodynamics law for the mixture is expressed by:

$$\sum_{\alpha=s,w,i}\left[\rho^\alpha \frac{D^\alpha \eta^\alpha}{Dt} + \operatorname{div}\frac{q^\alpha}{T} - \rho^\alpha \frac{r^\alpha}{T}\right] \geq 0, \tag{8}$$

where η^α is the entropy density of α-phase, and T is the absolute temperature of the mixture. By the energy equation (6) this inequality can be written in terms of Helmholtz free energies:

$$\sum_{\alpha=s,w,i}\left[-\rho^\alpha\left(\frac{D^\alpha A^\alpha}{Dt} + \eta^\alpha \frac{D^\alpha T}{Dt}\right) + \operatorname{tr}(\sigma^\alpha L^\alpha) - \frac{1}{T} q^\alpha \cdot \nabla T - v^\alpha \cdot \pi^\alpha\right] \geq 0. \tag{9}$$

where the Helmholtz energy density is defined by

$$A^\alpha = e^\alpha - T\eta^\alpha. \tag{10}$$

For a triphasic medium with an elastic matrix containing fixed charges undergoing finite deformation, we make the following constitutive assumption on A^α for cartilage and other hydrated soft tissues:

$$A^\alpha = A^\alpha(T, \mathbf{C}, \rho^w, \rho^i, c^F), \tag{11}$$

where **C** is the right Cauchy-Green deformation tensor of the solid matrix. We note that the "immobile" counter-ions always stay with the solid matrix so that c^F is solely determined by its value c_o^F at the reference configuration for deformation and the current volume determined by det(**C**), thus we have

$$c^F = c_o^F f(\det \mathbf{C}) , \tag{12}$$

where f is a monotonic decreasing function of det(**C**) only.[1]

The variables $\mathbf{L}^s$, $\mathbf{L}^w$, $\mathbf{L}^i$, $v^s - v^w$, $v^w - v^i$, and $v^i - v^s$ appearing in the entropy inequality (9) are subjected to two constraints: i) the incompressibility assumption expressed by equation (3), which can be written as

$$\phi^s \operatorname{tr}(\mathbf{L}^s) + \phi^w \operatorname{tr}(\mathbf{L}^w) + (v^s - v^w)\cdot\nabla\phi^s = 0, \tag{13}$$

and ii) the relation between the three relative velocities:

---

[1]For example, if c^F is concentration per unit tissue volume, then $f(\det\mathbf{C}) = (\sqrt{\det\mathbf{C}})^{-1}$.

$$(\boldsymbol{v}^s-\boldsymbol{v}^w) + (\boldsymbol{v}^w-\boldsymbol{v}^i) + (\boldsymbol{v}^i-\boldsymbol{v}^s) = \boldsymbol{0}. \tag{14}$$

With these constraints the entropy inequality (9) becomes:[2]

$$\begin{aligned}
&\sum_{\alpha=s,w,i} -\rho^\alpha\left(\frac{\partial A^\alpha}{\partial t}+\eta^\alpha\right)\frac{D^\alpha T}{Dt} - \frac{1}{T}(\boldsymbol{q}^s+\boldsymbol{q}^w+\boldsymbol{q}^i)\cdot\nabla T \\
&+ \mathrm{tr}\Bigg[\Bigg(\sigma^s + \phi^s\lambda\mathbf{I} - 2\mathbf{F}\left(\rho^s\frac{\partial A^s}{\partial \mathbf{C}} + \rho^w\frac{\partial A^w}{\partial \mathbf{C}} + \rho^i\frac{\partial A^i}{\partial \mathbf{C}}\right)\mathbf{F}^T \\
&\quad - 2c_0^F(\det\mathbf{C})g\left(\rho^s\frac{\partial A^s}{\partial c^F} + \rho^w\frac{\partial A^w}{\partial c^F} + \rho^i\frac{\partial A^i}{\partial c^F}\right)\mathbf{I}\Bigg)\mathbf{L}^s\Bigg] \\
&+ \mathrm{tr}\left[\left(\sigma^w + \phi^w\lambda\mathbf{I} + \rho^w\left(\rho^s\frac{\partial A^s}{\partial \rho^w} + \rho^w\frac{\partial A^w}{\partial \rho^w} + \rho^i\frac{\partial A^i}{\partial \rho^w}\right)\mathbf{I}\right)\mathbf{L}^w\right] \\
&+ \mathrm{tr}\left[\left(\sigma^i + \rho^i\left(\rho^s\frac{\partial A^s}{\partial \rho^i} + \rho^w\frac{\partial A^w}{\partial \rho^i} + \rho^i\frac{\partial A^i}{\partial \rho^i}\right)\mathbf{I}\right)\mathbf{L}^i\right] \\
&+ \rho^s\frac{\partial A^s}{\partial \rho^w}(\boldsymbol{v}^w-\boldsymbol{v}^s)\cdot\nabla\rho^w + \rho^i\frac{\partial A^i}{\partial \rho^w}(\boldsymbol{v}^w-\boldsymbol{v}^i)\cdot\nabla\rho^w \\
&+ \rho^s\frac{\partial A^s}{\partial \rho^i}(\boldsymbol{v}^i-\boldsymbol{v}^s)\cdot\nabla\rho^i + \rho^w\frac{\partial A^w}{\partial \rho^i}(\boldsymbol{v}^i-\boldsymbol{v}^w)\cdot\nabla\rho^i \\
&+ \rho^w(\boldsymbol{v}^s-\boldsymbol{v}^w)\cdot[\nabla\mathbf{C}]\frac{\partial A^w}{\partial \mathbf{C}} + \rho^i(\boldsymbol{v}^s-\boldsymbol{v}^i)\cdot[\nabla\mathbf{C}]\frac{\partial A^i}{\partial \mathbf{C}} \\
&+ c_0^F(\det\mathbf{C})g\left[\rho^w\frac{\partial A^w}{\partial c^F}(\boldsymbol{v}^s-\boldsymbol{v}^w) + \rho^i\frac{\partial A^i}{\partial c^F}(\boldsymbol{v}^s-\boldsymbol{v}^i)\right]\cdot[\nabla\mathbf{C}]\mathbf{C}^{-1} \\
&- (\boldsymbol{\pi}^s - \lambda\nabla\phi^s)\cdot\boldsymbol{v}^s - (\boldsymbol{\pi}^w - \lambda\nabla\phi^w)\cdot\boldsymbol{v}^w - \boldsymbol{\pi}^i\cdot\boldsymbol{v}^i \\
&+ \boldsymbol{\eta}\cdot[(\boldsymbol{v}^s-\boldsymbol{v}^w) + (\boldsymbol{v}^w-\boldsymbol{v}^i) + (\boldsymbol{v}^i-\boldsymbol{v}^s)] \geq 0,
\end{aligned} \tag{15}$$

where $\mathbf{F}$ is the deformation gradient, $g=f'(\det\mathbf{C})$, and λ and $\boldsymbol{\eta}$ are Lagrangian multipliers. This inequality must be satisfied for all thermodynamic processes, thus, we obtain, under the assumption of elastic solid matrix and inviscid interstitial fluid, the constitutive relations for the stresses and momentum

[2]Here $[\nabla\mathbf{C}]\mathbf{B}$ defines a vector $\partial_i C_{mn} B_{mn} \boldsymbol{i}$ for any two second order tensors $\mathbf{C}$ and $\mathbf{B}$.

supplies:

$$\sigma^s = -\phi^s\lambda\mathbf{I} + 2\mathbf{F}\left(\rho^s\frac{\partial A^s}{\partial \mathbf{C}} + \rho^w\frac{\partial A^w}{\partial \mathbf{C}} + \rho^i\frac{\partial A^i}{\partial \mathbf{C}}\right)\mathbf{F}^T$$
$$+ 2c_0^F(\det\mathbf{C})g\left(\rho^s\frac{\partial A^s}{\partial c^F} + \rho^w\frac{\partial A^w}{\partial c^F} + \rho^i\frac{\partial A^i}{\partial c^F}\right)\mathbf{I}, \tag{16}$$

$$\sigma^w = -\phi^w\lambda\mathbf{I} - \rho^w\left(\rho^s\frac{\partial A^s}{\partial \rho^w} + \rho^w\frac{\partial A^w}{\partial \rho^w} + \rho^i\frac{\partial A^i}{\partial \rho^w}\right)\mathbf{I}, \tag{17}$$

$$\sigma^i = -\rho^i\left(\rho^s\frac{\partial A^s}{\partial \rho^i} + \rho^w\frac{\partial A^w}{\partial \rho^i} + \rho^i\frac{\partial A^i}{\partial \rho^i}\right)\mathbf{I}, \tag{18}$$

$$\pi^s = \lambda\nabla\phi^s - \rho^s\frac{\partial A^s}{\partial \rho^w}\nabla\rho^w + \rho^w[\nabla\mathbf{C}]\frac{\partial A^w}{\partial \mathbf{C}} - \rho^s\frac{\partial A^s}{\partial \rho^i}\nabla\rho^i$$
$$+ \rho^i[\nabla\mathbf{C}]\frac{\partial A^i}{\partial \mathbf{C}} + c_0^F(\det\mathbf{C})g\left(\rho^w\frac{\partial A^w}{\partial c^F} + \rho^i\frac{\partial A^i}{\partial c^F}\right)[\nabla\mathbf{C}]\mathbf{C}^{-1}$$
$$+ \mathbf{K}_{sw}(\boldsymbol{\nu}^w - \boldsymbol{\nu}^s) + \mathbf{K}_{is}(\boldsymbol{\nu}^i - \boldsymbol{\nu}^s), \tag{19}$$

$$\pi^w = \lambda\nabla\phi^w + \rho^s\frac{\partial A^s}{\partial \rho^w}\nabla\rho^w - \rho^w[\nabla\mathbf{C}]\frac{\partial A^w}{\partial \mathbf{C}} + \rho^i\frac{\partial A^i}{\partial \rho^w}\nabla\rho^w$$
$$- \rho^w\frac{\partial A^w}{\partial \rho^i}\nabla\rho^i - c_0^F(\det\mathbf{C})g\rho^w\frac{\partial A^w}{\partial c^F}[\nabla\mathbf{C}]\mathbf{C}^{-1}$$
$$+ \mathbf{K}_{sw}(\boldsymbol{\nu}^s - \boldsymbol{\nu}^w) + \mathbf{K}_{wi}(\boldsymbol{\nu}^i - \boldsymbol{\nu}^w), \tag{20}$$

$$\pi^i = \rho^s\frac{\partial A^s}{\partial \rho^i}\nabla\rho^i - \rho^i[\nabla\mathbf{C}]\frac{\partial A^i}{\partial \mathbf{C}} - \rho^i\frac{\partial A^i}{\partial \rho^w}\nabla\rho^w + \rho^w\frac{\partial A^w}{\partial \rho^i}\nabla\rho^i$$
$$- c_0^F(\det\mathbf{C})g\rho^i\frac{\partial A^i}{\partial c^F}[\nabla\mathbf{C}]\mathbf{C}^{-1} + \mathbf{K}_{is}(\boldsymbol{\nu}^s - \boldsymbol{\nu}^i) + \mathbf{K}_{wi}(\boldsymbol{\nu}^w - \boldsymbol{\nu}^i), \tag{21}$$

where $\mathbf{K}_{\alpha\beta}$ (α,β=s,w,i) are semi-positive definite tensors whose elements are the drag coefficients between the α- and β-phases. They satisfy $\mathbf{K}_{\alpha\beta}=\mathbf{K}_{\beta\alpha}$ and for isotropic mixtures, $\mathbf{K}_{\alpha\beta}=K_{\alpha\beta}\mathbf{I}$.

Equations of Motion in Terms of Chemical Potentials

The chemical potential tensor of each phase is defined as follows

$$\mathbf{K}^s = A^s\mathbf{I} - \sigma^s/\rho^s, \tag{22}$$

$$\mathbf{K}^w = \mu^w\mathbf{I} = A^w\mathbf{I} - \sigma^w/\rho^w, \tag{23}$$

$$\mathbf{K}^{i} = \mu^{i}\mathbf{I} = A^{i}\mathbf{I} - \sigma^{i}/\rho^{i}. \tag{24}$$

We note from equations (17) and (18), σ^w and σ^i are isotropic tensors so that the chemical potentials $\mathbf{K}^w$ and $\mathbf{K}^i$ reduce to scalar potentials denoted by μ^w and μ^i. In terms of these chemical potentials, the quasi-static momentum equations ($\mathrm{div}\sigma^\alpha + \pi^\alpha = \mathbf{0}$) take the following forms:

$$-\rho^s \mathrm{div}\mathbf{K}^s + \frac{1}{2}\rho^s\mathbf{K}^s([\nabla\mathbf{C}]\mathbf{C}^{-1}) - \frac{1}{2}\rho^s[\nabla\mathbf{C}]\left(\mathbf{F}^{-1}\mathbf{K}^s\mathbf{F}^{-T}\right)$$
$$+ K_{sw}(\nu^w - \nu^s) + K_{is}(\nu^i - \nu^s) = \boldsymbol{0}\,, \tag{25}$$

$$-\rho^w\nabla\mu^w + K_{sw}(\nu^s - \nu^w) + K_{wi}(\nu^i - \nu^w) = \boldsymbol{0}, \tag{26}$$

$$-\rho^i\nabla\mu^i + K_{is}(\nu^s - \nu^i) + K_{wi}(\nu^w - \nu^i) = \boldsymbol{0}. \tag{27}$$

These equations show that the chemical potentials are the sole driving forces for water and mobile ions to overcome the frictional drag of relative motion. For the solid matrix, the driving force also involves deformation described by $\mathbf{C}$. From the continuity and the momentum equations, one obtains a diffusion equation for the mobile ions:

$$\mathrm{div}\left(\frac{\rho^{i2}}{K_{is}+K_{wi}}\nabla\mu^i\right) - \mathrm{div}\left(\rho^i\frac{K_{is}\nu^s + K_{wi}\nu^w}{K_{is}+K_{wi}}\right) = \frac{\partial\rho^i}{\partial t}. \tag{28}$$

For isothermal conditions, the changes of these chemical potentials are related to the changes of the deformation in the solid matrix by the following Gibbs-Duhem equation:

$$\frac{1}{2}\rho^s\left[\mathbf{K}^s([\nabla\mathbf{C}]\mathbf{C}^{-1}) - [\nabla\mathbf{C}](\mathbf{F}^{-1}\mathbf{K}^s\mathbf{F}^{-T})\right] + \rho^s\mathrm{div}\mathbf{K}^s + \rho^w\nabla\mu^w\mathbf{I} + \rho^i\nabla\mu^i\mathbf{I} + \mathrm{div}\sigma = \boldsymbol{0}, \tag{29}$$

where the total stress σ is defined as:

$$\sigma = \sigma^s + \sigma^w + \sigma^i\,. \tag{30}$$

In the absence of the solid phase, the above equation reduces to the well known Gibbs-Duhem equation for a binary liquid solution:

$$\rho^w d\mu^w + \rho^i d\mu^i - dp = 0. \tag{31}$$

Summing the momentum equations ($\mathrm{div}\sigma^\alpha + \pi^\alpha = \boldsymbol{0}$) for all three phases, we obtain the simple equation for the stress of the total mixture:

$$\mathrm{div}\,\sigma = \boldsymbol{0}\,. \tag{32}$$

The Boundary of the Triphasic Mixture and Boundary Conditions

It is natural to define the boundary of our triphasic mixture to be fixed to the solid matrix. When a triphasic mixture interfaces with an external bathing solution, either directly or through a idealized porous wall, this boundary allows free exchange of the interstitial fluid and ions with the external solution. For quasi-static conditions, the interface boundary conditions for the total mixture stress σ and the chemical potentials μ^w and μ^i can be derived from the jump conditions. The jump conditions corresponding to the balances of mass, momentum, energy and entropy, with inertia neglected, on a boundary of a three-component mixture defined above, are (Hou et al 1989; Lai et al 1990)

$$[[\ \rho^w(\boldsymbol{v}^w - \boldsymbol{v}^s)\ ]]\cdot\boldsymbol{n} = 0, \tag{33}$$

$$[[\ \rho^i(\boldsymbol{v}^i - \boldsymbol{v}^s)\ ]]\cdot\boldsymbol{n} = 0, \tag{34}$$

$$[[\ \sigma\ ]]\cdot\boldsymbol{n} = \boldsymbol{0}, \tag{35}$$

$$[[\boldsymbol{q}^s + \boldsymbol{q}^w + \boldsymbol{q}^i + \sigma^s\boldsymbol{v}^s + \sigma^w\boldsymbol{v}^w + \sigma^i\boldsymbol{v}^i + \rho^w e^w(\boldsymbol{v}^w - \boldsymbol{v}^s) + \rho^i e^i(\boldsymbol{v}^i - \boldsymbol{v}^s)\ ]]\cdot\boldsymbol{n} = 0, \tag{36}$$

$$[[\ \frac{1}{T}(\boldsymbol{q}^s + \boldsymbol{q}^w + \boldsymbol{q}^i) + \rho^w\eta^w(\boldsymbol{v}^w - \boldsymbol{v}^s) + \rho^i\eta^i(\boldsymbol{v}^i - \boldsymbol{v}^s)\ ]]\cdot\boldsymbol{n} = 0. \tag{37}$$

For isothermal process, one obtains, with the definition of chemical potentials, from equations (35) - (37):

$$[[\ \mu^w\rho^w(\boldsymbol{v}^w - \boldsymbol{v}^s) + \mu^i\rho^i(\boldsymbol{v}^i - \boldsymbol{v}^s)\ ]]\cdot\boldsymbol{n} = 0. \tag{38}$$

Since the chemical potentials μ^w and μ^i are independent of the relative velocities $\boldsymbol{v}^w - \boldsymbol{v}^s$ and $\boldsymbol{v}^i - \boldsymbol{v}^s$; also $\boldsymbol{v}^w - \boldsymbol{v}^s$, $\boldsymbol{v}^i - \boldsymbol{v}^s$, ρ^w and ρ^i are independent variables, so that μ^w is independent of $\rho^w(\boldsymbol{v}^w - \boldsymbol{v}^s)$ and μ^i is independent of $\rho^i(\boldsymbol{v}^i - \boldsymbol{v}^s)$. Thus from equations (33) and (34) one can conclude that

$$[[\ \mu^w\ ]] = 0, \tag{39a}$$

$$[[\ \mu^i\ ]] = 0. \tag{39b}$$ [3]

Thus, for the triphasic theory, it is natural to express the momentum equations in terms of the total stress σ, equation (32), and of the two chemical potentials μ^w and μ^i, equations (26) and (27).

[3] For the case where the boundary is between two mixture, each of which has a solid component, equation (39) is also valid if $[[\boldsymbol{v}^s]] = \boldsymbol{0}$ across the boundary.

Constitutive Equations

Reference Configurations and Infinitesimal Deformation Theory

A reference configuration must be specified in order that deformation can be described. Although any configuration may serve as a reference, two are of particular interest: 1) unloaded equilibrium configuration in the hypothetical limit of infinite salt concentration; and 2) unloaded equilibrium configuration in a physiological saline bath. The physiological saline reference is often used for experimental measurements of cartilage swelling and deformation. In other experiments performed in bathing solutions with a specifically given salt concentration, the unloaded configuration of the tissue is often used as its reference. However, for constitutive modeling of tissue swelling behaviors, the reference corresponding to the infinite salt concentration is preferred, because at this reference the osmotic pressure and the chemical expansion pressure are negligibly small and the solid matrix may be considered to be stress free. In the triphasic theory, all deformations are measured relatively to this unloaded hypertonic state.[4]

For cartilage, deformations due to ion-induced swelling are generally small (Myers et al 1984; Mow and Schoonbeck 1984). Thus, for the present theory, we shall use the infinitesimal strain tensor **E**. Further, we assume the solid matrix to be isotropic and all deformations occur in an isothermal manner. However, in this present development, we shall allow for large variations of ionic environment–from a hypertonic condition to deionized water state. Under these assumptions, the total mixture stress and the chemical potentials for the interstitial water and salt are in the forms of:

$$\sigma = -p\mathbf{I} - T_c\mathbf{I} + \lambda_s \mathrm{tr}(\mathbf{E})\mathbf{I} + 2\mu_s\mathbf{E}, \tag{40}$$

$$\mu^w = \frac{1}{\rho_T^w}p + R_w + \frac{B_w}{\rho_T^w}\mathrm{tr}(\mathbf{E}), \tag{41}$$

$$\mu^i = R_i + B_i \mathrm{tr}(\mathbf{E}), \tag{42}$$

where all the coefficients T_c, λ_s, μ_s, R_w, R_i, B_w and B_i depend on ρ^w, ρ^i and c^F. In equations (40), the term $-T_c$ is a phenomenological continuum representation of the chemical-expansion stress due to the charge-to-charge electrostatic repulsion. The last two terms in equation (40) give the elastic stress for the solid matrix. Equations (41) and (42) give the general forms of the chemical potentials for the water and ion phases. Specific constitutive equations for T_c, R_w and R_i will be given in the following.

---

[4]Change of reference configuration can be easily made. We shall do so later to relate our experimental measurements made in the physiological saline reference state.

Chemical Potentials for the Triphasic Medium

The determination of R_i and R_w is guided by the physicochemical theory for polyelectrolytic solutions, to which our theory must reduce in the absence of a solid phase. Thus we take as the constitutive functions for the chemical potentials for the NaCl ions and the interstitial water as follows:

$$\mu^i = \mu_o^i + \frac{RT}{M_i}\ln\left[\gamma_\pm^2 c(c+c^F)\right], \tag{43}$$

$$\mu^w = \mu_o^w + \frac{1}{\rho_T^w}[p - RT\phi(2c+c^F) + B_w \mathrm{tr}\mathbf{E}], \tag{44}$$

where c and c^F are moles of the mobile NaCl and immobile Na^+ per unit interstitial water volume in the tissue respectively, and $\mu_o^w = \mu_o^{w*}$. The activity coefficient $\gamma_\pm$ is in general a function of c and c^F. The relation between the fixed charge density c^F and the infinitesimal solid matrix deformation **E** is

$$c^F = c_o^F\left(1 - \frac{1}{\phi_o^w}\mathrm{tr}\mathbf{E}\right), \tag{45}$$

where c_o^F and ϕ_o^w are the FCD and porosity at the reference configuration for the deformation **E**.

The external NaCl bathing solution can be considered to be a reduced triphasic medium, where there are no solid component and FCD. The chemical potentials for the solute (NaCl) and solvent (water) thus are given by

$$\mu^{i*} = \mu_o^{i*} + \frac{RT}{M_i}\ln\left(\gamma_\pm^{*2} c^{*2}\right), \tag{46}$$

$$\mu^{w*} = \mu_o^{w*} + \frac{1}{\rho_T^w}(p^* - 2RT\phi^* c^*), \tag{47}$$

where "*" denotes the external bathing solution. In general we also assume that the bathing solution is not pressurized, so that $p^*=0$.

Application of Triphasic Theory for Cartilage Swelling[5]

Equilibrium Free-Swelling — Change of Dimension

Consider a cylindrical specimen of tissue placed inside a circular confining ring, as shown in Figure 2. No load is applied onto the specimen in the axial

[5]More details may be found in reference by Lai et al (1990).

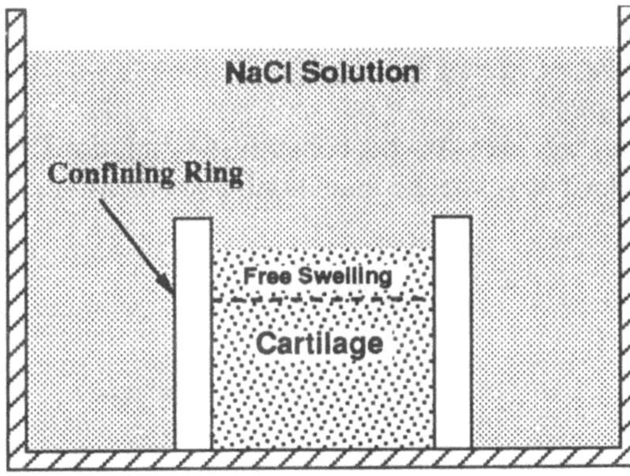

Figure 2. Schematic diagram of one-dimensional free-swelling of articular cartilage specimen. Dotted line indicates the free surface at hypertonic reference configuration.

direction z. The specimen is equilibrated in a NaCl solution with concentration c*. Thus, the boundary conditions on the free surface of the tissue are:

$$\sigma_{zz} = 0, \quad \mu^i = \mu^{i*}, \quad \text{and} \quad \mu^w = \mu^{w*}. \tag{48}$$

These conditions, together with equations (43) (47) and the fact that μ^i, μ^w and σ_{zz} are constant throughout the tissue (from the momentum equations), yield the following three equations for the mobile salt concentration c, the fluid pressure p, and the swelling strain e_{zz} (relative to its hypertonic reference configuration):

$$c(c+c^F) = \left(\frac{\gamma_\pm^*}{\gamma_\pm}\right)^2 c^{*2}, \tag{49}$$

$$p = RT[\phi(2c+c^F) - 2\phi^* c^*] + P_\infty - B_w e_{zz}, \tag{50}$$

$$(\lambda_s+2\mu_s)e_{zz} = p + T_c, \tag{51}$$

where c^F is related to e_{zz} through equation (45), and in equation (50), $P_\infty = \rho_T^w(\mu_o^{w*}-\mu_o^w)$. We see from equation (49) that the present triphasic theory yields the Donnan equilibrium ion distribution equation. Equation (49) (in molality form) has been used extensively to determine the physicochemical properties of articular cartilage (Maroudas 1975, 1979; Maroudas and Bannon 1981).

From equation (50), we see three sources contributing to the total pressure in the fluid: 1) the Donnan osmotic pressure $RT[\phi(2c+c^F)-2\phi^*c^*]$; 2) the osmotic pressure due to the presence of the proteoglycan particles, P_∞; and 3) the pressure due to deformation of the collagen-proteoglycan solid matrix given by $-B_w e_{zz}$. The latter two sources embody the so-called "excluded volume effect". In the absence of the solid matrix effect, i.e., $B_w=0$, equation (50) yields the osmotic pressure for a proteoglycan solution in equilibrium with a NaCl solution (Maroudas and Bannon 1981; Urban and Maroudas 1979, 1981). The term P_∞, arising from a difference of the reference chemical potentials of water between the internal (μ_o^w) solution and the external (μ_o^{w*}) solution, can be considered to depend on, among other things, the concentration of the proteoglycans in the tissue, and thus can be simply expressed as:

$$P_\infty = \phi_{pg} RT \frac{c_{pg}}{M_{pg}} + O\left(\frac{c_{pg}}{M_{pg}}\right)^2, \tag{52}$$

where c_{pg} is the proteoglycan concentration (in g/ml), M_{pg} is the mean molecular weight and ϕ_{pg} is the osmotic coefficient.

Osmotic pressures of PG solutions, as a function of FCD, have been measured by Urban and co-workers (1981). The measurements were made through an equilibration of the PG-NaCl solution (internal) with a PEG-NaCl solution (external) of known osmotic pressure. These investigators found, for example at FCD=0.4 mEq/(g water), p=0.25 MPa in a 0.15 M NaCl solution and p=0.12 MPa at 1.5 M NaCl. They also found that the Donnan (ionic) contribution to the osmotic pressure (i.e, the first term of equation (50)) is over 85% of the total measured osmotic pressure.

For articular cartilage, a solid matrix exists. The description of its swelling behavior (changes in dimensions, volume and pressures) thus must also incorporate the deformation of the solid matrix. Equation (51) of our equilibrium free-swelling problem states that a balance must exist between the fluid pressure p, the chemical-expansion pressure T_c, and the elastic stress in solid matrix due to deformation $(\lambda_s+2\mu_s)e_{zz}$. This equation suggests that we define a total swelling pressure P_s to be the sum of the fluid pressure p and the chemical-expansion pressure T_c, i.e.:

$$P_s = p + T_c. \tag{53}$$

Equilibrium Confined-Swelling — Change of Stress

In the confined isometric swelling experiment with the specimen equilibrated in c*, the volume of the cylindrical sample is prevented from changing by prescribing the fixed axial compressive offset strain ε $(= -e_{zz})$, as shown in Figure 3. The platen compressing the specimen is permeable to the ion and fluid phases. At equilibrium, the momentum equations and boundary conditions again yield the Donnan equilibrium ion distribution, i.e., equation (49), and the fluid pressure:

$$p = RT[\phi(2c+c^F) - 2\phi^* c^*] + P_\infty + B_w\varepsilon. \tag{54}$$

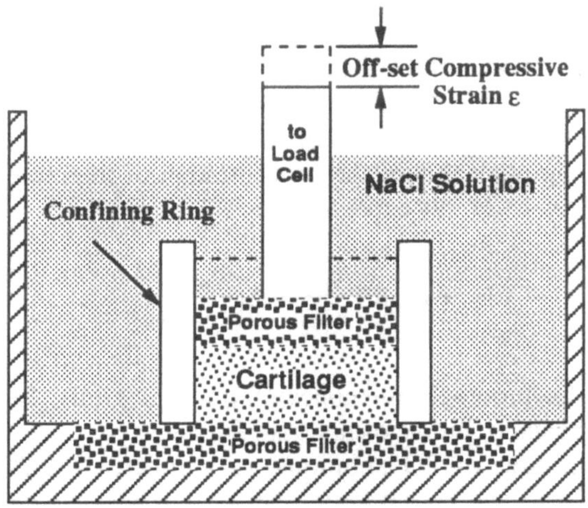

Figure 3. Schematic diagram of one-dimensional isometric confined-swelling of articular cartilage specimen. The specimen is kept at a constant thickness with an off-set strain ε and the force needed to keep it from swelling is measured with a load cell.

Now, from the boundary condition $\sigma_{zz} = -P_{app}$ and the constitutive relation equation (50), we obtain:

$$P_{app} = (\lambda_s + 2\mu_s)\varepsilon + P_s. \tag{55}$$

This equation states that the total applied compressive stress required to keep the tissue at the isometric configuration is the sum of the elastic compressive stress $(\lambda_s+2\mu_s)\varepsilon$ and the total swelling pressure, $P_s = p + T_c$. When the offset strain $\varepsilon = 0$, $P_{app} = P_s$ from equation (54). This means that for a tissue bathed in an external salt solution of concentration c^*, the applied compressive stress needed to keep the tissue at the unloaded hypertonic reference configuration dimensions is completely balanced by the total swelling pressure; and there is no elastic stress. This swelling pressure has been reported to be 0.17 MPa for a plug of cartilage from a human femoral head (Maroudas 1975, 1979). However, it should be noted again that in general the total swelling pressure P_s is the sum of two components: 1) the fluid pressure (which includes the Donnan osmotic pressure, the solid matrix coupling term $B_w e$ and P_∞), and 2) the chemical-expansion stress $-T_c$. We also note that provided P_∞ is negligible, and the tissue is kept at the volume corresponding to the unloaded hypertonic reference configuration, the fluid pressure is the same as the Donnan osmotic pressure.

Equilibrium Donnan Ion Distribution

Equation (49) defines the mobile NaCl concentration c in the tissue as a

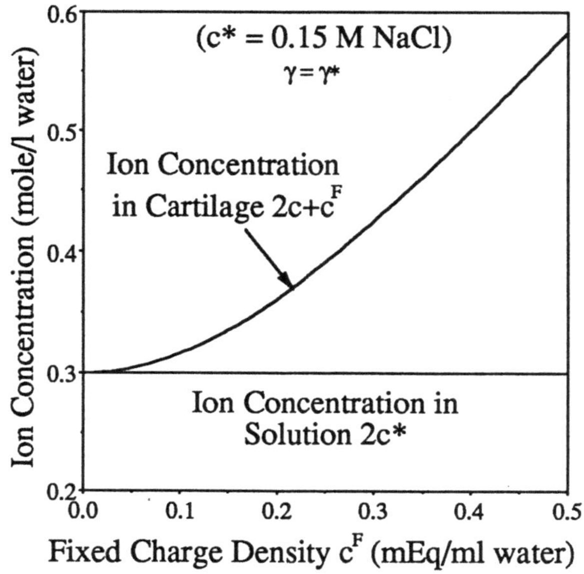

Figure 4. Ion concentration in the interstitium ($2c+c^F$) vs FCD (c^F), with the activity coefficients $\gamma_\pm/\gamma_\pm^* = 1$. The external bathing solution NaCl concentration $c^*=0.15$ M.

function of c^F and c^*. The ion concentration (Na^+ and Cl^-) inside the cartilage is $2c+c^F$, and the ion concentration in the external bath is $2c^*$. The difference between these two concentrations may be calculated for given values of c_o^F, ϕ_o^w and e_{zz}. Figure 4 gives the values of the ion concentration in the tissue ($2c+c^F$) for $c^*=0.15$ M (total concentration of the ions in the bathing solution is 0.3 M), and for values of c_o^F ranging from 0 to 0.5 mEq/(ml water) and the ratio $\gamma_\pm/\gamma_\pm^*$ is taken to be unity (Maroudas 1975, 1979). Further, the tissue is kept at the reference configuration (e=0, i.e. at the volume of the unloaded tissue in the hypertonic solution). The curves show that the ion concentration $2c+c^F$ in the tissue increases nonlinearly as c^F increases and is always larger than the concentration $2c^*$ in the bath. This imbalance of ion concentrations inside and outside the tissue gives rise to the Donnan ionic osmotic pressure.

Donnan Osmotic Pressure

Figure 5 shows the variation of Donnan osmotic pressure for a tissue equilibrated in a 0.15 M NaCl solution as a function of c^F. The tissue volume is kept fixed at its reference configuration (e=0). For these calculations, the osmotic coefficient ϕ is assumed to be the same as ϕ^* for the NaCl bath. The value of ϕ^* was taken from available data (Robinson and Stokes 1968), and P_∞ was assumed to be negligible. We see that the Donnan (ionic) osmotic pressure increases nonlinearly with c^F to approximately 0.6 MPa at $c^F=0.5$ (mEq/ml water).

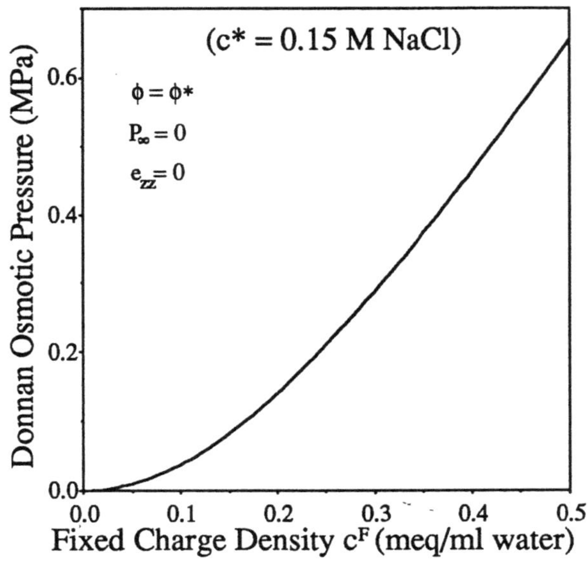

Figure 5. Donnan osmotic pressure (p) vs FCD (c^F) for an external solution of 0.15 M NaCl. The specimen is kept at its hypertonic reference configuration (e_{zz} =0). The activity and osmotic coefficients are assumed to satisfy $\gamma_\pm/\gamma_\pm^* = 1$ and $\phi/\phi^*=1$, with the value of ϕ^* taken from Robinson and Stokes (1968), and the colligative contribution of PG is neglected, i.e., $P_\infty=0$.

Contribution of Physicochemical Factors to Cartilage Stiffness

Here we derive a "stress-strain" relation from our triphasic theory to show how the osmotic pressure and chemical-expansion stress contribute to the total confined compressive stiffness of the tissue. For a tissue specimen which is laterally confined at its hypertonic reference configuration, a linear axial stress-strain relation for the tissue in a solution with constant salt concentration c* has been derived from the linear biphasic theory as

$$P_{app} = H_A \varepsilon', \tag{56}$$

where the stiffness H_A is called the aggregate modulus (Mow et al 1980). In equation (56), the compressive axial strain ε' is measured from the unloaded configuration of cartilage in a bathing solution with NaCl concentration c*. Under infinitesimal deformation, ε' is related to ε by the simple linear transformation

$$\varepsilon = \varepsilon' - e_{zzo} , \tag{57}$$

where e_{zzo} is the free-swelling axial strain measured from the hypertonic reference configuration (so that ε'=0) and is determined by equation (51).

The relation between the stiffness H_A and the intrinsic material coefficients $\lambda_s+2\mu_s$, the fluid pressure p and the chemical-expansion stress T_c can be derived as following. Using equations (51) and (57), equation (55) can be written as

$$P_{app} = (\lambda_s+2\mu_s)\varepsilon' + (p+T_c)\Big|_{\varepsilon=\varepsilon'-e_{zz0}} - (p+T_c)\Big|_{\varepsilon=-e_{zz0}} \quad . \tag{58}$$

By Taylor series expansion of $p+T_c$ in terms of the infinitesimal strain ε', equation (58) can be approximated with a linear function of ε':

$$P_{app} = \left[(\lambda_s+2\mu_s) + \frac{\partial(p+T_c)}{\partial\varepsilon'}\Big|_{\varepsilon=-e_{zz0}} \right]\varepsilon' \; . \tag{59}$$

Compare equation (56) with (59), we see that

$$H_A = (\lambda_s+2\mu_s) + \frac{\partial(p+T_c)}{\partial\varepsilon'}\Big|_{\varepsilon=-e_{zz0}} \quad . \tag{60}$$

Hence cartilage stiffness H_A comes from two contributions: (i) The elastic part of the solid matrix stiffness $\lambda_s+2\mu_s$ and (ii) the slope of the total swelling pressure due to deformation. The aggregate modulus H_A has been measured in many experiments and it is shown to decrease with increasing c* (Parsons and Black 1979; Mow and Schoonbeck 1984).

Chemical-Expansion Stress T_c

The chemical-expansion stress $-T_c(c,c^F)$ in equation (40) is a continuum representation of the charge-to-charge repulsive forces developed by the fixed charge groups on the GAG chains of the PG molecules. The general formulation of the triphasic theory indicates that the chemical-expansion stress contributes to cartilage swelling together with the Donnan osmotic pressure. Table 1 shows the data for H_A in a confined compression experiment and strain e' in a one-dimensional free-swelling experiment of bovine articular cartilage for six NaCl concentrations c* (Mow and Schoonbeck 1985), where e' is measured from the unloaded configuration at c*=0 (water). Both H_A and e' decrease with c* in an exponential manner. Thus, it is natural to expect T_c to also decrease exponentially with c* and so we assume

$$T_c(c,c^F) = a_0 c^F e^{-\kappa(\gamma_\pm/\gamma_\pm^{*})\sqrt{c(c+c^F)}} - P_\infty . \tag{61}$$

We note that (i) in equilibrium, the ion concentration in the tissue is related to c* by equation (49), so that equation (61) indeed reduces to the desired exponential dependence of T_c on c*, (ii) T_c is assumed to be proportional to c^F

so that $T_c \to 0$ as $c^F \to 0$, and (iii) the term P_∞ is included so that $e_{zz}=0$ as $c^* \to \infty$, as required by our choice of reference configuration.

c* (M NaCl)	0.00	0.15	0.30	0.75	1.50	2.50
Aggregate modulus H_A (MPa)	2.00	1.00	0.80	0.58	0.50	0.48
Axial free-swelling strain (measured from unloaded configuration in water) e'	0.0	−0.145	−0.208	−0.245	−0.250	−0.265

Table 1. Experimental measurements (Mow and Schoonbeck 1984) of aggregate modulus H_A and free-swelling axial strain e' (measured from the unloaded configuration in water) of confined cartilage specimen.

A Numerical Result

The free-swelling strain e_{zz} in a bathing solution with NaCl concentration c* is given by equation (51), where $p=p(c,c^F(e_{zz}),e_{zz})$ and $T_c=T_c(c,c^F(e_{zz}))$. By Taylor series expansion, the total swelling pressure can be written as a linear function of e_{zz}:

$$p+T_c = p(c,c_0^F,0) + T_c(c,c_0^F) + \left(\frac{\partial(p+T_c)}{\partial e_{zz}}\bigg|_{e_{zz}=0}\right)e_{zz}. \qquad (62)$$

Thus equation (51) can be written as

$$\left(\lambda_s + 2\mu_s - \frac{\partial(p+T_c)}{\partial e_{zz}}\bigg|_{e_{zz}=0}\right)e_{zz} = p(c,c_0^F,0) + T_c(c,c_0^F)\,. \qquad (63)$$

For infinitesimal strain, $\partial(p+T_c)/\partial e_{zz}$ is virtually constant for a given c*. Therefore by equations (60), (50) and (61), equation (63) can be written as

$$H_A e_{zz} = RT\left[\phi\sqrt{c_0^{F2}+4(\gamma_\pm/\gamma_\pm^*)^2c^{*2}} - 2\phi^*c^*\right] + a_0 c_0^F e^{-\kappa c^*}. \qquad (64)$$

With equation (64), using the experimental measurements of H_A and e' ($=e_{zz}-e_{zzo}$, where e_{zzo} is the free-swelling strain in water measured from the hypertonic configuration), one can determine the parameters in the chemical-expansion stress $-T_c$, for known physicochemical values of $\gamma_\pm/\gamma_\pm^*$, ϕ, ϕ^* and c_0^F. With the experimental data for H_A and e' given in Table 1, assuming $c_0^F = 0.1$ mEq/(ml

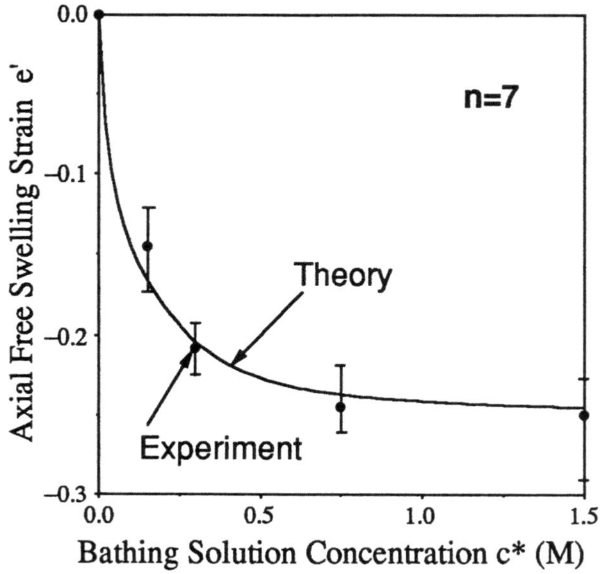

Figure 6. Experimental (Mow and Schoonbeck 1984) result and theoretical calculation of a specimen of cartilage in free-swelling as functions of bathing solution NaCl concentration, as described in Figure 2. The axial swelling strain e' is measured from the unloaded configuration of cartilage in water.

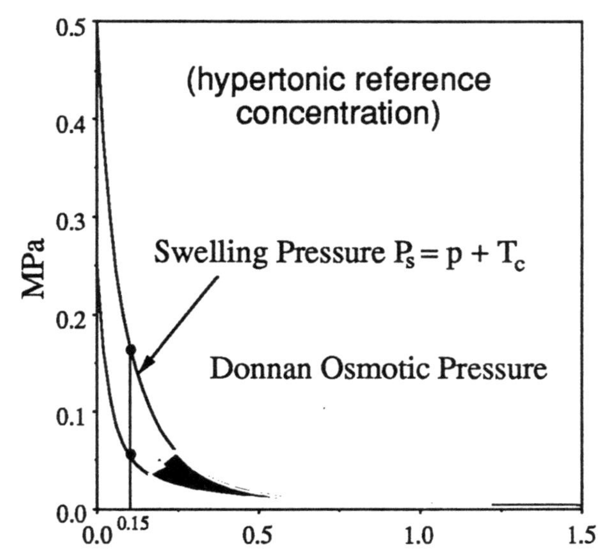

Figure 7. Theoretical calculations of Donnan osmotic pressure and total swelling pressure of a specimen of cartilage in confined-swelling as functions of the bathing solution NaCl concentration, as described in Figure 3. The specimen is kept at its hypertonic reference configuration.

water), $\gamma_{\pm}/\gamma_{\pm}^{*}=1$ and $\phi/\phi^{*}=1$ with $\phi^{*}(c^{*})$ given by Robinson and Stokes (1968), the parameters in T_c were found from curve-fitting to be $a_0c_0^F=2.5$ MPa and k=7.5. The theoretical curve of the free-swelling strain calculated from the above parameters is shown in Figure 6 for a comparison with the experimental measurement.

When the tissue is kept at its hypertonic reference configuration, $e_{zz}=0$, the fluid pressure p at any c* is the Donnan (ionic) osmotic pressure, see equation (54) (with negligible P_{∞}). From our results of parameters for p and T_c, we may now calculate their relative contributions in producing the total swelling pressure P_s. This calculation is shown in Figure 7. For our assumed physicochemical coefficients, at c*=0.15 M NaCl, we find that the Donnan (ionic) osmotic pressure and the chemical-expansion stress contribute in nearly equal proportions to the total swelling pressure P_s.

The role of physicochemical factors in determining cartilage compressive stiffness may also be calculated. Figure 8 shows a linear stress-strain curve for the confined compression problem when the specimen is equilibrated in a 0.15 M NaCl solution, using H_A=1 MPa (Table 1), and the assumed physicochemical coefficients. In this figure, the compressive strain ε' is measured with reference to the unloaded configuration at c*=15 M. The stress-strain curve is P_{app} vs ε'. Also the normalized total swelling pressure, $\overline{P} = P_s - P_{so}$, and the normalized fluid pressure, $\overline{p} = p - p_o$, are presented, where P_{so} and p_o are evaluated at $\varepsilon'=0$.

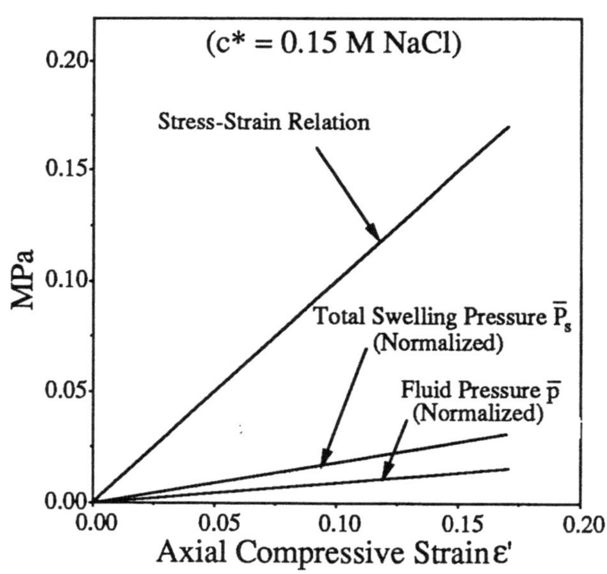

Figure 8. The stress-strain curve for the tissue (Mow and Schoonbeck 1984) in 0.15 M NaCl bathing solution, whose slope is the aggregate modulus H_A. The axial compressive strain ε' is measured from the unloaded configuration. Also shown are the predicted and normalized total swelling pressure and Donnan osmotic pressure as functions of the compressive strain.

From equation (60), we see that the total swelling pressure P_s contributes to the tissue stiffness H_A through its slope $dP_s/d\varepsilon'$. Figure 8 shows the slope of P_s is relatively small in comparison with the slope of the stress-strain relationship (aggregate modulus H_A=1 MPa). Thus for this set of bovine articular cartilage specimens, assuming c_0^F=0.1 mEq/(ml water), the elastic part of the stiffness of the solid matrix makes major contribution to the overall compressive stiffness of cartilage.

Isometric Transient Swelling

The kinetics of swelling, as measured either by the dimensional change or by the isometric constraint force, depends on the rate of ion diffusion into or out of the tissue (Maroudas 1979; Maroudas and Bannon 1981; Myers et al 1984), as well as the rate of interstitial fluid flow (Myers et al 1984; Eisenberg and Grodzinsky 1985, 1987). One of the most interesting swelling phenomenon may be seen in the isometric tensile experiment. In going from H_20 to 0.15M NaCl, isometrically constrained cartilage will exhibit a bimodal force response. The experimental results show that the isometric constraint force will increase or decrease depending on the magnitude of offset tensile strain [Myers et al 1984; Akizuki et al 1986).

Consider a sample of cartilage, with radius R_o and length L_o in a hypertonic solution. The same unloaded sample swells to a larger length L_1 in pure water. In the isometric experiment, this specimen is held at a fixed axial length L larger than L_1 so that there is an offset tensile axial strain, which is denoted by e_c, when measured from L_1 or by e_o when measured from L_o. Both e_c and e_o will be assumed to be infinitesimal. Prior to the beginning of the experiment, the sample is bathed in pure water. At t=0, the bathing solution in contact with the specimen surface is suddenly changed from H_20 to 0.15 M NaCl solution. Subsequently, the time history of the isometric constraint tensile force is observed. Here we use the triphasic theory to predict this time history. We assume that L_o is much larger than R_o so that we may assume all displacements, flow and ion diffusion occur in the radial direction only.

For this axisymmetric problem with the conditions that $v_r^s=v_r^w=0$ at r=0, the integration of the continuity equation for the mixture (3) yields:

$$v_r^w = -\frac{\phi^s}{\phi^w} v_r^s \,. \tag{65}$$

For infinitesimal radial displacement u,

$$v_r^s = \frac{\partial u}{\partial t} \,. \tag{66}$$

Thus the ion diffusion equation (28) can be written as, with the relation $\rho^i = M_i \phi^w c$,

$$\frac{1}{r}\frac{\partial}{\partial r}\left(\frac{M_i\phi^{w2}c^2}{K_{is}+K_{wi}}r\frac{\partial\mu^i}{\partial r}\right)-\frac{1}{r}\frac{\partial}{\partial r}\left(\phi^w c\frac{K_{is}-(\phi^s/\phi^w)K_{wi}}{K_{is}+K_{wi}}\frac{\partial u}{\partial t}\right)=\frac{\partial(\phi^w c)}{\partial t}, \tag{67}$$

Also, from the momentum equations (26), (27) and (32), one obtains the following equation

$$\frac{1}{\phi^{w2}}\left(K_{sw}-\frac{K_{is}K_{wi}}{K_{is}+K_{wi}}\right)\frac{\partial u}{\partial t}-\frac{\partial}{\partial r}\left[(\lambda_s+2\mu_s+B_w)\frac{1}{r}\frac{\partial(ru)}{\partial r}\right]+2\frac{u}{r}\frac{\partial\mu_s}{\partial r}-e_o\frac{\partial(\lambda_s+B_w)}{\partial r}$$

$$=-\frac{\partial T_c}{\partial c}-RT\rho^w_T\frac{\partial}{\partial r}(\phi(2c+c^F))+\frac{RTK_{wi}c}{K_{is}+K_{wi}}\frac{\partial}{\partial r}\left[\ln\left(\gamma_\pm^2 c(c+c^F)\right)\right], \tag{68}$$

Equations (67) and (68) form a set of coupled diffusion equations for determining the solid matrix displacement u and the salt concentration c. These equations are highly nonlinear. In the following we shall make the following simplification by neglecting the higher order terms induced by the changes in ϕ^s, ϕ^w and c^F due to the infinitesimal deformation, so that in equations (67) and (68) they are taken to be constants ϕ^s_o, ϕ^w_o and c^F_o. We also take $\gamma_\pm/\gamma^*_\pm=1$ and assume an ideal condition that $\phi=\phi^*=1$. We also assume that the diffusive drag between the mobile ions and other components is mainly the friction between the ions and the interstitial water, i.e., $K_{is}<<K_{wi}$, so that K_{is} can be taken to be zero in these equations. Under these approximations, the aggregate modulus $H_A=\lambda_s+2\mu_s+B_w$, and equations (67) and (68) can be written as

$$\frac{\partial c}{\partial t}=\frac{1}{r}\frac{\partial}{\partial r}\left(Dr\frac{\partial c}{\partial r}\right)-\frac{1-\phi^w_o}{\phi^w_o}\frac{1}{r}\frac{\partial}{\partial r}\left(rc\frac{\partial u}{\partial t}\right), \tag{69}$$

$$\frac{1}{k}\frac{\partial u}{\partial t}-\frac{\partial}{\partial r}\left[H_A\frac{1}{r}\frac{\partial(ru)}{\partial r}\right]+2\frac{u}{r}\frac{\partial\mu_s}{\partial r}-e_o\frac{\partial(\lambda_s+B_w)}{\partial r}=-\left(\frac{\partial T_c}{\partial c}+RT\frac{c^F_o}{(c+c^F_o)}\right)\frac{\partial c}{\partial r}, \tag{70}$$

where

$$D=\frac{RT\phi^w c}{K_{wi}}\left(1-\frac{c^F_o}{2(c+c^F_o)}\right)=D_o\left(1-\frac{c^F_o}{2(c+c^F_o)}\right), \tag{71}$$ [6]

and

$$k=\frac{\phi^{w2}}{K_{sw}}. \tag{72}$$

---

[6] $K_{wi}/(\phi^w_o c)$ is the diffusive resistance coefficient per unit mass of salt which may be assumed to be a constant.

We note that in the absence of deformation, equation (69) reduces to the classical diffusion equation and if concentration effect is absent, then equation (70) reduces to the biphasic gel diffusion equation. Thus D is the diffusivity and k is the permeability (Lai and Mow 1980). Notice that if the tissue contains neither FCD, i.e., $c_0^F = 0$, nor solid matrix, then D ($=D_o$) is the diffusivity of the mobile salt in the interstitial water. Thus we take the value of D_o to be that of the diffusivity of NaCl in an aqueous solution.

The coupled diffusion equations (69) and (70) are to be solved with the following boundary conditions:

$$u\Big|_{r=0} = 0, \qquad \frac{\partial c}{\partial r}\Big|_{r=0} = 0, \tag{73,74}$$

$$c(c+c_0^F)\Big|_{r=R_o} = c^{*2}, \tag{75}$$

$$(\lambda_s+B_w)\left(\frac{\partial u}{\partial r}+\frac{u}{r}+e_o\right) + 2\mu_s\frac{\partial u}{\partial r}\Big|_{r=R_o} = RT\left(\sqrt{4c^{*2}+c_0^{F2}}-2c^*\right) + a_o c_0^F e^{-\kappa c^*}, \tag{76}$$

where conditions (73) and (74) are from axisymmetry, condition (75) is the continuity of ion chemical potential and (76) is from the stress-free condition $\sigma_{rr}=0$ at the boundary $r=R_o$. In obtaining (76), the continuity of the water chemical potential was used. The initial conditions are:

$$c(r,0) = 0, \tag{77}$$

$$u(r,0) = \left[\frac{(RT+a_o)c_0^F - (\lambda_s+B_w)e_o}{2(\lambda_s+\mu_s+B_w)}\right]r. \tag{78}$$

Equation (78) is obtained from solving the equilibrium problem where the tissue is bathed in pure water with the axial offset strain e_o.

Figure 9 shows the schematic description of an isometric tensile swelling experiment. The cartilage specimen initially is equilibrated in water with an axial pre-strain e_c (measured from its unloaded configuration in water). The step change of the bathing solution concentration c* at t=0+ is provided by switching the shower from H_2O to 0.15 M NaCl. The transient tensile force (F) change is measured via a load cell. The transient behavior of the tensile force is the combination of three effects: (i) The increase in tensile force caused by a decrease of the osmotic pressure (equation (40)) due to the increase of salt concentration; (ii) the increase in tensile force caused by the decrease of the chemical-expansion pressure, T_c; and (iii) the decrease in tensile force caused by the decrease of the tensile modulus E, (Akizuki et al 1986). These investigators found a decrease of tensile modulus from 5 MPa in H_2O to 3 MPa in 0.15 M NaCl solution.

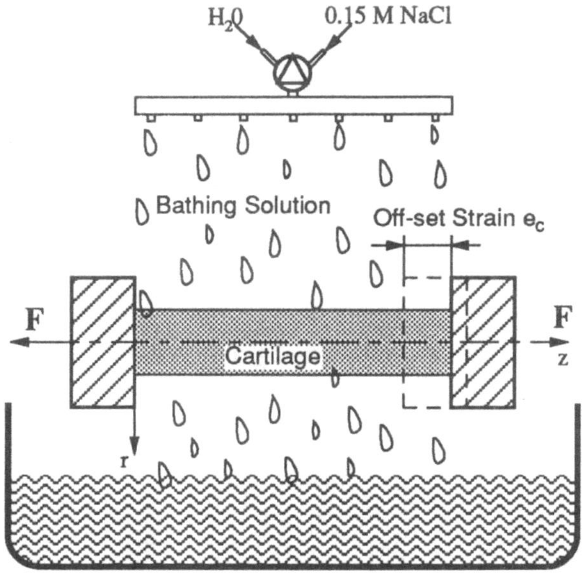

Figure 9. Schematic description of an isometric tensile swelling experiment. The cartilage specimen initially is equilibrated in water with an axial offset strain e_c (measured from the unloaded configuration in water). The concentration of the bathing solution c* is changed to 0.15 M NaCl at t=+0. The transient tensile force change is measured via a load cell.

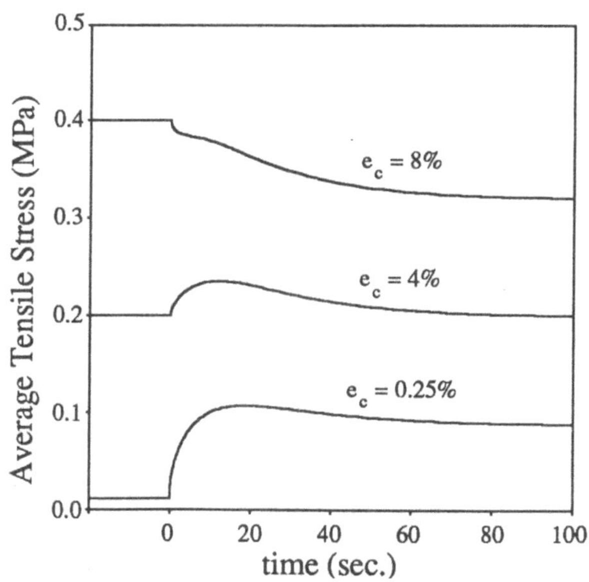

Figure 10. Predicted transient tensile force by the triphasic model of a cartilage specimen in an isometric swelling experiment, as described in Figure 9. Three curves are plotted for low (0.25%), medium (4%) and high (8%) offset strain.

Figure 10 depicts the transient average tensile stress (total tensile force divided by the cross-section area) for the cartilage tissue under low (0.25%), medium (4%) and high (8%) pre-strains. In the numerical calculations, the permeability k is taken to be $0.3\text{x}10^{-15}$ m^4/Ns, the diffusivity coefficient D_o, the diffusivity for the NaCl diffusion in an uncharged (c^F=0) hydrated tissue, is taken to be the diffusivity of NaCl in H_2O, i.e. 10^{-9} m^2/s, the volume fraction ϕ^w is assumed to be 0.8, and the specimen radius is 250 μm. The tensile modulus E_s is taken to be a linear function of the bathing solution concentration c*, which decreases from 5 MPa in water to 3 MPa in 0.15 M NaCl solution (Akizuki et al 1986). By using the equilibrium ion distribution equation (49), it can be written as the following function of c:

$$E_s = 5 - \frac{2}{0.15}\sqrt{c(c+c^F)} \; . \tag{79}$$

The Poisson's ratio is taken to be 0.2. The material coefficients in the chemical-expansion stress are $a_o c_o^F$=0.2 MPa and κ=5. For small strain e_c (0.25% from the unloaded configuration in water), the tensile force shows a nearly monotonic increase, because at this low strain, the predominant concentration effect is the decrease of the swelling pressure (the sum of the fluid pressure and the chemical-expansion pressure) which causes an increase in the tensile force, while the decrease of the tensile stress due to the decrease of the tensile modulus is small in comparison. For larger strain (8%), the decrease of the tensile modulus causes a much larger drop in tensile stress than the increase due to the effect of the decreasing osmotic pressure and chemical-expansion pressure, thus the tensile force exhibits a monotonic decrease. For intermediate strain (4%), the tensile force exhibits a peak value, then relaxes before reaching equilibrium. The specific shape of the curves also depends on other material properties, such as the permeability, fixed charge density, Poisson ratio, and etc. This bimodal pattern agrees very well with what observed experimentally (Myers et al 1984, Akizuki et al 1986).

Figure 11 shows the pressure distribution in the cartilage specimen, at different time. When the bathing solution changes from H_2O to 0.15 M NaCl, the fluid pressure tends to drop as the salt gradually diffuses into the tissue from the boundary. Thus the pressure near the boundary is lower than that in the middle region. Thus pressure gradient contributes to driving the interstitial water out of the tissue as NaCl diffuses into the tissue. When reaching equilibrium, the fluid pressure in the tissue drops from the initial 0.25 MPa to about 0.04 MPa. The corresponding radial r-fluid flux ($l/m^2/s$) is plotted in Figure 12.

Figure 13 illustrates the effect of different values of permeability k on the transient behavior of the average tensile stress of the cartilage specimen. These curves are calculated for the specimen with an offset strain e_c=4%, and the values of other parameters are the same as used for Figure 10. It shows that higher permeability k results in a higher peak tensile force before it decreases due to the decrease in tensile modulus. Higher permeability provides less diffusive drag

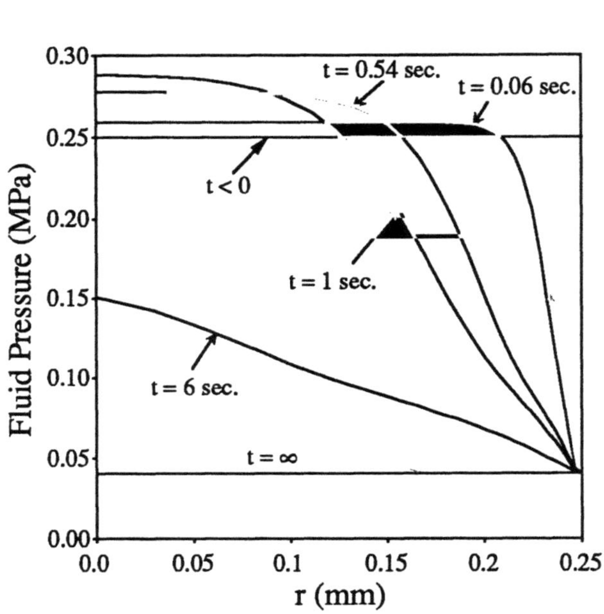

Figure 11. Pressure distribution in the cartilage at different time.

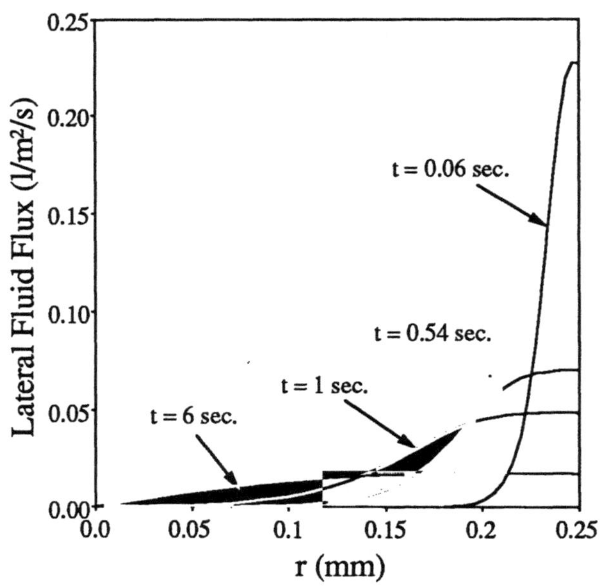

Figure 12. Radial (r) interstitial water flux in the cartilage specimen at different time.

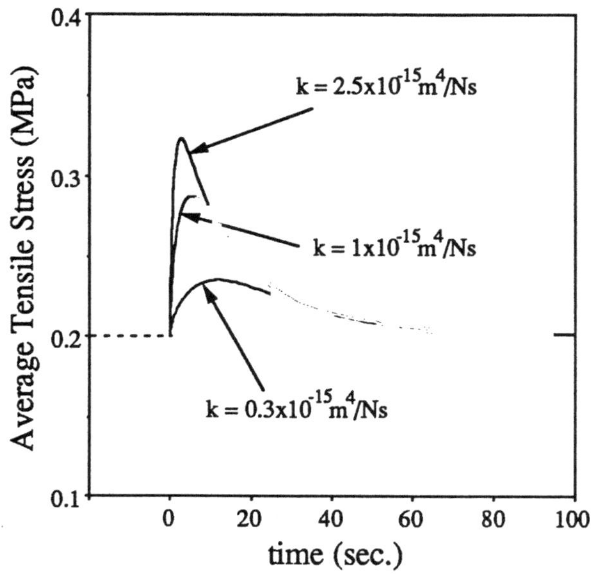

Figure 13. Effect of different values of permeability k on the transient behavior of the tensile force of the cartilage specimen, as described in Figure 9.

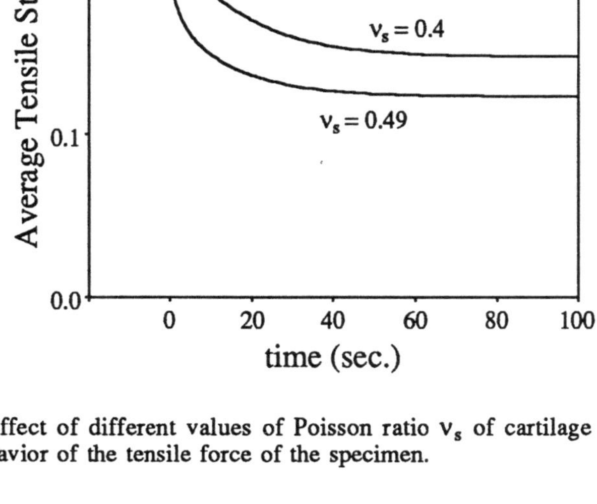

Figure 14. Effect of different values of Poisson ratio ν_s of cartilage matrix on the transient behavior of the tensile force of the specimen.

resistance to the radial fluid flow as indicated in Figure 12, so that the pressure in the tissue drops quicker than in the case for lower permeability. This lower pressure results in a higher tensile stress.

Figure 14 shows the effect of Poisson's ratio ν_s of cartilage matrix on the transient behavior of the average tensile stress of the specimen for a fixed offset strain (e_c=4%). For this calculation, the tensile modulus E_s is taken to be the same for all curves. It is interesting to note that the equilibrium stresses are different for these four curves, even though they have the same tensile modulus and the same offset tensile strain. This is quite different from the behavior of a single phase or biphasic material. In a triphasic medium, the increase in salt concentration induces a decrease in swelling pressure as well as a decrease in the tissue's tensile modulus. Clearly, from the constitutive equation for the total stress, equation (40), we see that a decrease in the swelling pressure induces an increase in the tensile force on the tissue since it is kept at a fixed length. This increase in tension is a maximum when the Poisson's ratio is zero and a minimum when the Poisson's ratio is 0.5. This is because a tissue with a smaller Poisson's ratio responds to the decrease in swelling pressure with a larger decrease in volume if it were free to do so. But, the tissue is restrained axially, therefore it responds with a rise in tension whose magnitude is largest when Poisson's ratio is zero. Thus, as seen in Figure 14, the equilibrium stress for ν_s=0 is the largest of the four curves. In this figure, the decrease in stiffness is the same for all the curves, the difference in equilibrium stress is entirely due to this Poisson's effect[7]. In transient responses, when the Poisson's ratio is large, the decrease in tensile modulus predominates so that the responses are monotonically decreasing functions of time (ν_s=0.4 and 0.49 in Figure 14). On the other hand when the Poisson's ratio is small, the two effects compete with each other and may result in a bimodel patterns as is seen in the curves for ν_s=0 and ν_s=0.2 in Figure 14.

Conclusion

A theory for a tertiary mixture has been developed to model articular cartilage swelling and deformational behaviors. This triphasic theory includes two immiscible fluid-solid phases (biphasic), and a third miscible ion phase. The momentum equations for the ions and the interstitial water are expressed in terms of their chemical potentials μ^i and μ^w. We have shown that this theory is capable of predicting the stress-strain fields in the solid matrix, interstitial fluid flow, along with the Donnan equilibrium ion distribution and osmotic pressure. An expression for the total equilibrium swelling pressure is derived, and this is the sum of two effects: 1) Osmotic pressure; and 2) chemical-expansion stress.

[7]The equilibrium tensile stress can be derived to be $\sigma_{zz} = Ee_c + (1-2\nu_s)\Delta P_s$, where $\Delta P_s = P_s$(in water)$-P_s$(in 0.15 M NaCl) is the total swelling pressure drop due to adding the salt in the bathing solution. Note for our calculations, the terms Ee_c and ΔP_s are the same for all values of Poisson's ratio ν_s in Figure 14.

Osmotic pressure derives predominantly from the Donnan ionic effect due to an excess of total ion concentration within the tissue with fixed charged density c^F over the ion concentration in the external solution. The chemical-expansion stress derives from the charge-to-charge repulsive force between the closely spaced charged groups along the glycosaminoglycan chains of the proteoglycans. Analytical terms for other factors, which may be interpreted as excluded-volume effects, have also been included in the theory. The theory is capable of predicting all field variables, equilibrium or transient, within the tissue when it is subjected to either a mechanical load and/or a chemical load. The triphasic theory provides a unified view for the physicochemical aspect of cartilage swelling and the biphasic aspects of solid matrix deformation and interstitial fluid flow.

Acknowledgements

This work was sponsored in part by grants from the National Science Foundation (EET-85-18501) and the National Institutes of Health (AR-38733). Any opinions, findings, and conclusions or recommendations expressed in this publication are those of the authors and do not necessarily represent the views of the National Science Foundation.

References

Akizuki S, Mow VC, Müller F, Pita JC, Howell DS, Manicourt DH: Tensile properties of human knee joint cartilage: I. Influence of ionic conditions, weight bearing, and fibrillation on the tensile modulus. J Orthop Res 1986;4:379-392.

Bowen RM: Incompressible porous media models by use of the theory of mixtures. Int J Eng Sci 1980;18:1129-1148.

Donnan FG: The theory of membrane equilibria. Chemical Review 1924;1: 73-90.

Eisenberg SR, Grodzinsky AJ: Swelling of articular cartilage and other connective tissues: electromechanochemical forces. J Orthop Research 1985;3:148-159.

Eisenberg SR, Grodzinsky, AJ: The kinetics of chemically induced nonequilibrium swelling of articular cartilage and corneal stroma. J Biomech Eng 1987;109:79-89.

Gabler R: Electrical Interactions in Molecular Biophysics, An Introduction. Academic Press, 1978.

Grodzinsky AJ, Roth V, Myers E, Grossman WK, Mow VC: The significance of electromechanical and osmotic forces in the nonequilibrium swelling behavior of articular cartilage in tension. J Biomech Eng 1981;103:221-231.

Hascall VC, Hascall GK: Proteoglycans, in Hay ED (ed): Cell Biology of Extracellular Matrix. Plenum ,1983, pp 39-60.

Hou JS, Holmes MH, Lai WM, Mow VC: Interface conditions between fluids, mixtures and solids: applications to biomechanics problems, in 1989 Adv in Bioeng, pp 175-176.

Katchalsky A, Curran PF: (1965), Nonequilibrium Thermodynamics in Biophysics. Cambridge, Harvard University Press, 1965.

Lai WM, Hou JS, Mow VC: A triphasic theory for swelling and deformation behavior of articular cartilage. Submitted to J Biomech Eng 1990.

Lai WM, Mow VC: Drag-induced compression of articular cartilage during a permeation experiment. Biorheology 1980;17:111-123.

Lanir Y: Biorheology and fluid flux in swelling tissues. I. Bicomponent theory for small deformations, including concentration effects. Biorheology 1987; 23:173-188.

Maroudas A: Swelling pressure versus collagen tension in normal and degenerate articular cartilage. Nature 1975;260:808.

Maroudas A: Biophysical chemistry of cartilaginous tissues with special reference to solute and fluid transport. Biorheology 1975;12:233-248.

Maroudas A: Physicochemical properties of articular cartilage, in Freeman MAR (ed): Adult Articular Cartilage, 2nd ed. Pitman Medical, 1979, pp 215-290.

Maroudas A, Bannon C: Measurement of swelling pressure in cartilage and comparison with the osmotic pressure of constituent proteoglycans. Biorheology 1981;18:619-632.

Mow VC, Kuei SC, Lai WM, Armstrong CG: Biphasic creep and stress relaxation of articular cartilage in compression: theory and experiment. J Biomech Eng 1980;102:73-84.

Mow VC, Holmes MH, Lai WM: Fluid transport and mechanical properties of articular cartilage. J Biomech 1984;17:377-394.

Mow VC, Schoonbeck JM: Contribution of Donnan osmotic pressure towards the biphasic compressive modulus of articular cartilage. Trans Orthop Res Soc 1984; 9:262.

Mow VC, Kwan MK, Lai WM, Holmes MH: A finite deformation theory for nonlinearly permeable soft hydrated biological tissues. in S L-Y Woo, G Schmid-Schönbein, B Zweifach (eds): Frontiers in Biomechanics. New York, Springer-Verlag, 1986, pp 153-179.

Muir H: Proteoglycans as organizers of the extracellular matrix. Biochem Soc Trans 1983;11:613-622.

Myers ER, Lai WM, Mow V C: A continuum theory and an experiment for the ion-induced swelling behavior of articular cartilage. J Biomech Eng 1984;106:151-158.

Parsons JR, Black J: Mechanical behavior of articular cartilage, quantitative changes with alteration of ionic environment. J Biomech 1979;12:765-773.

Robinson RA, Stokes RH: Electrolyte Solutions. London, Butterworths, 1968.

Tombs MP, Peacocke AR: The Osmotic Pressure of Biological Macromolecules. Oxford, Clarendon Press, 1974.

Urban JPG, Maroudas A, Bayliss MT, Dillon J: Swelling pressures of proteoglycans at the concentrations found in cartilaginous tissues. Biorheology 1979;16:447-464.

Urban JPG, Maroudas A: Swelling of the intervertebral disc in vivo. Connect Tissue Res 1979;9:1-10.

Chapter 11

Viscometric Properties of Proteoglycan Solutions at Physiological Concentrations

W.B. Zhu, V.C. Mow

Introduction

Proteoglycans are important components of the extracellular matrix of articular cartilage and other soft tissues. The structural organization of these macromolecules is believed to be significant for maintaining the cohesion of the extracellular matrix, and thus influences the material properties of the tissue as a whole (Pottenger et al. 1982; Muir 1983). Recent studies have shown that the structure of proteoglycans varies with cartilage age and pathology (Hjertquist and Wasteson 1972; Bayliss and Ali 1979; Muir 1977, 1980, 1983; Roughley and White 1980; Pal et al. 1981; Buckwalter et al. 1983; Buckwalter and Rosenberg 1985). In general, as cartilage ages and degenerates, proteoglycan size decreases (i.e. lower molecular weight) and the percentage of non-aggregated forms increases. The decrease in proteoglycan size and percentage aggregation has been shown to be important factors in increased mobility of the proteoglycan within the collagen meshwork (Pottenger et al. 1982; Muir 1983). Link proteins serve to stabilize proteoglycan aggregates by joining the proteoglycan monomers to a linear hyaluronate chain (Hardingham 1979, 1981). Changes in proteoglycan aggregation may involve abnormalities in the hyaluronate binding region of the monomer or the link protein (Muir 1977, 1983; Hardingham 1979, 1981; Plaas and Sandy 1984; Poole 1986; Ratcliffe et al. 1986). These changes tend to alter the collagen-proteoglycan and proteoglycan-proteoglycan interactions (Obrink 1973; Myers et al. 1984b; Mow et al. 1989), causing possible migration of proteoglycan fragments through, and loss from, the extracellular matrix (Brandt 1974; Muir 1977; Bayliss and Ali

1979; Ratcliffe et al. 1986). Loss of proteoglycans from the matrix will change the intrinsic biomechanical properties of the whole tissue, as well as the ability of the tissue to continue its load bearing function in the joint (Mow and Lai 1980; Armstrong and Mow 1982b; Mow et al. 1984a; Schmidt et al. 1986).

To gain insight into the roles proteoglycans play in organizing the extracellular matrix of cartilaginous tissues, we must know whether proteoglycans in aqueous solutions at physiological concentrations can form networks, and if so, what are the physical characteristics of these networks. In this chapter we present an overview of the methodology we have used to determine these proteoglycan network characteristics, and the density and strength of proteoglycan-proteoglycan interaction sites in these networks at physiological concentrations. The influences of proteoglycan molecular size, percentage aggregation, and link protein stabilization, on the stiffness and strength of these proteoglycan networks are examined.

Composition and Structure of Extracellular Matrix

The details of articular cartilage biology, composition and structure have been provided in the chapter by Mow and co-workers in these volumes. The reader is referred to that chapter for a more complete discussion of this material. In the present chapter, we shall focus our attention on the roles played by proteoglycans in articular cartilage organization and function. Articular cartilage is composed of a sparse population of specialized cells, the chondrocytes, distributed throughout a large, highly hydrated extracellular matrix. The matrix is predominately formed by a high concentration of proteoglycans enmeshed in a fine network of collagen fibrils. The collagen network is composed of mainly type II collagen fibrils formed through intramolecular and intermolecular covalent crosslinks (Eyre et al. 1984; Nimni and Harkness 1988; Yamauchi and Mechanic 1988). At least two other collagens, type IX and XI, which interact covalently with type II collagen, have been identified in the matrix. The existence of these interactions may influence the strength and stability of the collagen network (Ricard-Blum et al. 1985; van der Rest and Mayne 1988), and is essential for maintaining high tensile stiffness and strength of the tissue (Woo et al. 1976; Kempson 1979; Roth and Mow 1980; Schmidt et al. 1986).

Proteoglycans are large macromolecules, trapped and immobilized in the tightly woven collagen network (Pottenger et al. 1982). The basic form of proteoglycans (M_r 1-4x10^6) is a type of glycoprotein and consists of a protein core to which are attached glycosaminoglycan chains, mainly, keratan sulfate and chondroitin sulfate chains, Fig. 1, (Muir 1980; Hardingham 1981). These chains contain many negatively charged sulfate and carboxyl groups (SO_4 and COOH), which provide large charge-charge repulsive forces and strong hydrophillic properties (Maroudas 1979; Myers et al. 1984a, 1984b; Eisenberg and Grodzinsky 1987; Lai et al. 1989). Non-covalent interactions are formed between the hyaluronic acid (M_r 0.5-2x10^6) and proteoglycan monomers at the

G_1 globular domain (Hardingham 1979, 1981; Paulsson et al. 1987) and each proteoglycan-hyaluronate bond is stabilized by a separate globular link protein (M_r 41,000-48,000), Fig. 1. The aggregation of proteoglycans promotes their immobilization within the fine collagen meshwork and adds to the structural rigidity of the matrix (Pottenger et al. 1982; Muir 1983). Other types of proteoglycans also exist, though much less is known of their structure and function in cartilage (Rosenberg et al. 1985; Poole 1986; Sampaio et al. 1988).

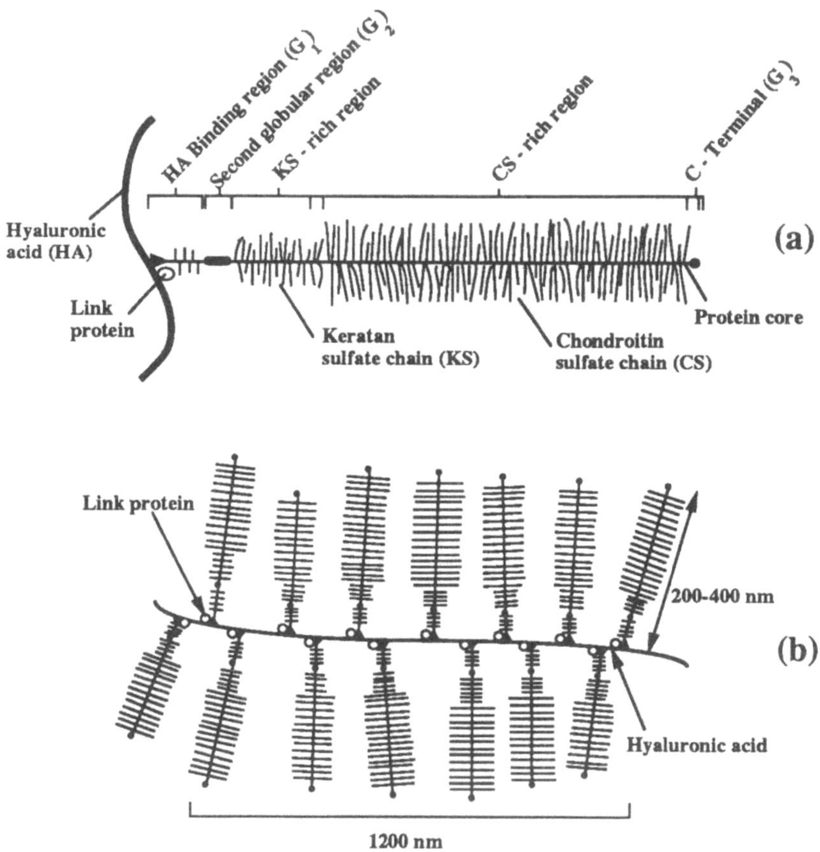

Figure 1. Schematic diagram of the structure of a proteoglycan monomer. The protein core contains three globular domains: the HA binding region (G_1), a second globular region (G_2), and C-terminal (G_3). The extended part of the protein core contains a keratan sulfate-rich region and a long chondroitin sulfate-rich region. The aggregate is composed of a linear hyaluronate filament associated with many monomers; the link protein stabilizes the association.

Proteoglycans in cartilage exist in a domain as small as 20% of their maximum free volume in dilute solution (Hascall and Hascall 1981; Muir 1983). The folding of proteoglycans into this highly compressed state provides extremely fine pores for interstitial fluid flow (Maroudas 1979; Mow et al. 1984a). The flow-induced interaction of the porous permeable solid matrix with the interstitial fluid generates significant frictional drag which governs the viscoelastic behaviors of cartilage in compression (see chapter by Mow et al. in these volumes for detailed discussions of this topic). The negatively charged groups on the proteoglycans also interact with the mobile ions in the interstitial water (e.g. Na^{+}, Cl^{-}) to generate a substantial osmotic (Donnan) swelling pressure (Maroudas 1979; Myers et al. 1984a, 1984b; Eisenberg and Grodzinsky 1987; Lai et al. 1989). The magnitude of this swelling pressure is related to the density of the charged groups on the proteoglycans, the concentration and valance of ions in the interstitial fluid, and the charge-charge repulsive forces between these charged groups (see chapter by Lai et al. in these volumes for detailed discussions on cartilage swelling). It is likely that proteoglycans also interact in the interfibrillar space to form a network. Thus, with the existing evidence, we hypothesize that the extracellular matrix of cartilage is composed of two interacting networks, a collagen network which is permanent, and a proteoglycan network which turns over and renewed with synthesis (Carney et al. 1984; Sandy et al. 1984; Schneiderman et al. 1986; Gray et al. 1988; Ratcliffe et al. 1989). The interactions between these to enmeshed networks produce a strong cohesive fiber-reinforced, porous-permeable solid matrix capable of supporting the high loads of normal joint articulation.

Age-related Changes of Proteoglycan

Recent biochemical studies have documented significant alterations in the molecular structures of proteoglycans for tissues in various biological states, such as aging or degeneration (Poole 1986). For example, under certain physiological conditions, the hyaluronic acid binding region on the protein core of these proteoglycan monomers may be missing. This would result in an incomplete monomer which is incapable of aggregating with hyaluronic acid. In the absence of link protein, the binding between proteoglycan monomer and hyaluronic acid is unstable (Ratcliffe et al. 1986). The monomers may be abnormally small because of a shortened protein core. In other situations, the glycosaminoglycan side chains may be unusually short. The packing density of these chains along the protein core can also vary (Bollet and Nance 1966; Brandt 1974; McDevitt and Muir 1976; Muir 1977, 1983; Adams 1979; Bayliss and Ali 1979; Vasan 1980; Poole 1986).

Many investigators have attempted to identify the causes of these structural changes in proteoglycans. For example, several studies have examined changes in the chemical composition of mature and immature cartilages (Pal et al. 1981; Rosenberg et al. 1973, 1976, 1982; Buckwalter and Rosenberg 1983; Buckwalter et al. 1985). In these investigations, proteoglycan monomers and aggregates from developing fetal epiphyseal cartilage were compared to those from analogous species isolated from mature articular cartilage. The two type of proteoglycans are generally similar in structure, but differ in chemical composition and molecular weight. Proteoglycan monomers from mature bovine articular cartilage are smaller in size but are much higher in keratan sulfate content (~16%), than the monomers from fetal epiphyseal cartilage (~2%). The increase in keratan sulfate content in mature cartilage proteoglycans is accompanied by a decrease in chondroitin sulfate content with age from ~70% in the inmature proteoglycan to 53% in the mature proteoglycan (Rosenberg et al. 1973, 1976).

Proteoglycan aggregates from fetal epiphyseal cartilage are much larger than aggregates from mature cartilage. The most important determinant responsible for the large size of the fetal aggregates is the longer length of the hyaluronate central filament; this allows more monomers to be attached, thus forming larger aggregates (Buckwalter and Rosenberg, 1983). Proteoglycan monomers are also more closely spaced along hyaluronate filaments in fetal epiphyseal cartilage aggregates. These monomers are also longer and more uniform in length than the monomers from mature bovine cartilage. With increasing age, the average monomer length decreases while the hyaluronate chain length, the number of monomers per aggregate and the spacing between monomers remain constant (Buckwalter and Rosenberg 1983).

Considerable changes in the structural organization of proteoglycans from human fetus and mature adult articular cartilages have also been observed (Roughley and White 1980; Santer et al. 1982). With increasing age, a decrease in the size of proteoglycan monomers and an increase in the ratio of keratan sulfate to chondroitin sulfate have also been noted. These changes occur gradually and are essentially completed by the end of skeletal growth. However, regardless of age, the majority of normal proteoglycan monomers possess the ability to interact with the hyaluronate chain. Although the hyaluronate binding region of proteoglycan monomers appear to be unchanging, tissue culture studies have shown that the percentage of total proteoglycan monomers present as link-stabilized aggregates synthesized by each culture decreases with age of the tissue (Plaas and Sandy, 1984). These results suggest that aging of chondrocytes *in vivo* may be accompanied by a decrease in their capacity for link protein synthesis.

Changes in Proteoglycan Structural Organization Associated with Osteoarthritis

Studies on changes of proteoglycan structure or properties of human and certain animal cartilages associated with osteoarthritis have been made. Osteoarthritic cartilage changes include surface fibrillation, fissuring, loss of proteoglycans, and focal erosion, as well as chondrocytic, biosynthetic, compositional and biomechanical material property changes. Increased hydration of osteoarthritic articular cartilage has been widely noted (Bollet and Nance 1966; Mankin and Thrasher 1975; Maroudas 1979; Bayliss and Ali 1979; Armstrong and Mow 1982a, 1982b; Muir 1977, 1983). The mechanisms responsible for this increase in water content are not well understood. One possible reason for increased tissue hydration during osteoarthritis may be the weakening or loosening of the collagen network. This would lead to an impaired ability of the collagen network to restrain the large swelling pressures exerted by proteoglycans (Maroudas 1981; Akizuki et al. 1986; Lai et al. 1989). Another reason may be the altered or decreased proteoglycan content and structure (Jaffe et al. 1974; McDevitt and Muir 1976; Armstrong and Mow 1982a, 1982b; Muir 1983; Sandy et al. 1984; Carney et al. 1985). In these studies, a decrease of chondroitin sulfate concentration in osteoarthritis cartilage was noted as compared to normal samples from the same individuals. A lower average chain length has been reported in the zone of decreased chondroitin sulfate concentrations (Bollet and Nance 1966). Also, proteoglycans in human osteoarthritic cartilage appear to be smaller and more heterogeneous than normal (Sweet et al. 1977; Adams 1979; Vasan 1980; Poole 1986). These molecules are more readily extracted from the tissue and exhibit a reduced capacity for aggregation than the proteoglycans from normal cartilage *in vitro* (Brandt 1974). A reduction in the keratan sulfate content of proteoglycans has been described in studies of osteoarthritic femoral head cartilage (Bayliss and Ali 1979; Vasan 1980). This decrease in keratan sulfate content is mirrored by the increase in serum keratan sulfate levels in osteoarthritic patients (Sweet et al. 1988).

Tissue culture studies of articular cartilage have shown that link protein is released at an elevated rate from degenerative cartilage (Ratcliffe et al. 1989). Studies of synovial fluid from the canine Pond Nuki model of osteoarthritis have shown elevated levels of link protein in the fluid from the osteoarthritic joints (Ratcliffe et al. 1986). These results indicate that at early stages of cartilage degeneration, there are biochemical events occurring within the tissue which specifically involve disruption of the proteoglycan aggregation resulting in an increased loss of link protein and other components of the proteoglycan aggregates from the matrix.

Changes in Mechanical Properties of Articular Cartilage

The intrinsic mechanical properties of cartilage and its function in diarthrodial joints depend on the characteristics of collagen and proteoglycan as well as the nature of the interactions between these two components (Kempson 1979; Maroudas 1979; Mow and Lai 1980; Armstrong and Mow 1982a; Muir 1983; Akizuki et al. 1986). Alterations of molecular structure and interactions between these components may cause degenerative changes in the organization of the extracellular matrix and hence the tissue (Muir 1977, 1983). These changes have been characterized, in part, by a loss of the mechanical stiffness and strength of the tissue, and its functional properties in joints (Maroudas 1981; Armstrong and Mow 1982a, 1982b; Myers et al. 1987; Schmidt et al. 1986, 1987). It has been shown that a loss of proteoglycans from cartilage and an increase of tissue hydration can cause a significant reduction of cartilage compressive stiffness as well as an increase in permeability (Armstrong and Mow 1982a, 1982b). Failure or loosening of the collagen network associated with fibrillation permits tissue swelling with significant increase of water content and decrease in tensile stiffness (Maroudas 1980; Muir 1983; Akizuki et al. 1986; Schmidt et al. 1987). These changes will greatly jeopardize the effectiveness of cartilage in providing load carriage and possibly the normal lubrication processes within diarthrodial joints. Recent studies of Simon et al. (1989) showed a one-third reduction in cartilage shear modulus induced by shear fatigue with no evidence of association with glycosaminoglycan content or structure difference of the collagen network. It was suggested that possible changes in proteoglycan aggregate size and interactions among proteoglycan-proteoglycan molecules and proteoglycan-collagen fibrils may be responsible for the weakening of the extracellular matrix of the tissue.

Viscoelastic Properties of Purified Proteoglycan Solutions

Knowledge of the viscometric properties of concentrated proteoglycan solutions (gels) provides insight into how proteoglycans might function in the extracellular matrix of cartilage. Many different techniques exist to measure the viscosity of a liquid (Coleman et al. 1966; Walters 1975). Capillary viscometry is one of the most popular techniques. It has been used to measure the viscosities of dilute proteoglycan solutions (Hardingham 1979) as well as for synovial fluids (Schurz and Ribitsch 1987). However, the capillary viscometry technique can only be used to measure easily the viscosity of Newtonian fluids. If the fluid is known to be non-Newtonian, the procedure for calculating the viscosity of the sample as a function of shear rate from the capillary viscometric data is so cumbersome that the method is of limited utility (Coleman et al. 1966). Thus, to determine the viscosity and other non-Newtonian properties of cartilage proteoglycan solutions at high concentrations (similar to those found *in situ*) a series of experiments have been carried out using a cone-on-plate viscometer (Mak et al. 1982, 1983; Mow et al. 1984b, 1989; Hardingham et al. 1987). These investigations demonstrated that flow properties of proteoglycan solutions were highly non-Newtonian. The viscosities of these proteoglycan solutions were shear-rate dependent for concentrations ranging from 10-50 mg/ml. Non-zero normal stress differences were also found for both proteoglycan aggregates and monomers. Furthermore, these viscometric properties of proteoglycan solutions were shown to be sensitive to changes in the proteoglycan structural organization, and were greatly influenced by the concentration and percentage of aggregation present in proteoglycan solutions.

From these studies, it has been shown that the relationships between composition and structure of proteoglycans, and their viscometric flow properties are complex and highly nonlinear. These viscometric flow properties have been analyzed using Oldroyd's four-parameter nonlinear viscoelastic fluid model (1950) to determine the apparent viscosity and nonlinear viscosity coefficients, and the relaxation and retardation times (Mow et al. 1984b; Hardingham et al. 1987). Also, analysis of the viscometric data to determine the density and strength of proteoglycan-proteoglycan interaction sites were made using statistical network models (De Kee and Carreau 1979; Zhu et al. 1988b).

The intent of this chapter is to present a precis of the experiments and theoretical analysis of viscometric properties of cartilage proteoglycan solutions.

Methodology

The viscometric flow measurements were performed on samples of precisely prepared and well characterized proteoglycan solutions (Hardingham et al. 1987; Mow et al. 1984b, 1989; Zhu et al. 1988a, 1988b). A wide spectrum properties, including steady-state and time-dependent transient behaviors, were determined. The structural and composition parameters studied included: 1) size of monomers and aggregates, 2) proportion of proteoglycans present as aggregates, 3) aggregation with and without link proteins, and 4) keratan sulfate to chondroitin sulfate ratio.

Preparation of Proteoglycan Solutions

The proteoglycans were extracted from cartilage in 4M guanidine HCl. This dissociated the proteoglycan aggregates, which were later reformed by lowering the guanidine HCl concentration (Hascall and Sajdesa 1969; Hardingham 1981). Preparations containing proteoglycan aggregates or monomers were obtained by CsCl density gradient centrifugation. The ability to isolate purified monomeric proteoglycan, separate from link protein and hyaluronate chains, enabled aggregates of different components in varying proportions to be reformed in associative conditions. Link-free aggregates were reformed by pooling the purified monomeric proteoglycans and hyaluronate under associative conditions. Link stable aggregates were obtained by adding link protein to this solution in stochiomtric proportions (Mow et al. 1989).

Using analytical ultracentrifugation, at concentrations below 1 mg/ml, the molecular size of the proteoglycans can be determined. For the proteoglycan solutions we studied, the sedimentation coefficient ($S°$) of the monomers ranged from 16 to 24, and that of the aggregates ranged from 80 to 140, depending on the source of the cartilages (Buckwalter and Rosenberg 1983; Zhu et al. 1988a). Link-free aggregates showed about 28% reduction in the value of $S°$ as compared to the link-stable aggregates (Mow et al. 1989). The proportion of proteoglycans present as aggregates in solution was determined by gel chromatography. These determinations showed a slightly lower percentage of aggregation in the link-free preparation (~59%) than in the link-stable preparation (~66%). The remaining 34-41% monomers in the solution were those proteoglycans incapable of aggregating with the hyaluronate chain, i.e. the non-aggregating proteoglycans.

Viscometric Flow Measurements

Solutions of proteoglycan monomers and aggregates were tested at various concentrations in a cone-on-plate viscometer, Fig. 2. The angle of the cone (α)

is 0.04 rad and the diameter of the plate (2a) is 50 mm. The vertex of the cone is truncated and is located 50 μm from the plate. The cone-on-plate configuration requires approximately 3 ml of the sample for each run. It allows for a relatively simple data reduction procedure when compared to other viscometric testing configurations. Uniform shear flows are produced in the specimen via a rotary motion of the plate driven by a precision d.c. motor. The angular speed of the rotating plate determines the shear rate. The upper plate is connected to a sensitive transducer which records the torque and normal force generated by the sheared solution in the cone-on-plate viscometer. To characterize the viscometric flow behaviors of proteoglycan solutions, a wide spectrum of flow properties were determined which includes: 1) dynamic complex shear modulus, 2) shear-rate dependent apparent viscosity and primary normal stress difference and 3) time-dependent transient responses such as stress growth, stress relaxation and hysteresis behaviors.

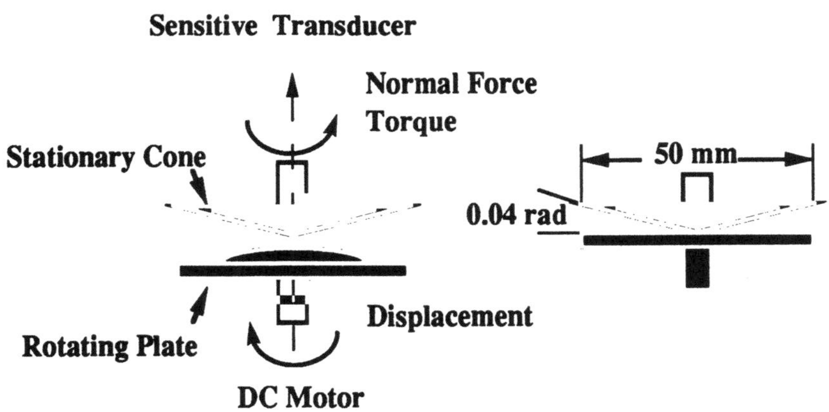

Figure 2 Diagram of the cone-on-plate viscometer showing the essential dimensions.

Dynamic Oscillatory Shear Experiment

The dynamic complex shear modulus G^*, characterizing the linear viscoelastic behavior of polymeric liquids, is measured by subjecting the proteoglycan specimen to a continuous sinusoidal shear oscillation of small amplitude, Fig. 3. The d.c. motor provides precise control of the angular displacement $\theta = \theta_0 \sin(\omega t)$, where θ_0 is the prescribed amplitude of motion. A sensitive transducer measures the torque $T=T_0\sin(\omega t+\delta)$. Here ω is the circular frequency in radian/sec ($f=\omega/2\pi$ in Hertz), δ is the phase shift angle between the sinusoidal displacement input and torque output, and T_0 is the amplitude of the measured torque. For the dynamic complex modulus, we performed the measurements at discrete frequency points on a $\log_{10}(\omega)$ scale. The viscoelastic spectrum, i.e. $G^*(\omega)$, of the solution was determined for the frequency range of $1 \le \omega \le 100$ rad/sec and a fixed amplitude ($\theta_0 = 0.02$ rad). The real and imaginary components of G^* are the storage modulus (G') and loss modulus (G''). The magnitude of the dynamic complex modulus $|G^*|$ and phase shift angle δ are related to G' and G'' by

$$|G^*| = \sqrt{G'^2 + G''^2}, \quad \delta = \tan^{-1}\{G''/G'\} \tag{1}$$

The storage modulus G' is proportional to elastically stored strain energy and the loss modulus G'' is proportional to dissipated strain energy in the sample over one cycle of periodic oscillation. The magnitude of dynamic shear modulus $|G^*|$ measures the overall stiffness of the proteoglycan solutions and the value of $\tan\delta$ measures the amount of energy dissipated (G'') relative to the energy stored (G') in the solution during a cycle of deformation. These quantities are shown in Fig. 4 for a 40 mg/ml proteoglycan aggregate solution. On this log-log scale, the magnitude of the dynamic modulus $|G^*|$ increases linearly with frequency (ω) which reflects a power-law relation between $|G^*|$ and frequency ω. The value of $|G^*|$ varied from 1.69 Pa to 35.4 Pa for frequency ranging from 1 to 100 rad/sec. The non-zero storage modulus G' indicates that proteoglycans at this concentration are capable of forming a molecular network in solution which can store energy elastically. This was true for all concentrations tested, 10 to 50 mg/ml, and for both monomer and aggregate solutions. The loss modulus G'' was always greater than the storage modulus G' for all proteoglycan solutions tested at all frequencies. It is therefore evident from this viscoelastic property that concentrated proteoglycan solutions tend more toward a fluid rather than solid. As frequency increases, the value of $\tan\delta$ always decreases, hence, less energy is dissipated and more energy is stored elastically in the networks at higher frequency. This behavior is common to many polymeric solutions (Ferry 1970).

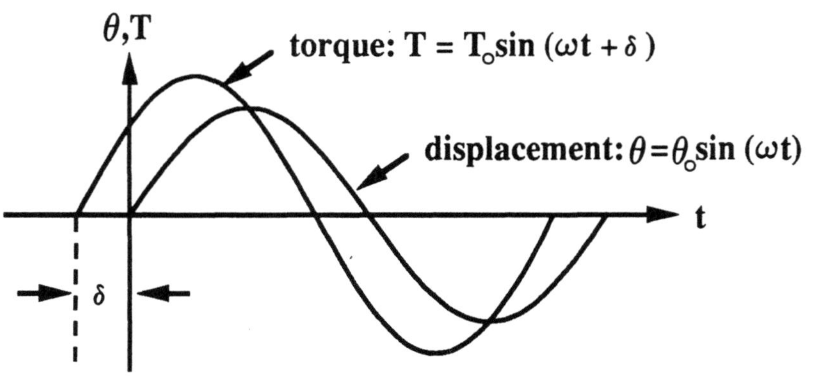

Figure 3 Schematics of a dynamic oscillatory shear experiment: A sinusoidal displacement of small amplitude θ_0 and frequency ω is imposed on the solution sample; the torque response T is measured from which the dynamic shear modulus may be calculated. For a linear viscoelastic response, the torque is also sinusoidal with frequency ω, amplitude T_0 and phase lag angle δ.

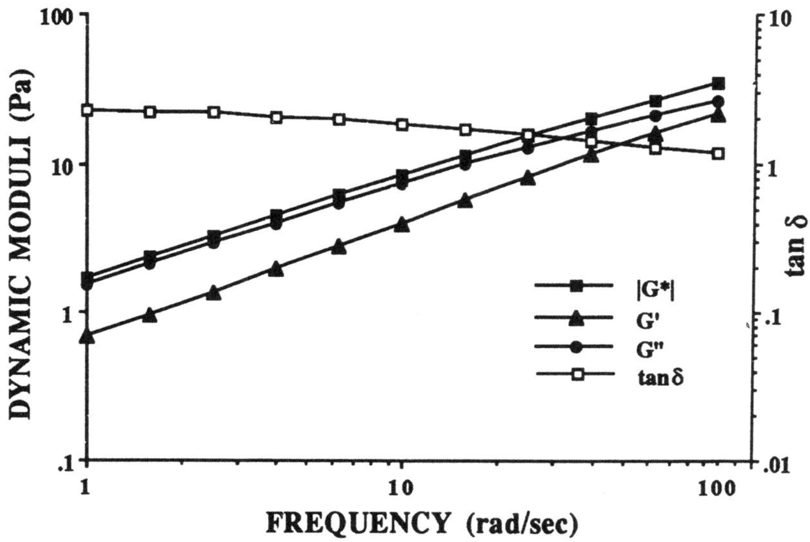

Figure 4 Frequency dependence of the magnitude of dynamic shear modulus $|G^*|$, tangent of phase shift angle δ, storage modulus G' and loss modulus G'' for a 40 mg/ml link-stable proteoglycan aggregate solution.

Steady Shear Flow Experiment

Steady shearing of polymeric solutions in the cone-on-plate viscometer yields a torque and normal force from which the apparent viscosity, η_{app}, and the primary normal stress difference, σ_1, may be calculated. For a given rotational speed of the plate (Ω rad/sec), one can determine the shear rate ($\dot{\gamma}$ s^{-1}) in the fluid specimen by the simple equation:

$$\dot{\gamma} = \frac{\Omega}{\alpha}. \tag{2}$$

The apparent viscosity η_{app} is related to the measured torque (T) and the shear rate ($\dot{\gamma}$) by

$$\eta_{app}(\dot{\gamma}) = \frac{3T}{2\pi a^3 \dot{\gamma}}, \tag{3}$$

and the primary normal stress difference is calculated by

$$\sigma_1(\dot{\gamma}) = \frac{2N}{\pi a^2} + \frac{3}{20}\rho\Omega^2 a^2, \tag{4}$$

where N is the measured normal force required to maintain a 50μm gap between the vertex of the cone and the plate, and ρ is the density of the specimen. The second term in equation (4) is a correction factor to account for the inertia effects (Bird et al. 1977a, 1977b). Shear rates $\dot{\gamma}$ ranging from 0.25 to 250 s^{-1} were used to determine the nonlinear shear-rate dependent apparent viscosity and normal stress difference. For our studies, a shear-rate sweep was performed at five discrete points per decade on the $\log_{10}(\dot{\gamma})$ scale.

For concentrated proteoglycan solutions, the η_{app} and σ_1 were found to depend nonlinearly on $\dot{\gamma}$. Figure 5 shows that proteoglycan solutions exhibited shear thinning effect, i.e. their apparent viscosities decreased with increasing shear rate. There was at least an order of magnitude change in apparent viscosity (3.2 - 0.3 Pa.s) over the shear rates ranging from 0.25 to 250 s^{-1} for a 40 mg/ml proteoglycan aggregate solution. At low shear rates, the viscosity approached a constant value. Note that for water, the viscosity is 0.01 Pa.s at room temperature. The zero-shear-rate viscosity, η_0, is defined as the value of η_{app} when $\dot{\gamma} \to 0$, and is determined by extrapolation. At high shear rates, the viscosity exhibited a leveling-off trend for all viscosity curves. The infinite-shear-rate viscosity, η_∞, is also determined by extrapolation. The primary normal stress difference, σ_1, increased monotonically with increasing shear rate and approached zero at low shear rates.

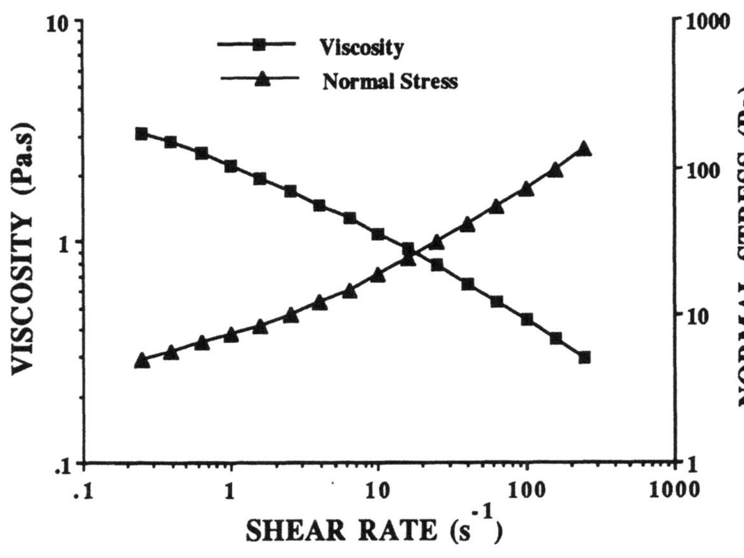

Figure 5 Shear-rate dependence of the apparent viscosity η_{app} and primary normal stress difference σ_1 for a 40 mg/ml link-stable proteoglycan aggregate solution.

Transient Stress-Growth Response

Many polymeric solutions exhibit transient responses upon initiation of shear from a resting state (Ferry 1970). The characteristic of the transient response is a rapid stress growth to τ_{max} followed by a slower decay until a steady stress response (τ_{∞}) is attained, Fig. 6. The area defined by the shear stress curve and the horizontal time axis up to the time of peak shear stress is denoted by A. The product of this area and the imposed shear rate, $A\dot{\gamma}_o$, provides the measure of the energy per unit volume required to change the conformational state of the proteoglycan network in a solution at rest to the conformational state at steady-shear flow.

Typical stress growth patterns of a 40 mg/ml proteoglycan aggregate solution for three magnitudes of shear rate is shown in Fig. 7. As can be seen, the proteoglycan aggregate solution exhibited a nonlinear stress growth effect which was strongly dependent upon the magnitude of the shear rate. There was a very gentle overshoot when the imposed shear rate is 25 s^{-1}. At smaller shear rates, there was no stress overshoot. For larger shear rates (100 and 250 s^{-1}), the shear stress attained a maximum value before approaching a steady-shear value. The magnitude of this stress overshoot increased as the imposed shear rate increased. These results suggest that the proteoglycan aggregate solutions are sensitive to acceleration effects. The primary normal stress difference also showed similar stress overshoot phenomena (Mow et al. 1989).

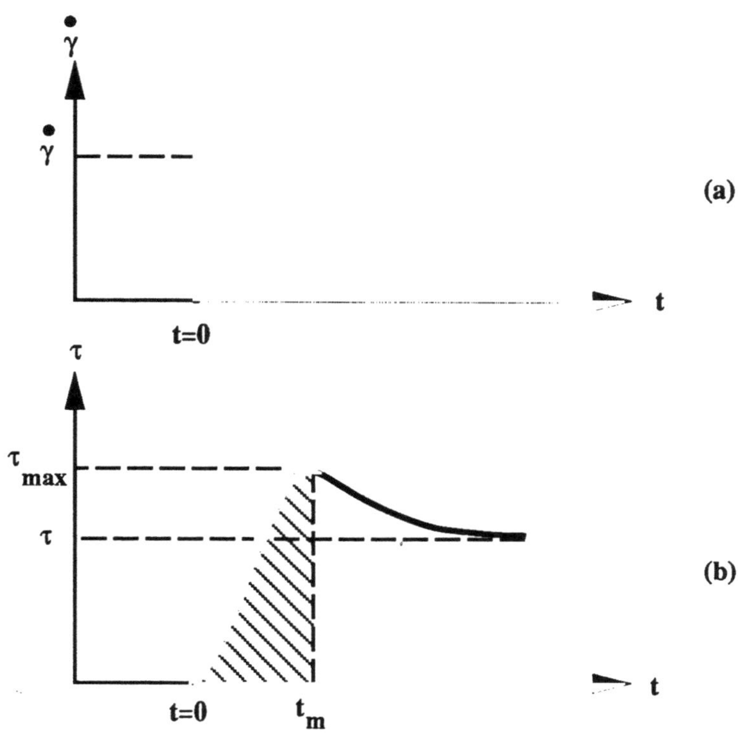

Figure 6 (a) Transient shear stress response following a sudden application of the shear rate $\dot{\gamma}_o$ at t=0. (b) Proteoglycan solutions exhibit stress overshoot effects prior to the attained steady-state response of τ_{∞}. The shaded area in the τ-t plane provides a measure of energy density required to disrupt the molecular network.

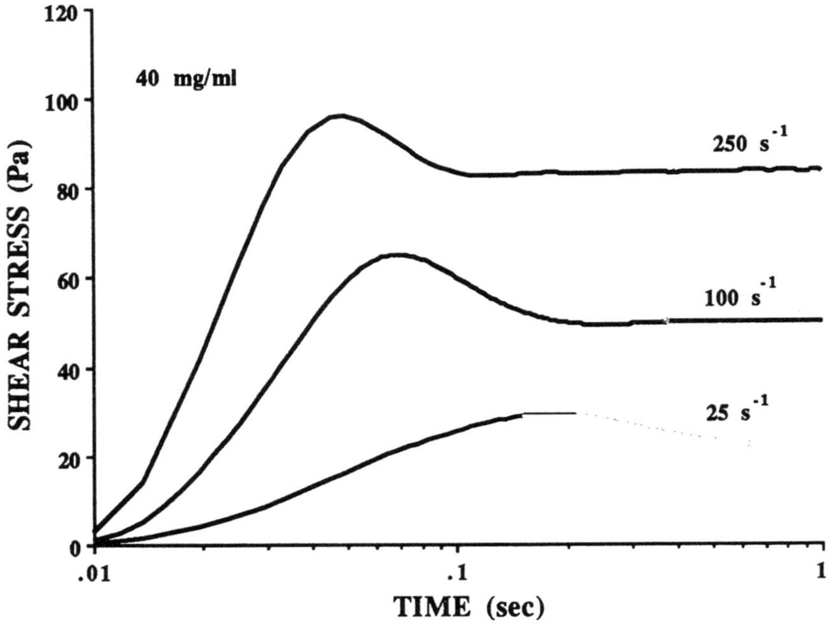

Figure 7 Transient shear stress overshoot effect following a sudden application of $\dot{\gamma}_0$ at three shear rates (250, 100, 25 s^{-1}) for a 40 mg/ml link-stable proteoglycan aggregate solution.

Transient Stress-Relaxation Response

The transient response after cessation of flow from a steady shear of $\dot{\gamma}_0$ is characterized by a rapid stress relaxation process from τ_0 to zero stress. The rate with which the stress decays is characterized by the relaxation time, or the relaxation spectrum in cases where the stress-relaxation process results from more than one relaxation mechanism. The relaxation time(s) provides information on the rate at which the molecular networks in solution can adjust from their streaming configurational state ($t<0$) to their resting state ($t>0$). The stress-relaxation process(es) is governed by the stiffness of the macromolecular network and viscous resistance against this network rearrangement in solution.

The stress relaxation curves of a 40 mg/ml proteoglycan aggregate solution for three magnitudes of shear rate are shown in Fig. 8 . The shear stress in this figure was presented in a normalized fashion, i.e. the current shear stress (τ) was divided by the shear stress during steady-shear flow (τ_0). Starting with unity at $t=0^+$ the shear stress relaxed monotonically with time to zero, which is a characteristic of a fluid. Thus, proteoglycans, by themselves, can not sustain a shear stress without flow. For most of the proteoglycan solutions tested, our results showed that the majority of the transient stress relaxation effect took place in less than one second. The shear stress tends to relax more rapidly with increasing shear rate.

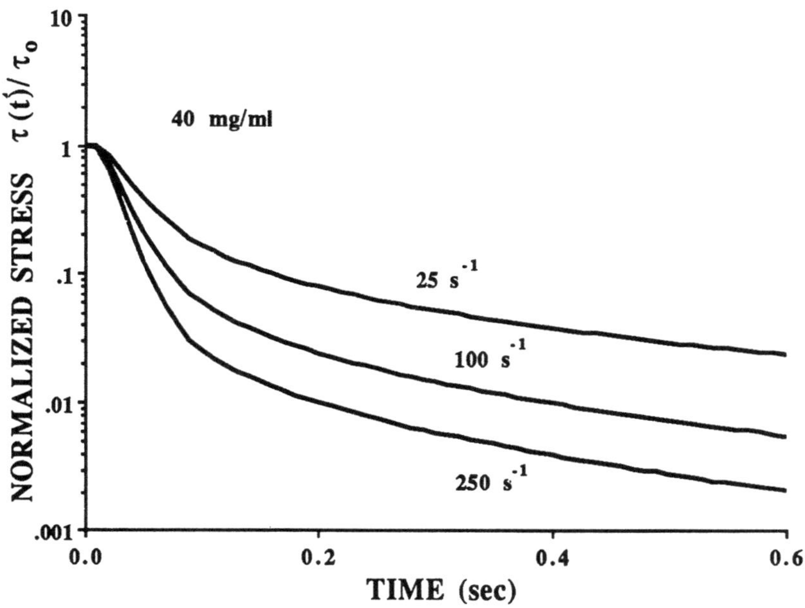

Figure 8 Normalized stress relaxation curves for a 40 mg/ml link-stable proteoglycan aggregate solution after cessation at t=0 from steady-shear flow at 250, 100 and 25 s^{-1}. The shear stresses in proteoglycan solutions always decay monotonically from τ_o to zero indicating their fluid-like behavior.

Acceleration Effects - Hysteresis Loop

In the hysteresis loop test, the imposed shear rate increases linearly from zero to a final shear rate, followed by a linear decrease to zero. In the ascending phase, a constant acceleration is thus imposed and in the descending phase, a constant deceleration is imposed. During the loop, resulting torque is registered as a function of shear rate. Some typical hysteresis loop responses for a fetal proteoglycan solution with two different magnitudes of acceleration are shown in Fig. 9. In the ascending phase, the shear stress increased drastically reaching a peak long before attaining the maximum shear rate. After reaching a peak, the shear stress decreased precipitously, followed by a gradual increase with increasing shear rate. This stress-surge effect is due to network rupture. In the descending phase, the shear stress decreases steadily, with a final residual stress remaining at zero shear rate.

The stress-surge phenomenon occurred during the early stage of the ascending phase of the hysteresis loop depends strongly upon the magnitude of the imposed acceleration and the concentration and structural organization of the proteoglycan present (Zhu et al. 1988a). As shown in Fig. 9, a relatively gentle stress surge occurred for the imposed acceleration of 0.25 s^{-2} when compared with that of 2.5 s^{-2}. For the 0.25 s^{-2} acceleration loop, the stress surge occurred at a lower shear rate and the residual stress at the end of the loop was lower. Stress-surge effects were only observed for proteoglycan solutions at higher concentrations (>30 mg/ml), and the effect was the greatest for fetal cartilage proteoglycans (Zhu et al. 1988a). Stress surge is typical of a rheopectic material, and occurs when the structure of the polymeric network in solutions has been disrupted by the shearing action (Walters 1975).

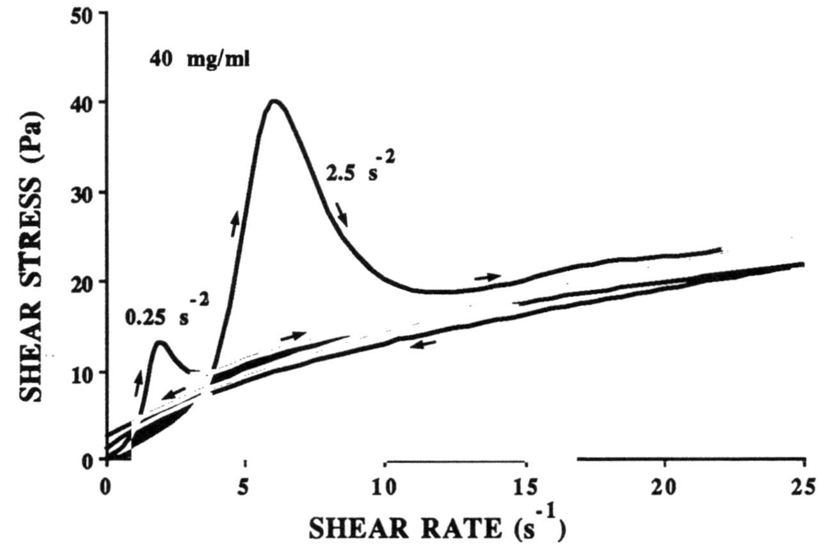

Figure 9 Stress surge effect during a hysteresis loop with the magnitudes of acceleration at 2.5 and 0.25 s^{-2} for a 40 mg/ml proteoglycan aggregate solution from bovine fetal epiphyseal cartilage.

Structure-Function Relationship of Proteoglycans

Monomer and Aggregate

Substantial differences in viscometric properties were observed between the aggregates and monomers of proteoglycan macromolecular solutions (Mow et al. 1984a). The aggregate solutions have consistently higher $|G^*|$ compared to monomer solutions at the corresponding frequency and concentration, Fig. 10. The value of $\tan\delta$ was generally higher for monomers (4.5-5.2) than for aggregates (2.2-3.2). Thus proteoglycan aggregate solutions tend to dissipate less energy relative to the energy stored than do proteoglycan monomer solutions. The greater capacity of aggregates to store energy could be due to their more highly ordered structure, which results in an increase in the density and/or strength of intermolecular interactions required to form networks in solution.

At high shear rates, the apparent viscosity of aggregate solutions was 1.5 to 2 times greater than that of monomer solutions at similar concentrations, Fig. 11.

This difference was more pronounced at low shear rates, where the viscosity of monomer solutions approached a limiting value while that of aggregates increased steadily. A nonlinear relationship existed between the limiting zero shear-rate viscosity η_0 and solution concentration (Mow et al. 1984), indicating the strong proteoglycan network interactions occurred when the molecules were at rest in solution. In addition, aggregation further enhanced the strength of the interactions in proteoglycan networks.

The differences observed between the two structural forms of proteoglycans demonstrate the sensitivity of the viscometric flow properties to the organization of the molecules. Such differences are most significant at physiological concentrations, thus indicating the limited applicability of viscosity measurements on dilute proteoglycan solutions. Variation in all measured flow properties with respect to different concentrations was greater for aggregates than for monomers. Hence, in the tissue, under disaggregating conditions or during pathological situations where proteoglycans are smaller or when they fail to aggregate, proteoglycans can flow out of the tissue much more easily than under normal situations. The loss of proteoglycans from the extracellular matrix is subject to the action of joint loading during articulation. Since cartilage compression is always associated with strong currents of interstitial fluid flow (Mow and Lai 1980; Mow et al. 1984a), the convective transport of proteoglycan fragments is expected to be even more significant when there is an increase of cartilage permeability during degeneration. As a result, the tissue would be even less stiff and more permeable, thereby initiating a vicious cycle toward cartilage degeneration.

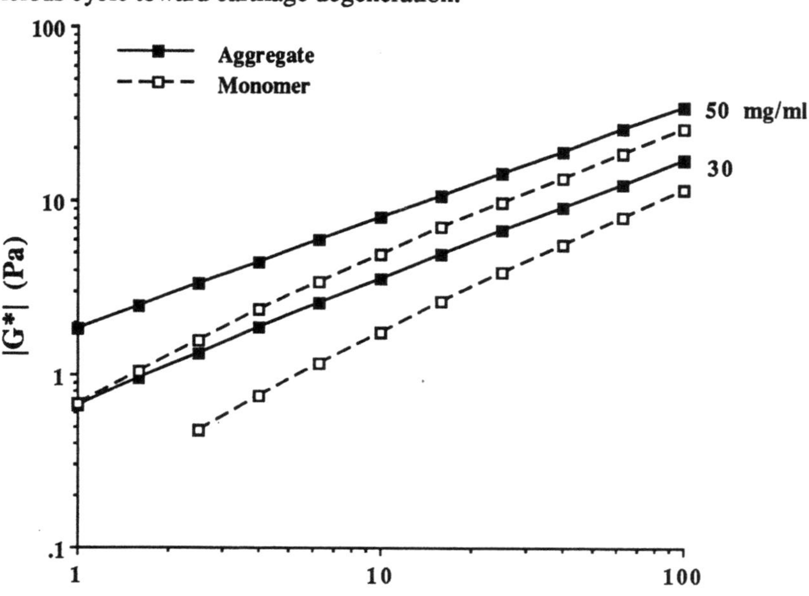

Figure 10 Variations of the magnitude of dynamic shear modulus with frequency and concentration for proteoglycan aggregate and monomer solutions.

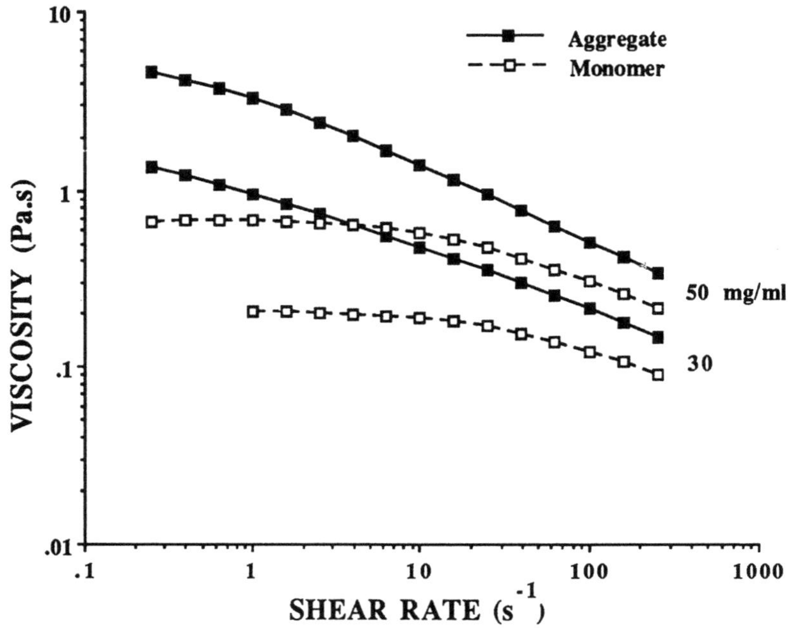

Figure 11 Variation of apparent viscosity with shear rate and concentration for proteoglycan aggregate and monomer solutions.

Varying Proportions of Proteoglycan Aggregates and Monomers

Having shown that there are major differences in the viscometric properties of aggregates and monomers, it is therefore important to assess the influence of the extent of aggregation present in solution on the viscometric flow properties. To do this, we examined a series of proteoglycan solutions at concentrations from 10 to 50 mg/ml, each containing 0, 3, 40, and 80% aggregation. We found that the flow behaviors of these solutions depend strongly on the percent aggregation, as well as solution concentration (Hardingham et al. 1987). Figure 12 shows the variation of the limiting zero-shear-rate viscosity η_0 and infinite-shear-rate viscosity η_∞ with percentage aggregation and concentration. The 0% aggregation corresponds to the monomeric solutions and the 100% aggregation is determined by extrapolation. These results show that the strength and elasticity of the networks formed by the proteoglycans in solution increased with concentration and extent of aggregation. There was a four-fold increase in the value of η_0 with increasing percentage aggregation from 3% to 80% (Fig. 12a). This indicates that aggregation of proteoglycans promotes strong network formation. Furthermore, there was a ten-fold reduction of viscosity from the limiting zero shear rate value, η_0, to that of high shear rate, η_∞.

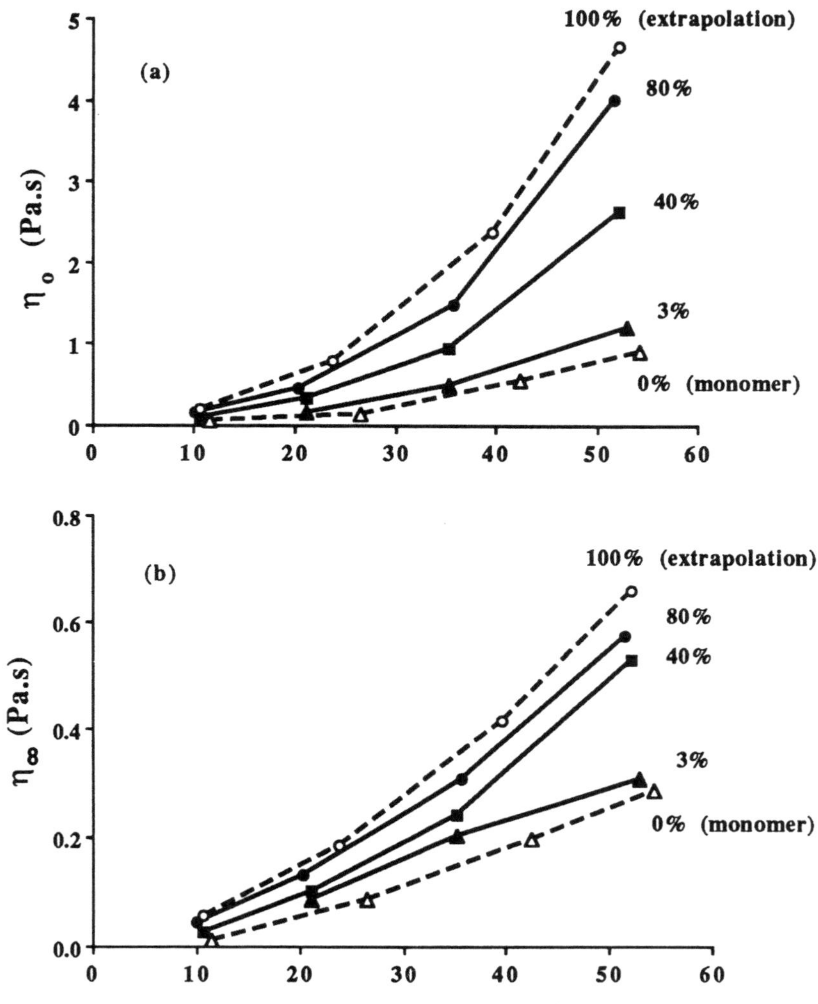

Figure 12 (a) Variation of the limiting zero-shear-rate viscosity with concentration and percentage aggregation. (b) Variation of the limiting infinite shear-rate viscosity with concentration and percentage aggregation.

Effect of Link Proteins

The binding of link protein to proteoglycan and hyaluronate greatly increases the strength of the association ($K_a \sim 5 \times 10^7 M$) between these two molecules (Hardingham 1979, 1981). Thus, the absence of link protein may cause significant changes in the viscometric flow behaviors of proteoglycans. To examine the effects of link protein on the viscometric flow behaviors, two identical proteoglycan aggregate preparations were made; one preparation was link stabilized and one was not (Mow et al. 1989). Over a concentration range of 10 to 50 mg/ml, which corresponds to a proteoglycan molarity of 6×10^{-6}M, we calculate that, at equilibrium, the binding of the monomers to hyaluronate would be about 99% efficient. There should therefore be a similar percentage of aggregation in each preparation.

Overall, link-free aggregate solutions showed lower values of $|G^*|$ than link-stable aggregate solutions. There was an approximately 20% reduction in $|G^*|$ with the absence of link protein. Link-free aggregate solutions appear to have larger values of $\tan\delta$ than link-stable aggregate solutions (Mow et al. 1989). The lower values of $|G^*|$ and higher values of $\tan\delta$ exhibited by link-free proteoglycan aggregates indicate that they form less stiff but more dissipative molecular networks in solution. When compared with link-stable proteoglycan aggregate networks, a larger portion of the deformational energy is dissipated than stored by the link-free proteoglycan networks. However, link-stable aggregate solutions have higher viscosities than link-free aggregate solutions. The differences were larger at low shear rates (~37%) than at high shear rates (~10%). The zero-shear-rate viscosity, η_0, and the infinite-shear-rate viscosity, η_∞, showed direct correlations with concentration. The values of η_∞ were about an order of magnitude lower than the values of η_0. The effect of link protein was found to have a much stronger influence on η_0 than on η_∞.

The stress overshoot and the stress-relaxation responses of both link-stable and link-free proteoglycan aggregate solutions at concentrations greater than 30 mg/ml depend strongly on the magnitude of imposed shear rate ($\dot{\gamma}_0$). Thus these proteoglycan solutions are also sensitive to acceleration and deceleration effects. Figure 13 shows the shear stress overshoot responses of 40 mg/ml solutions of the link-stable and the link-free aggregates at 100 s^{-1}. Clearly, the

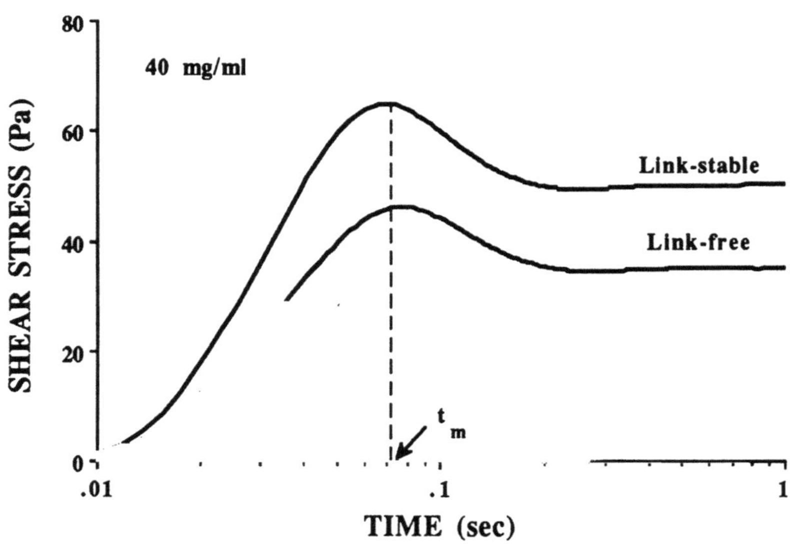

Figure 13 Transient shear stress overshoot effect following a sudden application of $\dot{\gamma}_0$ at 100 s^{-1} for 40 mg/ml link-stable and link-free proteoglycan aggregate solutions.

link-stable proteoglycan aggregate solution exhibited greater shear stress overshoot effect when compared to the link-free proteoglycan solution. These results demonstrate that the transient flow properties of proteoglycan solutions also depend on link protein stabilization of the aggregates. Link-stable proteoglycan aggregates appear to form stronger intermolecular interactions in solution, thus more energy is required to overcome their resistance during shear flow. The stress-relaxation results for both link-stable and link-free aggregate solutions showed a rapid decay in shear stress to zero shear stress upon cessation of steady flow. The rate of stress-relaxation seems to depend on $\dot{\gamma}_0$ but the dependence does not appear to be dramatically altered by the presence of link protein. However, the molecular networks formed by link-stable proteoglycan aggregates always relaxed at a slower rate than that formed by link-free aggregates (Mow et al. 1989).

Changes of Flow Properties with Age

A significant increase in the keratan sulfate to chondroitin sulfate ratio is found in proteoglycans from mature cartilage as compared to those from immature cartilage (Rosenberg et al. 1976, 1982). With increasing cartilage age the molecular size of proteoglycans also changes significantly, generally becoming much smaller in aging cartilage. These compositional and structural changes of proteoglycans may result in changes in their viscometric flow properties. When the flow properties between proteoglycan monomers from bovine fetal epiphyseal and mature articular cartilages were compared, we found the differences in apparent viscosity η_{app} to be very small, Fig. 14. The difference in the magnitude of dynamic shear modulus was also not significant between these two types of proteoglycan solutions (Zhu et al. 1988). This was true for all concentrations, frequencies and shear rates tested. The similar flow properties of these monomeric solutions may be due to their very similar molecular sizes.

Significant differences were, however, observed between proteoglycan aggregate solutions from fetal and mature articular cartilages, Fig. 14. The proteoglycan aggregate solutions from fetal cartilage always exhibited higher viscosities as well as greater shear moduli than the proteoglycan aggregate solutions from mature articular cartilage. This effect was particularly pronounced at high concentrations. It appears that the molecular size of proteoglycans is the dominant factor controlling the viscometric flow behavior of these solutions. The greater network stiffness and higher viscosity exhibited by fetal aggregate solutions are likely to be due to the fact that there are more intermolecular interactions formed in the solution by larger fetal proteoglycans.

Kinetics of Proteoglycan-Hyaluronate Interaction

The kinetics of the interactions forming proteoglycan aggregates from monomers and hyaluronate chains were determined by viscosity measurements utilizing our cone-on-plate viscometer. For each experiment, a bovine nasal

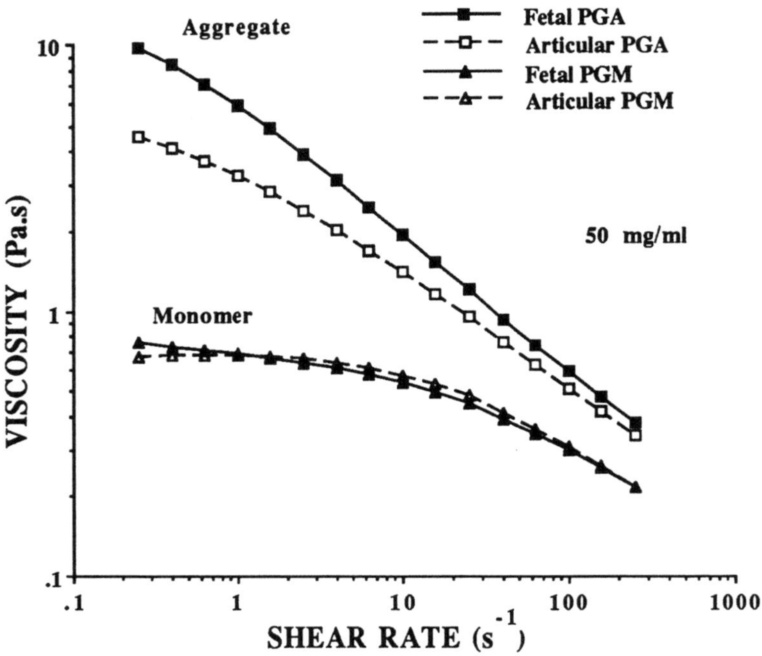

Figure 14 Shear-rate dependence of the apparent viscosity η_{app} for fetal and articular proteoglycan aggregates (PGA) and monomers (PGM), 50 mg/ml.

proteoglycan monomer solution was laid onto the plate of the cone-on-plate viscometer. Onto this layer of monomer solution was placed, in a stratified manner, a hyaluronate solution. A weight ratio of 0.8% hyaluronate/proteoglycan was used for optimal aggregate formation in each experiment. Concentrations of monomeric solutions ranging from 10 to 50 mg/ml were studied. Figure 15 shows the viscosity, normalized by its own control steady-state aggregate viscosity, as a function of time for shear rates of 1, 10, 100 s^{-1}. The figure clearly shows that the kinetics of monomers-hyaluronate interaction depends on the rate of shear. At the high shear rate of 100 s^{-1}, the viscosity approached monotonically to its control value, while at the low shear rate of 1.0 s^{-1}, an overshoot phenomenon occurred. The linear hyaluronate chain in a solution at rest assumes a random spherical state (Balazs and Gibbs, 1970). During shearing, this linear chain was stretched. Thus the viscosity overshoot phenomenon occurring during the monomer-hyaluronate interaction at the slow shear might be due to a supra-optimal packing of proteoglycan monomers on the stretched hyaluronate chain. At higher shear rates, there was not sufficient time for extra proteoglycans to be associated with hyaluronate; thus no overshoot occurred. It was also evident that the rate of monomer-hyaluronate association was slower at low shear rates.

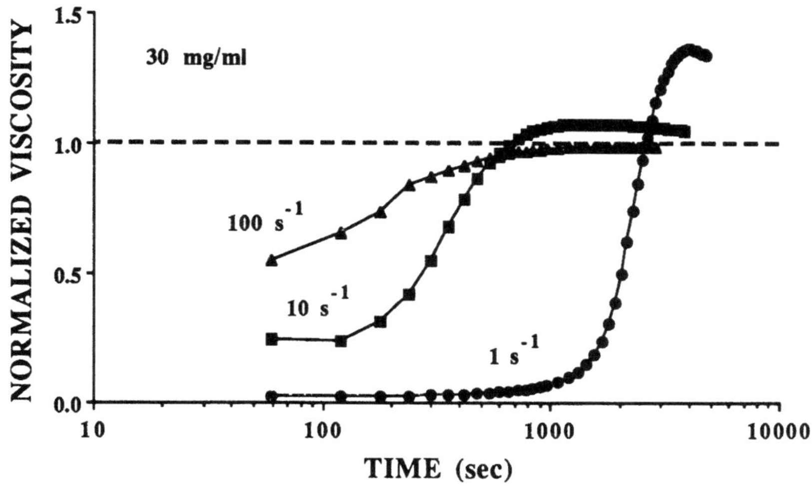

Figure 15 Kinetics of proteoglycan-hyaluronate interaction as measured by the normalized viscosity curves vs time under steady-shear flow (1, 10 and 100 s^{-1}); 30 mg/ml.

Statistical Network Theory for Proteoglycan Solutions

In the previous sections, we described both linear and nonlinear viscometric flow behaviors exhibited by proteoglycan solutions. These flow behaviors were obtained under both steady-state and transient conditions. In this section we summarize a new nonlinear second order statistical network theory which we recently developed to model these flow properties (Zhu et al. 1988b). This statistical network theory is an extension of the network theory developed by De Kee and Carreau (1979) for macromolecular solutions. From our theory, we have developed a method to relate the flow properties of the proteoglycan solutions to structural parameters defining an idealized molecular network modeling the proteoglycan network in solution.

In the statistical network theory, we first assume that a macromolecular network is formed by the proteoglycans in solution. We assume that this network is composed of chain segments and junction sites, Fig. 16a. Each chain segment is connected by two neighboring junction sites. A junction site is a common point where two molecules meet and where a force may be transferred from one molecule to the other. These forces may arise from mechanical entanglement of the two neighboring molecules, electrostatic interactions amongst charge groups along the molecules, frictional effects from one molecule sliding over another, etc. Fundamental to the statistical network theory is the assumption that the interactions amongst molecules are confined to local attractions at isolated points along the chains. Finally, we assume that these junction sites, the common point for the two molecules, are constrained to move as if they were material particles of an equivalent macroscopic continuum. It is important to note that the junction sites are not permanent, but rather they may be created or lost during flow. Clearly, during steady-state flow of these polymeric network solutions, the rate of creation of junction sites and the rate of loss of junction sites are in equilibrium.

With the above assumptions, we define a chain segment of a proteoglycan to be a freely jointed bead-rod chain of N masses connected by (N-1) stiff rods of length L, Fig. 16b. The end-to-end length of this flexible chain may vary between zero when two-ends coincide and (N-1)L when the chain is fully extended. For such a model, the statistical time average end-to-end length of the chain segment is $(N-1)^{1/2}L$ (Lodge 1968). In the molecular network, the two ends of this chain segment are constrained at the junction sites. The effect of the random motion of the chain segment gives rise to a time average tension in the segment which can be shown to be equivalent to a spring with a force constant $H=3kT/(N-1)L$, where k and T are the Boltzmann constant and absolute temperature, respectively (Bird et al. 1979a, 1979b). A collection of these network springs provides the molecular network with potential energy.

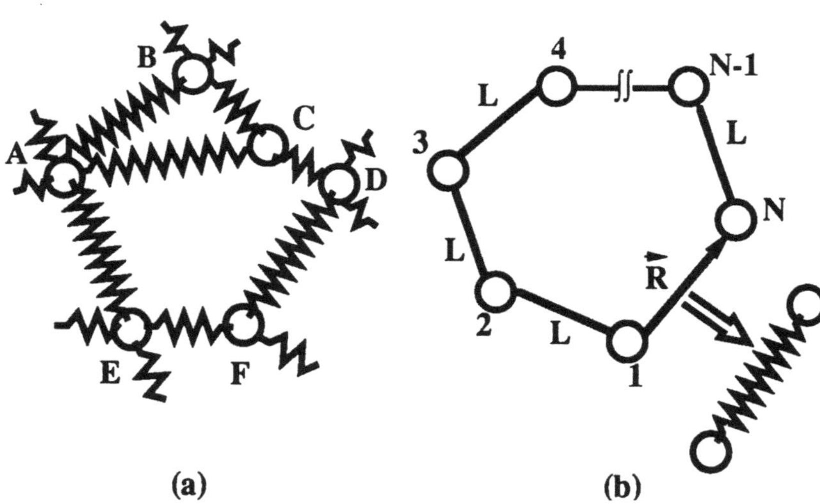

Figure 16 (a) Idealized network model for proteoglycan aggregates in solution. (b) A network segment is modeled as a freely jointed chain of N beads connected with N-1 rigid rods of length L. The force constant of the spring model is given by $H=3kT/(N-1)L$.

During flow, the network chain segments may be stretched and junction sites may be created and lost. In general, we would expect the statistical distribution of the chain segments to be a function of the flow history of the polymeric solution, i.e., it depends on the memory of the fluid. The memory function is in turn a function of rate of creation and loss probability of segment interactions. For example, if the junction sites are permanent and the equivalent spring segment is perfectly elastic, then the material would have a perfect memory, i.e.

an elastic material. In early models developed by Lodge (1968), the creation rate and loss probability of these junction sites were assumed to be constants. With this assumption, the network model was not capable of describing the observed shear rate dependent apparent viscosity and normal stress difference for viscoelastic fluids. De Kee and Carreau (1979) advanced Lodge's theory by assuming that these two rates may be depend on the flow history; specifically, they assumed that the rates depend on the second invariant of the rate of deformation tensor (the first Rivlin-Erickson tensor). [1] To account for our observed acceleration effects (hysteresis loop) on concentrated proteoglycan solutions, we assume that the memory function depends on even the higher order terms, i.e. the second invariant of the second Rivlin-Erickson tensor (Zhu et al. 1988b). Thus the constitutive equation for a second order macromolecular network model takes the form:

$$\tau = \int_{-\infty}^{t} m(t-t', II_1(t'), II_2(t'))\, \Gamma(t,t')dt' \tag{5}$$

where τ is the extra stress tensor, Γ is the Finger strain tensor, II_1 and II_2 are the second invariants of the first and second Rivlin-Erickson tensor, respectively, and m(t,t') is the memory function. From the statistical network model described above, the expressions for the dynamic complex shear moduli (storage modulus, G' and loss modulus G'') are given by:

$$G'(\omega) = \int_0^{\infty} \frac{\eta(s)\lambda(s)\omega^2}{1+\{\lambda(s)\omega\}^2} ds, \tag{6a}$$

$$G''(\omega) = \int_0^{\infty} \frac{\eta(s)\omega}{1+\{\lambda(s)\omega\}^2} ds \tag{6b}$$

with ω being the frequency of the oscillation. For the constant steady-state shear-flow experiment, the expression for the apparent viscosity η_{app} and normal stress function σ_1 are given by:

$$\eta_{app}(\dot{\gamma}) = \int_0^{\infty} \eta(s)\exp(-t_1(s)\dot{\gamma})ds, \tag{7a}$$

1 The second invariant, II, of a tensor, **A**, is defined as $II=(I^2-tr(\mathbf{A}^2))/2$.

$$\sigma_1(\dot{\gamma}) = 2\dot{\gamma}^2 \int_0^\infty \eta(s)\lambda(s)\exp\{-ct_1(s)\dot{\gamma}\}ds, \tag{7b}$$

where $\dot{\gamma}$ is the shear rate. Similarly, the expressions for the transient stress growth, stress relaxation and hysteresis loop can be obtained.

We have shown that this second order statistical network theory can be used to describe all the measured viscoelastic flow properties of concentrated proteoglycans solutions (Zhu et al. 1988b). The parameters obtained from curvefitting of the viscometric flow data to our theory have provided insights into how proteoglycans might function in the extracellular matrix of articular cartilage. For example, the theory allows the determination of the number of segments per unit volume, N(t), as a function of flow history. This information tells us how many network junction sites per unit volume of solution are created or lost during flow. When the proteoglycan solution is at rest, the network segments are randomly distributed, and the total number of chain segments is expected to be maximum. The maximum number of chain segments per unit volume, denoted by N_o, is given by (Zhu et al. 1988b):

$$N_o = \frac{\eta_o s_o}{kT\lambda_o} \frac{\ln(\eta_o/\eta_\infty)}{\ln(1+s_o)}. \tag{8}$$

We have shown that we can measure the energy required to deform the resting molecular network in solution, upon initiation of steady shear, from the stress overshoot curve, i.e. Figs. 6 and 7. This energy must depend on the strength of the interaction at junction sites. Thus the average strength (S) of interaction of the junction sites may be defined as the energy required to disrupted $N(0)-N(t_m)$ segments. This is given by the following relation:

$$S = \frac{E}{N(0)-N(t_m)}, \tag{9}$$

where E is the total energy per unit volume determined in the stress overshoot experiment, and N(0) and $N(t_m)$ are the number of segments per unit volume in the network at the initial state when time t=0 and at the state corresponding to the peak stress, respectively. The values of N_o calculated for link-stable and link-free proteoglycan solutions demonstrated that there was a direct correlation with proteoglycan solution concentration, Fig. 17a. This indicates that proteoglycan solutions at higher concentrations form more interaction sites than those at lower concentrations. However, there was no significant difference in N_o between link-stable and link-free aggregate solutions. Thus, the difference in viscosity between the link-stable and link-free proteoglycan solutions could be due to the difference in the strengths of interaction at the junction sites. In fact, the network strength determined from transient stress overshoot curves (Fig. 7) showed that link-stable aggregates form much stronger interactions than link-free aggregates in solution. As shown in Fig. 17b, more energy is required to overcome the shear resistance offered by the strong interactions at the junction sites formed by link-stable aggregate proteoglycans. This higher resistance is due to the greater structural rigidity of the link-stable aggregates. Indeed, the rigidity of proteoglycans molecules may be a principal determinant of solution viscosity and dynamic shear modulus, and their functional relationships in the extracellular matrix of cartilage.

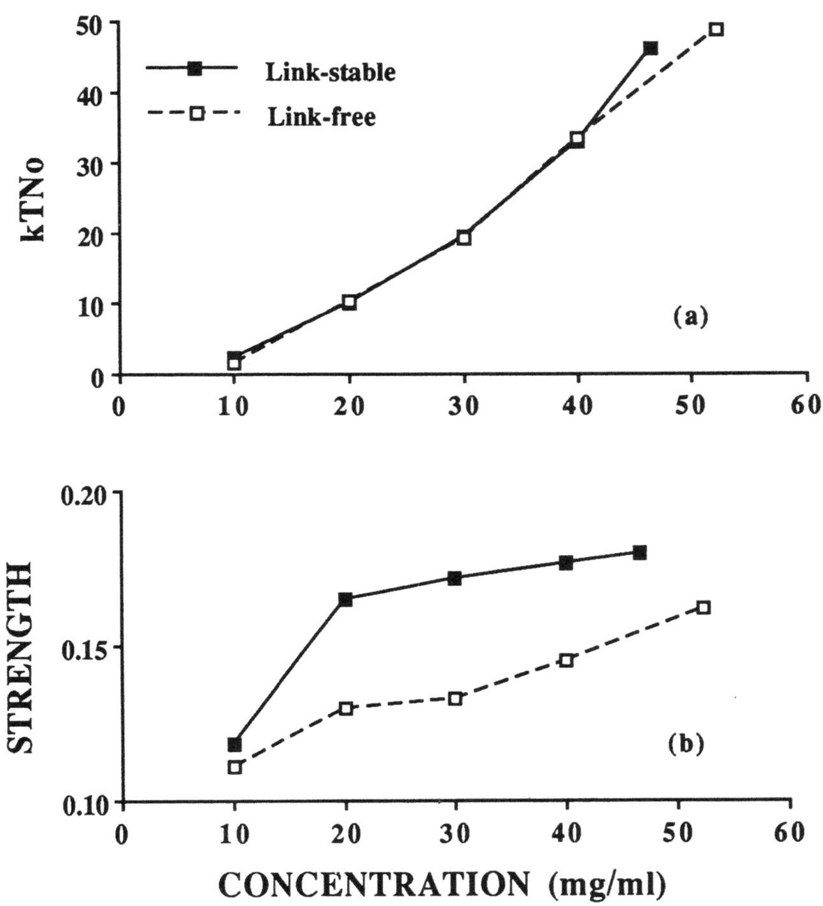

Figure 17 (a) The idealized junction sites per unit volume of solution formed by proteoglycans in solution at rest (kTN_0). For all concentrations, network formed by link-stable and link-free aggregate solutions have same number of junction sites. (b) Variation of network junction site strength (S) with concentration for link-stable and link-free aggregate solutions. Link-stable proteoglycans form much stronger networks in solution.

SUMMARY

Proteoglycans are major components of the extracellular matrix of articular cartilage and other soft tissues. Their structural organization is important for maintaining the cohesion of the extracellular matrix and the material properties of these tissues. To gain insight into the roles proteoglycans play in organizing the extracellular matrix of cartilaginous tissues, we studied the viscometric properties of: 1) proteoglycan monomers, 2) proteoglycan aggregates, 3) percentage of proteoglycans present as aggregates, 4) link-stable and link-free proteoglycan aggregates, and 5) chondroitin sulfate to keratan sulfate ratio. All solutions were studied at the concentrations ranging from 10 to 50 mg/ml. Our experiments show that the viscometric flow properties of proteoglycan solutions are highly non-Newtonian and time-dependent. These proteoglycan solutions exhibit shear-rate dependent viscosities and significant non-zero normal stress effects. The linear viscoelastic storage modulus and loss modulus data demonstrate that proteoglycans are capable of forming molecular networks in solution. All viscometric flow properties were shown to be very sensitive to proteoglycan structural organization. These data have significant physiological implications in terms of normal cartilage function and etiology of osteoarthritis. A second order statistical network theory has been developed to describe the entire spectrum of the linear and nonlinear viscoelastic properties of proteoglycan solutions including both steady-state and transient flow phenomena. Using our viscometric data, this theory provides a method to determine the density and strength of the physical interactions at junction sites in the proteoglycan network. The most important result from this analysis is that link-protein stabilization of proteoglycans significantly increases the rigidity of proteoglycan aggregates and the strength of the network formed by these molecules in solution.

Acknowledgment

This research was sponsored by a grant from the National Institutes of Health (AR-38742), a grant from the National Science Foundation (EET-85-18501), and a grant from the Whitaker Foundation (WZ). Any opinions, findings, conclusions or recommendations expressed in this publication are those of the authors and do not necessarily represent the views of the National Science Foundation.

References

Adams M: Cartilage and osteoarthritis: changes of collagen and proteoglycans. Czech Med 1979; 2:64-68.

Akizuki S, Mow VC, Muller F, Pita JC, Howell DS, Manicourt DH: The tensile properties of human knee joint cartilage: I. Influence of ionic conditions, weight bearing, and fibrillation on the tensile modulus. J Orthop Res 1986; 4(3):379-392.

Armstrong CG, Bahrani AS, Gardner DL: *In vitro* measurement of articular cartilage deformation in the intact human hip joint under load. J Bone Joint Surg 1979; 61-A:744-755.
Armstrong CG, Mow VC: Variations in the intrinsic mechanical properties of human cartilage with age, degeneration and water content. J Bone Joint Surg 1982a; 64-A:88-94.
Armstrong CG, Mow VC: Biomechanics of normal and osteoarthrotic articular cartilage, in Wilson PD, Straub LR (eds): Clinical Trends in Orthopaedics. New York, Thieme-Stratton, Inc, 1982b, pp 189-197.
Balazs EA, Gibbs DA: In Chemistry and Molecular Biology of the Intercellular Matrix, Balazs EA (eds), Academic Press, 1970, pp. 1241-1257.
Bayliss MT, Ali SY: Age-related changes in the composition and structure of human articular cartilage proteoglycans. Biochem J 1979; 176:683-693.
Bird RB, Armstrong RC, Hassager O: Dynamics of Polymeric Liquids: Fluid Mechanics, John Wiley & Sons, Ins, New York 1977a.
Bird RB, Hassager O, Armstrong RC, Curtiss CF: Dynamics of Polymeric Liquids: Kinetic theory, John Wiley & Sons, Ins, New York 1977b.
Bollet AJ, Nance JL: Biochemical findings in normal and osteoarthritic articular cartilage, II. chondroitin sulfate concentration and chain length, water and ash content. J Clinical Investigation 1966; 45(7):1170-1177.
Brandt KD: Enhanced extractability of articular cartilage proteoglycans in osteoarthrosis. Biochem J 1974; 143:475-478.
Buckwalter JA, Kuettner KE, Thonar EJ-M: Age-related changes in articular cartilage proteoglycans: electron microscopic studies. J Orthop Res 1985; 3:251-257.
Buckwalter JA, Rosenberg LC: Structural changes during development in bovine fetal epiphyseal cartilage: Electron microscopic studies of proteoglycan monomers and aggregates. Collagen Rel Res 1983; 3: 489-504.
Carney SL, Billingham MEJ, Muir H, Sandy JD: Demonstration of increased proteoglycan turnover in cartilage explants from dogs with experimental arthritis. J Orthop Ser 1984; 2:201-206.
Coleman BD, Markowitz H, Noll W: Viscometric flows of non-Newtonian Fluids, Springer- Verlag, New York, 1966.
De Kee D, Carreau PJ: A Constitutive Equation Derived from Lodge's Network Theory. J Non-Newtonian Fl Mech 1979; 6:127-143.
Eisenberg SR, Grodzinsky AJ: The kinetics of chemically induced nonequilibrium swelling of articular cartilage and corneal stroma. J Biomech Eng 1987; 109:79-89.
Eyre DR, Koob TJ, Van Ness KP: Quantitation of hydroxypyridinium crosslinks in collagen by high-performance liquid chromatography. Analytical Biochem 1984; 137:308-388.
Ferry JD: Viscoelastic Properties of Polymers, Wiley, New York, Second Edition 1970.
Gray ML, Pizzanelli AM, Grodzinsky AJ, Lee RC: Mechanical and physicochemical determinants of the chondrocyte biosynthetic response. J Orthop Res 1988; 6:777-792.
Hardingham TE: The role of link protein in the structure of cartilage proteoglycan aggregates. Biochem J 1979; 177:237-247.
Hardingham TE: Proteoglycans: Their structure, interactions and molecular organization in cartilage. Biochem Soc Trans 1981; 9:489-497.
Hardingham TE, Meardmore-Grey M, Dunham DG: Protein domain structure of the aggregating proteoglycan from cartilage. Trans Orthop Res Soc 1987a; 12:61.

Hardingham TE, Muir H, Kwan MK, Lai WM, Mow VC: Viscoelastic properties of proteoglycan solutions with varying proportions present as aggregates. J Orthop Res 1987b; 5:36-46.

Hascall VC, Hascall GK: Proteoglycans, in Hay ED (ed) Cell Biology of Extracellular Matrix, Plenum Press, New York, 1981, pp 39-63.

Hascall VC, Sajdesa F: Proteinpolysaccharide complex from bovine nasal cartilage, the function of glycoprotein in the formation of aggregates. J Biol Chem 1969, 244:2384-2396.

Hjertquist SO, Wasteson A: The molecular weight of chondroitin sulfate from human articular cartilage: effect of age and of osteoarthritis. Calcif Tissue Res 1972; 10:31-37.

Jaffe FF, Mankin HJ, Weiss C, Zarins A: Water binding in the articular cartilage of rabbits. J Bone Joint Surg 1974; 56A:1031-1039.

Kempson GE: Mechanical properties of articular cartilage, in Freeman MAR (ed) Adult Articular Cartilage, Tunbridge Wells, England, Pitman Medical, 1979, pp 333-414.

Lai WM, Hou J, Mow VC: Triphasic theory for articular cartilage swelling, in Torzill PA, Friedman MH (eds) Proc Biomech Symp, San Diego, ASME, 1989, pp 33-36.

Lodge AS: Constitutive equations from molecular network theories for polymer solutions. Rheol Acta 1968; 7:379-392.

Mak AF, Mow VC, Lai WM, Hardingham TE, Muir H, Eyre DR: Assessment of proteoglycan-proteoglycan interactions from solution biorheological behavior. Trans Orthop Res Soc 1982; 7:169.

Mak AF, Mow VC, Lai WM, Hardingham TE, Muir H: Predictions of the Number and Strength of the Proteoglycan-Proteoglycan Interactions from Viscometric Data. Trans Orthop Res Soc 1983; 8:3.

Mankin HJ, Thrasher AZ: Water content and binding in normal and osteoarthritic human cartilage. J Bone Joint Surg 1975; 57A:76-80.

Maroudas A: Physicochemical properties of articular cartilage, in Freeman MAR (ed) Adult Articular Cartilage, Tunbridge Wells, England, Pitman Medical, 1979, pp 215-290.

Maroudas A: Physical chemistry of articular cartilage and the intervertebral disc, in Sokoloff L (ed) The Joint and Synovial Fluid, II, New York Academic Press, 1980, pp 239-291.

Maroudas A: Proteoglycan osmotic pressure and collagen tension in normal, osteoarthritic human cartilage, in Huskisson EC, Katona G (eds) Int Symp New Trends in Osteoarthritis, 1981, pp. 36-39.

McDevitt CA, Muir H: Biochemical changes in the cartilage of the knee in experimental and natural osteoarthrosis in the dog. J Bone Joint Surg 1976; 58-B:94-101.

Mow VC, Lai WM (1980): Recent developments in synovial joint biomechanics. SIAM Rev 1980; 22(3): 275-317.

Mow VC, Holmes MH, Lai WM: Fluid transport and mechanical properties of articular cartilage: A review. J Biomech 1984a; 17:377-394.

Mow VC, Mak AF, Lai WM, Rosenberg LC, Tang LH: Viscoelastic properties of proteoglycan subunits and aggregates in varying solution concentrations. J Biomech 1984b; 17:325-338.

Mow VC, Zhu WB, Lai WM, Hardingham TE, Hughes C, Muir H: The influence of link protein stabilization on the viscometric properties of proteoglycan aggregate solutions. Biochim Biophys Acta 1989; 992:201-208.

Muir H: A molecular approach to the understanding of osteoarthrosis. Ann Rheum Dis 1977; 36:199-208.

Muir H: The chemistry of the ground substance of joint cartilage, in Sokoloff L (ed) The Joints and Synovial Fluid, Vol II. New York, Academic Press, 1980, pp 27-94.
Muir H: Proteoglycans as organizers of the extracellular matrix. Biochem Soc Trans 1983; 11:613-622.
Myers ER, Zhu WB, Mow VC: Viscoelastic properties of articular cartilage and meniscus, in Nimni ME (ed) Collagen, Biochemistry, Biology and Biotechnology, Vol II. CRC Press, Boca Raton, FL, 1987, pp 267-288.
Myers, E.R. Lai, W.M. and Mow, V.C.: A continuum theory and an experiment for the ion-induced swelling behavior of articular cartilage. J. Biomech. Eng. 106:151-158, 1984a.
Myers, ER, Armstrong, CG, Mow, VC. Swelling pressure and collagen tension. In Connective Tissue Matrix. ed. DWL Hukins, MacMillan Press, Ltd, 1984;161-168, 1984b.
Nimni ME, Harkness RD: Molecular structure and function of collagen, in Nimni ME (ed) Collagen: Biochemistry, Vol I. CRC Press, Boca Raton, Florida, 1988, pp 1-78.
Obrink B: A study of the interactions between sununitic tropocollagen and glycosaminoglycan. Euro J Biochem 1973; 33:387-400.
Oldroyd JG: On the formulation of rheological equations of state. Proc R Soc 1950; A-250:523-541.
Pal S, Tang LH, Choi H, Habermann E, Rosenberg LC, Roughley P, Poole AR: Structural changes during development in bovine fetal epiphyseal cartilage. Coll Res 1981; 1:151-176.
Paulsson M, Morgelin M, Wiedemann H, Beardmore-Gray M, Dunham D, Hardingham TE, Heinegard D, Timpl R, Engel JHH: Extracted and globular protein domains in cartilage proteoglycans. Biochem J 1987; 245:763-772.
Plaas AHK, Sandy JD: Age-related decrease in the link-stability of proteoglycan aggregates formed by articular chondrocytes. Biochem J 1984; 220:337-340.
Poole AR: Proteoglycans in health and disease: structure and functions. Biochem J 1986; 236:1-14.
Pottenger LA, Lyon NB, Hecht JD, Neustadt PM, Robinson RA: Influence of cartilage particle size and proteoglycan aggregation on immobilization of proteoglycans. J Biol Chem 1982; 257:11479-11485.
Ratcliffe A, Tyler J, Hardingham TE: Articular Cartilage Cultured with Interleukin 1: Increase release of Link Protein, Hyaluronate-Binding Region and Other Proteoglycan Fragments. Biochem J 1986; 238:571-580.
Ratcliffe A, Billingham MEJ, Muir H, Hardingham TE: Experimental canine osteoarthritis and cartilage explant culture: increased release of specific proteoglycan components. Trans Orthop Res Soc 1989; 14.
Ricard-Blum S, Tiollier J, Garrone R, Herbage D: Further Biochemical and physicochemical characterization of minor disulfide-bonded (Type IX) collagen, extracted from foetal calf cartilage. J Cellular Biochem 1985; 27:347-358.
Rosenberg LC, Pal S, Beale R: Proteoglycans from bovine proximal humeral articular cartilage. J Biol Chem 1973; 218:3681-3690.
Rosenberg LC, Wolfenstein-Todel C, Margolis R, Pal S, Strider W: Proteoglycans from bovine proximal humeral articular cartilage: structural basis for the polydispersity of proteoglycan subunit. J Biolo Chem 1976; 251(20):6439-6444.
Rosenberg LC, Choi HU, Tang LH, Johnson TL, Pal S: Isolation of dermatan sulfate proteoglycans from mature bovine articular cartilages. J Biol Chem 1985; 260:6304-6313.

Rosenberg LC, Mow VC, Buckwalter JA, Poole AR: Structure and function of proteoglycans in developing cartilage, in Akeson WH, Bornstein P, Glimcher MJ (eds) American Academy of Orthop Surg Symp on Heritable Disorders of Connective Tissue. CV Mosby Co, St Louis, 1982, pp 285-306.

Roth V, Mow VC: The intrinsic tensile behavior of the matrix of bovine articular cartilage and its variation with age. J Bone Joint Surg 1980; 62-A:1102-1117.

Roughley PJ, White RJ: Age-related changes in the structure of the proteoglycan subunits from human articular cartilage. J Biolo Chem 1980; 255(1):217-224.

Sampaio UD, Bayliss MT, Hardingham TE, Muir H: Dermatan sulphate proteoglycan from human articular cartilage. Biochem J 1988; 254:757-764.

Sandy JD, Adams ME, Billingham MEJ, Plaas A, Muir H: *In vivo* and *in vitro* stimulation of chondrocyte biosynthetic activity in early experimental osteoarthritis. Arthritis Rheum 1984; 27:388-397.

Santer V, White RJ, Roughley PJ: O-linked oligosaccharides of human articular cartilage proteoglycan. Biochim Biophys Acta 1982; 716:277-282.

Schmidt MB, Schoonbeck JM, Mow VC, Eyre DR, Chun LE: Effects of enzymatic extraction of proteoglycans on the tensile properties of articular cartilage. Trans Orthop Res Soc 1986; 11:450.

Schmidt MB, Schoonbeck JM, Mow VC, Eyre DR, Chun LE: The relationship between collagen cross-linking and the tensile properties of articular cartilage. Trans Orthop Res Soc 1987; 12:134.

Schneiderman R, Keret D, Maroudas A: Effects of mechanical and osmotic pressure on the rate of glycosaminoglycan synthesis in the human adult femoral head cartilage: an *in vitro* study. J Orthop Res 1986; 4:393-408.

Schurz J, Ribitsch V: Rheology of synovial fluid. Biorheology 1987; 24:385-399.

Simon WH, Mak A, Spirt A: The effect of shear fatigue on bovine articular cartilage. J Orthop Res 1989; 8:86-93.

Sweet MBE, Thonar E J-M, Immelman AR, Solomon L: Biochemical changes in progressive osteoarthrosis. Ann Rheum Dis 1977; 36:387-398.

Sweet MBE, Coelho A, Schnitzler CM, Schnitzer TJ, Lenz ME, Jakim I, Kuettner KE, Thonar E J-MA: Serum keratan sulfate levels in osteoarthritis patients. Arthritis and Rheum 1988; 31(5):648-652.

van der Rest M, Mayne R: Type IX collagen proteoglycan from cartilage is covalently cross-linked to type II collagen. J Biol Chem 1988; 263:1615-1618.

Vasan N: Proteoglycans in normal and severely osteoarthritic human cartilage. Biochem J 1980; 187:781-787.

Walters K: Rheometry. Halsted Press, New York, 1975.

Woo SL-Y, Akeson WH, Jemmott GF: Measurements of nonhomogeneous directional mechanical properties of articular cartilage in tension. J Biomech 1976; 9:785-791.

Yamauchi M, Mechanic G: Cross-linking of collagen, in Nimni ME (ed) Collagen: Biochemistry, Vol I. CRC Press, Boca Raton, Florida, 1988, pp 157-172.

Zhu WB, Lai WM, Mow VC, Tang LH, Rosenberg LC, Hughes C, Hardingham TE, Muir H: Influence of composition, size and structure of cartilage proteoglycans on the strength of molecular network formed in solution. Trans Orthop Res Sci 1988a; 13:67.

Zhu WB, Lai WM, Mow VC: A second order rheological model to predict the time-dependent behavior of proteoglycan solutions. 1988 Advances in Bioengineering, Trans ASME 1988b; 8:187-190.

Chapter 12

Osmotic and Hydraulic Flows in Proteoglycan Solutions

W.D. Comper

Introduction

Articular cartilage is an integral component of diarthrodial joints where it functions as the covering of articulating bone surfaces to provide a bearing interface which has both compressive resistance and viscoelasticity. The tissue itself is avascular in which chondrocytes are sparsely distributed in an extracellular matrix which is synthesized by these cells. The physical properties of the cartilage are determined by its extracellular matrix. The matrix is a multicomponent system. Notwithstanding the compositional and topographical heterogeneity of matrix macromolecules, its major components are water with dissolved NaCl and other salts, type II collagen and proteoglycan.

These components have been considered to exist in a biphasic arrangement (Gersh and Catchpole 1960; Mow et al 1980) consisting of a porous network of insoluble collagen fibres filled with a soluble phase of water and proteoglycan up to 50-80 mg ml^{-1} in concentration (Maroudas 1980).

The major proteoglycan population has an hierarchical branching and entrapment organisation that ensures the retention of the highly anionic but relatively small glycosaminoglycan chains (mainly chondroitin -4 and -6 sulfate together with keratan sulfate) within the tissue. The chains are covalently attached at one end, to a protein core to give rise to a bottle brush type structure. Such a structure in articular cartilage is referred to as a proteoglycan subunit (PGS). Proteoglycans are normally present in the extracellular matrix as proteoglycan aggregates (PGA) in which 20-50 PGS molecules are bound through noncovalent interactions to an hyaluronate core; these interactions being stabilised by glycoproteins called link proteins (for reviews see Carney and Muir 1988; Hascall 1988). The aggregates, by virtue of their size, are thought to be retained, by a physical entrapment mechanism, within the coarse collagen network of the tissue. Weak electrostatic and hydrogen-bonding interactions between proteoglycans and collagen, which may be facilitated by the relatively lower NaCl concentration in proteoglycan compartments (due to the Donnan equilibrium) may augment the retention of the proteoglycans in this composite structure.

In relation to the mechanical properties of cartilage its most dominant and important component is water. The load-bearing properties of cartilage result largely from its ability to retain water (an essentially incompressible fluid) under the application of load; both equilibrium and dynamic factors will be involved in this retentive capacity.

The types of processes that govern water concentration and movement in cartilage are osmotic and hydraulic flows. These are transport processes that take place at the molecular level and therefore will be controlled by soluble components in the matrix, particularly the soluble proteoglycans. Interpretations of these flows should therefore be made primarily in relation to the hydrodynamic properties of the proteoglycan and proteoglycan-containing collagen networks. This study then focuses on the various aspects of water-proteoglycan interaction in simple ternary systems that results in net movement of water relative to the proteoglycan. The following discussion will encompass detailed experimental and theoretical studies of osmotic flow and hydraulic conductivity in free solution and in membrane systems that retain the proteoglycan. These studies will also highlight the structure-function relationships of the proteoglycan on these hydrodynamic processes. Another feature of this approach is the appreciation of the microorganisation of cartilage hydrodynamic determinants in terms of the distance function embodied in the flow processes. Overall, this reductionist approach should actively complement the biomechanical studies on whole cartilage under different biomechanical regimes (Kwan et al 1984; Mow et al 1980,1984) or other chemically-induced nonequilibrium regimes (Grodzinsky et al 1981; Eisenberg and Grodzinsky 1987, 1988; Lai et al 1990). The phenomenological basis of whole cartilage behaviour has been successfully interpreted by various electromechanical models yet there is a paucity of data which relates biomechanical properties to molecular composition and structure. These efforts have been confined to osmotic activity (Maroudas and Bannon 1981; Urban et al 1979) and viscoelasticity of proteoglycans (Mow et el 1984).

Status of Concentrated Proteoglycan Solutions

An important aspect of proteoglycan hydrodynamics is the effective size, composition, and molecular interactions that the molecule undergoes in concentrated solution. In the simple case of a dilute solution the proteoglycans are non-interacting individual molecules. They can be regarded as microscopic gels with characteristic kinetic segments of chondroitin sulfate chains (this unit will be featured as an important dynamic component *vide infra*) which undergo the elastic restriction of the covalently linked proteoglycan structure. The tendency of the chondroitin sulfate segments to move is strong (due to their diffusional motion) so that each individual proteoglycan molecule is highly hydrated in dilute solution. The PGS has an effective hydrodynamic radius in the range of 50-80nm and that of the aggregate 1000-1600nm (Comper and Williams 1987). Water properties are not altered in their domain (Comper and Laurent 1978; Comper and Williams 1987) nor in proteoglycan compartments in cartilage (Maroudas and Venn 1977; Maroudas 1980). There is no evidence of significantly bound water or structured water in the proteoglycan domain.

In concentrating proteoglycans there will be a concentration where their hydrodynamic domains will consistently make contact. This is called the critical concentration, which corresponds to 5 mg ml $^{-1}$ for PGS and 0.06 mg ml $^{-1}$ for PGA (Comper and Williams 1987). For concentrations above the critical concentration it is necessary, purely through space filling requirements, that the proteoglycan occupy a reduced volume as compared to its hydrodynamic volume at infinite dilution (as unrestricted molecular interpenetration is unlikely). The nature of the required conformational changes in the proteoglycan are not clear. On the basis of osmotic considerations the initial conformational change from the dilute regime will be one forming a stiffer core structure and a more elongated molecule (Comper and Williams 1987). This is consistent with the restricted flexibility of the protein core of PGS units in cartilage as measured by ^{13}C nmr (Torchia et al 1977). In these concentrated states the proteoglycan forms a transient network structure in which supermacromolecular aggregates may form and dissipate relatively quickly. In contrast to the commonly expressed view that concentration-dependant proteoglycan conformation has some role in compressive resistance (Hascall 1977, 1988; Muir 1983) (see also Comper 1990) it will be shown *vide infra* that factors that determine the relative movement of water to the proteoglycan are independent of these concentration-dependent conformational changes. There is some evidence, however, that in membrane systems supermacromolecular aggregates may be active in affecting osmotic flow (Comper and Williams 1990).

Volume Flow Associated With Translational Diffusion

Matrix molecules, like proteoglycans move through collisions with water in the tissue. The thermal energy of solvent is transduced to kinetic energy of the matrix molecules; the most important, in terms of tissues' biomechanical properties, is the energy associated with translational motion relative to water. The translational diffusional process in an isothermal system is related to the concentration gradient of the molecules described by Fick's equation,

$$J_1 = -D_1(\text{grad } c_1) \quad (1)$$

where J_1 is the flux of component 1 (which is the proteglycan in most cases considered here) and c_1 the concentration of component 1 (moles per unit volume). The relationship between the molecular flux of component 1 and its concentration gradient is given by the translational (or mutual) diffusion coefficient D_1. The diffusion coefficient in a binary system for a volume - fixed frame (designated by the subscript v) has been derived by Bearman (1961) for component 1 and component 2 (solvent) as

$$(D_1)_v = (D_2)_v = (1-\phi_1)(c_1/f_{12})(\partial\mu_1/\partial c_1)_{T,p} \quad (2)$$

where ϕ_1 is the volume fraction of 1, T is the temperature, p the pressure, μ_1 the chemical potential of 1 and f_{12} is the frictional factor between 1 mole of proteglycan and water defined as (Spiegler 1958)

$$-(\partial\mu_1/\partial x) = f_{12}(u_1 - u_2) \quad (3)$$

where u_1 is the velocity of i.

Derivation of the translational diffusion coefficient corresponding to common experimental standard conditions of constant temperature and chemical potential of solvent μ_2 is (Comper et al 1986)

$$(D_1)_v = RT(1-\phi_1)^2(M_1/f_{12})[(1/M_1)+2A_2C_1+3A_3C_1^2...] \quad (4)$$

where R is the universal gas constant, M_1 is the molecular weight of component 1 and A_2 and A_3 are the standard osmotic second and third virial coefficients respectively. The diffusion coefficient in equation 4 is a composite function of an hydrodynamic parameter associated with the frictional coefficient and a thermodynamic equilibrium parameter of osmotic pressure as embodied in the virial expansion.

The volume flux associated with this diffusional process will be exactly balanced by an opposite volume flux of solvent (Figure 1) so that

$$J_1V_1 = -J_2V_2 \quad (5)$$

where V_i is the partial molar volume of i. The right hand term of equation 5 could be thought of as an osmotically driven flow in free solution. The diffusion coefficients defined by equation 4 for PGS, PGA and individual chondroitin sulfate chains, as measured by ultracentrifugal techniques (Comper and Williams, 1987) are markedly different in dilute solution but show molecular weight independence above a concentration of 5-10 mg ml^{-1} (Figure 2). The marked increase in the diffusion coefficient with concentration is due to the predominance of the osmotic term over the hydrodynamic frictional term in equation 4. The compelling feature of this data is that at concentrations >10 mg ml^{-1}, PGA with a molecular weight of 10^8 diffuses at the same rate as its constituent chondroitin sulfate chains (MW ~ 30000). The molecular weight independence of the individual parameters of equation 4 have been established previously. Molecular weight independence of osmotic pressure has been demonstrated by Urban et al (1979) and that of the frictional term M_1/f_{12} demonstrated *vide infra.*

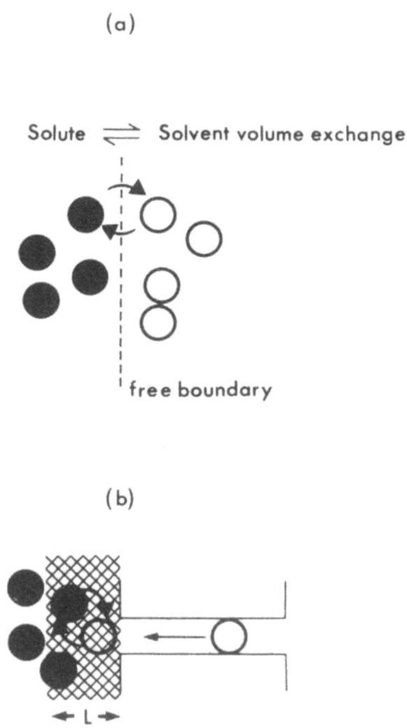

Figure 1. Schematic diagram of long time averaged solute (filled circles) - solvent (empty circles) volume exchange a) across a free boundary (dashed line) and b) in a thin layer on the solution side of the semipermeable membrane.

The Frictional Factor and Specific Hydraulic Conductivity

Independent estimates of the frictional interaction of proteoglycans with water can be made directly from sedimentation velocity experiments. In this technique water is made to move relative to the proteoglycan by sedimentation of the proteoglycan. The viscous dissipation of water over the surface of the proteoglycan will then govern the sedimentation coefficient (S_1) which can be directly related to the specific hydraulic conductivity (k) of the solution. The following equations apply (Mijnlieff and Jaspers 1971; Comper et al 1986)

$$k = \eta_2 (S_1)_v / C_1 (1-(v_1/v_2)) \quad (6)$$

where η_2 is the dynamic viscosity of solvent, C_1 the concentration of 1 in mass per volume units and v_i the partial specific volume of i. The sedimentation coefficient is directly related to f_{12} through the equation

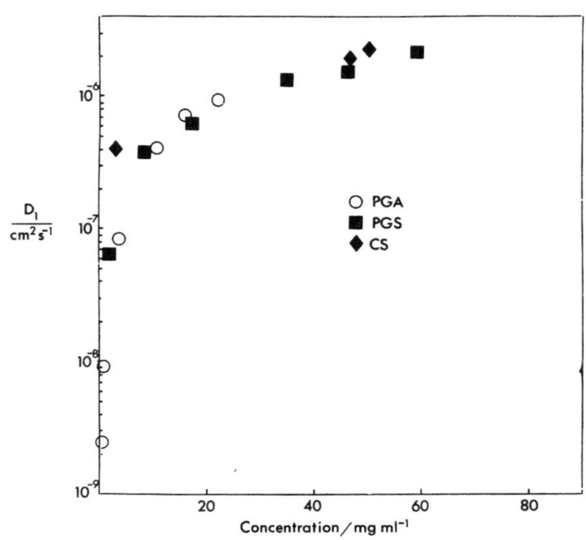

Figure 2. Variation of the mutual diffusion coefficient D_1 as a function of concentration for native Swarm rat chondrosarcoma aggregate (PGA) , its constitutent monomer (PGS) and chondroitin sulfate chains . All solutions were in thermodynamic equilibrium with phosphate buffered saline, ionic strength = 0.15, pH7.4. Data compiled from Comper and Williams (1987) and Comper and Zamparo (1990).

$$(S_1)_v = (1-\rho v_1)(1-\phi_1)M_1/f_{12} \tag{7}$$

where ρ is the solution density. The term M_1/f_{12} represents the frictional coefficient between unit mass of proteoglycan and water.

Specific hydraulic conductivities of various preparations including PGA, PGS, and chondroitin sulfate are shown in Figure 3. Hydraulic conductivities have been measured up to 80 mg ml^{-1} of chondroitin sulfate, which is comparable to concentrations found in some extracellular matrices. The data shown in Figure 3 reveal that the specific hydraulic conductivities are molecular weight independent. Therefore, for the chondroitin sulfate proteglycans, their core structures and macroscopic viscosities do not influence the relative movement of water to proteoglycan. Rather, this movement is governed by the interaction of water with a critical segment of the chondroitin sulfate chain. Translational movement as embodied in equation 1 of such enormous molecules like PGA and PGS is governed by, and behaves like, chondroitin sulfate chain segments.

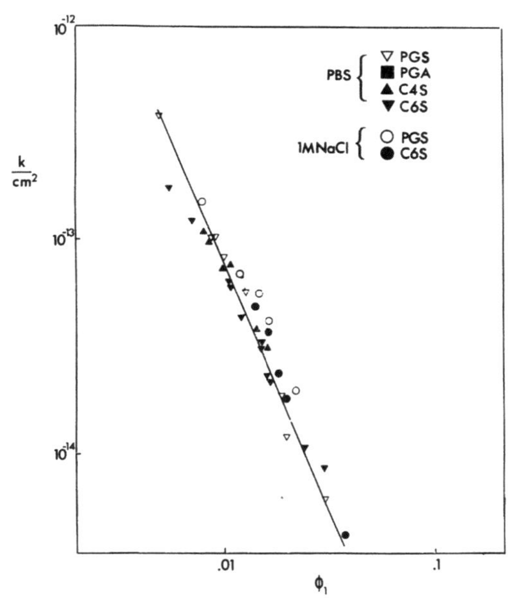

Figure 3. Specific hydraulic conductivities (k) of Swarm rat chondrosarcoma aggregate, its constitute proteoglycan monomer , chondroitin 4-sulfate , and chondroitin 6-sulfate. All solutions were in thermodynamic equilibrium with phosphate buffered saline pH7.4. Chondroitin sulfate and PGS were also analysed in 1M NaCl. Data compiled from Comper and Williams (1987) and Zamparo and Comper (1989).

In other words, water displacement relative to the proteoglycan occurs genuinely within the proteoglycan hydrodynamic domain. This type of behaviour then clearly distinguishes this functional property of the proteoglycan on water transport from the role of the proteoglycan in the viscoelastic motion of the tissue. We also note that all the glycosaminoglycans associated with PGS or PGA namely chondroitin 4 - sulfate chondroitin 6 - sulfate, keratan sulfate and hyaluronate have similar k values whether compared on a mass or volume basis(Comper and Zamparo 1990). This insensitivity to chemical composition, particularly in relation to the hyaluronate and chondroitin sulfate, has been confirmed in other studies including the use of desulfated chondroitin sulfate (chondroitin) (Zamparo and Comper 1989). And also by the fact that the ionic strength dependence of k for these polyions is low (Zamparo and Comper 1989)(Figure 3). It is primarily the surface to volume ratio of the polysaccharide critical segment which will govern k. The use of the Happel-Brenner model (1983) however, derived for the flow of water through a random distribution of neutral fibers whose variable parameters are fiber radius and volume fraction, offers a poor prediction for the experimental data although it does qualitatively show the same trend (Comper and Zamparo 1989). Previous attempts to estimate k for proteoglycans from this model therefore have severely underestimated its value(Maroudas et al, 1987; Levick, 1987).

Comparative studies of k for various polysaccharides (Comper and Williams, 1987; Zamparo and Comper, 1989; Comper and Zamparo, 1990) have demonstrated that the nature of the glycosidic linkage is of major importance in governing the magnitude of k. Hyaluronate, chondroitin sulfate and keratan sulfate with alternating β1,4 and β1,3 linkages have considerably lower k values as compared to heparin-like polysaccharides with α1,4 and β1,4 linkages and dextrans with α1,6 linkages and carboxymethyl celluloses with β1,4 linkages. In fact, the glycosaminoglycan group with β1,4 and β1,3 linkages, including the chondroitin sulfates, exhibit the lowest specific hydraulic conductivity per unit volume or mass of any polymer material that we have measured (Comper and Zamparo, 1989, 1990). This identifies a structure-function relationship that would make chondroitin sulfate/keratan sulfate particularly suitable for systems required to resist the flow of water under applied load ie.the compressive resistance of cartilage.

Tritiated Water Diffusion

Tritiated water (HTO) will undergo exchange with normal water at a very fast rate with a diffusion coefficient of ~$200 \times 10^{-7} cm^2 s^{-1}$. This compares with the mutual diffusion coefficient of water associated with chemical potential gradients in solutions in the range of 0.01×10^{-7}-$15 \times 10^{-7} cm^2 s^{-1}$ (Figure 2). Therefore, in using tritiated water one has to take into account the marked influence of HTO-H_2O exchange; in cartilage this will be significant as the tissue contains 80%

water. For HTO movement in polymer systems with no solute concentration gradients the diffusion coefficient can be derived as (Comper et al 1982)

$$D_{2*} = RT/(f_{2*2} + f_{2*1}) \quad (8)$$

where HTO is designated as component 2*. Using the Onsager reciprocal relationship (Onsager and Fuoss, 1932) this equation may be reduced to the form

$$D_{2*} = RT/(f_{2*2}+(c_1f_{12}/c_2)) \quad (9)$$

where f_{12} is the frictional coefficient associated with the relative movement of water to component 1 as used in diffusion and sedimentation.

The value of the frictional coefficient cannot be absolutely obtained by HTO diffusion measurements as the effective molecular weight (or molar concentration) of component 1 is not known ie the size of the critical segments. Studies on HTO diffusion in dextran solutions (Comper et al 1982) have given concentration dependent effective molecular weights in the range of 200 - 10000. This may give some idea the range of sizes of critical segments that may be associated with chondroitin sulfate in the proteoglycan.

We have also demonstrated (Comper and Zamparo 1989) using HTO diffusion analysis that the concentration dependent reduction in HTO diffusion was similar, as expected, to the decrease in k obtained from dextran sedimentation studies. This was not found to be the case of chondroitin sulfate where the concentration dependent decrease in k is greater than that found for HTO diffusion. This has been rationalised on the basis of the existance of significant osmotic fields around the chondroitin sulfate polymer chain which may restrict flow under mechanical pressure (Comper and Zamparo, 1989).

Membrane - Related Phenomena

We are interested now in applying the concepts of macromolecular diffusion and hydraulic conductivity of water to systems with membranes which are impermeable to macromolecules. This is analogous to the physically entrapped polysaccharides in collagen matrices in cartilage. We regard that in the solution in contact with the membrane there will be a very thin layer, extending from the membrane pore to a distance L into the solution where the solute concentration (or chemical potential) drops from its solution value to zero at the membrane pore/solution interface (Figure 1). It is the relative movement of water in relation to solute within this layer that will govern osmotic flow and ultrafiltration. This model forms the basis for a new interpretation of membrane hydrodynamics (Williams and Comper 1987, 1990; Zamparo and Comper 1989; Comper and Williams 1990).

Osmotic Flow

Osmotic flow in an important process in cartilage hydrodynamics. Apart from offering resistance to mechanical pressure that tends to drive water out of the tissue, it provides the only mechanism by which water can be reimbibed into a compressed tissue once the mechanical load is released.

In a membrane system, osmotic flow occurs when a solute dissolved in water (a solution) is separated from solvent by a membrane permeable to solvent but not solute. Flow of solvent will spontaneously occur from the solvent compartment into the solution compartment. The driving force for solvent flow will be the tendency of the solute concentration gradient to relax in the thin layer adjacent to the membrane. It is exactly the same force that governs mutual diffusion in free solution as discussed *vide supra*. In this case it was pointed out that a solute concentration gradient across a free liquid boundary will give rise to a solute diffusion which could equally well be described by water diffusion (volume flow) in the opposite direction. This water flow is driven by identical osmotic pressure gradients that drive osmotic flow across membranes. Yet we know that in the free boundary system the diffusion coefficient of water and that of the solute in a volume fixed frame of reference are identical (Bearman, 1961) ie the rate of osmotic flow across a free boundary is governed by solute diffusion.

Osmotic flow across a membrane has been modelled in our studies on a series of flows consisting of 1) water flow across the membrane, and 2) the diffusional exchange of osmotically active solute with solvent in the thin layer on the solution side of the membrane - it is the exchange process that draws water through the membrane. Considerable controversy has previously existed as to the mechanism of osmosis with most interpretations recognising (1) but not (2) as the effective kinetic process. There was, however, early qualitative recognition by some investigators of the importance of the solution - exchange layer adjacent to the membrane (Ray 1960; Dainty 1965; Soodak and Iberall 1978).

The usual relationship between osmotic volume flow, J_v, of water and the osmotic pressure difference ($\Delta\Pi$) across the membrane is

$$J_v = - L_p^{\circ}\Delta\Pi \tag{10}$$

where L_p° is the osmotic permeability coefficient which has formerly been regarded as a constant describing the interaction of water with the membrane. Prior to our studies, there had been no account made of the influence of the strong concentration dependent dynamic properties of the osmotically active solute on the magnitude of L_p^o Rather, any deviation from ideal behavior of water - membrane interaction was commonly ascribed to 'unstirred boundary layer effects' (Heyer et al 1969). We have derived (Williams and Comper 1990) the following expression for L_p^o which takes into account the series interaction model of water with the membrane and solute such that

$$L_p^o = 1/[(1/L_p) + (L/v_1(1-\phi_1)^2 AM_1/f_{12})] \tag{11}$$

where L_p is the hydraulic permeability coefficient in the absence of solute and embodies the water-membrane interaction term. The water-solute interaction will

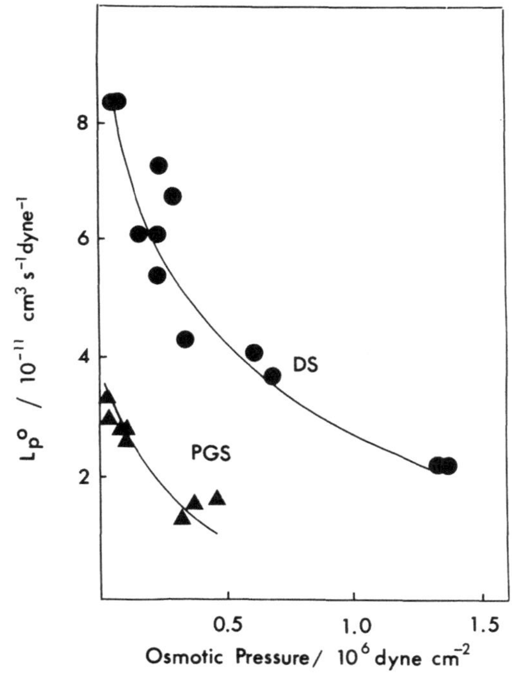

Figure 4. The variation of the osmotic permeability coefficient L_p^o measured for osmotic flows across semipermeable polyester membranes as a function of osmotic pressure for PGS and dextran sulfate in thermodynamic equilibrium with phosphate buffered saline pH7.4. L_p for the membrane in solvent only was 10.97×10^{-11} cm^3 $dyne^{-1} s^{-1}$ (data from Williams and Comper 1990).

be included in the M_1/f_{12} term which notably is the same parameter that governs specific hydraulic onductivity. The membrane area A is the effective area of the pores in the membrane and L represents the distance over which the osmotic solute-solvent exchange process takes place in front of the pore. Any involvement of solute-membrane interaction in modifying the exchange process will be included in the A/L term. For osmotically active polymer solutions at concentrations greater that 10 mg ml^{-1} the second term on the rhs of equation far outweighs the first term governing water-membrane interactions for all types of commercially available membranes studied (Williams and Comper 1987; 1990) (Figure 4).

This demonstrates that the limiting factor governing the rate of osmotic flow is the frictional term M_1/f_{12}. The data in Figure 4 also demonstrates that L_p^o decreases rapidly with osmotic pressure and that this is mirrored in a similar fashion in the variation of the frictional factor (as determined from sedimentation studies) with osmotic pressure (Figure 5). The relative differences

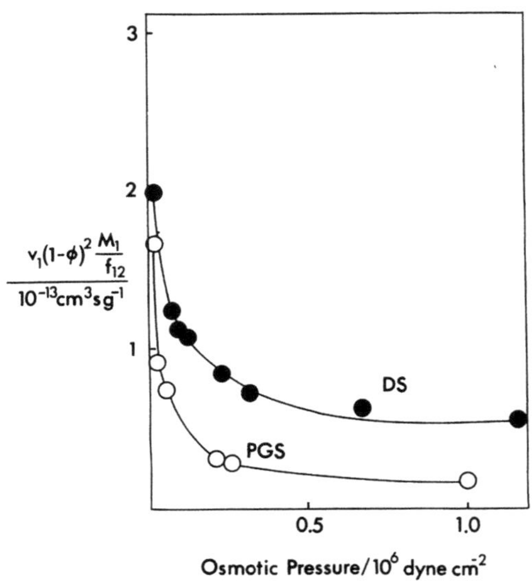

Figure 5. Variation of $v_1(1-\phi_1)^2M_1/f_{12}$ from equation 11 as determined from sedimentation studies as a function of osmotic pressure for dextran sulfate and PGS . From Williams and Comper (1990).

between dextran sulfate and PGS in terms of L_p^o are also exemplified in the M_1/f_{12} function in Figure 5.

A number of important conclusions can be derived at this stage. While it is commonly recognised that the colligative properties of the proteoglycan solution are governed mainly be its constituent micro-counterions, the kinetics of osmotic flow is determined by the frictional factor of the proteoglycan which, as shown *vide supra*, resides essentially with the dynamic interaction of water with segments of the chondroitin sulfate chain. These segments, characterised by their glycosidic linkage, chain conformation and relatively independent electrostatic nature, therefore are critical in the manifestation of osmotic pressure; reducing the mobility of these units will have a significant influence on the osmotic properties of the proteoglycan.

In studies of osmotic flow across membranes with straight cylindrical pores of known effective area, the thin layer distance L for a 20 mg ml $^{-1}$ PGS solution was estimated to be the order of a molecular dimension namely 40nm (Comper and Williams 1990). This value was consistently obtained for membranes of different pore size that were impermeable to the proteoglycan (Figure 6). The

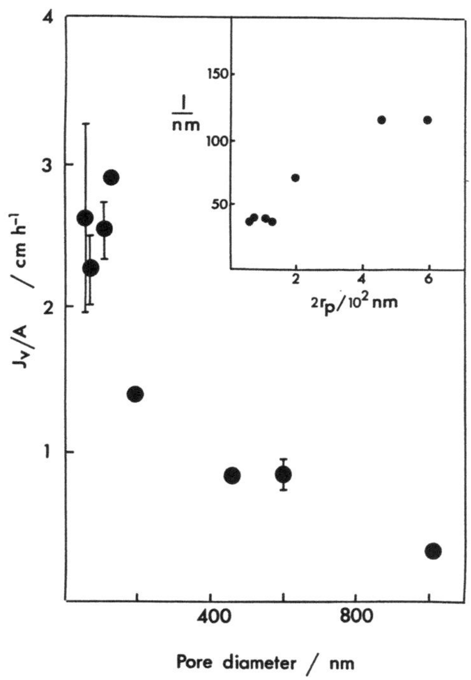

Figure 6. The osmotic flow J_v/A obtained over a 1h period generated by 19.8 mg ml $^{-1}$ PGS across well characterised Nuclepore straight capillary pore membranes of known pore diameter($2r_p$) and effective pore area. The corresponding distance L in front of the pore ,calculated from equation 11, is shown in the inset. From Comper and Williams (1990).

finite dimension of the thin layer would also indicate that in collagen fiber networks in tissues that retain proteoglycan, this range of dimensions be available for the proteoglycan to move about in order to generate osmotic flow. Therefore in understanding the mechanism of osmotic flow recognition must be made of matrix microorganisation of proteoglycans that enable segmental mobility and finite distances over which solute-solvent exchange takes place. Clearly a recognition of the role of collagen and its coexistance with proteoglycans must be made although not much is known yet of the dynamic properties of collagen network.

Osmotic Activity in Microenvironments

It is of interest to pursue the significance of the mechanism of osmotic flow to the microenvironment that may possibly exist in the cartilage extracellular matrix. The osmotic flow model requires an effective concentration of solute (osmotic pressure) and a characteristic kinetic unit of the solute to move in relation to water. If this kinetic unit is immobilised then there will be no osmotic flow and under certain conditions this may apply to proteoglycans in tissues. It is convenient at this stage to introduce the concept of effective osmotic pressure in a multicomponent system. This is the swelling pressure which is described as

swelling pressure = internal osmotic pressure - elastic (or restraining contribution) (12)

The swelling pressure of the multicomponent system is its normal osmotic pressure or internal pressure which is counteracted by forces which confine the system. These may be internal forces associated with covalent linkages within a macromolecule or intermolecular cross-links within a gel or even a membrane impermeable to the osmotically active solute. External forces may include a mechanical force of some one kind. Osmotic flow in gel, a familiar system, results in gel imbibition of water through the osmotic pressure difference between the gel phase and the solvent phase. It has been demonstrated that the rate of osmotic flow into the gel is governed by the diffusion of the gel-polymer network and this is identical with polymer diffusion is semiconcentrated polymer solutions(for review Candau et al 1982). The gel will swell until the swelling pressure is zero where restraints of the cross linked network balance the internal osmotic pressure. In a similar way, a proteoglycan or even a chondroitin sulfate chain can be regarded as a gel with an internal osmotic pressure derived essentially from electrostatic contributions and have effective kinetic units of critical segments of the chondroitin sulfate chain and elastic restraints due to intramolecular cross linking. This model also realises the important function of distance over which the internal osmotic pressure can operate in relation to the swelling pressure of the whole system. It was shown *vide supra* that in a membrane-constrained system a distance of 40nm was required for the proteoglycan chondroitin sulfate segments to move. Further restraints that could be considered are immobilisation of the hyaluronate core or protein core of the aggregate and subunit respectively. This would severely reduce the distance over which the osmotic behaviour of the chondroitin sulfate segments could have an influence. Any immobilisation of the chondroitin sulfate chain segments themselves would have a drastic influence on the osmotic activity of the proteoglycan.

Ultrafiltration (Compressive Resistance)

The load - bearing and filtration properties of cartilage result largely from the interaction of the tissues' components with water under the influence of a number of forces. At the molecular level this has to be interpreted in relation to the balance of osmotic and mechanical forces on the proteoglycan containing system. This can be described by an equation analogous to that describing sedimentation-diffusion in the ultracentrifuge (Williams and Comper, 1990) in the form of D'Arcy's law such that for solute impermeable systems,

$$J_v = L_p^o(\Delta P - \Delta \Pi) \tag{13}$$

where ΔP is the net mechanical pressure difference and L_p^o is given by equation 11. For concentrated polymers in free solution the L_p^o coefficient has been demonstrated in the ultracentrifuge to be very similar under both conditions of $\Delta P >> \Delta \Pi$ and $\Delta \Pi >> \Delta P$.

For ultrafiltration (or compressive load) in polysaccharide systems we would have $\Delta P >> \Delta \Pi$. Efforts to examine the volume flow under this condition have met with considerable difficulties, such as time dependent flows and concentration polarisation near the membrane interface. We note, however, that the factors governing ultrafiltration are essentially the same as those governing osmotic flow as embodied in the righthand bracket of equation 11 particularly the M_1/f_{12} term and the distance L over which the relative displacement of water and solute must take place. As the distance L is difficult to quantitate it does indicate that ultrafiltration measurements are of semi-quantitative value only as they involve both solution-dependent and membrane-dependent parameters (Zamparo and Comper, 1989).

However, we can compare the hydraulic conductivity of proteoglycan solutions with conductivity measurements made on cartilage. Maroudas (1975) had established an inverse correlation between articular cartilage proteoglycan content and cartilage hydraulic conductivity. Direct evidence for the major role of proteoglycan in tissue conductivity from comes from the sedimentation studies described earlier (Comper and Williams, 1987; Zamparo and Comper, 1989). For example cartilage slices have a range of k extending from 8×10^{-15} - 2×10^{-15} cm^2 corresponding to a proteoglycan concentration of 35 - 100 mg ml^{-1}. These values show close correspondence of hydraulic conductivity on proteoglycan in solutions (Figure 3). The differences may correspond to inaccuracies in the estimate of proteoglycan concentration, the role of the collagen network (Levick, 1987) and the distribution of proteoglycan in cartilage. Further, this comparison is based on the average proteoglycan concentration in unstressed tissue whereas hydraulic flow measurements may correspond to higher proteoglycan concentrations due to stress effects on the distribution of proteoglycan in the tissue (see also Mow et al 1984). This may be an important factor considering the marked concentration dependence of k; for a 10 fold change in k from 10^{-13} cm^{-2} to 10^{-14} cm^2 corresponds to a 2.7 fold change in proteoglycan concentration from 18.8 mg ml^{-1} to 50 mg ml^{-1} (Figure 3).

The high concentration increment in k also raises the question then on the microorganisation of the proteoglycan in terms of what is its most effective distribution to maximise resistance to flow?. The balance is between the concentration of proteoglycan where water displacement occurs and the distance over which displacement takes place; permeability with $\Delta P >> \Delta\Pi$ is given by

$$J_v = kA\Delta P/L\eta_2 \qquad (14)$$

Mobile proteoglycans can undergo concentration polarisation which will increase the concentration to decrease k but this will be offset by a lower effective distance L over which the relative movement of water and proteoglycan can take place. Immobile proteoglycans (at the level of protein or hyaluronate core) will not undergo concentration polarisation but may offer relatively long distances over which molecular displacement occurs.

Summary

In semidilute solutions of proteoglycan the effective unit that governs the movement of water relative to the proteoglycan in both diffusion and hydraulic conductivity is a critical segment of the chondroitin sulfate chain. The important characteristics of this segment is its chain conformation and the nature of its glycosidic linkage. In relation to water transport the charge properties of the proteoglycan are important only in terms of the osmotic activity of the molecule. Therefore, in considering different pressure regimes associated with equation 13 we have at high mechanical pressures ($\Delta P >> \Delta\Pi$) the major resistance of the proteoglycan system being offered by will be the frictional term which shows low ionic strength dependence, whereas electromechanical effects would only be expected at relatively low pressures ($\Delta P \approx \Delta\Pi$) as the osmotic pressure does show ionic strength dependence. Viscoelasticity and its dependence on overall proteoglycan molecular weight and conformation appears to be a separate property that is independent of considerations associated with net water movement.

Acknowledgements

I gratefully acknowledge the important contribution to this work by students and associates who have worked with me. This work was supported by grants from the Australian Research Council and Monash University Special Research Section.

References

Bearman RJ: On the molecular basis fo some theories of diffusion. J. Phys. Chem. 1961; 73: 1961-1968

Candau S, Bastide J, Delsanti M: Structural,elastic, and dynamic properties of swollen polymer networks. Adv. Polym. Sci. 1982; 44: 27-71

Carney SL, Muir H: The structure and function of cartilage proteoglycans. Physiol. Rev. 1988; 68: 858-910

Comper WD: Physicochemical aspects of cartilage extracellular matrix, in Hall BK, Newman SA (eds): Cartilage Molecular Aspects, New Hampshire, Telford Press 1990 (in press).

Comper WD, Laurent TC: Physiological function of connective tissue polysaccharides. Physiol. Rev. 1978; 58: 255-315

Comper WD, Preston BN, Daivis P: The approach of dextran mutual diffusion coefficients to molecular weight independence in semi dilute solutions of polydisperse dextran fractions. J. Phys. Chem. 1986; 90: 128-132.

Comper WD, Van Damme M-P, Preston BN: Diffusion of tritiated water (HTO) in dextran and water mixtures. J. Chem Soc. Faraday Trans. I. 1982; 78: 3369-3378

Comper WD, Williams RPW: Hydrodynamics of concentrated proteoglycan solutions. J. Biol Chem. 1987; 262: 13464-13471

Comper WD, Williams RPW: Osmotic flow caused by chondroitin sulfate proteoglycan across well defined Nuclepore membranes Biophys. Chem. 1990 (in press)

Comper WD, Zamparo O: Hydraulic conductivity of polymer matrices. Biophys. Chem. 1989, 34: 127-135.

Comper WD, Zamparo O: The hydrodynamic properties of connective tissue polysaccharides. Biochem. J. 1990 (in press).

Dainty J: Osmotic flow. Federation Proc. 1965; 19: 75-85

Eisenberg SR, Grodzinsky AJ: The kinetics of chemically induced nonequilibrium swelling of articular cartilage and corneal stroma. J. Biomech. Eng. 1987; 109:79-89

Eisenberg SR, Grodzinsky AJ: Electrokinetic micromodel of extracellular matrix and other polyelectrolyte networks. PCH Physicochem Hydrodynamics 1988; 10: 517-539

Gersh I, Catchpole HR: The nature of the ground substance of connective tissue. Perspect. Biol. Med. 1960; 3: 282-319.

Grodzinsky AJ, Roth V, Myers ER, Grossman W,Mow VC: The significance of electromechanical and osmotic forces on the nonequilibrium swelling behaviour of articular cartilage in tension. J. Biomech. Eng. 1981; 103:221-231

Happel J, Brenner H: Low Reynolds Number Hydrodynamics, Englewood, N.J. Prentice-Hall, 1983.

Hascall VC: Interaction of cartilage proteoglycans with hyaluronic acid. J. Supramol. Struct. 1977; 7: 101-120.

Hascall VC: Proteoglycans: The chondroitin sulfate/keratan sulfate proteoglycan of cartilage ISI Atlas of Science: Biochemistry 1988: 189-198. Heyer E, Cass A, Mauro A: A demonstration of the effect of permeant and impermeant solutes, and unstirred boundary layers of osmotic flow. Yale J. Biology and Med. 1969-70; 42: 139-153.

Kwan MK, Lai MW, Mow VC: Fundamentals of fluid transport through cartilage in compression. Ann. Biomed. Eng. 1984; 12: 537-558.

Lai WM, Hou JS, Mow VC: A triphasic theory for the swelling and deformation behaviors of articular cartilage (submitted for publication).

Levick JR: Flow through interstitium and other fibrous matrices. Quart. J. Exp. Physiol. 1987; 72: 409-438

Maroudas A: Biophysical chemistry of cartilagenous tissues with special reference to solute and fluid transport. Bioheology 1975; 12: 233-248.

Maroudas A: Physical chemistry of articular cartilage and the intervertebral disc in Sokoloff L (ed): The Joints and Synovial Fluid. Vol. II, London, Academic Press, 1980, pp 239-291.

Maroudas A, Bannon C: Measurement of swelling pressure in cartilage and comparison with the osmotic pressure of constituent proteoglycans. Bioheology, 1981; 18: 619-632.

Maroudas A, Mizrahi J, Ben Haim E, Ziv I: Swelling pressure in cartilage in Staub NC, Hogg JC, Hargens AR (eds): Interstial-Lymphatic Liquid and Solute Movement (Advances in Microcirculation Vol. 13) Basel, Kargen 1987, pp 203-212.

Maroudas A, Venn M: Chemical composition and swelling of normal and osteoarthritic femoral head cartilage. Ann. Rheum Dis. 1977; 36: 399-403.

Mijnlieff PF, Jaspers WJM: Solvent permeability of dissolved polymer material. The direct determination from sedimentation measurements. Trans. Faraday Soc. 1971; 67: 1837-1854.

Mow VC, Holmes MK, Lai WM: Fluid transport and mechanical properties of articular cartilage. A review J. Biomech. 1984; 17: 377-394

Mow VC, Kuei SC, Lai WM, Armstrong CG: Biphasic creep and stress relaxation of articular cartilage in compression: Theory and experiments. J. Biomech. Eng. 1980; 102: 73-84.

Mow VC, Mak AF, Lai WM, Rosenberg LC, Tang L-H: Viscoelastic properties of proteoglycan subunits and aggregates in varying solution concentrations. J. Biomech. 1984: 17: 325-338

Muir H: Proteoglycans as organisers of the extracellular matrix. Biochem. Soc. Trans 1983; 11: 613-622.

Onsager L, Fuoss RM: Irreversible processes in electrolytes. Diffusion, conductance, and viscous flow in arbitrary mixtures of strong electrolytes. J. Phys. Chem. 1932; 36: 2689-2778.

Ray P: On the theory of osmotic water movement. Plant Physiol. 1960; 35: 783-797.

Soodak H, Iberall A: Osmosis, diffusion, convection, Am. J. Physiol. 1978; 235: R3-R17.

Spiegler KS: Transport processes in ionic membranes. Trans Faraday Soc. 1958; 54: 1408-1426.

Torchia DA, Hasson MA, Hascall VC: Investigation of molecular motion of proteoglycans in cartilage by ^{13}C magnetic resonance. J. Biol. Chem 1977;252: 3617-3625.

Urban JPG, Maroudas A, Bayliss MT, Dillon J: Swelling pressures of proteoglycans at the concentrations found in cartilagenous tissues. Biorheology 1979; 16: 447-464.

Williams RPW, Comper WD: Osmotic flow caused by non-ideal macromolecular solutes. J. Phys. Chem. 1987; 91: 3443-3448.

Williams RPW. Comper WD: Osmotic flow caused by polyelectrolytes. Biophys. Chem. 1990 (in press).

Zamparo O, Comper WD: Hydraulic conductivity of chondroitin sulfate proteoglycan solutions. Arch. Biochem. Biophys. 1989; 274: 259-269.

Chapter 13

Water Content and Solute Diffusion Properties in Articular Cartilage

P.A. Torzilli, E. Askari, J.T. Jenkins

Introduction

All living tissues depend on solute transport for proper physiological function. Articular cartilage is no exception. Articular cartilage is, however, unique compared to most other biological tissues in that it lacks a vascular supply. All solute transport into and out of mature tissue must occur across the articular surface (in immature tissue vascular communication occurs at the subchondral junction)(Ogata et al., 1978). Nutrients enter across the articular surface and move through the tissue's interstitial fluid space to nourish the chondrocytes. Deprive the cells of this mechanism and they will quickly die. Solute transport is not only important for nutrition but also essential for proper physicochemical balance and biomechanical function. Metabolic waste products are removed from the tissue by excretion across the articular surface. Other cellular products, such as those necessary for collagen and proteoglycan construction, must also move freely throughout the tissue matrix to repair and replenish the tissue's structural matrix.

Solute movement through articular cartilage's interstitial fluid space is a complex and not well understood phenomena.

In fact, solute movement through most homogeneous, synthetic polymeric materials is a very complicated phenomena (Paul, 1985). In cartilage this process is further complicated by its inhomogeneous and anisotropic characteristics, and the unknown molecular characteristics of most organic molecules. This clearly poses a challenge to anyone studying this highly non-linear transport phenomena.

Solute movement occurs at both the microstructural level, where solutes move across cell membranes, and at the macrostructural level where tissue organs control the mass flux processes necessary for health. While there are numerous physical and biological mechanisms governing solute movement at all levels, diffusion, electrochemical and fluid convection are probably the primary ones for mass transport. Unfortunately, little is known about how these mechanisms control solute transport or of the relative contribution from each. Only diffusion has been studied by direct methods (Allhands et al., 1984; Bernich et al., 1972,1976; Lotke and Granda, 1971,1972; Maroudas, 1970,1975,1976; Torzilli et al., 1987; Urban et al., 1978,1982), where the actual spatial movement of solute is followed. Attempts have been made to determine solute transport rates using indirect mechanochemical and mechanoelectrical methods (Grodzinsky et al., 1981; Mow et al., 1981; Myers et al., 1984). However, these indirect methods do not yield actual solute transport rates but only the rate limiting interaction between the three mechanisms.

What is well recognized is that a large variety of solutes move through cartilage's interstitial fluid space. These solutes are of different size, conformation and charge. Molecular sizes range from small salt (58 MW) and glucose (180 MW) molecules all the way up to proteoglycan aggregate macromolecules (200 million MW). Anionic and cationic solutes range from univalent and bivalent molecules, such as Na (+1), Cl (-1) and Ca (+2), to highly negative, charged multivalent molecules such as chondroitin and keratin sulfate and proteoglycans. Molecular conformations can range from compact flexible globular shapes to rigid extended rod like structures. Not only will the molecule's characteristics affect its transport properties but so will the tissue's characteristics. A unique feature of many solutes and the tissue is that they can independently change their size, conformation and charge depending on the physicochemical and mechanical environment (e.g., pH, ionic concentration, matrix deformation). Thus, the transport properties are easily modified.

In healthy tissue the movement of large molecules, on the order of 60,000 MW and larger, are restricted, to a large extent, by the tissue's matrix structure. However, in pathological tissue the normal pathways are changed. Larger molecules, such as enzymes, have easier access and movement through the tissue. More important, the tissue's own constituents, principally the proteoglycan subunits, are not restrained and can escape, resulting in tissue softening.

Water Content

Whatever the transport mechanism, solutes must move through the interstitial fluid medium filling the non-solid matrix spaces. In cartilage this fluid is water. Water comprises almost 80% of cartilage's total volume. The amount of water, its spatial distribution and location relative to the other solid constituents (proteoglycans and collagen) are important factors to consider when studying solute transport. They are especially important when determining the spatial distribution of solutes, that is, spatial concentrations.

Fluid content is easily measured by removing the cartilage layer from its subchondral bone and measuring the difference between the wet and dry weights. Several investigators have studied the variation in water content as a function of depth from the articular surface (Brockelhurst et al., 1984; Lemperg et al., 1971, 1974; Lipshitz et al., 1976; Maroudas and Venn, 1977; Sweet et al., 1977; Torzilli, 1988; Venn, 1978; Venn and Maroudas, 1977), as a function of age (Lemperg et al., 1971, 1974; Maroudas 1980; Torzilli, 1988; Venn, 1978), and in osteoarthritic tissue (Brockelhurst et al., 1984; Maroudas and Venn, 1977; McDevitt and Muir, 1976; Venn and Maroudas, 1977).

In mature tissue water content is highest at the articular surface and decreases with depth, Figure 1. For bovine articular cartilage the spatial variation in water content, $\beta(\xi)$, is given by

$$\beta(\xi) = 0.852 - 0.210\,\xi + 0.745\,\xi^2 - 0.817\,\xi^3 \qquad (1)$$

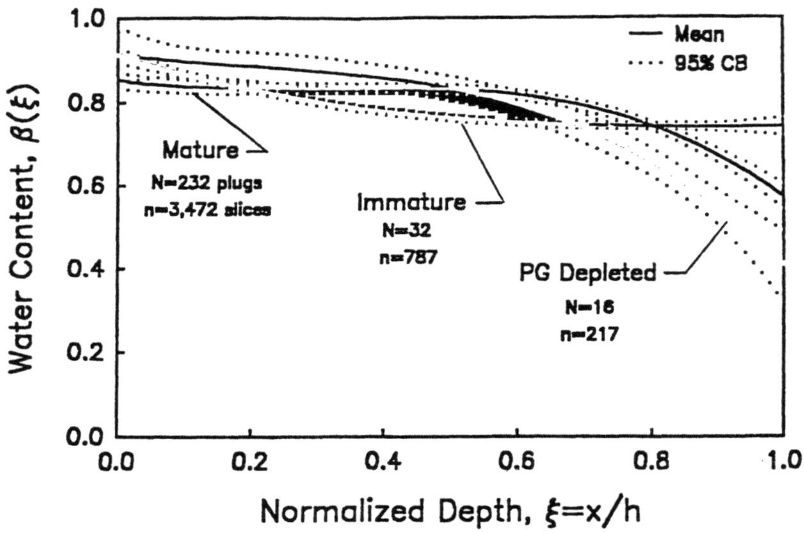

Figure 1. Variation in water content with depth for mature, immature and proteoglycan depleted (98%) mature bovine articular cartilage.

where $\xi = x/h$, the depth, x, being normalized with respect to tissue thickness, h. Mean bulk fluid content, calculated by averaging over all spatial positions, is 79.2 $\pm$ 9.0%. In general, spatial variations in hydration appear independent of species (human, bovine, canine) and age. In immature tissue water content is also highest at the articular surface and decreases with depth (Figure 1). For bovine cartilage this is given by

$$\beta(\xi) = 0.913 - 0.504\,\xi + 0.489\,\xi^2 - 0.157\,\xi^3 \qquad (2)$$

with an average bulk value of 78.8 $\pm$ 6.9%. While no significant difference is found between mature and immature bulk fluid contents, immature cartilage does have a significantly higher fluid content in the superficial and deep regions (Lemperg et al., 1971, 1974; Torzilli, 1988). Furthermore, in tissue ranging in age from 3 to 86 years, Venn (1978) reported a linear decrease in bulk water content with increasing age, approximately 3.2% per decade. Again, hydration was found highest at the surface with a gradual decrease with depth.

Several investigators have reported elevated water content in osteoarthritic cartilage (Brockelhurst et al., 1984; Maroudas and Venn, 1977; McDevitt and Muir, 1976). Brockelhurst et al. (1984) found that in tissue having only surface fibrillation water content was increased in the superficial regions but unchanged in the middle and deep regions. However, deeply fibrillated tissue had increased water throughout the tissue thickness, a result also reported by Maroudas and Venn (1977). In a canine osteoarthritic model, McDevitt and Muir (1976) reported increased hydration in areas showing mild tissue fibrillation, with or without an intact articular surface. In addition, Maroudas and Venn (1977) were able to increase hydration by degrading the collagen matrix enzymatically. These findings appear to indicate that increased water content may be a result of collagen fiber disruption, where the tissue can swell and imbibe additional water.

On the other hand, the increased hydration may be a direct result of proteoglycan loss, the later a common finding in osteoarthritic tissue. In tissue having 98% of its proteoglycan component enzymatically removed, there was a significant difference in the spatial distribution of the water even though no significant change was found in the bulk water content (78.5 $\pm$ 15.7%), Figure 1. However, bulk water loss has been reported by Wurster and Lust (1986) following proteoglycan removal. The spatial variation in hydration for proteoglycan depleted mature bovine cartilage is given by

$$\beta(\xi) = 0.914 - 0.215\,\xi + 0.507\,\xi^2 - 0.803\,\xi^3 \qquad (3)$$

In the deeper regions, an area normally high in proteoglycan content in intact tissue, there was a significant decrease in water content. This decrease probably reflects the loss of the proteoglycan's hydrophilic capacity. However, there was a significant increase in hydration in the superficial region, an area normally high in collagen but low in proteoglycan content. This finding is probably a result of increased collagen intrafibrillar water imbibition. Collagen has been reported to contain significant amounts of intrafibrillar water (Grynpas et al., 1980; Maroudas and Bannon, 1981; Torzilli, 1985). In intact tissue the collagen fibers are under tension as a result of proteoglycan swelling. This results in a minimum intrafibrillar

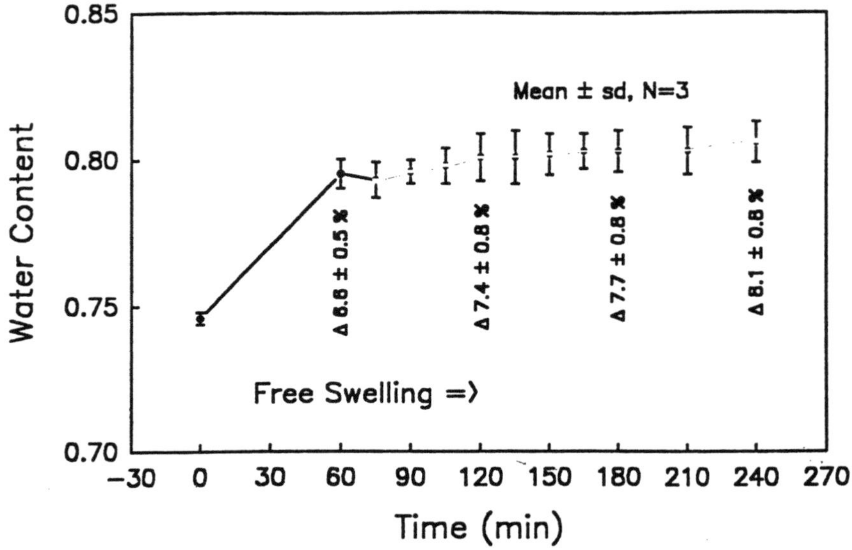

Figure 2. Changes in water content due to tissue swelling.

water space. With proteoglycan loss the tension in the collagen fibers is relaxed and intrafibrillar water increases (Torzilli, 1985). In addition, an overall volumetric increase probably occurs as the collagen matrix relaxes and expands. Thus, following proteoglycan removal areas with a high relative collagen content (superficial region) would increase in water content while areas with initially high proteoglycan content (deeper region) would decrease water content.

Increased water imbibition also results when cartilage is allowed to swell. This is often an unrecognized source of error when measuring tissue fluid content. Unless laterally constrained and attached to the subchondral bone, articular cartilage will swell and imbibe water. Most investigators measure water content by first equilibrating removed cartilage slices in a bath solution (normally phosphate bufferred saline) before wet weighing. However, this method will result in a significant and artificial increase in fluid content, Figure 2. Increases could be as high as 10% and easily mask both bulk and spatial changes. This is especially important when determining local water position within the tissue and when determining fluid volumes available for solute movement.

Water and Solute Partition

Solute equilibrium partition is defined as the relative concentration of solute between two communicating volumes at equilibrium or infinite diffusion time. For porous media such as cartilage, the partition coefficient, K, is the ratio of the concentration within the media, C, to the concentration in a bathing solution, Co, where K = C/Co. The partition coefficient is usually measured by counting the number of molecules per unit volume of solvent in each space using radioactively tagged molecules. Coefficients can be different from unity. When less than unity the solute is effectively excluded from a finite portion of the interstitial space, while values greater than unity usually mean the solute is entrapped or absorbed within the matrix itself.

Partition coefficients for a variety of solutes in cartilage and in different solute-solvent systems (simulating cartilage) have been widely reported (Dunston, 1966; Maroudas, 1970,1975,1976; Preston et al. 1972; Snowdon and Maroudas, 1976). Coefficients less than unity are common and usually a result of steric or geometric exclusion, where the physical interaction between the molecule and the matrix limits the molecular packing or closeness compared to the packing in free solution. Tissue composition also affects solute partition, as shown in Figure 3 for glucose where the partition changes significantly from the superficial to the middle and deep regions. This is similar to changes in collagen and proteoglycan content. In general, larger molecules will have smaller partition coefficients due to increased and more complex solute-matrix steric interactions, as illustrated in Figure 4 for different sized molecules in hyaluronate solution (Laurent, 1964). Finally, solute partition is dependent on the net charge of the solute and matrix, resulting in either attraction or repulsion. For instance, serum albumin, a large 69,000 MW molecule with a net negative charge of -18, has a partition coefficient in cartilage which decreases more than two orders of magnitude, from approximately 0.7 to 0.001, for only a nine-fold increase in tissue fixed charge density (glycosaminoglycan content) (Maroudas and Bannon, 1981).

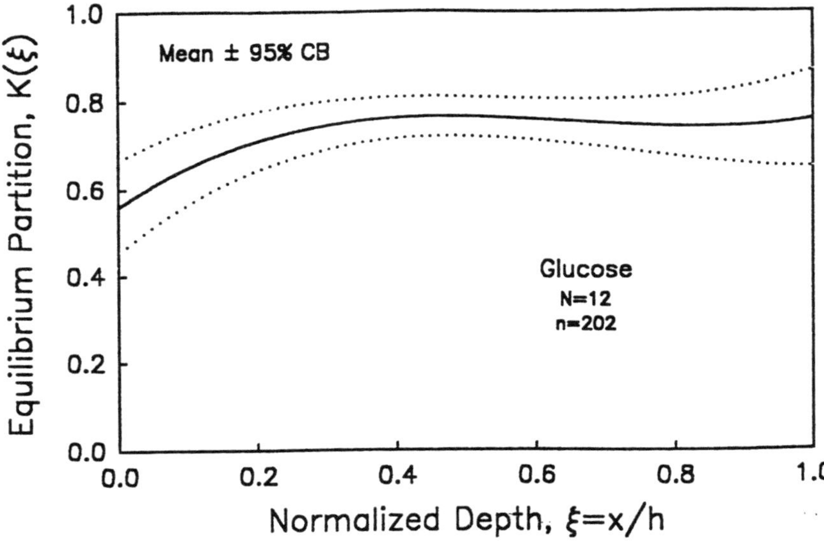

Figure 3. Variation in glucose equilibrium partition as a function of depth.

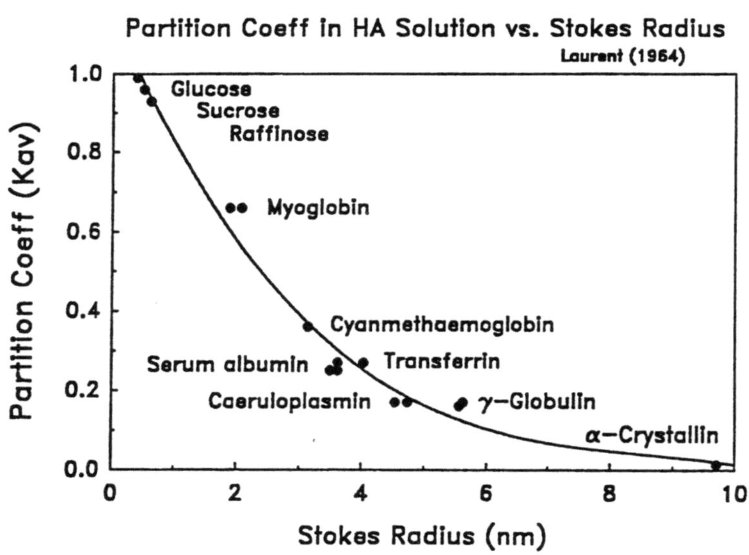

Figure 4. Solute partition for different size molecules in hyaluronate.

Solute partition and transport is also effected by the solute's access to the interstitial water. Both the amount of water available for transport, and whether the water is itself 'free' or 'trapped' within the matrix, is controversial (Maroudas and Venn, 1977; Maroudas and Schneiderman, 1987; Torzilli, 1982,1985,1988). Clearly, there are interstitial spaces not accessible to large molecules due to steric exclusion. This is only a geometric exclusion. There is also some evidence to suggest the existence of water not available to even small molecules. This even includes water molecules. Inaccessible water can take two forms, so called 'bound water', where the water molecules are strongly bound to the solid matrix components (Mathews and Decker, 1977; Tasaka et al., 1988), and as 'trapped water' within the collagen intrafibrillar network (Grynpas et al., 1980; Torzilli, 1985; Viswanadham et al., 1976). Maroudas and co-workers (1977,1987) calculated that all or most of the interstitial water is freely exchangeable, while Torzilli and co-workers (1982,1985) found approximately 70-80% free, Figure 5.

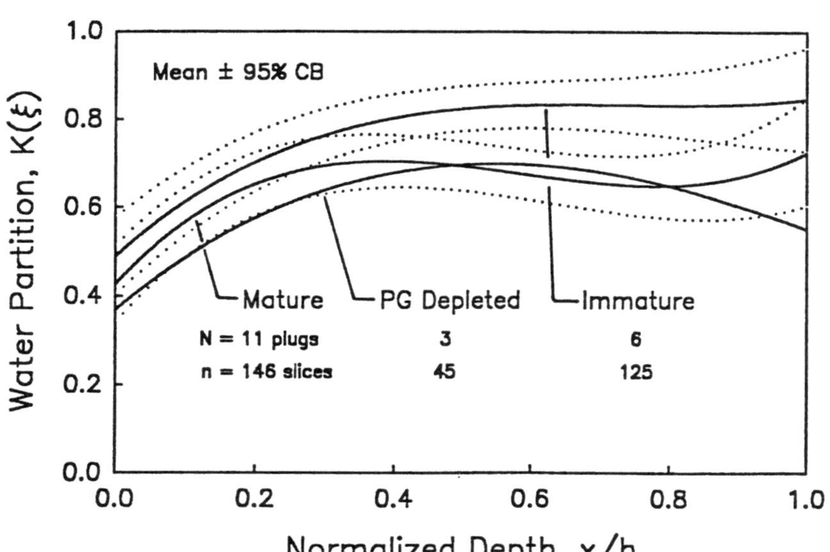

Figure 5. Variation in water partition with depth for mature, immature and proteoglycan depleted (98%) mature bovine articular cartilage.

What is important, however, is the accessibility of the water to solutes and whether the interstitial space can be changed. This is especially important when attempting to deliver a 'local' solute concentration, for instance, at the chondrocyte location. Whatever the exact amount of free and trapped water, clearly the water partition can be varied. Torzilli (1987) found a 52% increase in water partition when the pH was decreased from 11.5 to 3.9, and calculated this resulted from a 54% increase in free water space and a 49% decrease in trapped space. He postulated that the water was trapped in the intrafibrillar collagen space, and that changes in the partition were due to local conformation changes in the collagen fibril structure. The increased water partition was attributed to lateral fibril swelling resulting from a relaxation in fibril tension as the proteoglycan macromolecules collapsed from charge shielding, and as the fibrils became charged away from neutral pH. In addition, water partition also increased 62% with a temperature increase from 6 to 42°C, a change of +28% and -53% in free and trapped space. This increase is probably a result of fibril expansion (soluble at 55°C) and a decrease in water binding resulting from increased thermal vibrations. Finally, there was a significant increase in water content (2.9%) and partition (6.8%) when the cartilage layer was removed from the bone before testing. However, the increase in partition was attributed solely to the increase in hydration, a result of tissue swelling, and not a change in the free and trapped space. This later finding further illustrates the importance of lateral confinement and subchondral bone attachment.

Finally, water partition in immature cartilage is significantly higher in the middle and deep regions but not different from mature tissue at the surface, Figure 5. Bulk water partition is also greater, 76.3% $\pm$ 15.7% vs. 64.3% $\pm$ 15.7%, respectively. However, in proteoglycan depleted mature tissue no difference was found, 61.0% $\pm$ 12.4%. The spatial variations in water partition for mature, immature and proteoglycan depleted bovine cartilage are given by, respectively,

$$K(\xi) = 0.427 + 1.728\,\xi - 3.346\,\xi^2 + 0.463\,\xi^3 \qquad (4)$$

$$K(\xi) = 0.490 + 1.432\,\xi - 1.977\,\xi^2 + 0.901\,\xi^3 \qquad (5)$$

$$K(\xi) = 0.369 + 1.329\,\xi - 1.539\,\xi^2 + 0.391\,\xi^3 \qquad (6)$$

Solute Diffusion

Diffusion is the process where one substance (solute) is transported through another substance (solvent) as a result of random Brownian (molecular) motion. This process is described by Fick's second law

$$dC/dt = \text{div}\,(D \text{ grad } C) \qquad (7)$$

where C is the concentration, D the diffusion coefficient, and t time. The diffusion coefficient is the rate of transfer of diffusing solute through the solvent. In general, D=D(C,x), a function of concentration and spatial position, x. However, for sufficiently dilute and uniform D is usually assumed constant. Fickian or linear diffusion, as defined by Eqn. (4), is valid for most solute-solvent systems but usually fails for more complex systems involving porous media or polymeric substrates. This is especially true when significant solute-matrix interactions occur, as with solute absorption, charged membranes, matrix relaxation, and strain (Berens and Hopfenberg, 1978; Idol and Anderson, 1986; Neogi et al., 1986; Osada et al., 1986; Trivant et al., 1983; Wan and Whittenberg, 1987).

The precise definition and measurement of the diffusion coefficient has, in the past, resulted in some confusion. When two different solutes of similar size and mass diffuse into one another, D is usually referred to as the mutual diffusion coefficient; if a solute is diffusing through itself, D is the self-diffusion or intradiffusion coefficient; and when two solutes have different size and mass, or when one solute diffuses alone, D is called the intrinsic or translational diffusion coefficient (Crank, 1975; Laurent et al., 1976). Another solute transport coefficient often referred to is the permeability constant, P. The permeability constant is only applicable when gas or vapor pressures are prescribed for the boundary conditions instead of concentration. Under certain conditions of linearity, P=SD, where S is the solute solubility (Crank and Park, 1968). With liquids, where the boundary concentrations are known, P=KD. Note that the permeability constant is a far less fundamental property than the diffusion coefficient, and should be avoided if possible. Unfortunately, the permeability-diffusion relationship has often been misused to calculate D using a Darcy's Law type permeability test, where the calculated coefficient is a combined diffusion and convection rate (Bernich et al., 1972,1976, Lotke and Granda, 1971,1972; Maroudas 1980).

Diffusion coefficients for a variety of small and large solutes diffusing through articular cartilage, water and several solute-solvent solution combinations are given in Table 1. The coefficients were determined using both steady state and transient (non-steady state) measurements.

Table 1

Solute	MW	Matrix	D*	Temp °C	Ref
H20		18	30.4	37	[1]
H20		PGS	18.2	20	[4]
H202			13.7	37	[2]
H20		Cart	12.0-14.0	37	[6]
Glucose	180		9.2	37	[2]
			5.9	20	[7]
		HA	4.4	20	[7]
		HA	2.1	20	[7]
		Cart	3.2-3.6	37	[6]
		Cart	4.0-7.4	37	[10]
NaCl	58		20.4	37	[2]
CaCl2	110		16.6	37	[2]
NaOH	40		27.7	37	[2]
Urea	60	Cart	8.0	37	[6]
Na(+1)	23	Cart	6.4-7.4	37	[6]
Ca(+1)	40	Cart	2.0	37	[6]
Cl(-1)	35	Cart	10.0-11.4	37	[6]
SO4(-2)	96	Cart	2.8-3.5	37	[6]
Inulin	5,000	Cart	0.33	37	[6]
	5,000	Cart	1.0-3.3	37	[10]
IgG	150,000	Cart	0.11	37	[6]

Solute	MW	Matrix	D*	Temp °C	Ref
Dextran	10,000	Cart	0.16	37	[6]
	10,000	Cart	2.7-5.7	37	[10]
	20,000	Cart	1.0-3.3	37	[10]
	40,000	Cart	0.022	37	[6]
	44,000		0.99	75	[3]
	77,000	Cart	0.5-3.7	37	[10]
	179,000		0.24		[3]
	864,000	Dex 20	0.11		[3]
Serum Albumin	69,000		0.03	37	[11]
			0.62		[3]
		Cart	0.21	37	[6]
			0.61	20	[7]
		HA (2g/l)	0.16	20	[7]
		HA (8g/l)	0.03	20	[7]
Chondroitin Sulfate		CS(1g/l)	0.40	20	[4]
		CS(50g/l)	2.0	20	[4]
		CS(10g/l)	5.2	20	[8]
		CS(50g/l)	7.5	20	[8]
		CS(15g/l)	24.6	20	[8]
		CS(15g/l)	3.4	20	[8]
PGsubunit		PGS(0.2g/l)	0.002	20	[5]
		PGS (50g/l)	1.5	20	[5]
Hyaluronate		HA(0.7mM)	0.2		[9]
		HA(4.4mM)	3.0		[9]

*D, 10^{-6} cm^2/sec HA=hyaluronate
PGS=Proteoglycan subunit CS=chondroitin sulfate

[1] Harris & Woolf (1980)
[2] Bretsznojder (1971)
[3] Phillies (1986)
[4] Comper & Williams (1987)
[5] Harper et al. (1985)
[6] Maroudas et al. (1970,1975,1976)
[7] Ogston and Sherman (1961)
[8] Tivant (1983)
[9] Wik & Comper (1982)
[10] Torzilli et al. (1987)
[11] Miller and Peppas (1988)

Steady State Diffusion

Diffusion coefficients are most often found using steady state methods (Maroudas, 1968,1970,1975; Maroudas and Evans, 1974; Norton et al., 1982; Preston and Snowdon, 1972, 1973). Steady state experiments are usually performed using a diffusion cell, in which a thin specimen, initially free of solute, is placed between two chambers, one containing a solute of concentration Co and the other at zero concentration, and the amount of solute passing through the specimen measured. The solute-solvent volumes are usually stirred to avoid a stagnant layer at the tissue boundaries. The solute concentration within the tissue, as a function of distance and time t, is given by

$$\frac{C}{C_0} = 1 - \frac{x}{l} - \frac{2}{\pi}\sum_{n=1}^{\infty}\frac{1}{n}\sin\frac{n\pi x}{l}\exp(-Dn^2\pi^2 t/l^2) \tag{8}$$

where l is the specimen thickness. The amount of diffusing solute per unit area in time t is found by integrating Eqn. (8)

$$Q = C_0 l\left[\frac{Dt}{l} - \frac{1}{6} - \frac{2}{\pi^2}\sum_{n=1}^{\infty}\frac{(-1)^2}{n^2}\exp(-Dn^2\pi^2 t/l^2)\right] \tag{9}$$

The concentration profile within the tissue, C(x,t), will continue to change (transient) until a steady state is reached. Once steady state has been reached the diffusion coefficient can be easily determined from Eqn. (9).

An advantage of the steady state method is in the simplicity of the test apparatus and the ease of measuring the solute flux as a function of time. However, for articular cartilage this method is probably not appropriate. First, the normal spatial architecture of the tissue is disrupted because the tissue must be removed from the subchondral bone and parallel surfaces cut to obtain a uniform thickness. Solute transport will not be similar to that occurring in-situ, that is, from the articular surface downward. Secondly, cutting the tissue will allow it to swell, effectively changing its porosity. Thirdly, the specimen is usually clamped around the edges using impermeable plates. For small aspect ratio (thickness/diameter less than 0.1) the one-dimensional diffusion assumption is reasonable and edge effects can be safely neglected. However, most studies used aspect ratios between 0.1 and 0.2, which introduces a 6% to 11% error, respectively (Crank, 1975). Unfortunately, using very thin specimens will introduce other artifacts, for instance, swelling and proteoglycan loss during the test. Finally, the time necessary to reach steady state, approximately $t=0.45\ l^2/D$, will be very long, especially for larger molecules (Crank, 1975; Siegal, 1986). As an example, a minimum of 75 minutes is necessary for glucose to reach steady state, while for dextran (77,000 MW) or serum albumin (69,000 MW) ten hours is required.

Non-Steady State Diffusion

On the other hand, transient experiments, while more difficult to perform, have several advantages for articular cartilage. In general, a concentration vs. distance profile is generated and the diffusion coefficient found by fitting a diffusion model to the profile. The advantage of this model is that short times can be used (15 minutes to 1 hour), the tissue can be tested in an in-situ configuration, and, most important, the exact spatial concentration profile is obtained. This later advantage is essential considering the tissue's spatial inhomogeneity and when using charged solutes, where adsorption can occur. Disadvantages include having to slice specimens into thin sections (100 microns) to obtain the profile and working with frozen specimens to stop solute diffusion while processing the tissue.

A typical transient diffusion test is performed as follows (Torzilli et al., 1985). A radioactively tagged solute of concentration Co is deposited on the articular surface and after a fixed period the specimen is removed, frozen and sliced. The tracer is desorbed and counted, and a concentration profile plotted, as shown schematically in Figure 6. Ideally, the solute concentration just inside the articular surface (x=+0) should be Co, but in cartilage, as in most polymeric materials, a solute partition exists such that the concentration is KCo. If purely Fickian (linear) diffusion governed the transport phenomena the concentration profiles would always begin at the same point just within the articular boundary, C(+0,t)=KCo, and continually rise with increasing diffusion times, Figure 6.

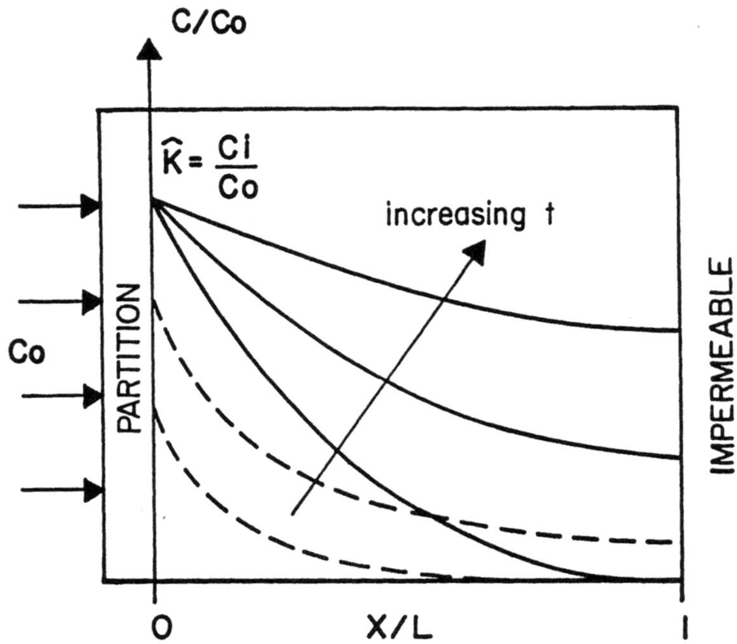

Figure 6. Schematic illustration of one-dimensional transient diffusion into articular cartilage.

The concentration profile for one-dimensional Fickian diffusion into a finite cartilage layer of thickness l is given by

$$\frac{C(x,t)}{C_0} = \frac{K\alpha}{1+\alpha}\left[1+\sum_{n=1}^{\infty}\frac{2(1+\alpha)\exp(-Dt\gamma_n^2/l^2)}{1+\alpha+\alpha^2\gamma_n^2}\times\frac{\cos\gamma_n(1-x/l)}{\cos\gamma_n}\right] \quad (10)$$

where $\alpha = V_0/KV_f$ is a modified fluid volume ratio between the external bath volume, V_0, and tissue fluid volume, V_f, and γ_n are the non-zero roots of

$$\tan\gamma_n + \alpha\gamma_n = 0 \quad (11)$$

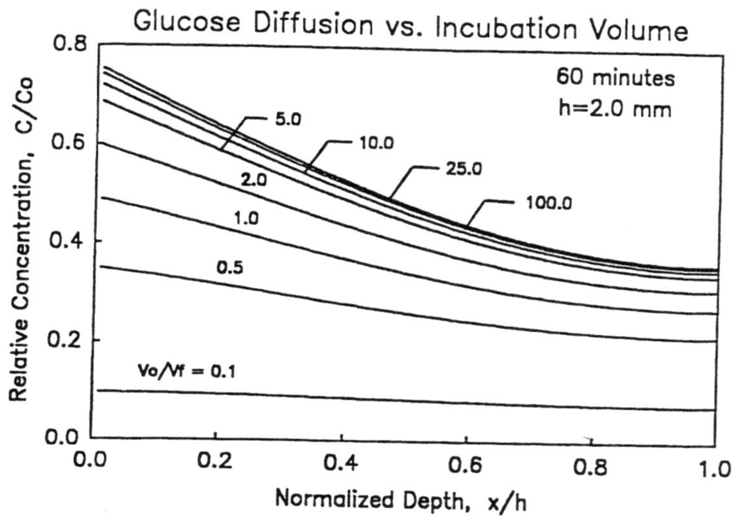

Figure 7. Effect of bathing solution volume, V_o, relative to tissue fluid volume, V_f, on solute concentration profiles. For ratios greater than 25:1, the bath volume appears infinite.

In most steady state diffusion experiments the external solution volume is very large (infinite) compared to the tissue's fluid volume, to avoid external solute depletion effects. However, this is not always practical, especially when using radioactive tracers in experiments or when considering drug delivery methodologies. Equation (7) assumes a finite external fluid volume. As diffusion proceeds, the solute concentration in the external solution will decrease, and the concentration profile within the tissue will on the volume ratio, Figure 7. This is an important consideration when designing a diffusion experiment and in analyzing the data. In general, for volume ratios greater than 25:1 the external volume may be considered infinite and depletion effects neglected.

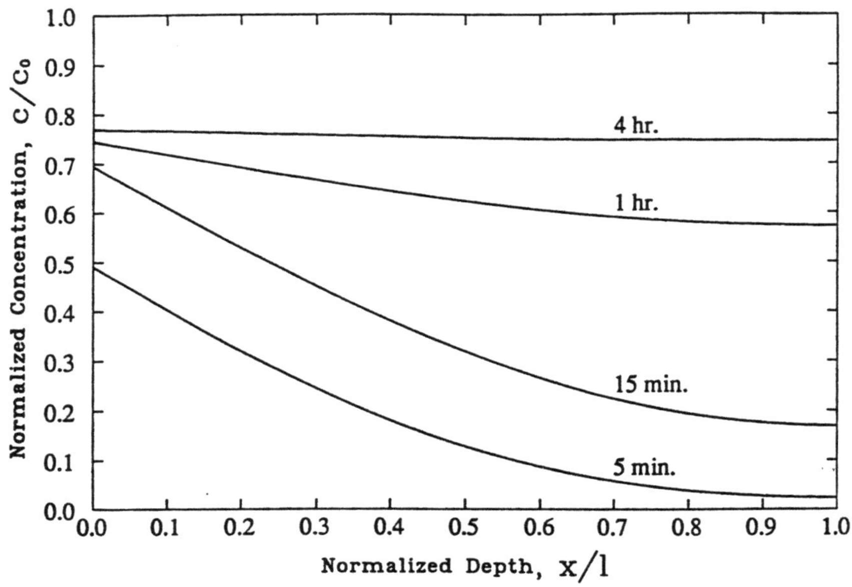

Figure 8. Normalized concentration-depth profiles for glucose diffusion into mature bovine articular cartilage. Curves are mean fits to experimental data using a dual diffusion model.

Solute Diffusion in Cartilage

Typical concentration-distance profiles for glucose are shown in Figure 8. Similar profiles were obtain for larger uncharged solutes, from 5,000 to 77,000 MW (Torzilli, et al., 1985) The diffusion rates were found to be inversely proportional to the Stokes radius, Rs, but not the molecular weights. An important finding from these transient experiments is the very long diffusion times necessary to achieve temporal and spatial equilibrium, even for a small molecule such as glucose. If drug delivery systems are eventually to be used, this must be taken into consideration to achieve a known concentration throughout the entire tissue thickness.

Diffusion transport rates were also found to depend on temperature and proteoglycan content, but not on solute concentration (unpublished data). As expected, increasing temperature increased the diffusion rate, in good agreement with the Stokes-Einstein relationship

$$D' = D\,(T'/T)\,(\eta/\eta') \tag{12}$$

where T is the temperature and η the solvent viscosity. Proteoglycan removal had an increasingly greater affect on the diffusion rates for larger solutes compared to smaller ones. Removal of 86% and 98% of the proteoglycan content resulted in a significant increase of 71% and 95% for dextran (70,000 MW, Rs=6.1 nm), a significant increase of 60% at 98% removal for inulin (5,000 MW, 3.4 nm), and no change for glucose (180 MW, 0.4 nm). Similar results were reported by Lotke and Granda (1971,1972) for solute permeability (diffusion + convection) in osteoarthritic and enzymatically treated cartilage.

These results indicate that in cartilage the proteoglycan macromolecule acts as a solute filter and the primary restraint to solute transport. Small solutes, such as glucose, are capable of moving freely through the tissue with little or no restraint, that is, through the proteoglycan macromolecule, Figure 9. However, as the size of the solute increases, so will the restriction to movement, until the solute is forced to move around the proteoglycan macromolecular or be trapped in the matrix. It is probably that in degenerative tissue, where the proteoglycan content is decreased, large molecules will now move more easily through the tissue's matrix. This would effect both enzyme and proteoglycan movement into, through and out of the tissue. Unless the solute transport restrictive properties of the proteoglycan macromolecule can be replaced, it will not be possible to stop further tissue degradation.

Multiple Diffusion Paths - A New Model

Comparison of the data from the transient diffusion experiments and the predictions of the simple linear diffusion model (Eqns. 10 & 11) resulted in two unusual findings. First, an apparent time-dependent value for the diffusion coefficient was found (Torzilli et al., 1987). Although this type of behavior can occur when concentration dependent parameters are present, the affect was considered negligible at the 'dilute' concentrations used. In addition, increasing the solute

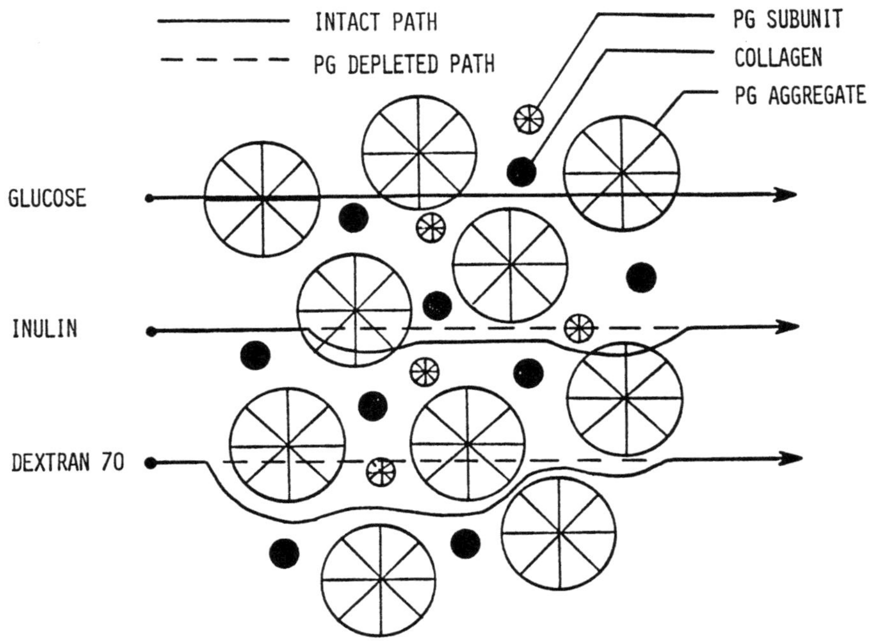

Figure 9. Schematic representation of selective diffusion of glucose (180 MW), inulin (5,000 MW) and dextran (70,000 MW) through the cartilage matrix. Glucose can move freely through all the available water, inulin is partially excluded from the proteoglycan intramolecular water, and dextran can only move through the bulk water space.

concentration did not change the diffusion coefficient (unpublished data), again ruling out these dependencies. Second, there was a characteristic time-dependent rise in the solute concentration at the interface between the tissue and the bathing solution, Figure 8. The failure of the linear diffusion theory to account for this phenomena, and the apparent time-dependent diffusion coefficient, led to various hypotheses aimed at resolving these discrepancies. The formation of a stagnant layer at the interface was first proposed as the probable cause. However, this was not found experimentally. Instead a new model was developed based on multiple diffusion pathways.

The proposed model is based on the hypothesis that

several distinct diffusion paths are present in articular cartilage, each with a different diffusion rate. The different diffusion paths are distinguished by the state of the water associated with them. The assumption is that water can exist in bound (trapped), interstitial and bulk states. Bound water is strongly associated with the collagen network and is not available for solute transport within the tissue. Interstitial water is associated with the proteoglycan-water gel and has selective transport properties dependent on the solute's characteristics. Finally, bulk water is the water through which the solute transport is governed by purely Fickean diffusion.

The theoretical analysis for the present model is based on a model developed for naturally fractured reservoirs by Barenblatt and Zheltov (1960). In cartilage it is assumed that two diffusion paths exist, one through the bulk water, with diffusion rate D_1, and the other through the proteoglycan-water gel with diffusion rate D_2. The regions associated with bound water are not available to the transport process. In addition, solute mass exchange can occur between the two paths with rate constants k_1 and k_2, respectively. Under the usual assumptions of conservation of mass flux and exchange, the governing diffusion equations for each path are given by

$$\begin{aligned} \frac{\partial c_1}{\partial t} &= D_1 \frac{\partial^2 c_1}{\partial x^2} - k_1 c_1 - k_2 c_2, \\ \frac{\partial c_2}{\partial t} &= D_2 \frac{\partial^2 c_2}{\partial x^2} + k_1 c_1 + k_2 c_2. \end{aligned} \tag{13}$$

where the c's are the apparent concentrations per unit volume of available water.

Assuming that the rate of diffusion through the bulk water is much faster than through the interstitial water, such that, $D_1 \gg D_2$, and that a solute partition ω exits between the bulk and interstitial spaces, the governing equations (13) can be combined to yield

$$\frac{\partial^2 c}{\partial t^2} + k_1\left[1 + \frac{f}{\omega(1-f)}\right]\frac{\partial c}{\partial t} = D_1 \frac{\partial}{\partial t}\frac{\partial^2 c}{\partial x^2} + \frac{f k_1 D_1}{\omega(1-f)}\frac{\partial^2 c}{\partial x^2}. \tag{14}$$

where c is the total concentration, $c = c_1 + c_2$, f is defined as the fraction of available volume occupied by the fast (bulk water) path, and k_1 is the rate of mass exchange from the bulk water into the interstitial water. Solution of Eqns. (13) at the interface between the bath solution and the tissue, x=0, yields the boundary condition for Eqn. (14), given by

$$c = f + \omega(1-f)\left[1 - e^{-\frac{f k_1}{\omega(1-f)}t}\right]. \tag{15}$$

It is apparent from Eqn. (15) that the solute concentration at the interface shows a steady rise to an equilibrium value characterized by the rate of exchange between the two paths, k_1, the solute partition coefficient in the interstitial region, ω, and the ratio of the volume fraction of the two paths, f/(1-f). Solution of Eqn. (14), subject to the usual boundary condition of impermeability at the cartilage-bone junction (x=l) and initial solute free tissue, yields

$$c(x,t) = \sum_{n=0}^{\infty}\left\{A_n e^{r_{n1}t} + B_n e^{r_{n2}t} + \frac{4w(1-f)}{(2n+1)\pi}e^{\frac{-f k_1}{\omega(1-f)}t}\right\}\sin\lambda_n x + f + \omega(1-f)\left[1 - e^{-\frac{f k_1}{\omega(1-f)}t}\right], \tag{16}$$

where

$$r_{n1,2} = -1/2[k_1(1+\frac{f}{\omega(1-f)}) + D_1\lambda_n^2]$$
$$\pm 1/2[(1+\frac{f}{\omega(1-f)})^2 k_1^2 + D_1^2\lambda_n^4 + 2(1-\frac{f}{\omega(1-f)})k_1 D_1 \lambda^2]^{1/2},$$

$$A_n = \frac{4\omega r_{n2}(1-f)}{(2n+1)\pi[r_{n1}-r_{n2}]}, \qquad (17)$$
$$B_n = -A_n - \frac{4\omega(1-f)}{(2n+1)\pi}.$$

In comparing the model with the experimental results discussed above, assumptions were made that the diffusion coefficient D_1 was the same as that of the solute in aqueous solution, and the concentration profiles from the experimental data were measured per total water content. Water partition data was used to modify the predicted concentration profiles so that they would reflect the observation that bound water was not available for solute transport.

The resulting exchange rate k_1, fast volume fraction f, and solute partition coefficient ω for glucose, obtained by least-squares fit of the model to the experimental data, are listed in Table 2. The mean concentration profiles are shown in Figure 8. The model accurately predicts the main features of the experimental observations, including those not accounted for in the linear Fickian diffusion model, Eqns. (10 & 11); specifically, the time dependent rise of the concentration at the articular surface. For glucose, approximately half of the available water (f=0.5) was predicted to be in the bulk diffusion pathway. The large calculated values for the exchange rate k_1 indicated that the glucose molecules are freely and instantaneously exchanged between the bulk and interstitial water.

Table 2

Time (min)	K_1 (min^{-1})	f	ω
5	>100	0.4664	0.1479
15	>100	0.4669	0.5711
60	>100	0.5166	0.6895
240	>100	0.2334	0.8114

The slight variation of f and ω over time is attributed to the inhomogeneity of the cartilage matrix. This inhomogeneity has not been taken into account in the current analysis. Note that at longer times the solutes move deeper into the tissue layer, where the ratio of proteoglycan to collagen content is higher compared to the surface regions, that is, more available water. Consequently, the increase in ω can be attributed to the increased presence of the proteoglycan-water gel in the deeper regions of the tissue and to its greater solute retention capacity.

Another attractive feature of this dual diffusion model over earlier ones is the elimination of the need to rely upon bulk or average parameters. The diffusion coefficient used is that of the solute in water. In addition, the partition coefficient ω is only dependent on the interaction of the solute with the proteoglycan-water gel. These quantities can be independently measured and used to gain advanced insight into the behavior of any given solute in articular cartilage.

Finally, the affects of a stagnant layer at the interfacial boundary was analyzed using the dual diffusion model. The stagnant layer was assumed to have a thickness comparable to that of the tissue layer, and the resulting governing equations solved. The results indicated that a significant effect on solute flux could result if inadequate solute-solvent mixing occurred at the interface. To further investigate whether a stagnant layer actually formed during the diffusion experiments, transient diffusion tests were repeated for 15 and 60 minutes with and without stirring of the external bathing solution. The concentration profiles are shown in Figure 10. No significant difference was found between the predicted coefficients with and without stirring. Thus, the effects of a stagnant layer were considered negligible.

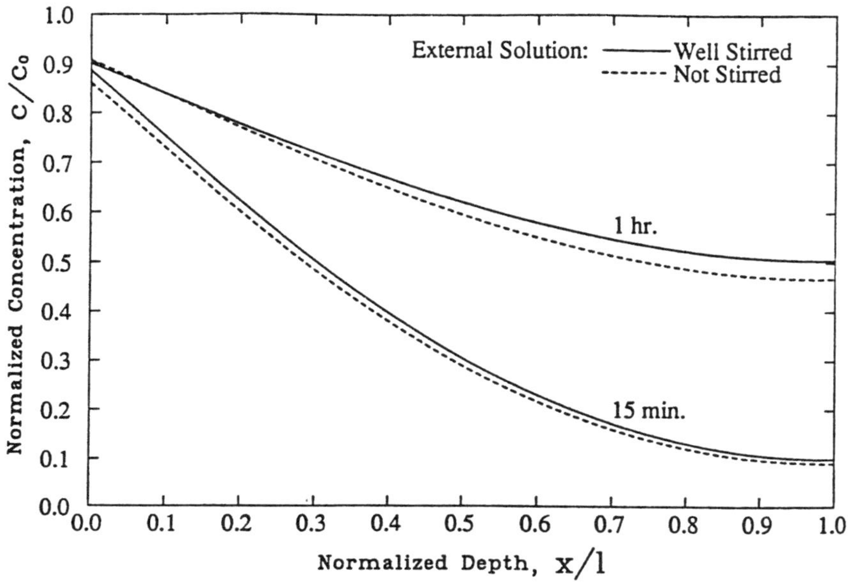

Figure 10

Comparison of glucose diffusion with and without stirring of the bath solution. No significant effect was observed.

In conclusion, the dual diffusion model accurately predicts the solute transport phenomena observed in articular cartilage. The model predicts the time-dependent concentration rise at the interface between the articular cartilage surface and bath solution, and the concentration profile within the tissue layer. It also has the capability of predicting where solute movement occurs, that is, relative to the bulk and interstitial water, and the solute partition between the solute and the proteoglycan-water gel.

Acknowledgement

The authors wish to express their appreciation to the National Institutes of Health, Grant AM28151, for its support of research in solute transport in articular cartilage.

References

Aifantis EC: A new interpretation of diffusion in high-diffusivity paths. A continuum approach. Acta Metallurgica 1979;27:683-691

Allhands RV, Torzilli PA, Kallfelz F: Measurement of diffusion of uncharged molecules in articular cartilage. Cornell Veterinarian 1984;74:111-123

Barenblatt GI, Zheltov IP, Kochina IN: Basic concepts in the theory of seepage of homogeneous liquids in fissured rocks (strata). PMM 1960;24:1286-1303

Berens AR, HopfenbergHB: Diffusion and relaxation in glassy polymer powders: 2. Separation of diffusion and relaxation parameters. Polymer 1978;19:489-496

Bernich E, Rubenstein R, Bellin JS: Membrane transport properties of bovine articular cartilage. Biochem Biophys Acta 1976;448:551-561

Bretsznajder S: Prediction of Transport and Other Physical Properties of Fluids. New York, Pergamon Press, 1971

Brocklehurst R, Bayliss MT, Maroudas A, Coysh HL, Freeman MAR, Revell PA, Ali SY: The composition of normal and osteoarthritic articular cartilage from human knee joints. J. Bone and Joint Surgery 1984;66A:95-106

Comper WD, Williams RPW: Hydrodynamics of concentrated proteoglycan solutions. The Journal of Biological Chemistry 1987;262:13464-13471

Crank J: The Mathematics of Diffusion. Oxford, Clarendon Press, 1975

Crank J, Park GS: Diffusion in Polymers. New York, Academic Press, 1968

Dunstone JR: Ion-exchange reactions between cartilage and various cations. Biochem J 1966;77:164-170

Grodzinsky AJ, Roth V, Myers E, Grossman WD, Mow VC: The significance of electromechanical and osmotic forces in the nonequilibrium swelling behavior of articular cartilage in tension. J Biomech 1981;103:221-231

Grynpas MD, Eyre DR, Kirschner DA: Collagen type II differs from type I in native molecular packing. Biochem Biophys Acta 1980;626:346-355

Handler-Bernich E, Lotke P, Rubenstein R: Membrane characteristics of human articular cartilage. Biochemica Biophysica Acta 1972;266:732-736

Harris K, Woolf LA: Pressure and temperature dependence of the self diffusion coefficient of water and oxygen-18 water. J.C.S. Faraday I 1980;76:377-385

Harper GS, Comper WD, Preston BN, Daivis P: Concentration dependence of proteoglycan diffusion. Biopolymers 1985;24:2165-2173

Idol WK, Anderson JL: Effects of adsorbed polyelectrolytes on convective flow and diffusion in porous membranes. J Mem Biol 1986;28:269-286

Laurent TC: The interaction between polysaccharides and other macromolecules. 9. The exclusion of molecules from hyaluronic acid gels and solutions. J Biochem 1964;93:106-111

Lemperg R, Larsson S-E: The glycosaminoglycans of bovine articular cartilage. I. Concentration and distribution in different layers in relation to age. Calc Tiss Res 1974;15: 237-251

Lemperg RK, Larsson SE, Hjertquist SO: Distribution of water and glycosaminoglycans in different layers of cattle articular cartilage. Biochem Biophys Aspects 1971;7:419-421

Lipshitz H, Etheredge R, Glimcher MJ: Changes in the hexosamine content and swelling ratio of articular cartilage as functions of depth from the surface. J Bone Jt Surg 1976; 58A:1149-1153

Lotke PA, Granda JL: Changes in the permeability of human articular cartilage in early degenerative osteoarthritis. Surgical Forum 1971;22:449-450

Lotke PA, Granda JL: Alterations in the permeability of articular cartilage by proteolytic enzymes. Arth Rheum 1972; 15:302-308

Maroudas A: Distribution and diffusion of solutes in articular cartilage. Biophysical Journal 1970;10:365-379

Maroudas A: Biophysical chemistry of cartilaginous tissues with special reference to solute and fluid transport. Biorheology 1975;12:233-248

Maroudas A: Transport of solutes through cartilage: permeability to large molecules. J Anat 1976;122:335-347

Maroudas A: Physical Chemistry of Articular Cartilage and the Intervertebral Disc., in L Sokoloff (ed.): The Joints and Synovial Fluid. New York, Academic Press, 1980, pp. 240- 293

Maroudas A, Bannon C: Measurement of swelling pressure in cartilage and comparison with the osmotic pressure of constituent proteoglycans. Biorheology 1981;18:619-632

Maroudas A, Bullough P: Permeability of articular cartilage. Nature 1968;219:1260-1261

Maroudas A, Evans H: Sulfate diffusion and incorporation into human articular cartilage. Biochem Biophys Acta 1974;338:265-279

Maroudas A, Schneiderman R: "Free" and "exchangeable" or "trapped" and "non-exchangeable" water in cartilage. J Orthop Res 1987;5:133-138

Maroudas A, Venn M: Chemical composition and swelling of normal and osteoarthritic femoral head cartilage. II. Swelling. Ann. Rheum. Dis. 1977;36:399-406

Mathews MB, Decker L: Comparative studies of water sorption of hyaline cartilage. Biochem Biophys Acta 1977;497:151-159

McDevitt CA, Muir H: Biochemical changes in the cartilage of the knee in experimental and natural osteoarthritis in the dog. J Bone Jt Surg 1976;58:94-101

Miller DR, Peppas NA: Diffusional effects during albumin adsorption on highly swollen poly(vinyl alcohol) hydrogels. European Polymer Journal 1988;24:611-615

Mow VC, Myers ER, Roth V, Lalik P: Implications for collagen-proteoglycan interactions from cartilage stess relaxation behavior in isometric tension. Seminars in Arthritis Rheum. 1981;11(1):41-43

Myers ER, Lai WM, Mow VC: A continuum theory and an experiment for the ion-induced swelling behavior of articular cartilage. J Biomech 1984;106:151-158

Neogi P, Kim M, Yang Y: Diffusion in solids under strain, with emphasis on polymer membranes. American Institutes of Chemical Engineers Journal (AIChE J) 1986;32:1146-1157

Norton J, Urban J, Maroudas A, Parker KH, Winlove CP: A failure to observe enhanced diffusivity of glucose in a matrix of hyaluronic acid. The Journal of Biological Chemistry 1982;257:14134-14135

Ogata K, Whiteside LA, Lesker PA: Subchondral route for nitrition to articular cartilage in the rabbit. J Bone Jt Surg 1978;60A:905-910

Ogston AG, Sherman TF: Effects of hyaluronic acid upon diffusion of solutes and flow of solvent. J Physiol 1961;156: 67-74

Osada Y, Honda K, Ohta M: Control of water permeability by mechanochemical contraction of poly(methacrylic acid)- grafted membranes. J Mem Biol 1986;27:327-338

Paul DR: Transport properties of polymers. Applied Polymer Science., American Chemical Society, 1985, pp. 253-275

Phillies GDJ: Universal scaling equation for self-diffusion by macromolecules in solution. Macromolecules 1986;19:2367-2376

Preston BN, Snowden JM: Model connective tissue systems: The effect of proteoglycans on the diffusional behavior of small non-electrolytes and microions. Biopolymers 1972;11:1627-1643

Preston BN, Snowden JM, Houghton KT: Model connective tissue systems: The effect of proteoglycans on the distribution of small non-electrolytes and micro-ions. Biopolymers 1972;11: 1645-1659

Preston BN, Snowden JMcK: Diffusion properties of model extracellular systems, in E Kulonen J Pikkarainen (eds.): Biology of Fibroblast. New York, Academic, 1973, pp. 215-230

Snowden JM, Maroudas A: The distribution of serum albumin in human normal and degenerate articular cartilage. Biochem Biophys Acta 1976;428:726-740

Tasaka M, Suzuki S, Ogawa Y, Kamaya M: Freezing and nonfreezing water in charged membranes. J Mem Biol 1988;38: 175-183

Tivant P, Turq P, Drifford M, Magdelenat H, Menez R: Effect of ionic strength on the diffusion coefficient of chondroitin sulfate and heparin measured by quasielastic light scattering. Biopolymers 1983;22:643-662

Torzilli PA: The influence of cartilage conformation on its equilibrium water partition. J Orthop Res 1985;3:473-483

Torzilli PA: Water content and equilibrium water partition in immature cartilage. J Orthop Res 1988;6:766-769

Torzilli PA, Adams TC, Mis RJ: Transient solute diffusion in articular cartilage. J Biomech 1987;20:203-214

Torzilli PA, Rose DE, Dethmers DA: Equilibrium water partition in articular cartilage. Biorheology 1982;19:519-537

Urban J, Holm S, Maroudas A, Nachemson A: Nutrition of the intervertebral disc. Effect of fluid flow and solute transport. Clin. Orth. Rel. Res. 1982;170:296-302

Urban JPG, Holm S, Maroudas A: Diffusion of small solutes into the intervertebral disc: an in vivo study. Biorheology 1978;15:203-223

Venn M, Maroudas A: Chemical composition and swelling of normal and osteoarthritic femoral head cartilage. I. Chemical composition. Ann. Rheum. Dis. 1977;36:121-129

Venn MF: Variation of chemical composition with age in human femoral head cartilage. Ann. Rheum. Dis. 1978;37:168-174

Viswanadham RK, Kramer EJ: Elastic properties of reconstituted collagen hollow fibre menbranes. J Mat Sci 1976;11:1254-1262

Wan W, Whittenburg SL: Concentration dependence of the polymer diffusion coefficient. Reversible Polymeric Gels and Related Systems, American Chemical Society 1987 pp. 4.46-4.56

Wik KO, Comper WD: Hyaluronate diffusion in semidilute solutions. Biopolymers 1982;21:583-599

Wurster NB, Lust G: Fibronectin and water content of articular cartilage explants after partial depletion of proteoglycans. J Orthop Res 1986;4:437-445

Chapter 14

Biomechanical Properties of Healing Cartilage

M.K. Kwan, S.L-Y. Woo

Introduction

Damage to articular cartilage frequently occur following trauma and pathology (Curtiss 1969; Mankin and Brandt 1984). The limited ability of cartilage to heal has presented a continuous challenge in the treatment of damaged articular surfaces (Haggart 1940; Furukawa et al. 1980; Mankin and Brandt 1984). Many procedures have been explored and implemented to remedy this problem (Coletti et al. 1972; Charnley and Cupic 1973; Coventry et al. 1974; Aston and Bentley 1986; Meyers 1989), and the popular one by far is artificial joint replacement (McKee and Farrar 1966). The long-term survival problems associated with artificial joint replacement (Miller et al. 1978), however, have contraindicated this procedure as an ideal treatment for cartilage resurfacing. Alternatives have thus been sought, and in recent years efforts have been focused on biological arthroplasty. The basic approach in biological arthroplasty is to repair the cartilage defect with an implantable biological graft containing a chondrogenic cell source which will promote growth of a new cartilaginous tissue and eventual functional healing of the defect. The joint surface regenerated this way may potentially last for longer periods of time than the artificial implants.

The interest in exploring biological grafting techniques for cartilage repair was started more than a century ago when Tizzone (1878) and Haas (1914) first observed the potential of perichondrium to induce cartilaginous growth. This interest was renewed much later when Skoog et al. (1972, 1975) demonstrated that the rapid growth of a cartilaginous tissue from ear perichondrium. In fact, cartilage formation had also been found following implantation of perichondrium into subcutaneous tissue, muscle, and liver. Several clinical applications of the perichondrial grafts were reported. Pastacaldi and Engkvist (1979) resurfaced wrist joints with perichondrial grafts and reported satisfactory results; however, results for finger joints were variable (Johansson 1979; Seradge et al. 1984).

The applications of chondrogenic tissues including perichondrium and periosteum to the repair of cartilage defects have been studied in various animal experiments (Engkvist et al. 1979; Engkvist 1979; Salter et al. 1980; Rubak 1982; Ohlsen et al. 1983; Coutts et al. 1984; O'Driscoll et al. 1986; Amiel et al. 1988; Kwan et al. 1989a). Engkvist et al. (1979) applied rib perichondrium to a rabbit femoral defect and found formation of cartilaginous tissue. They showed the new tissue grew from the perichondrium and resembled closely hyaline articular cartilage. They also evaluated perichondrial grafts implanted on canine patellar surface and found again cartilage formation shortly after the surgery (Engkvist 1979). Wasteson et al. (1977) demonstrated that the cartilaginous tissue grown from perichondrium contained chondroitin-4 and chondroitin-6 sulfate. Some variable results from perichondrial grafting in rabbit knee joints had also been reported (Kon 1981). The use of periosteum, another source material has also been studied (Salter et al. 1980; Rubak 1982). Salter et al. (1980) and O'Driscoll et al. (1986) showed that articular defects in patellar groove grafted with periosteum were filled with a new tissue histologically and biochemically similar to articular cartilage, particularly when continuous passive motion was applied. However, for grafting large defect over the patellar surface, the results were clinically unsuccessful (O'Driscoll et al. 1989). There have been, nonetheless, little information concerning the biomechanical properties of the new tissue grown from biological grafts. To a large extent, it is not clearly understood whether the new tissues can function as normal articular cartilage, and yet this information is crucial for evaluating the success of the repair.

Perichondrium-Autologus Bone Graft and Post-operative Passive Motion Treatment

The efficacy of using biological grafts to repair large articular defects in rabbit knee joint has been demonstrated in our laboratory. Previously, we had studied an autograft composed of rib perichondrium sutured to autologus bone (Coutts et al. 1984). This autograft, when placed in the rabbit knee joint, introduced a new cell population which proliferated to fill a full thickness defect in the rabbit femur condyle. The newly grown tissue was shown to contain significantly more type II collagen and proteoglycans than perichondrium, similar to hyaline articular cartilage (Amiel et al. 1988). The arthroplasty surface survived up to one year, demonstrating a time-dependent improvement. Biomechanically, the neocartilage exhibits viscoelasticity which is not an apparent characteristic of the perichondrium. The complex shear modulus of the neocartilage, indicating its ability to resist shear load, was found to increase with healing time and approach that for normal articular cartilage at one year (Figure 1) (Kwan et al. 1989a).

It was further shown that post-operatively applied passive motion (PM) might enhance the quality of the new tissue growth by improving the nutritional supply to the graft and providing mechanical stimulation, particularly during the early stage of the repair (Figure 1). However, this enhancement effect might not last over time, as difference in quality of the repair tissue between PM-treated and nontreated groups became diminished at one year.

The success rate of the perichondrium-autologus bone autografts, however, was not satisfactory. The overall acceptance rate was about 65% (Table 1), with high instances of graft detachment. Detachment occurred particularly when post-operative treatment of passive motion was applied. It is thus important for the success of the graft to have firm fixation in the defect, particularly during the early stage of the repair when the regeneration process begins. Improved surgical techniques are certainly needed for initial fixation of the graft. Further investigations into other composite biological grafts which allow higher success rates are also necessary.

Weeks (postop.)	PM*	CAGE**
6	10/14	9/15
12	9/17	10/17
26	5/7	5/7
52	8/14	7/9

* PM-treated; ** Cage activity

Table 1. Incidence of biological acceptance (expressed as no. of acceptable samples/ no. of examined).

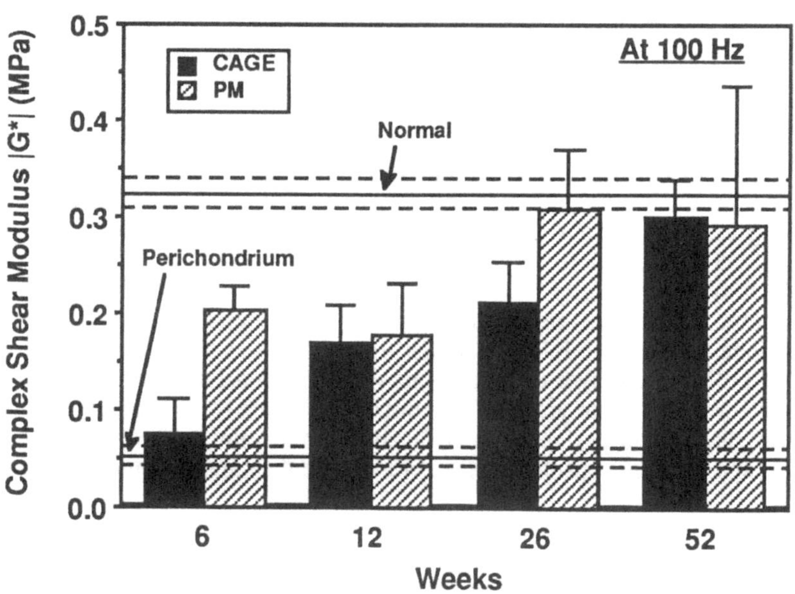

Figure 1. The magnitude of the complex shear modulus for neocartilage grown from perichondrium-autologus bone grafts, plotted as a function of postoperative time. Two treatment groups are indicated: CAGE -- allowed *ad lib* cage activity; PM - undergone two weeks of passive motion treatment after surgery.

Perichondrium - Demineralized Bone Autograft

To achieve a higher success rate, we have recently studied a composite graft of autologus perichondrium sutured to a supporting matrix of demineralized bone (DBM). The DBM is a softer and easier-to-handle material for graft fixation. It has osteoinductive properties (Kohler et al. 1987; Wittbjer et al. 1982) and has been effectively used in many surgical reconstructions (Olkarinen 1982; Lane et al. 1987). In this recent study, the implantation of DBM 1) with and 2) without perichondrium in a rabbit model for growth of cartilage repair tissue.

Experimental Model

Skeletally mature New Zealand white rabbits were used in this study. The demineralized bone matrix (DBM) was sterilely harvested from the femurs and tibias of several donor rabbits. The femurs and tibias were cleaned in deionized water at 4°C to remove all soft tissues, bone marrow and periosteum. The bones were defatted in a mixture of chloroform and methanol for one hour and then placed in 0.6 N HCl at 4°C for 24 hrs for demineralization. The bones were then rinsed with sterile deionized water and stored at -4°C.

For the *in vivo* study, the rabbits were anesthetized with a mixed solution of ketamine (100 mg/kg) and xylazine (8 mg/kg). Under sterile surgical conditions, a 2.0 cm cartilaginous portion of the most inferior attached rib was obtained from each rabbit through a 3.0 cm longitudinal incision made on the anterior left chest. The perichondrium was removed and placed in sterile saline. A medial parapatellar incision was then made on both knees, the patellar was dislocated laterally, and the medial femoral condyle was exposed. Surgical drill bits measuring 1, 2.5, and 4 mm in diameter were sequentially used to create a 4 mm diameter by 5 mm deep defect on each medial femoral condyle, as far posterior as possible with the knee fully flexed. The right knee defect was filled with two discs (4 mm in diameter) of allogeneic DBM sewn together using 7-0 vicryl (DBM-alone graft). The left defect was filled with a composite graft of two layers of DBM and a layer of autologous rib perichondrium harvested earlier (DBM-and-perichondrium graft). These three layers were sewn together with the cambium side of the perichondrium faced into the joint. The patellar was relocated and the joint capsule was then closed, and the animals returned to cage activity.

The animals were euthanized at 12 weeks after the surgery, and gross examination of the joint surfaces was made to determine the biological acceptability of the repair site. The term "biological acceptability" was used to identify specimens that were adequate for histological and biomechanical evaluation. Biologically acceptable repair tissues were defined as having firm, cohesive neocartilage growth that made contact with the periphery and had reasonable continuity with the surrounding articular cartilage (Amiel et al. 1988; Kwan et al. 1989a).

Histological and Biomechanical Assessments

For histological examination, the specimens were decalcified in EDTA and fixed in Bouin's solution. The medial femoral condyles were then embedded in paraffin and cut along the sagittal plane. The sections were stained with hematoxylin and eosin (H&E) for structural detail and with safranin o/fast green for assessment of glycosaminoglycan distribution in the neocartilage.

Biomechanically, the repair tissues were evaluated by two independent compression tests: an *in situ* indentation test and a uniaxial confined compression test. The indentation test was used to assess the mechanical behavior of the tissue under a three-dimensional loading configuration, and the confined compression test was used to assess the aggregate modulus and apparent permeability of the cartilage matrix (Kwan et al. 1989b). These two properties are important properties controlling the viscoelastic behavior of articular cartilage under compression (Mow et al. 1980; Kwan et al. 1984). For the indentation test, the repair articular surfaces were mounted in the testing apparatus and oriented such that the loading shaft would be perpendicular to the surface and directly over the center of the repair site. A 1.5 mm diameter porous indenter tip is attached to the end of the loading shaft to allow fluid exudation from the tissue during compression. After a small pre-load was applied and equilibrated, a step-load of 0.05 N was applied onto the cartilage surface. The instantaneous and creep deformation was measured with time until equilibrium was established, over a period of 45-60 minutes. Specimens from both knees were tested in the same manner.

After the indentation test, 4 mm diameter cylindrical osteochondral plugs encompassing the entire repair area were harvested from the femoral condyles and tested in confined compression. The cylindrical plugs were compressed in rigid confining chamber allowing uniaxial deformation by a porous plate. A constant stress of approximately 0.01 MPa was applied to the tissue through the porous plate, and the resulting time-dependent deformation of the cartilage surface was measured. The data were curve-fitted by using a theoretical equation derived from the linear biphasic model (Mow et al. 1980; Kwan et al. 1989b) to determine the aggregate modulus and apparent permeability.

Results

Gross examination indicated that growth of repair tissue occurred in all specimens regardless of the presence or absence of the perichondrial grafts. Repair using DBM-alone grafts had a biological acceptance rate of 88% (i.e. 15/17), while those with DBM-and-perichondrium grafts had an acceptance rate of 82% (i.e. 14/17). The neocartilage grown from DBM-alone grafts had an appearance ranging from smooth to convoluted. In both cases, the repair tissue was in generally good confluence with the surrounding cartilage, and the bone underlying the repair area was firm as determined from the drilled osteochondral specimens used for the confined compression tests. The repair tissue was securely attached to the underlying bone, and the demarcation between the repair tissue and the bone was clearly evident. Histologically, the repair tissue demonstrated cells appearance, organization, and orientation similar to normal cartilage tissue.

Indentation creep curves for the DBM-alone and DBM-and-perichondrium groups are shown in Figure 2. Shown also is the creep curve for normal articular cartilage from the same location on the rabbit femoral condyle. The repair tissues from both groups exhibited similar viscoelastic behavior, and took a long time (more than 3,000 seconds) to reach equilibrium as normal articular cartilage. The two groups appeared to creep at slightly different rates but attained similar normalized displacements (i.e., displacement/thickness) at equilibrium. The repair tissues from both groups crept significantly more than normal articular cartilage under the same indenting load.

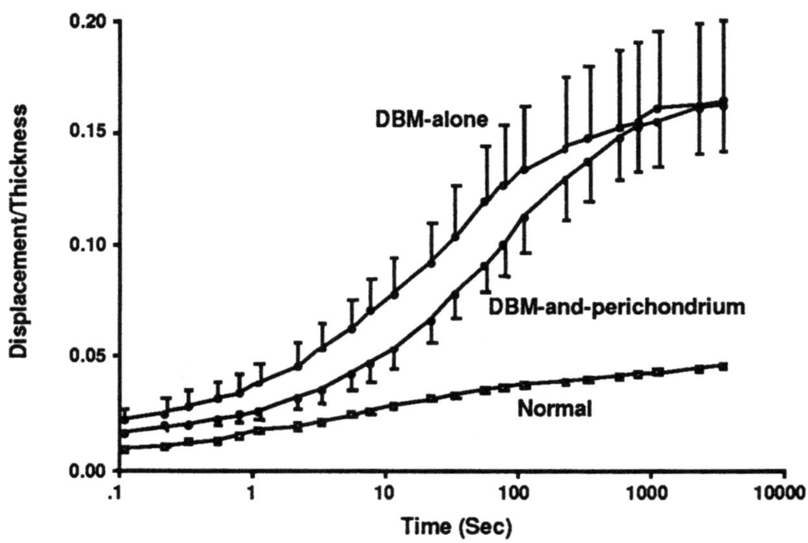

Figure 2. Indentation creep curves for repair tissues grown from DBM-alone and DBM-and-perichondrium grafts, and normal articular cartilage.

The aggregate modulus and apparent permeability for the repair tissues obtained from the confined compression tests are shown in Figure 3. The repair tissues from both groups had similar moduli and permeabilities. Their moduli were lower than those reported in the literature for normal articular cartilage, while their permeabilities were higher. At this time point (12 weeks) after the surgery, the extracellular matrix might not be fully organized, appearing to be softer and more permeable. Further investigation will be necessary for evaluating the long-term development of the repair tissue.

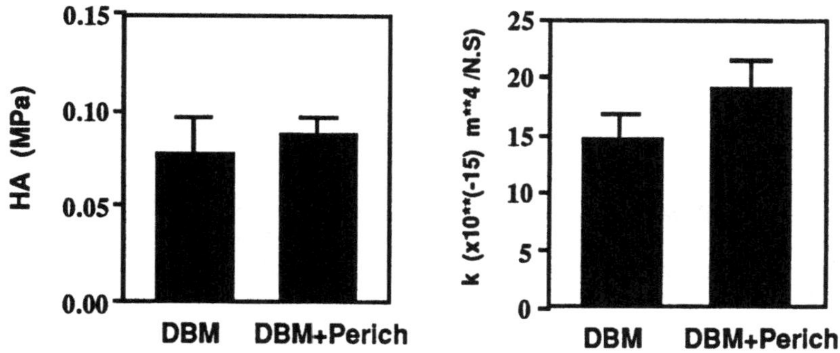

Figure 3. The aggregate modulus (HA) and apparent permeability (k) for repair tissues grown from DBM-alone and DBM-and-perichondrium grafts.

Discussion

Implantable composite grafts composed of chondrogenic tissue, such as autologus perichondrium or periosteum, and an osteoinductive supporting matrix such as demineralized bone matrix are potential, important alternative for the repair of articular cartilage defects. This repair technique has the advantage that only the damaged site on the joint surface needs be replaced, thus allowing the possibility of salvaging much of the normal joint.

The efficacy of using perichondrial grafts for cartilage repair is again demonstrated. The perichondrial cells were able to differentiate and grow into cartilage-like tissues filling the defects. It was interesting to observe that a similar cartilaginous tissue grew also from the repair with only the demineralized bone matrix. Chondrogenic cells possibly might have migrated from the synovial fluid, bone, or neighboring cartilage, and augmented by the growth factors in the demineralized bone matrix (Sampath et al. 1982; Hauschka et al. 1986; Reddi 1983). The precise effects of the growth factors on the cartilaginous growth is not yet fully understood, and studies in this area need to be pursued. Nonetheless, the demineralized bone matrix was found to be a suitable material for filling osteochondral defects. The success rate of the perichondrium-demineralized bone autografts represents a significant improvement over our previous models. The survival of the chondrogenic aautografts, however, must be further evaluated in long-term experiments. Other potential composite grafts also need to be explored in the continuous quest for higher success rate.

References

Amiel D, Coutts RD, Harwood FL, et al.: The chondrogenesis of rib perichondrial grafts for repair of full-thickness articular cartilage defects in the rabbit model: A one-year postoperative assessment. Conn Tissue Res 1988;18:27-39.

Aston JE, Bentley G: Repair of the articular surface by allografts of articular and grow-plate cartilage. J Bone Joint Surg 1986;68B:29-35.

Charnley J, Cupic F: The nine and ten year results of how friction arthroplasty of the hip. Clin Orthop 1973;95:9.

Coletti JM Jr, Akeson WH, Woo SL-Y: A comparison of the physical behavior of normal articular cartilage and the arthroplasty surface. J Bone Joint Surg 1972;54A:147-160.

Coventry MB, Beckenbaugh RO, Nolan DR, et al.: 2012 total hip arthroplasties: A study of postoperative cause and early complications. J Bone Joint Surg 1974;56A:273.

Coutts RD, Amiel D, Woo SL-Y, et al.: Technical aspects of perichondrial grafting in the rabbit. Eur Surg Res 1984;16:322-328.

Curtiss PH Jr: Cartilage damage in septic arthritis. Clin Orthop 1969;64:87-90.

Engkvist O: Reconstruction of patellar articular cartilage with free autologous perichondrial grafts. An experimental study in dogs. Scand J Plast Reconstr Surg 1979;13:361.

Engkvist O, Wilander E: Formation of cartilage from rib perichondrium grafted to an articular defect in the femur condyle of the rabbit. Scand J Plast Reconstr Surg 1979;13:371-376.

Furukawa T, Eyre DR, Koide S, et al.: Biochemical studies on repair cartilage resurfacing experimental defects in the rabbit knee. J Bone Joint Surg 1980;62A:79-89.

Haas SL: Regeneration of cartilage and bone with a special study of these processes as they occur at the chondrocostal junction. Surg Gynecol Obstet 1914;19:604-617.

Haggart GE: The surgical treatment of degenerative arthritis of the knee joint. J Bone Joint Surg 1940;22A:717-729.

Hanschka PV, Mavrakos AE, Iafrati MD, et al.: Growth factors in bone matrix: Isolation of multiple types by affinity chromatograph on heparinsepharose. J Biol Chem 1986;261:12665-12764.

Johansson S: Perichondrial graft resurfacing of articular joints clinical applications, in M Meyers (ed): Proc Conf Rehab Articular Joint by Biol Resurfacing, Dallas, Texas, 1979;60-70.

Kohler P, Krekberg A: Incorporation of autoclaved antogeneic bone supplemented with allogeneic demineralized bone matrix: An experimental study in the rabbit. Clin Orthop 1987;218:247-258.

Kon M: Cartilage formation from perichondrium in a weight-bearing joint. Eur Surg Res 1981;13:387-396.

Kwan MK, Lai WM, Mow VC: Fundamentals of fluid transport through articular cartilage i n compression. Ann Biomed Eng 1984;12:537-558.

Kwan MK, Coutts RD, Woo SL-Y, Field FP: Morphological and biomechanical evaluation of neocartilage from the repair of full-thickness articular cartilage defects using rib perichondrium autografts: A long-term study. J Biomech 1989a;22:921-930.

Kwan MK, Wayne JS, Woo SL-Y, et al.: Histological and biomechanical assessment of articular cartilage from stored osteochondral shell allografts. J Orthop Res 1989b;7:637-644.

Lane JM: Current approaches to experimental bone grafting. Orthop Clin N America 1987;18:213.

Mankin HJ, Brandt KD: In Moskowiz et al. (eds): Osteoarthritis: Diagnosis and management. WB Saunders, 1984;43-80.

McKee GK, Farrar JW: Replacement of arthritic hips by the McKee-Farrar prosthesis. J Bone Joint Surg 1966;48B:245.

Meyers MH, Akeson WH, Convery FR: Resurfacing of the knee with fresh osteochondral allografts. J Bone Joint Surg 1989;71A:704-713.

Miller J, Burke DL, Stachiewicz JW, et al.: Pathophysiology of loosening of femoral components in total hip arthroplasty. Clinical and experimental study of cement fracture and loosening of cement-bone interface, in Hip, Proc Sixth Open Sci Mtg Hip Soc, CV Mosby Co, 1978.

Mow VC, Kuei SC, Lai WM, Armstrong CG: Biphasic creep and stress relaxation of articular cartilage in compression: Theory and experiments. J Biomech Eng 1980;102:73-84.

O'Driscoll SW, Keeley FW, Salter RB: The chondrogenic potential of free autogenous periosteal grafts for biological resurfacing of major full-thickness defects in joint surfaces under the influence of continuous passive motion: An experimental study in rabbit. J Bone Joint Surg 1986;68A:1017-1035.

O'Driscoll SW, Delaney JP, Salter RB: Experimental patellar resurfacing using periosteal autografts: Reasons for failure. Trans Orthop Res Soc 1989;14:145.

Ohlsen L, Widenfalk B: The early development of articular cartilage after perichondrial grafting. Scand J Plast Reconstr Surg 1983;17:163-177.

Olkarinen J: Experimental spinal fusion with decalcified bone matrix and deep frozen allogeneic bone in rabbits. Clin Orthop 1982;162:211-218.

Pastacaldi P, Engkvist O: Perichondrial wrist arthoplasty in rheumatoid patients. Hand 1979;11:184-190.

Reddi AH: Extracellular bone matrix dependent local induction of cartilage and bone. J Rheumatol 1983;10(suppl 11):67-69.

Rubak JM: Reconstruction of articular cartilage defects with free periosteal grafts: An experimental study. Acta Orthop Scand 1982;53:175-180.

Salter RB, Simmonds DF, Malcolm BW, et al.: The biological effect of continuous passive motion on the healing of full-thickness defects in articular cartilage. An experimental investigation in the rabbit. J Bone Joint Surg 1980;62A:1232-1251.

Sampath TK, DeSimone DP, Reddi AH: Extracellular bone matrix-derived growth factor. Exp Cell Res 1982;142:460-464.

Seradge H, Kutz JA, Kleinert HE, et al.: Perichondrial resurfacing arthroplasty in the hand. J Hand Surg 1984;9A:880-886.

Skoog T, Ohlsen L, Sohn SA: Perichondrial potential for cartilaginous regeneration. Scand J Plast Reconstr Surg 1972;6:123-125.

Skoog T, Ohlsen L, Sohn SA: Chondrogenic potential of perichondrium. Chir Plast (Berl) 1975;3:91-103.

Tizzone G: Sulla istologia normale e pathologisa delle cartilagini ialine. Arch Sci Med 1878;2:27-105.

Wasteson A, Ohlsen L: Biosynthesis of chondroitin sulphate in cartilage regenerated from perichondrium. Scand J Plast Reconstr Surg 1977;11:17-22.

Wittbjer J, Palmer B, Thorngren KG: Osteogenetic properties of reimplanted decalcified and undecalcified autologous bone in the rabbit radius. Scand J Plast Reconstr Surg 1982;16:239-244.

Chapter 15

Alternate Hybrid, Mixed, and Penalty Finite Element Formulations for the Biphasic Model of Soft Hydrated Tissues

R.L. Spilker, J-K. Suh, M.E. Vermilyea, T.A. Maxian

Introduction

It is widely accepted that soft connective tissues such as tendon, ligament, intervertebral disc, articular cartilage, and meniscus, are multiphasic materials, i.e. a mixture of collagen/elastin fibrils, water, glycosaminoglycans, glycoproteins, and cells. Based on this concept, Kenyon (1979) and Simon et al. (1985) used a classical consolidation theory of soil mechanics (Biot, 1962) to describe aortic tissue and intervertebral disk, respectively. As a more rigorous and theoretically versatile approach, Mow et al. (1980) used mixture theory (Truesdell and Toupin, 1960) to describe the deformation of articular cartilage. In their model, called the *biphasic theory*, Mow et al. assumed that soft hydrated tissue such as cartilage is a mixture of two immiscible constituents: an incompressible solid matrix and an incompressible interstitial fluid. This model has been shown to accurately describe both the stress distribution and interstitial fluid flow within soft hydrated tissue such as cartilage under various loading conditions (Armstrong, et al., 1984; Mow, et al., 1984; Mak, et al., 1987; Hou, et al., 1989). Moreover, the interaction between the solid and fluid phases has been identified to be responsible for the apparent viscoelastic properties in the compression of hydrated soft tissue (Mow, et al., 1984). The biphasic model has been extended to include nonlinear behaviors such as strain dependent permeability (Lai and Mow, 1980; Lai, et al., 1981; Holmes, et al., 1985) and finite deformation (Holmes, 1985; Mow, et al., 1986). Recently, Lai et al. (1989) have presented an extended version of the theory, called the *triphasic model*, to include the dissolved solute concentration which is known to be responsible for the Donnan osmotic pressure and swelling effect of the soft tissue.

These biphasic and triphasic models provide a versatile and rigorous framework to simulate the response of hydrated soft tissues. However for practical geometries and load distributions (indeed, for all but the most specialized geometries, load distributions, and boundary conditions), analytic solution is intractable, and numerical solutions are required. The finite element method is the most appropriate choice for such a formulation. Early development of finite element formulations for multiphase systems modeled using consolidation theory are found in the literature on soil mechanics. For example, Ghaboussi et al. (1973, 1978), Zienkiewicz et al. (1982, 1984), and Simon et al. (1986a, 1986b) have constructed finite element formulations corresponding to the linear poroelastic theory of Biot (1962), for the study of dynamic behavior of saturated soils. Simon et al. (1985) have also applied these formulations to the deformational behavior of the intervertebral disc and arterial walls with large deformations (Simon and Gaballa, 1988). Some applications of the finite element method to the theory of mixtures have also been reported. Among them, Prevost (1982, 1984, 1985) developed a fluid velocity - solid displacement formulation of a fluid-saturated soil mixture, in which the solid skeleton is assumed to be piecewise linear elasto-plastic so as to obey a rate-type constitutive equation. In the limit of incompressibility, that formulation is equivalent to a penalty method. Oomens et al. (1987) recently developed a mixed formulation of nonlinear mixture theory for the study of porcine skin, utilizing the continuity equation with the momentum equation of the fluid substituted, and the total momentum equation for the mixture.

In this chapter, we will examine three alternate finite element formulations for the biphasic equations that we have developed as part of our ongoing analysis of soft tissue components. A *penalty* formulation will be presented in which the continuity equation is replaced by a penalty form and used to eliminate the pressure variable prior to construction of the weak form. A *mixed-penalty* method is described in which the penalty form of the continuity equation is introduced into the weighted residual statement and the pressure is independently interpolated. Finally, a *hybrid* formulation is presented in which the momentum equation for the mixture is satisfied exactly and corresponding equilibrated weighting functions are used. Pressure variables are eliminated at the element level in the latter two approaches and the general form of the resulting matrix equations is identical in all three approaches. We will show via selected example problems that each of these approaches can produce accurate solutions. However, the mixed-penalty method is preferred over the penalty method for higher order elements, and the hybrid method has advantages overall (particularly for nonlinear problems) in that no penalty parameter need be specified.

Governing Equations for a Nonlinear Biphasic Mixture

The theory of mixtures can be applied to a multi-phase continuum with an arbitrary number of phases. However, for present purposes we focus on a two-phase mixture of solid and fluid, and define the governing equations accordingly. Consider two continuum bodies Ω^s and Ω^f in three dimensional space, where the superscripts s and f denote the solid and the fluid constituents, respectively. Let $\mathbf{X}^\alpha$ be the position of a particle of the α phase in its reference configuration (α = s, f). The current configuration of each body at the time t can be represented by the *deformation function* $\mathcal{X}^\alpha$; the current spatial position $\mathbf{x}^\alpha$ of the particle $\mathbf{X}^\alpha$ at the time t can be expressed as (Truesdell and Toupin, 1960),

$$\mathbf{x}^\alpha = \mathcal{X}^\alpha(\mathbf{X}^\alpha, t), \qquad \alpha = s, f. \tag{1}$$

Consider an apparent domain Ω of the soft tissue at time t in three dimensional space which coincides with the domain Ω^s of the solid phase (Figure 1). Let Γ denote the boundary of Ω, and let V denote the volume of Ω. Using the same reference axes for both $\mathbf{x}^\alpha$ and $\mathbf{X}^\alpha$, the deformed configuration of the solid phase can be written as

$$\mathbf{x}^s = \mathcal{X}^s(\mathbf{X}^s, t) = \mathbf{X}^s + \mathbf{u}^s(\mathbf{X}^s, t), \tag{2}$$

where $\mathbf{u}^s$ is the displacement of the solid phase. The velocity of a particle of each phase can be defined as the time derivative of the corresponding deformation function of Eq. (1).

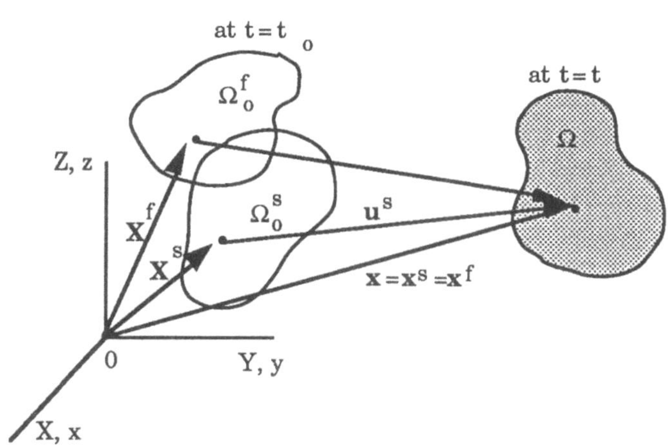

Figure 1. The kinematics of a biphasic material.

If we assume that the biphasic mixture is chemically inert, each phase is intrinsically incompressible, the solid phase is hyperelastic, and the fluid phase is inviscid, then the problem for a biphasic soft tissue can be posed for a given domain Ω as follows (Kwan, 1985; Holmes, 1985; Mow et al., 1986)
Continuity equation,

$$\nabla\bullet(\phi^s\mathbf{v}^s + \phi^f\mathbf{v}^f) = 0\,. \tag{3}$$

Momentum equations, neglecting inertia terms and body forces,

$$\nabla\bullet\boldsymbol{\sigma}^\alpha + \boldsymbol{\pi}^\alpha = \mathbf{0},\quad \alpha = s, f \tag{4}$$

Constitutive equations,

$$\boldsymbol{\sigma}^s = -\,\phi^s p\mathbf{I} + \boldsymbol{\sigma}_E^s\,, \tag{5}$$

$$\boldsymbol{\sigma}^f = -\,\phi^f p\mathbf{I}, \tag{6}$$

$$\boldsymbol{\pi}^s = -\,\boldsymbol{\pi}^f = -\,p\nabla\phi^f + K(\mathbf{v}^f - \mathbf{v}^s). \tag{7}$$

Here, ∇ is the gradient operator with respect to the current configuration, ϕ^α is the volume fraction of the α phase ($=V^\alpha/V$), $\mathbf{v}^\alpha$ is the velocity of the α phase, $\boldsymbol{\sigma}^\alpha$ is the Cauchy stress tensor for the α phase, $\boldsymbol{\pi}^\alpha$ is the diffusive momentum exchange between the two phases, p is the apparent pressure, $\mathbf{I}$ is the identity tensor, $\boldsymbol{\sigma}_E^s$ is the elastic Cauchy stress tensor of the solid phase, K is the scalar diffusive drag coefficient, and $\phi^s + \phi^f = 1$ is assumed corresponding to a saturated mixture. For a general nonlinear model, $\boldsymbol{\sigma}_E^s$ and K are defined as;

$$\boldsymbol{\sigma}_E^s = 2\rho^s\mathbf{F}^s\bullet\frac{\partial\Psi^s}{\partial\mathbf{C}^s}\bullet{\mathbf{F}^s}^T, \tag{8}$$

and

$$K = \frac{(\phi^f)^2}{\kappa}, \tag{9}$$

respectively, where Ψ^s is the Helmholtz free energy function of the solid phase, ρ^s is the apparent density of the solid phase, $\mathbf{F}^s = (\nabla_X \mathcal{X}^s)^T$ is the deformation gradient of the solid phase, $\mathbf{C}^s = {\mathbf{F}^s}^T\bullet\mathbf{F}^s$ is the right Cauchy-Green tensor of the solid phase, and κ is the permeability function. Here ∇_X denotes the gradient operator with respect to the reference configuration, and standard dyadic notation is used for tensorial operations.

The choice of the free energy function is not unique. Based upon experiments on bovine and human articular cartilage (Kwan, 1985) as well as certain constitutive requirements in multi-dimensional stress states (Truesdell and Noll, 1965), the free energy and the permeability functions† chosen for the present study are (Holmes, 1985; Holmes and Mow, 1990)

$$\Psi^s = \gamma\,\frac{\exp[\alpha_1(I_1-3)+\alpha_2(I_2-3)]}{I_3^n}, \tag{10}$$

and

$$\kappa = \kappa_o\left(\frac{J^s}{J^f}\right)^2 \exp[M(I_3-1)/2]\,, \tag{11}$$

† The notation used here for the permeability function differs from that used in Holmes (1986) and Holmes and Mow (1990) where k is used.

respectively, where I_1, I_2, and I_3 are the strain invariants; α_1, α_2, γ, n, κ_o, and M are material parameters; and J^s and J^f are the volume changes of each phase. From the intrinsic incompressibility of each phase, it can be shown that

$$\phi_o^\alpha = J^\alpha \phi^\alpha \ , \quad \alpha = s, f, \tag{12a}$$

and

$$\frac{1}{J^f} = \frac{1}{J^s} + \frac{1}{\phi_o^f}\left(1 - \frac{1}{J^s}\right), \tag{12b}$$

where the subscript $(\ )_o$ is used to denote a quantity at the reference configuration£.

The infinitesimal version of Eqs. (5-7) is referred to as the linear biphasic or KLM model, and can be written as follows (Mow, et al., 1980);

$$\boldsymbol{\sigma}^s = - \phi^s p\mathbf{I} + \lambda_s e^s \mathbf{I} + 2\mu_s \boldsymbol{\varepsilon}^s, \tag{13}$$

$$\boldsymbol{\sigma}^f = - \phi^f p\mathbf{I}, \tag{14}$$

$$\boldsymbol{\pi}^s = - \boldsymbol{\pi}^f = K(\mathbf{v}^f - \mathbf{v}^s), \tag{15}$$

where ϕ^f and ϕ^s have been assumed constant. λ_s and μ_s are Lamé constants of the solid phase, and e^s and $\boldsymbol{\varepsilon}^s$ are the dilatation and the infinitesimal strain tensor, respectively, of the solid phase. The permeability, κ in Eq. (11), can be reduced to either of the following;

Linear KLM model:

$$\kappa = \kappa_o, \tag{16a}$$

Nonlinear KLM model (Lai and Mow, 1980):

$$\kappa = \kappa_o \exp(Me^s). \tag{16b}$$

To complete the initial-boundary value problem, the following boundary conditions are added:

$$\mathbf{x}^s(\mathbf{X}^s,t) = \bar{\mathbf{h}}^s \quad \text{for } \mathbf{x}^s \in \Gamma_{h^s} \tag{17}$$

$$\mathbf{v}^f(\mathbf{X}^f,t) = \dot{\bar{\mathbf{h}}}^f \quad \text{for } \mathbf{x}^f \in \Gamma_{h^f} \tag{18}$$

$$\mathbf{n}\cdot\boldsymbol{\sigma}^s = \bar{\mathbf{t}}^s \quad \text{for } \mathbf{x}^s \in \Gamma_{t^s} \tag{19}$$

$$\mathbf{n}\cdot\boldsymbol{\sigma}^f = \bar{\mathbf{t}}^f \ (\text{ or } p = \bar{p}\ ) \quad \text{for } \mathbf{x}^f \in \Gamma_{t^f} \tag{20}$$

and a set of appropriate initial conditions can be defined for each phase at time t=0. Here, $\overline{(\ )}$ represents a prescribed value of the quantity ( ), so that $\bar{\mathbf{h}}^s$, $\dot{\bar{\mathbf{h}}}^f$, $\bar{\mathbf{t}}^s$, and $\bar{\mathbf{t}}^f$ represent prescribed solid displacement, fluid velocity, traction on the solid phase, and traction on the fluid phase, respectively. The outward normal

£ An exception to this convention is found in the parameters used to describe the applied ramp displacement in stress relaxation.

vector to Γ is denoted by $\mathbf{n}$, and Γ_{hs}, Γ_{hf}, Γ_{ts}, and Γ_{tf} are portions of the boundary, Γ, on which solid displacement, fluid velocity, solid traction, and fluid traction (or fluid pressure), respectively, are prescribed.

Mixed-Penalty and Penalty Methods for Nonlinear Biphasic Analysis

In the mixed-penalty and penalty formulations, the continuity equation, Eq. (3), is replaced by

$$\nabla \cdot (\phi^s \mathbf{v}^s + \phi^f \mathbf{v}^f) + \frac{p}{\beta} = 0 \,, \tag{21}$$

where β is a user-specified penalty parameter. Notice that as β approaches infinity, the continuity equation is satisfied exactly, and p calculated from Eq. (21) is the correct pressure -- β could be interpreted as the bulk modulus. Since the actual value of β cannot be infinite in the context of a numerical computation, this penalty expression amounts to allowing a perturbed compressibility. This form of the penalty method has been applied to single phase materials such as Stokes flow (Bercovier and Engelman, 1979; Hughes, et al., 1979; Oden, et al., 1982) and incompressible elasticity (Bercovier, et al., 1981), and to multiphase materials such as soil (Prevost, 1985).

We can implement the penalty formulation of Eq. (21) in two ways. One approach is to substitute p from Eq. (21) directly into the constitutive equations, Eqs. (5-7) or (13-15), to eliminate the pressure p from the governing equations. This approach requires special treatment of the penalty term in the element matrix expressions using methods such as selectively reduced integration (Malkus and Hughes, 1978). We refer to this approach as the *penalty* method. The other is to use a mixed formulation in which the penalty form of the continuity equation and the momentum equations are introduced via the weighted residual method (Engelman, et al., 1982; Spilker and Maxian, 1990), and the pressure becomes an independent variable. Because the pressure in this approach can be discontinuous between elements, the coefficients in the pressure interpolation can be eliminated at the element level. Therefore, this approach will require more computational effort at the element level than the standard penalty method with selective reduced integration. Engelman *et al.* (1982) have shown that the latter approach, which they call a consistent mixed-penalty method, is more accurate in general. We refer to this approach as the *mixed-penalty* method.

Derivation of the Finite Element Equations for the Mixed-Penalty Method

We will derive in this subsection the finite element equations corresponding to the mixed-penalty method. In a later subsection, the equations corresponding to the penalty method will be easily extracted by modification of the results to be derived here. The weak form of the biphasic problem, which forms the starting point for the construction of the finite element equations, will be derived using the weighted residual method; details of this approach can be found in many texts on finite element methods (e.g. Hughes, 1987).

Let $\mathcal{V}^s$ and $\mathcal{V}^f$ be spaces of arbitrary admissible test functions ($\in \mathbb{R}^3$) for the solid and fluid phases, which are C^0 continuous over Ω, and zero on Γ_{hs} and Γ_{hf}, respectively (i.e., they satisfy boundary conditions equivalent to the homogeneous part of the essential boundary conditions, Eqs. (17) and (18)). Let $\mathcal{V}^p$ be the space of arbitrary admissible test functions ($\in \mathbb{R}^3$) for the pressure, which are C^{-1} continuous over Ω. The momentum equation, Eq. (4), penalty form of the continuity condition, Eq. (21), and natural boundary conditions, Eqs. (19) and (20), are introduced into the weighted residual statement to give

$$\int_\Omega \delta\mathcal{X}^s \cdot [\nabla \cdot \sigma_E^s - \phi^s \nabla p - K(\mathbf{v}^s - \mathbf{v}^f)]\, d\Omega + \int_{\Gamma_{ts}} \delta\mathcal{X}^s \cdot (\bar{\mathbf{t}}^s - \mathbf{n} \cdot \sigma^s)\, d\Gamma$$

$$+ \int_\Omega \delta\mathcal{X}^f \cdot [- \phi^f \nabla p + K(\mathbf{v}^s - \mathbf{v}^f)]\, d\Omega - \int_{\Gamma_{tf}} \delta\mathcal{X}^f \cdot \phi^f (\bar{p} - p)\, \mathbf{n}\, d\Gamma$$

$$+ \int_\Omega \delta w^p [\nabla \cdot (\phi^s \mathbf{v}^s + \phi^f \mathbf{v}^f) + \frac{p}{\beta}]\, d\Omega = 0 \qquad (22)$$

where, in the Galerkin weighted residual method, the variation in the deformation function defined in Eq. (1) is chosen to be the test function, or weighting function, so that $\delta\mathcal{X}^s \in \mathcal{V}^s$ and $\delta\mathcal{X}^f \in \mathcal{V}^f$. The weighting function of the continuity equation is chosen so that $\delta w^p \in \mathcal{V}^p$.

Since Ω and Γ in the above weighted residual statement correspond to the current configuration, they are time-dependent and, therefore, unknown. In this case, the total Lagrangian formulation can be used (e.g. Bathe, 1982), where the integrations in Eq. (22) are referred to the reference configuration at initial time t=0 by the relationships;

$$d\Omega = J^s\, d\Omega_o, \quad \text{and} \quad \mathbf{n} d\Gamma = J^s\, \mathbf{n}_o \cdot (\mathbf{F}^s)^{-1}\, d\Gamma_o. \qquad (23)$$

Here, $\mathbf{n}_o$ is the outward normal vector to Γ_o. Also it is preferable to use the Lagrangian strain, $\mathbf{E}^s$, and the second Piola-Kirchhoff stress, $\mathbf{S}_E^s$, defined as

$$\mathbf{E}^s = \frac{1}{2}[\mathbf{C}^s - \mathbf{I}] \text{ and } \mathbf{S}_E^s = J^s (\mathbf{F}^s)^{-1} \cdot \sigma_E^s \cdot (\mathbf{F}^s)^{-T} = \rho_o^s \frac{\partial \Psi^s}{\partial \mathbf{E}^s}, \qquad (24)$$

respectively.

With the use of the divergence theorem, the relations that $\delta\mathcal{X}^s = \delta\mathbf{u}^s$ from Eq. (2), and the above definitions and transformations, the following *weak form* can be obtained (Suh, 1989):

$$\int_{\Omega_o} \delta \mathbf{u}^s \cdot \mathrm{K}(\mathbf{v}^s - \mathbf{v}^f)\, J^s\, d\Omega_o - \int_{\Omega_o} p[(\mathbf{F}^s)^{-T} \cdot \nabla_{\mathbf{X}}] \cdot (\phi^s \delta \mathbf{u}^s) J^s\, d\Omega_o$$

$$- \int_{\Omega_o} \delta \mathcal{X}^f \cdot \mathrm{K}(\mathbf{v}^s - \mathbf{v}^f)\, J^s\, d\Omega_o - \int_{\Omega_o} p[(\mathbf{F}^s)^{-T} \cdot \nabla_{\mathbf{X}}] \cdot (\phi^f \delta \mathcal{X}^f) J^s\, d\Omega_o$$

$$+ \int_{\Omega_o} \delta w^p \{ [(\mathbf{F}^s)^{-T} \cdot \nabla_{\mathbf{X}}] \cdot (\phi^s \mathbf{v}^s + \phi^f \mathbf{v}^f) + \frac{p}{\beta} \}\, d\Omega_o + \int_{\Omega_o} \delta \mathbf{E}^s : \mathbf{S}_E^s\, d\Omega_o$$

$$= \int_{\Gamma_{t^s_o}} \delta \mathbf{u}^s \cdot \bar{\mathbf{t}}^s J_a^s\, d\Gamma_o - \int_{\Gamma_{t^f_o}} \delta \mathcal{X}^f \cdot \phi^f \bar{p}\, \mathbf{n}_o \cdot (\mathbf{F}^s)^{-1} J^s\, d\Gamma_o\,, \tag{25}$$

where J_a^s is the area ratio defined from Eq. (23) as

$$d\Gamma = J_a^s\, d\Gamma_o = J^s \sqrt{\mathbf{n}_o \cdot (\mathbf{C}^s)^{-1} \cdot \mathbf{n}_o}\; d\Gamma_o \tag{26}$$

The corresponding finite element weak form of Eq. (25) can be obtained by subdividing the continuum into elements of domain Ω_n and boundary Γ_n. Within a typical element, the deformation functions for the solid and fluid phases are interpolated in matrix form§ in terms of corresponding sets of nodal values. The pressure and corresponding weighting function, w^p, are interpolated in terms of pressure and weighting parameters. These interpolations are in the form;

$$\mathcal{X}^s = \mathbf{N}^s \hat{\mathcal{X}}_n^s \;(\text{ or } \mathbf{u}^s = \mathbf{N}^s \hat{\mathbf{u}}_n^s\,)\,, \quad \mathbf{v}^s = \mathbf{N}^s \hat{\mathbf{v}}_n^s\,,$$

$$\mathcal{X}^f = \mathbf{N}^f \hat{\mathcal{X}}_n^f\,, \quad \mathbf{v}^f = \mathbf{N}^f \hat{\mathbf{v}}_n^f\,,$$

$$p = \mathbf{N}^p \hat{\mathbf{p}}_n\,, \quad w^p = \mathbf{N}^p \hat{\mathbf{w}}_n^p\,, \tag{27}$$

where $\hat{(\,)}_n$ denotes the vector of corresponding nodal quantities for the typical element n, and $\mathbf{N}^s$ and $\mathbf{N}^f$ are matrices of C^o interpolation functions. For our applications we utilize the same order of approximation for the solid and fluid phases: that is, $\mathbf{N}^s = \mathbf{N}^f = \mathbf{N}$ in Eq. (27). Notice that the interpolation functions, $\mathbf{N}^p$, for the C^{-1} pressure and weighting function are identical. With the use of Eqs. (27), the finite element weak form, Eq. (25), can be discretized in

§ Subsequent equations associated with the finite element approximation will be presented in a matrix/vector notation: first and second order tensors can be represented by the equivalent vectors and matrices, respectively.

terms of the solid and fluid nodal displacements (or deformations) and velocities, and the pressure coefficients as follows:

$$\sum_{n=1}^{n_{et}} \{ [\delta\hat{\mathbf{u}}_n^{\,T}, \delta\hat{\mathbf{w}}_n^{pT}] \begin{bmatrix} \Xi_{2n} & \mathbf{0} \\ -\mathbf{A}_n & \mathbf{0} \end{bmatrix} \begin{Bmatrix} \dot{\hat{\mathbf{v}}}_n \\ \hat{\mathbf{p}}_n \end{Bmatrix} +$$

$$[\delta\hat{\mathbf{u}}_n^{\,T}, \delta\hat{\mathbf{w}}_n^{pT}] \begin{bmatrix} \mathbf{0} & -\mathbf{A}_n^T \\ \mathbf{0} & -\frac{1}{\beta}\mathbf{k}_n^p \end{bmatrix} \begin{Bmatrix} \hat{\mathbf{u}}_n \\ \hat{\mathbf{p}}_n \end{Bmatrix} + \int_{\Omega_{no}} \delta\mathbf{E}^s : \mathbf{S}_E^s \, d\Omega_o \}$$

$$= \sum_{n=1}^{n_{et}} [\delta\hat{\mathbf{u}}_n^{\,T}, \delta\hat{\mathbf{w}}_n^{pT}] \begin{Bmatrix} \mathbf{f}_n^e \\ \mathbf{0} \end{Bmatrix} , \tag{28}$$

where

$$\hat{\mathbf{u}}_n = [\ \hat{\mathbf{u}}_n^s\ ,\ \hat{\mathcal{X}}_n^f\ ]^T , \quad \hat{\mathbf{v}}_n = [\ \hat{\mathbf{v}}_n^s\ ,\ \hat{\mathbf{v}}_n^f\ ]^T, \tag{29}$$

$$\Xi_{2n} = \begin{bmatrix} \Xi_4 & -\Xi_4 \\ -\Xi_4 & \Xi_4 \end{bmatrix} , \quad \Xi_4 = \int_{\Omega_{no}} K\, \mathbf{N}^T \mathbf{N}\, J^s\, d\Omega_o \, , \tag{30a,b}$$

$$\mathbf{A}_n = [\ \mathbf{A}^s , \mathbf{A}^f\ ] , \quad \mathbf{A}^\alpha = \int_{\Omega_{no}} \mathbf{N}\mathrm{p}^T \mathbf{B}^\alpha\, J^s\, d\Omega_o, \quad \alpha = s\ , f \tag{31a,b}$$

$$\mathbf{k}_n^p = \int_{\Omega_{no}} \mathbf{N}\mathrm{p}^T \mathbf{N}\mathrm{p}\, J^s\, d\Omega_o \, , \tag{32}$$

$$\mathbf{f}_n^e = \begin{Bmatrix} \displaystyle\int_{\Gamma_{ts_{no}}} \mathbf{N}^T\, \bar{\mathbf{t}}^s\, J_a^s\, d\Gamma_o \\ \displaystyle -\int_{\Gamma_{tf_{no}}} \phi^f\, \bar{p}\, \mathbf{N}^T\, (\mathbf{F}^s)^{-T}\, \mathbf{n}_o\, J^s\, d\Gamma_o \end{Bmatrix} . \tag{33}$$

Here n_{et} is the total number of elements, and $\mathbf{B}^\alpha$ is the equivalent row vector associated with the gradient operator $(\mathbf{F}^s)^{-1}:\nabla_{\mathbf{X}}(\phi^\alpha \mathbf{v}^\alpha)$ and has the form

$$\mathbf{B}^\alpha = [\ \mathbf{B}_1^\alpha, \mathbf{B}_2^\alpha, \ldots\ , \mathbf{B}_a^\alpha, \ldots], \qquad a = 1, 2, \ldots\ , N_{npe} \tag{34a}$$

where N_{npe} is the number of nodes per element. The row vector, $\mathbf{B}^{\alpha}_{a}$, corresponds to the ath node in an element so that

$$[\mathbf{B}^{\alpha}_{a}]_i = \frac{\partial X^s_I}{\partial x^s_i} \frac{\partial(\phi^{\alpha} N_a)}{\partial X^s_I} . \tag{34b}$$

The subscripts i and I refer to the current and reference configurations, respectively.

Because pressure is discontinuous between elements, we can eliminate the pressure coefficients, $\hat{\mathbf{p}}_n$, at the element level by using the last equation in Eq. (28) :

$$\hat{\mathbf{p}}_n = -\beta\, [\mathbf{k}^p_n]^{-1} \left[\mathbf{A}^s \hat{\mathbf{v}}^s_n + \mathbf{A}^f \hat{\mathbf{v}}^f_n \right] \tag{35}$$

Substituting Eq. (35) into Eq. (28) produces the final set of matrix equations for the mixed-penalty formulation:

$$\sum_{n=1}^{n_{el}} \{\delta\hat{\mathbf{u}}_n^T [\beta\Xi_{1n} + \Xi_{2n}]\, \hat{\mathbf{v}}_n + \int_{\Omega_{no}} \delta\mathbf{E}^s{:}\mathbf{S}^s_E\, d\Omega_o\} = \sum_{n=1}^{n_{el}} \delta\hat{\mathbf{u}}_n^T \mathbf{f}^e_n , \tag{36}$$

where

$$\Xi_{1n} = \mathbf{A}_n^T [\mathbf{k}^p_n]^{-1} \mathbf{A}_n . \tag{37}$$

Standard assembly operations can be performed to sum up the contribution of each element. Since $\delta\mathbf{u}^s$ and $\delta\chi^f$, and therefore $\delta\hat{\mathbf{u}}_n$ and $\delta\mathbf{E}^s$, can be arbitrary (and nonzero except on $\Gamma_{h^s_o}$ and $\Gamma_{h^f_o}$, respectively), the following global system of matrix equations is produced

$$\Xi\, \hat{\mathbf{v}} + \mathbf{g} = \mathbf{f}^e, \tag{38}$$

where $\Xi=[\beta\Xi_1 + \Xi_2]$, $\hat{\mathbf{v}}$ is the global vector of the velocities defined in Eq. (29), and Ξ_1, Ξ_2, and $\mathbf{f}^e$ are the assembled matrices for the soft tissue continuum. The assembled vector function, $\mathbf{g}$, is the contribution of the nonlinear elasticity of the solid phase. A detailed expression for $\mathbf{g}$ will be presented in the next subsection. The equilibrium relation, Eq. (38), for the tissue must be satisfied at all times throughout the deformation.

Incremental Linearization of the Solid-Phase Elasticity

The terms defined in Eq. (38) (or Eq. (36)) cannot be directly evaluated because the integrals for Ξ_1, Ξ_2, and $\mathbf{f}^e$ are functions of the current configuration, which in turn should satisfy the equilibrium relation, Eq. (38), throughout the response history. However, the integrations can be approximated within each time increment with the use of alternative numerical methods (Oden, 1972).

With the assumption that the solution at time t is known, the solid displacement at time t+Δt can be estimated as

$$\mathbf{u}^{s}_{t+\Delta t} = \mathbf{u}^{s}_{t} + \Delta\mathbf{u}^{s} \ . \tag{39}$$

The contributions to the nonlinear solid phase strains and stresses, Eq. (36), can be linearized within a small time increment between t and t+Δt as follows :

$$\mathbf{E}^{s}_{t+\Delta t} = \mathbf{E}^{s}_{t} + \Delta\mathbf{E}^{s}, \text{ and } \mathbf{S}^{s}_{E_{t+\Delta t}} \approx \mathbf{S}^{s}_{E_t} + \mathcal{L} :\Delta\mathbf{E}^{s} , \tag{40a,b}$$

where

$$\mathcal{L} = \rho^{s}_{o} \frac{\partial^2 \Psi^s}{\partial \mathbf{E}^s \partial \mathbf{E}^s} \ . \tag{40c}$$

Here $\mathcal{L}$ is the fourth order tensor of instantaneous tangent stiffness moduli, which is symmetric and positive-definite if Ψ^s is a convex function.

In order to relate $\Delta\mathbf{E}^s$ in Eqs. (40) to $\Delta\mathbf{u}^s$, we can decompose the strain into the linear and nonlinear components as follows :

$$\Delta\mathbf{E}^{s} = \Delta\mathbf{E}^{s}_{L} + \Delta\mathbf{E}^{s}_{NL} , \tag{41}$$

where

$$\Delta\mathbf{E}^{s}_{L} = \frac{1}{2}\left[\nabla_{\mathbf{X}}\Delta\mathbf{u}^{s} + (\nabla_{\mathbf{X}}\Delta\mathbf{u}^{s})^{T} + \nabla_{\mathbf{X}}\Delta\mathbf{u}^{s}\cdot(\nabla_{\mathbf{X}}\mathbf{u}^{s}_{t})^{T} + \nabla_{\mathbf{X}}\mathbf{u}^{s}_{t}\cdot(\nabla_{\mathbf{X}}\Delta\mathbf{u}^{s})^{T}\right] ,$$

$$\Delta\mathbf{E}^{s}_{NL} = \frac{1}{2}\nabla_{\mathbf{X}}\Delta\mathbf{u}^{s}\cdot(\nabla_{\mathbf{X}}\Delta\mathbf{u}^{s})^{T} \ . \tag{42a,b}$$

Using the same interpolation functions as Eq. (27), $\Delta\mathbf{E}^{s}_{L}$ and $\nabla_{\mathbf{X}}\Delta\mathbf{u}^{s}$ in Eqs. (42) can be related to the vector of nodal displacement increments through the linear and nonlinear strain-displacement matrices, $\mathbf{B}_L$ and $\mathbf{B}_{NL}$, as defined in Bathe (1982);

$$\Delta\mathbf{E}^{s}_{L} = \mathbf{B}_{L}\,\Delta\hat{\mathbf{u}}^{s}_{n} , \text{ and } \nabla_{\mathbf{X}}\Delta\mathbf{u}^{s} = \mathbf{B}_{NL}\,\Delta\hat{\mathbf{u}}^{s}_{n} \ . \tag{43}$$

Now that the solution at time t is assumed to be known, $\delta\mathbf{E}^{s}_{t+\Delta t} = \delta\Delta\mathbf{E}^{s}$ and $\delta\hat{\mathbf{u}}^{s}_{t+\Delta t} = \delta\Delta\hat{\mathbf{u}}^{s}$. Therefore, substitution of Eqs. (40-43) into Eq. (36) and standard assembly operation yields the incrementally linearized version of Eq. (38) at time t+Δt as follows:

$$\Xi_{t+\Delta t}\,\hat{\mathbf{v}}_{t+\Delta t} + \mathbf{g}_{t} + \mathbf{K}_{t}\,\Delta\hat{\mathbf{u}} = \mathbf{f}^{e}_{t+\Delta t} \tag{44}$$

where

$$\mathbf{g} = \begin{Bmatrix} \mathbf{g}^{s} \\ \mathbf{0} \end{Bmatrix} , \text{ and } \mathbf{K} = \begin{bmatrix} \mathbf{K}^{s}_{L} + \mathbf{K}^{s}_{NL} & \mathbf{0} \\ \mathbf{0} & \mathbf{0} \end{bmatrix} . \tag{45a,b}$$

$$\mathbf{g}_n^s = \mathbf{g}_n^s(\mathbf{S}_E^s) = \int_{\Omega_{no}} \mathbf{B}_L^T \mathbf{S}_E^s \, d\Omega_o , \tag{45c}$$

$$\mathbf{K}_{Ln}^s = \int_{\Omega_{no}} \mathbf{B}_L^T \mathcal{L} \mathbf{B}_L \, d\Omega_o , \text{ and } \mathbf{K}_{NLn}^s = \int_{\Omega_{no}} \mathbf{B}_{NL}^T \, \tilde{\mathbf{S}}_E^s \mathbf{B}_{NL} \, d\Omega_o . \tag{45d,e}$$

Here, $\Delta\hat{\mathbf{u}}$ is the assembled incremental displacement vector, and $\mathbf{g}^s$, $\mathbf{K}_L^s$, and $\mathbf{K}_{NL}^s$ are the assembled matrices of the corresponding element matrices, $\mathbf{g}_n^s$, $\mathbf{K}_{Ln}^s$, and $\mathbf{K}_{NLn}^s$, respectively. $\mathbf{g}_n^s$ is a vector function of the second Piola-Kirchhoff stress at time t, which corresponds to the contribution of the solid phase elasticity at time t. $\mathbf{K}_{Ln}^s$ and $\mathbf{K}_{NLn}^s$ are the contributions from the linear instantaneous tangent stiffness moduli and the geometrical nonlinearity associated with finite deformation of the solid phase, respectively. Notice that the solid phase elasticity terms, $\mathbf{g}^s$, are evaluated at the previous time step.

Solution of the Governing Equations

The system of first order differential equations in time, given by Eq. (44), can be solved using finite difference techniques. Given a known solution at time t, we use the generalized trapezoidal family of first order difference rules to estimate the velocity and displacement at time t+Δt as follows ;

$$\hat{\mathbf{v}}_{t+\Delta t} = \hat{\mathbf{v}}_t + \Delta\hat{\mathbf{v}} , \tag{46a}$$

$$\hat{\mathbf{u}}_{t+\Delta t} = \hat{\mathbf{u}}_t + \Delta\hat{\mathbf{u}} \tag{46b}$$

where

$$\Delta\hat{\mathbf{u}} = \Delta t \, \hat{\mathbf{v}}_t + \omega \, \Delta t \, \Delta\hat{\mathbf{v}} , \tag{46c}$$

The parameter ω is chosen by the user in the range $0 \le \omega \le 1$: for example, the case ω=0.5 is called the central difference (or Crank-Nicolson) scheme.

Substituting Eqs. (46) into Eq. (44) leads to the following predictor-corrector iterative scheme, by which the equilibrium solution can be obtained iteratively within each time increment between t and t+Δt (i is the iteration number). When i=1,

$$\hat{\mathbf{v}}_{t+\Delta t}^{(i-1)} \equiv \hat{\mathbf{v}}_t . \tag{47}$$

Predictor stage :

$$\hat{\mathbf{v}}_{t+\Delta t}^{(i)} = \hat{\mathbf{v}}_{t+\Delta t}^{(i-1)}, \tag{48}$$

$$\hat{\mathbf{u}}^{(i)}_{t+\Delta t} = \hat{\mathbf{u}}_t + \Delta t\, \hat{\mathbf{v}}^{(i-1)}_{t+\Delta t} . \tag{49}$$

Solution stage :

$$[\Xi_t + \omega\, \Delta t\, \mathbf{K}_t]\, \Delta\hat{\mathbf{v}}^{(i)} = \mathbf{f}^{e}_{t+\Delta t} - \Xi^{(i)}_{t+\Delta t}\, \hat{\mathbf{v}}^{(i)}_{t+\Delta t} - \mathbf{g}^{(i)}_{t+\Delta t}. \tag{50}$$

Corrector stage :

$$\hat{\mathbf{v}}^{(i)}_{t+\Delta t} = \hat{\mathbf{v}}^{(i)}_{t+\Delta t} + \Delta\hat{\mathbf{v}}^{(i)} , \tag{51}$$

$$\hat{\mathbf{u}}^{(i)}_{t+\Delta t} = \hat{\mathbf{u}}^{(i)}_{t+\Delta t} + \omega\, \Delta t\, \Delta\hat{\mathbf{v}}^{(i)}. \tag{52}$$

Notice that the right hand side of Eq. (50) is equivalent to the out-of-balance residual prior to calculation of the equilibrium solution, Eq. (38), at the ith iteration. Also notice that a modified Newton-Raphson method is used in Eq. (50) for computational efficiency. The iteration continues until the following convergence criterion is satisfied;

$$\frac{|\, \Delta\hat{\mathbf{v}}^{(i)} |}{|\, \Delta\hat{\mathbf{v}}^{(1)} |} < \mathrm{TOL} , \tag{53}$$

where TOL is a user specified tolerance, e.g. $\mathrm{TOL}=10^{-2}$.

Finite Element Equations for the Penalty Method

In the *penalty* finite element method, the penalty form of the continuity equation, Eq. (21), can be solved for pressure, p, and substituted into the constitutive equations to eliminate the pressure as an independent variable (Suh et al., 1990). The derivation of the weak form based on the weighted residual method, and subsequent finite element formulation, leads to a resultant matrix equation which is identical to Eq. (36) except that

$$\Xi_{1n} = \begin{bmatrix} \Xi^{ss}_3 & \Xi^{sf}_3 \\ \Xi^{fs}_3 & \Xi^{ff}_3 \end{bmatrix} , \tag{54a}$$

$$\Xi^{\alpha\beta}_3 = \int_{\Omega_{no}} \mathbf{B}^{\alpha T}\, \mathbf{B}^{\beta} \mathbf{J}^{s}\, d\Omega_o , \quad \alpha, \beta = s, f , \tag{54b}$$

and all other terms are as defined previously.

Treatment of the Constraint Conditions

In any constrained media problem it is important that the proper set of constraints be imposed on the approximate solution, but that these conditions not produce excessive constraint (a phenomenon usually referred to as locking). In the mixed-penalty formulation, the number and form of the constraints corresponding to the continuity equation is controlled by the pressure interpolation. If the order of the interpolation is too high, then excessive constraints on the velocity fields will lead to an unacceptable velocity solution. Using incompressible flow problems as a guide, we expect that an appropriate pressure interpolation will be about one order lower than the velocity interpolation.

When penalty methods are used for constrained media problems, the number of constraints is related to the number of integration stations used to evaluate the penalty terms. Often, the use of an "exact" integration rule leads to locking. For the present application of the penalty method, selective reduced integration is used (reduced integration applied only to the penalty term -- in this case, Ξ_{1n}). When selective reduced integration is used for a plane 2-D or 3-D element, it can be shown that the constraint condition is enforced at the numerical integration stations, and that the constraint is satisfied in the mean sense for the element. For an axisymmetric element, however, the constraint condition can be satisfied in the mean sense by the mean dilatation formulation (Suh et al., 1990), analogous to that given by Nagtegaal *et al.* (1974);

$$\Xi_3^{\alpha\beta} = \frac{\tilde{\mathbf{B}}^{\alpha T}\,\tilde{\mathbf{B}}^{\beta}}{V_{no}}, \tag{55a}$$

where

$$\tilde{\mathbf{B}}^{\alpha} = \int_{\Omega_{no}} \mathbf{B}^{\alpha}\, J^s d\Omega_o \quad \text{and} \quad V_{no} = \int_{\Omega_{no}} J^s\, d\Omega_o\,. \tag{55b}$$

The equivalence between the mixed-penalty method and the penalty method with the mean dilatation formulation was examined for an axisymmetric four node quadrilateral element in Spilker and Maxian (1990).

In principle, the user-specified penalty parameter should be an arbitrarily large number. For a computer with a finite number of digits, however, it should be large enough to enforce the constraint condition, but not so large that the governing equations become ill-conditioned. For 64 bit double precision calculations, it has been generally suggested that the ratio, Θ, of the penalty term, $\beta\Xi_1$, to the other terms be in the range $\Theta=10^6$-10^{10}. An initial estimate of the magnitude of β can be obtained as (Spilker and Suh, 1990) $\beta=\Theta\tau_o H_A/\phi$, where $\phi=\phi^s$ or ϕ^f, H_A is the equivalent aggregate modulus, and τ_o is a characteristic time such as the ramp time. Alternately, we can estimate the required magnitude of β using a round-off parameter which is calculated during the triple-factorization of the coefficient matrix $[\Xi_t + \omega \Delta t \mathbf{K}]$ in Eq. (50). In the present program, the ratio of the diagonal term in the triple factored coefficient matrix to the value of the corresponding diagonal term in the original coefficient matrix is calculated for each row of the coefficient matrix. The round-off parameter indicates the minimum value of these ratios. Our numerical experience suggests that a properly chosen β produces a round-off parameter of the order of Θ^{-1}. Thus β can be automatically adjusted in the program until this condition is approximately satisfied; this is particularly useful in the solution of finite deformation problems.

Mixed-Penalty and Penalty Methods for Biphasic Mixtures with Infinitesimal Strains

In some problems it may be adequate to use the infinitesimal biphasic model, Eqs. (13-15), for a hydrated soft tissue. In this case, the governing finite element equation can be significantly simplified to

$$\Xi\ \hat{\mathbf{v}} + \mathbf{K}\ \hat{\mathbf{u}} = \mathbf{f}^e. \tag{56}$$

The matrices Ξ and $\mathbf{K}$ for the mixed-penalty method are defined in Spilker and Maxian (1990); from Eqs. (16), Ξ is either constant for the linear KLM model, or dependent on the strain of the solid phase for the nonlinear KLM model, and $\mathbf{K}$ is constant for both cases. The matrices Ξ and $\mathbf{K}$ for the penalty method are defined in Spilker and Suh (1990).

Using the same finite difference scheme, Eq. (56) can be written in a recursive form between time t and t+Δt as before. For the linear KLM model, Eq. (16a),

$$[\Xi + \omega\, \Delta t\, \mathbf{K}]\, \Delta\hat{\mathbf{v}} = \mathbf{f}^{e}_{t+\Delta t} - \Xi\, \hat{\mathbf{v}}_t - \mathbf{K}\, \hat{\mathbf{u}}_t. \tag{57}$$

Here, Eq. (57) can be solved for each time step without iteration. For the nonlinear KLM model, Eq. (16b), a predictor-corrector iterative scheme similar to Eqs. (47-52) can be constructed

$$[\Xi_t + \omega\, \Delta t\, \mathbf{K}]\, \Delta\hat{\mathbf{v}}^{(i)} = \mathbf{f}^{e}_{t+\Delta t} - \Xi^{(i)}_{t+\Delta t}\, \hat{\mathbf{v}}^{(i)}_{t+\Delta t} - \mathbf{K}\, \hat{\mathbf{u}}^{(i)}_{t+\Delta t}. \tag{58}$$

Notice that Eqs. (50), (57), and (58) are identical in form; we can take advantage of this fact to combine the finite deformation, nonlinear strain-dependent permeability, and linear models into a single program.

The Hybrid Model for Biphasic Mixtures with Infinitesimal Strains

Hybrid finite element formulations for constrained media problems such as incompressible materials (Lee and Pian, 1976; Spilker, 1981), incompressible flows (Atluri, et al., 1981; Bratianu and Atluri, 1983; Ying and Atluri, 1983), and plate theories including transverse shear (e.g. Mau, et al., 1972; Nishioka and Atluri, 1980; Spilker, 1982) have been quite successful and are generally found to be more accurate and less susceptible to numerical ill-conditioning than penalty methods. This advantage is especially important in nonlinear problems where the constraint condition (e.g. incompressibility) can lead to difficulties in convergence in some cases. To date, we have had no difficulties with the penalty formulations of the biphasic problem. However, the care which must be exercised in selecting an appropriate value for the penalty parameter for nonlinear problems suggests that the elimination of the penalty parameter is advantageous. We therefore believe that the most robust formulation for the biphasic problem will be of the hybrid type.

All hybrid formulations are multi-field approximations, usually involving both a kinetic variable (e.g. stress) and a kinematic variable (e.g. displacement). One of the distinguishing characteristics of a hybrid formulation, which differentiates it from a mixed formulation, is the fact that the kinetic variable satisfies the appropriate governing differential equation (e.g. the linear momentum equation). In addition, the kinetic parameters (e.g. stress parameters) can be eliminated at the element level. Most formulations of hybrid methods are based on weak forms which are derived from variational principles. The equations defining such formulations can also be derived using the weighted residual method by proper choice of the weighting functions. We will present in this section a hybrid formulation for the linear biphasic equations, Eqs. (3), (4), (13-15), which is derived from a weighted residual formulation.

Derivation of the Finite Element Equations

In deriving the final matrix equations for a typical time-dependent problem, a spatial approximation is constructed using the finite element method, and the temporal approximation is then obtained using the finite difference method. In order to derive the present hybrid formulation, we have *reversed* this order. First, the finite difference rule is applied to the solid phase displacement. Using the Generalized Trapezoidal family of finite difference rules (rearranged from Eqs. (46)), the displacement at time t_m in terms of the displacement at time t_{m-1} and the velocities at these times may be represented as:

$$\mathbf{u}^s = \hat{\mathbf{u}}^s + (1-\omega)\,\Delta t\,\hat{\mathbf{v}}^s + \omega\,\Delta t\,\mathbf{v}^s \tag{59}$$

In the notation used in this section, variables refer to the current time, t_m, except for those with an over-strike ($\hat{\ }$) which denote values at the previous time step, t_{m-1}. The parameter ω will be constrained to lie between 0.5 and 1.0 for this analysis; this range leads to implicit methods which are known to ensure unconditional stability of the time solution.

The weighted residual statement of the governing equations is made next. In order to obtain the equations to which a weighted residual method will be applied, the linear biphasic equations are manipulated as follows. First, substitute

Eqs. (13), (14), and (15), which will be exactly satisfied, into Eqs. (4) to obtain modified momentum equations

$$-\phi^s \nabla p + \nabla \cdot (\lambda_s e^s \mathbf{I} + 2 \mu_s \boldsymbol{\varepsilon}^s) + K(\mathbf{v}^f - \mathbf{v}^s) = 0 \tag{60}$$

$$-\phi^f \nabla p - K(\mathbf{v}^f - \mathbf{v}^s) = 0 \tag{61}$$

Now add Eqs. (60) and (61) to obtain the total momentum equation:

$$\nabla \cdot \boldsymbol{\sigma}_E^s - \nabla p = 0, \tag{62}$$

where $\boldsymbol{\sigma}_E^s = \lambda_s e^s \mathbf{I} + 2\mu_s \boldsymbol{\varepsilon}^s$ represents the elastic part of the solid phase stress. The two momentum equations are now replaced by the modified fluid momentum, Eq. (61), and total momentum, Eq. (62).

The weighted residual statement of the governing equations is formed next. We will choose the pressure and elastic stress fields so that they *satisfy the total momentum equation*, Eq. (62), exactly, and introduce the remaining governing equations - (3) and (61), and the natural boundary conditions, Eqs. (19) and (20) - into a weighted residual statement. Essential boundary conditions, Eqs. (17) and (18), will be satisfied exactly. We include in the weighted residual statement the strain - displacement relation for the solid phase since the strains from stress and those from the gradient of solid phase displacement are independent. The strain-displacement equation is modified by eliminating the displacement using Eq. (59) and dividing through by $\omega \Delta t$. Note that the intended range of ω will allow this division; further, the final form of the equations will allow use of the explicit method ($\omega = 0$) if so desired. The scalar, first order tensor, and second order tensor weighting functions which are required will be called g, **r** (having contributions $\mathbf{r}^s$ and $\mathbf{r}^f$, in order to correspond to the velocities $\mathbf{v}^s$ and $\mathbf{v}^f$), and **h**, respectively.

The finite element statement of this equation is obtained by subdividing the domain Ω into elements Ω_n and locally interpolating the velocity, pressure, and stress fields appropriately. Since the interelement continuity of traction and pressure is difficult to guarantee, that condition will be relaxed and introduced using weighting functions $\mathbf{r}^f$ for the pressure term and $\mathbf{r}^s$ for the traction term, and integrals evaluated over the interelement boundaries. The notations $\Gamma_{i_n^s}$ and $\Gamma_{i_n^f}$ represent the portion of an element boundary which is shared with adjacent elements but on which no traction or displacement condition is set for the solid and fluid phases, respectively. The finite element weighted residual statement of the governing equations for the n_{et} elements may therefore be written

$$\sum_{n=1}^{n_{et}} \left\{ \int_{\Omega_n} g \, \nabla \cdot [\phi^f \mathbf{v}^f + \phi^s \mathbf{v}^s] \, d\Omega \right. +$$

$$\int_{\Omega_n} \mathbf{h}:[\frac{\boldsymbol{\varepsilon}^s}{\omega\Delta t} - (\nabla \mathbf{v}^s)^s - \frac{(\nabla \hat{\mathbf{u}}^s)^s}{\omega\Delta t} - \frac{(1-\omega)}{\omega}(\nabla \hat{\mathbf{v}}^s)^s]\, d\Omega \; -$$

$$\int_{\Omega_n} \mathbf{r}\bullet[-\phi^f \nabla p - K(\mathbf{v}^f - \mathbf{v}^s)]\; d\Omega \; -$$

$$\int_{\Gamma_{t^s_n}} \mathbf{r}^s \bullet (\mathbf{t}^s - \bar{\mathbf{t}}^s)\, d\Gamma + \int_{\Gamma_{t^f_n}} \mathbf{r}^f \bullet \phi^f (p - \bar{p})\, \mathbf{n}\, d\Gamma \; -$$

$$\left. \int_{\Gamma_{i^s_n}} \mathbf{r}^s \bullet \mathbf{t}^s\, d\Gamma + \int_{\Gamma_{i^f_n}} \mathbf{r}^f \bullet \phi^f p \mathbf{n}\, d\Gamma \right\} = 0 \qquad (63)$$

In deriving the weak form of this boundary value/initial value problem it is important to note that g, $\mathbf{r}$, and $\mathbf{h}$ will be interpolated using the same element shape functions as p, $\mathbf{v}$, and $\boldsymbol{\sigma}_E^s$, respectively. Therefore, since the stress and pressure satisfy Eq. (62), the weighting functions $\mathbf{h}$ and g will satisfy the condition $\nabla \bullet \mathbf{h} = \nabla g$ After manipulations described in Vermilyea and Spilker (1990), and transformation from tensor notation to matrix notation, Eq. (63) may be written as the weak form

$$\sum_{n=1}^{n_{el}} \left\{ \int_{\Omega_n} g \mathbf{D}_\nabla [\phi^f (\mathbf{v}^f - \mathbf{v}^s)]\, d\Omega + \int_{\Omega_n} p \mathbf{D}_\nabla [\phi^f (\mathbf{r}^f - \mathbf{r}^s)]\, d\Omega \; - \right.$$

$$\int_{\Omega_n} (\mathbf{r}^f - \mathbf{r}^s)^T K (\mathbf{v}^f - \mathbf{v}^s)\, d\Omega + \frac{1}{\omega\Delta t} \int_{\Omega_n} \mathbf{h}^T \mathbf{S} \boldsymbol{\sigma}_E^s\, d\Omega \; -$$

$$\left. \int_{\Omega_n} (\mathbf{D}_\varepsilon \mathbf{v}^s)^T (\mathbf{h} - g\mathbf{m}^T)\, d\Omega - \int_{\Omega_n} (\mathbf{D}_\varepsilon \mathbf{r}^s)^T (\boldsymbol{\sigma}_E^s - p\mathbf{m}^T)\, d\Omega \right\}$$

$$= \sum_{n} \left\{ \frac{1}{\omega\Delta t} \int_{\Omega_n} \mathbf{h}^T (\mathbf{D}_\varepsilon \hat{\mathbf{u}}^s)\, d\Omega + \frac{(1-\omega)}{\omega} \int_{\Omega_n} \mathbf{h}^T (\mathbf{D}_\varepsilon \hat{\mathbf{v}}^s)\, d\Omega \; - \right.$$

$$\left. \int_{\Gamma_{t^s_n}} (\mathbf{r}^s)^T \bar{\mathbf{t}}^s\, d\Gamma + \int_{\Gamma_{t^f_n}} (\mathbf{r}^f)^T \phi^f \bar{p} \mathbf{n}\, d\Gamma \right\} \qquad (64)$$

where $\mathbf{D}_\nabla$ and $\mathbf{D}_\varepsilon$ are the matrix representations of the divergence and symmetric gradient operators, respectively; $\mathbf{S}$ is the compliance matrix of the solid phase, i.e. $\boldsymbol{\varepsilon}^s = \mathbf{S}\boldsymbol{\sigma}_E^s$; and $\mathbf{m}$ = [1 1 1 0 0 0] and [1 1 0] in three and two dimensions, respectively. Note that $\mathbf{m}\mathbf{D}_\varepsilon = \mathbf{D}_\nabla$. Since g, $\mathbf{r}$, and $\mathbf{h}$ are to be interpolated using the same functions as p, $\mathbf{v}$, and σ_E^s, respectively, and since $\mathbf{S}$ is a symmetric tensor, this equation can be seen to lead to a symmetric matrix form in the global degrees of freedom upon substitution of shape functions and degrees of freedom for each interpolated quantity. Of the left hand side integrals, integrals 1 and 2, as well as integrals 5 and 6, will lead to matrix pairs which are the transposes of each other, while integrals 3 and 4 will lead to symmetric matrices.

The field variables to be interpolated are the solid and fluid phase velocities $\mathbf{v}^s$ and $\mathbf{v}^f$, the solid elastic stress σ_E^s, and the pressure p. The respective weighting functions for these variables are $\mathbf{r}^s$ and $\mathbf{r}^f$, $\mathbf{h}$, and g. The shape functions for the solid elastic stress and those for the solid and fluid velocities will be denoted $\mathbf{P}$ and $\mathbf{N}$, respectively. The coefficients in element n are β_n for stress, $\mathbf{s}_n$ for solid velocity, and $\mathbf{q}_n$ for fluid velocity[¥]. The requirement that the pressure and elastic stress satisfy the total momentum equation, Eq. (62), leads to a relation between their interpolations. However, since Eq. (62) contains the gradient of the pressure, the constant term in the pressure interpolation will not be related to the elastic stress and must be included separately. The pressure interpolation thus contains a constant term in each element, denoted as α_n, and higher order terms using the coefficients β_n. The weighting function for these higher order terms is denoted as $\mathbf{D}$. Thus, the interpolations may be written

$$\sigma_E^s = \mathbf{P}\beta_n \;;\; \mathbf{h} = \mathbf{P}\tilde{\beta}_n \;;\; p = \mathbf{D}\beta_n + \alpha_n \;;\; g = \mathbf{D}\tilde{\beta}_n + \tilde{\alpha}_n$$

$$\mathbf{v}^s = \mathbf{N}\mathbf{s}_n \;;\; \mathbf{r}^s = \mathbf{N}\tilde{\mathbf{s}}_n \;;\; \mathbf{v}^f = \mathbf{N}\mathbf{q}_n \;;\; \mathbf{r}^f = \mathbf{N}\tilde{\mathbf{q}}_n \tag{65}$$

where (~) denotes a weighting function coefficient. $\mathbf{N}$ are standard C^0 continuous shape functions, and $\mathbf{P}$ and $\mathbf{D}$ must be chosen so that the interpolated stress and pressure fields satisfy the equilibrium relation, Eq. (62). Since there are no derivatives of stress or pressure in Eq. (64), functions $\mathbf{P}$ and $\mathbf{D}$ can be discontinuous between elements.

After substituting these interpolations into Eq. (64), we group terms with $\tilde{\beta}_n$, $\tilde{\alpha}_n$, $\tilde{\mathbf{s}}_n$, and $\tilde{\mathbf{q}}_n$ as coefficients. Since the weighting functions must be arbitrary, so will be their coefficients. Further, since $\tilde{\beta}_n$ and β_n are independent from element to element, the equations obtained for arbitrary nonzero $\tilde{\beta}_n$ may be solved for β_n in terms of $\mathbf{s}_n$, $\mathbf{q}_n$, and α_n at the element level to yield

$$\beta_n = \omega\Delta t\, \mathbf{H}^{-1}\, [\mathbf{G}^s\mathbf{s}_n - \mathbf{G}^f\mathbf{q}_n] \;+ \mathbf{H}^{-1}\, [\mathbf{F}_u + (1\text{-}\omega)\Delta t\, \mathbf{F}_v] \tag{66}$$

and substituted into the remaining equations. For arbitrary nonzero $\tilde{\alpha}_n$, $\tilde{\mathbf{s}}_n$, and $\tilde{\mathbf{q}}_n$, the following matrix equations are thus obtained:

$$[\mathbf{C} + \omega\Delta t\, \mathbf{K}] \begin{Bmatrix} \mathbf{s} \\ \mathbf{q} \\ \boldsymbol{\alpha} \end{Bmatrix} = \mathbf{F} \tag{67}$$

Note that since there is only one pressure constant α_n per element, the element variable is a scalar, while the global variable $\boldsymbol{\alpha}$ is a vector of length n_{et}. Here,

---

¥ The vector of stress parameters, β_n, is not to be confused with the penalty parameter β referred to in the previous sections.

the global capacity matrix **C**, stiffness matrix **K**, and force vector **F** are formed by standard assembly of the corresponding element matrices $\mathbf{c}_n$, $\mathbf{k}_n$, and $\mathbf{f}_n$, which are defined as follows:

$$\mathbf{c}_n = \begin{bmatrix} \mathbf{M}_d & -\mathbf{M}_d & (\mathbf{C}_1 - \mathbf{C}_2)^T \\ -\mathbf{M}_d & \mathbf{M}_d & -\mathbf{C}_1^T \\ (\mathbf{C}_1 - \mathbf{C}_2) & -\mathbf{C}_1 & 0 \end{bmatrix} \tag{68a}$$

$$\mathbf{k}_n = \begin{bmatrix} \mathbf{G}^{s^T}\mathbf{H}^{-1}\mathbf{G}^s & -\mathbf{G}^{s^T}\mathbf{H}^{-1}\mathbf{G}^f & 0 \\ -\mathbf{G}^{f^T}\mathbf{H}^{-1}\mathbf{G}^s & \mathbf{G}^{f^T}\mathbf{H}^{-1}\mathbf{G}^f & 0 \\ 0 & 0 & 0 \end{bmatrix} \tag{68b}$$

$$\mathbf{f}_n = \begin{Bmatrix} \mathbf{F}_t - \mathbf{G}^{s^T}\mathbf{H}^{-1}[\mathbf{F}_u + (1-\omega)\Delta t\mathbf{F}_v] \\ \mathbf{G}^{f^T}\mathbf{H}^{-1}[\mathbf{F}_u + (1-\omega)\Delta t\mathbf{F}_v] - \mathbf{F}_p \\ 0 \end{Bmatrix} \tag{68c}$$

and the assembly operation simply places the terms of the element matrices and force vector into the proper places in the corresponding global arrays according to the numbering of the element and global degrees of freedom. The element matrices in Eqs. (68a) - (68c) are:

$$\mathbf{H} = \int_{\Omega_n} \mathbf{P}^T\mathbf{S}\mathbf{P}\, d\Omega \tag{69a}$$

$$\mathbf{G}^f = \int_{\Omega_n} \mathbf{D}^T\, [(\mathbf{D}_\nabla \phi^f)\mathbf{N} + \phi^f(\mathbf{D}_\nabla \mathbf{N})]\, d\Omega \tag{69b}$$

$$\mathbf{G}^S = \int_{\Omega_n} \mathbf{D}^T\, [(\mathbf{D}_\nabla \phi^f)\mathbf{N} + \phi^f(\mathbf{D}_\nabla \mathbf{N})]\, d\Omega$$

$$+ \int_{\Omega_n} \mathbf{P}^T(\mathbf{D}_\varepsilon \mathbf{N})\, d\Omega - \int_{\Omega_n} \mathbf{D}^T\mathbf{m}(\mathbf{D}_\varepsilon \mathbf{N})\, d\Omega \tag{69c}$$

$$\mathbf{C}_1 = \int_{\Omega_n} [(\mathbf{D}_\nabla \phi^f)\mathbf{N} + \phi^f(\mathbf{D}_\nabla \mathbf{N})]\, d\Omega \tag{69d}$$

$$\mathbf{C}_2 = \int_{\Omega_n} \mathbf{m}(\mathbf{D}_\varepsilon \mathbf{N})\, d\Omega \tag{69e}$$

$$\mathbf{M}_d = \int_{\Omega_n} \mathbf{N}^T\mathbf{K}\mathbf{N}\, d\Omega \tag{69f}$$

$$\mathbf{F}_u = \int_{\Omega_n} \mathbf{P}^T(\mathbf{D}_\varepsilon \hat{\mathbf{u}}^s)\, d\Omega \quad ; \quad \mathbf{F}_v = \int_{\Omega_n} \mathbf{P}^T(\mathbf{D}_\varepsilon \hat{\mathbf{v}}^s)\, d\Omega \tag{69g}$$

$$\mathbf{F}_t = \int_{\Gamma_{t^s_n}} \mathbf{N}^T \bar{\mathbf{t}}^s\, d\Gamma \quad ; \quad \mathbf{F}_p = \int_{\Gamma_{t^f_n}} \mathbf{N}^T \phi^f \bar{p} \mathbf{n}\, d\Gamma \tag{69h}$$

It should be noted that for the linear case with constant constituent fractions ϕ^s and ϕ^f, integrals $\mathbf{G}^f$, $\mathbf{G}^s$, and $\mathbf{C}_1$ may be simplified by elimination of the $\mathbf{D}_\nabla\phi^f$ terms.

The solution algorithm consists of initializing the displacement and velocity at time zero, computing $\mathbf{F}_t$ and $\mathbf{F}_p$, and solving the assembled system, Eqs. (67), for all elements subject to constraints on velocities. The values of $\mathbf{s}_n$, $\mathbf{q}_n$, and α_n for each element are then substituted into Eq. (66) to obtain the stress and pressure parameters $\boldsymbol{\beta}_n$, from which the stresses and pressure can be computed. The displacement vector is then updated using Eq. (59), and the new $\mathbf{F}_u$ and $\mathbf{F}_v$ vectors computed for the next time step. This recursive process continues for as many time increments, Δt, as desired.

Some comments on the choice of the stress and pressure fields are appropriate. As with most hybrid elements, the constraints imposed in a constrained media problem and the rank of the element matrices are controlled by the stress/pressure field. Detailed discussion of these issues is found in Vermilyea and Spilker (1990). In summary, the number of constraints corresponding to the continuity condition is related to the number of independent parameters in the pressure field. If n_β denotes the number of independent stress/pressure parameters β, too small a value of n_β will lead to inadequate enforcement of the constraints, while too large a value can lead to excessive constraint and possible "locking" of the solution. Proper element matrix rank can be obtained provided that n_β satisfies

$$n_\beta \geq n_q - n_R + n_e - 1 \tag{70}$$

where n_q is the number of nodal degrees of freedom for the solid phase, n_R is the number of anticipated rigid body modes for the element, and n_e is the number of independent polynomial contributions in the divergence of the fluid velocity. The last contribution (-1) accounts for the constant term α_n, which is not included in the count of stress/pressure parameters but which leads to a single equation related to the continuity constraint. Note that this condition on n_β is necessary but not sufficient for correct rank, and that correct rank does not ensure an accurate element.

Choice of Stress/Pressure Fields for a 6-Node Triangle

The hybrid method has been applied to *plane strain* problems using a 6 node triangular element. The process of selecting a stress field for this element will be described briefly here; see Vermilyea and Spilker (1990) for further details.

First, solving Eq. (70) for this element, with $n_q = 12$, $n_R = 3$, and $n_e = 3$, yields $n_\beta \geq 11$. Complete linear stress and pressure fields contain a total of 11 parameters (constant, x, and y for each of 3 stress terms; x and y for pressure), and the 2 equilibrium relations will each remove a single parameter, yielding a net of 9 independent parameters. An element with such fields would therefore exhibit some form of under-constraint and rank deficiency. Complete quadratic fields contain 23 parameters (6 from each stress and 5 from pressure), and the 2 equilibrium relations each lead to 3 equations (in x, y, and a constant), so the net is 17 independent parameters. An element with such fields would be expected to properly enforce the constraints, but could also over-constrain the solution in some cases. Some intermediate set of fields with exactly 11 independent terms would lead to a more computationally efficient element and eliminate over-constraint concerns, but any such element would have to be tested to ensure proper enforcement of the constraints and matrix ranks.

In the present study we will restrict attention to the 17 β quadratic stress and pressure field since our experience on highly constrained problems suggests that this element will provide an accurate solution which is *not* over-constrained. More extensive studies of more efficient intermediate stress fields, closer to the minimum number of β's, are presented in Vermilyea and Spilker (1990). Finally, it should be noted that the stress field is defined in a local coordinate system (triangular coordinates) to avoid the potential difficulties of ill-conditioning due to element location or aspect ratio.

Example Problems and Numerical Results

Description of Elements

We will use the example problems of confined and unconfined compression of a soft hydrated tissue to illustrate the accuracy of the formulations and the effects of nonlinearity. Different element types may be used with each of the formulations. For the *penalty* method, including linear and nonlinear applications, a 4-node isoparametric quadrilateral element is used. The element can be used in either an axisymmetric version or a plane strain version. If the 4-node isoparametric element was formulated using the mixed-penalty method, a constant pressure interpolation would be used. Spilker and Maxian (1990) have shown that the final equations for this element are identical to those of the penalty element with mean dilatation. Thus there is no need to pursue this mixed-penalty method for the 4-node element.

To illustrate the accuracy of the *mixed-penalty* method, we will use a 6-node triangular 2-D element, in either an axisymmetric version or a plane strain version. This choice was motivated by the desire to link the biphasic analyses with automated and adaptive finite element mesh generation programs for three-dimensional analysis. Shephard et al. (1988, 1990) suggest that, particularly in 3-D, tetrahedral elements are to be preferred because meshes with reasonable shaped elements can be constructed for arbitrary 3-D domains without resorting to the use of special element shapes. The 6-node 2-D element is a precursor to the 10-node tetrahedral element we will develop for 3-D biphasic analyses. It is also of interest to note that the penalty formulation of a 6-node triangular element, with reduced integration of the penalty terms, produced unacceptable behavior in selected example problems; see Spilker and Maxian (1990) for details of this behavior and the derivation of the 6-node element.

A 6-node triangular isoparametric element has also been developed using the *hybrid* formulation, as described in an earlier subsection. This element is limited to use as a plane 2-D element; a different set of stress/pressure interpolations would be required for an axisymmetric version of the element. Since a major motivation of this study is an evaluation of the hybrid formulation, and we ultimately plan to extend the preferred scheme to 3-D, the formulation of an axisymmetric element is not required at the present time. In the example problems which follow, we will indicate whether the analysis is an axisymmetric or plane strain representation.

Confined Compression

In a confined compression problem, a cylindrical plug of soft tissue (diameter 2r and height h) is confined laterally and at the lower surface in a chamber and subjected to a prescribed ramp displacement through a porous free-draining platen at the upper surface (Figure 2). The interface between the specimen and confining chamber walls is assumed to be perfectly lubricated and frictionless. A maximum displacement of $u_o = \varepsilon_o h$ is imposed in a ramp time of t_o. The simulation of this test reduces to a one-dimensional analysis for which analytic and/or independent numerical solutions are available, and thus serves as a useful problem for validation of the formulation. For this example, the linear and nonlinear *penalty* finite element formulation will be used with a 4-node axisymmetric biphasic element to predict the deformational behavior of the tissue, showing the important nonlinear effects of strain-dependent permeability (with infinitesimal strain) and finite deformation. Some of these nonlinear effects have been investigated by others (Lai, et al., 1981; Holmes, 1985; Holmes, et al., 1985; Mow, et al., 1985; Spilker, et al., 1988), and we will use those numerical solutions for comparison where possible. Note that the accuracy of this formulation and element have been validated against analytic solutions for the linear problem (Spilker and Suh, 1990) and against independent finite difference solutions (Holmes, 1986) for the nonlinear and finite deformation analyses (Suh, et al., 1990).

For the case considered here, the specimen dimensions are r=3.175 mm and h=1.78 mm. The initial solid content and permeability are $\phi^s_o=0.2$, $\kappa_o=2.65\times10^{-14}$ $m^4/N{\cdot}s$, respectively, and M=10 for strain-dependent permeability. The equivalence between the KLM model and the finite deformation model can be established at infinitesimal strain levels through the aggregate modulus

$H_A = \lambda_s + 2\mu_s$ for the KLM model and the equivalent aggregate modulus $H_M = 4\rho_o^s\gamma(\alpha_1 + 2\alpha_2)$ for the finite deformation model (Suh, 1989). The aggregate modulus used in this study is 0.44 (λ_s=0.1 MPa and μ_s =0.17 MPa for the KLM model, and ρ_o^s =0.38×10^3 kg/m^3, γ=9.65×10^2 N·m/kg, and α_1=α_2=0.1 for the finite deformation model). The imposed equilibrium strain is ε_o=0.15 (*i.e.*, large strain) with t_o=350 secs so that a relatively large deformation is expected.

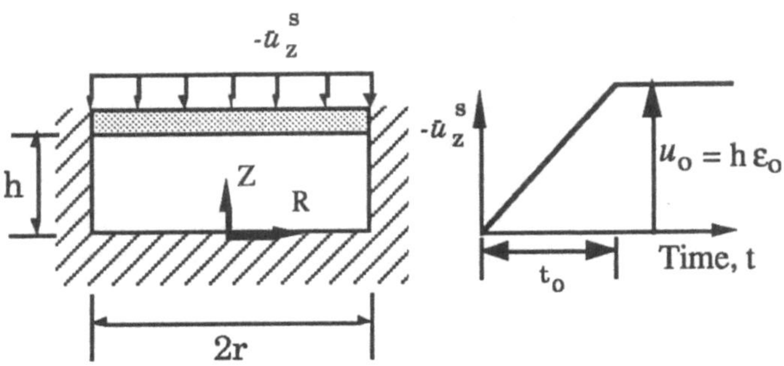

Figure 2. The confined compression problem subjected to prescribed ramp displacement.

Since the deformation of soft tissue in the confined compression is one dimensional and is independent of r, one element is used in the radial direction. The total number of elements is 22 in the axial direction. Since a severe deformational gradient is expected near the loaded surface, smaller elements are used over the upper region - 10 elements in the top 10% depth from the upper surface, 4 in the next 10% depth, 4 in the next 30% depth, 4 in the bottom 50% depth. The time increment Δt is manually controlled (where necessary) in order to achieve convergence. The value Δt=1 sec is used for the linear and nonlinear KLM models. For the finite deformation model, Δt=0.5 secs is used for $0 \le t \le 350$ secs, 0.1 secs for $350 \le t \le 360$ secs, and 0.5 secs for 360 secs $\le t$. In a fully automated code, however, the selection of Δt can be automatically controlled in the program (e.g. ABAQUS, 1987). In the results which follow, "linear KLM" refers to the linear biphasic analysis, "nonlinear KLM" refers to infinitesimal biphasic analysis including nonlinear strain-dependent permeability, and "finite deformation" refers to the nonlinear biphasic analysis with finite deformation.

Figures 3a-e show that the effects of finite deformation become significant even with a moderate level of applied strain (15%) over a long period of time (350 s). Figure 3a shows the stretch, λ_z, near the loaded surface (0.5% from the upper surface). It is observed that the linear KLM model produces a small strain (the maximum compressive strain at t_o is 18.8%), that the nonlinear KLM model predicts quite large strains (the maximum compressive strain at t_o is 54.3%), and that the finite deformation model produces an intermediate peak compressive strain at t_o of 34.8%. The ratio of the peak stretch to the equilibrium stretch is 1.25, 3.62, and 2.32, for the linear KLM, nonlinear KLM, and finite deformation models, respectively.

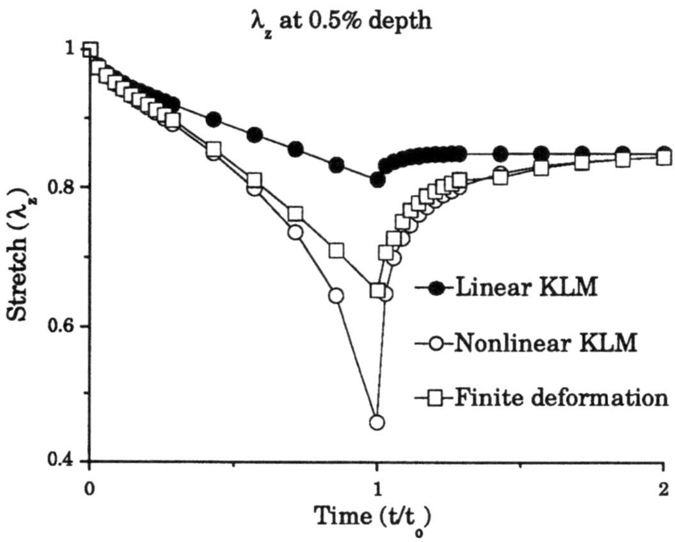

Figure 3a. The temporal changes of the stretch, λ_Z, near the loaded surface (0.5% depth) for the biphasic confined compression problem.

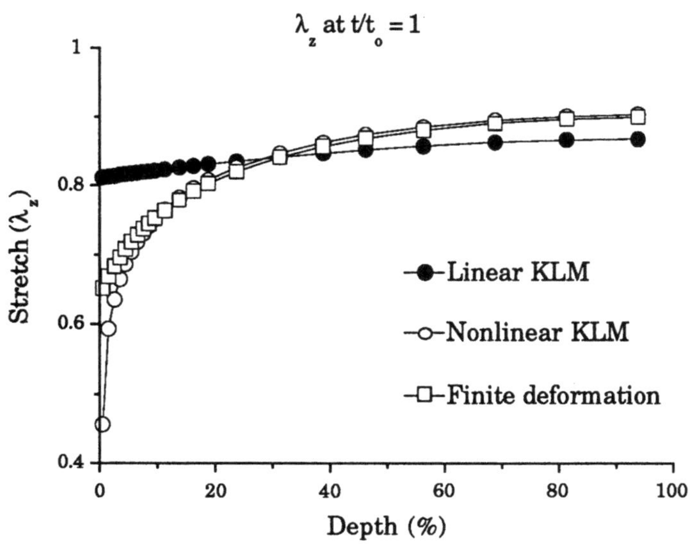

Figure 3b. The distribution of the stretch, λ_Z, versus % depth at $t/t_o=1$ for the biphasic confined compression problem.

The stretch versus % depth at $t/t_0=1$ is shown in Figure 3b. Differences in the three solutions are most prominent near the loaded surface (within approximately 20% of the loaded surface). While little change is observed for the linear solution in this region, significant variation is observed when strain-dependent permeability is included. The finite deformation model is in close agreement with the nonlinear KLM result except within the 5% depth closest to the loaded surface, where the nonlinear KLM model yields a more severe gradient. The distribution of relative velocity at $t/t_0=1$, shown in Figure 3c, is slightly different for each of the three models, and only the nonlinear KLM model predicts a steep gradient at the loaded surface. The pressure distributions at $t/t_0=1$, Figure 3d, show the previously observed trend of lowest values for the linear biphasic model, and largest values and steepest gradients for the nonlinear KLM model. The finite deformation model yields values that are about half those of the nonlinear KLM model. The reaction forces normalized with respect to the equilibrium force are shown in Figure 6e for the three models. The overshoot ratio for the nonlinear KLM model is 4.4, whereas this ratio is 1.26 and 3.0 for the linear and finite deformation models, respectively.

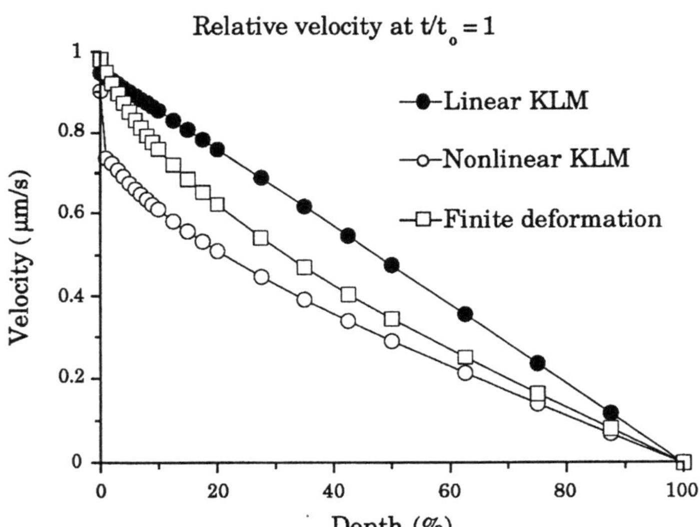

Figure 3c. The distribution of the relative velocity $v_z^f - v_z^s$, versus % depth at $t/t_0=1$ for the biphasic confined compression problem.

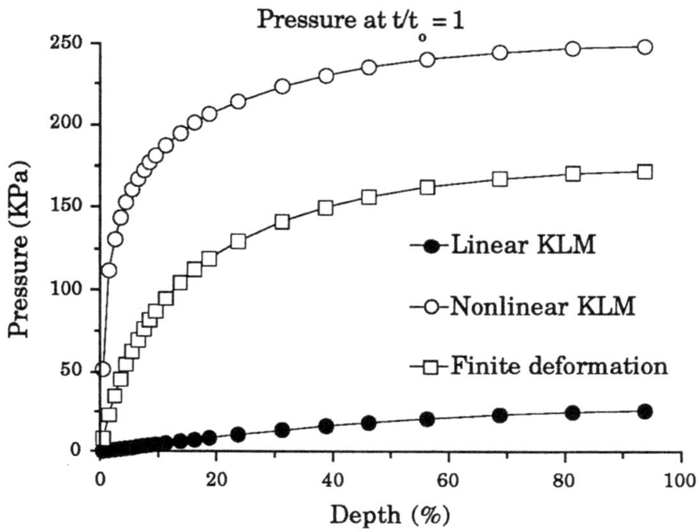

Figure 3d. The distribution of the pressure, p, versus % depth at $t/t_0=1$ for the biphasic confined compression problem.

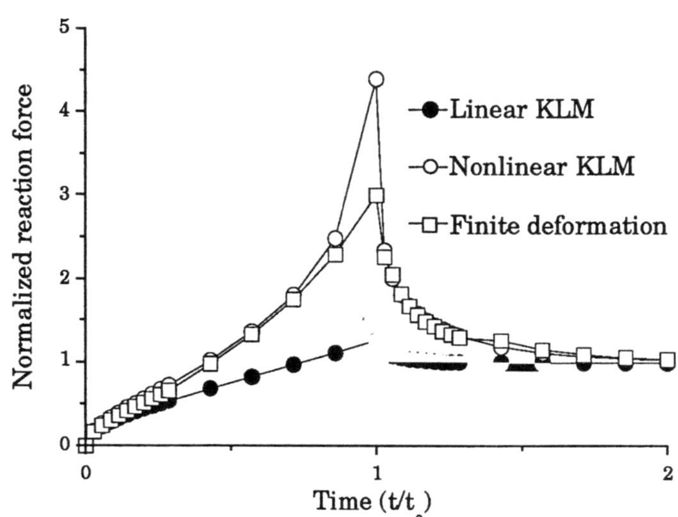

Figure 3e. The temporal change of the reaction force normalized with respect to the equilibrium reaction force for the biphasic confined compression problem.

In order to understand this phenomena, it should be pointed out that a local compressive deformation of the solid phase makes the permeability small in that region, and thus produces a larger diffusive drag force. This larger drag force will in turn result in a further increase of the local compressive deformation of the solid phase. With a large compressive deformation, this nonlinear permeability effect can be dramatic unless the nonlinear elasticity of the solid phase compensates for the larger drag force. A finite deformation model which accounts for the nonlinear elasticity of the solid phase helps to control the nonlinear permeability effect, and keeps the solid phase deformation within a physically reasonable bound (see Figures 3). In an extreme case, the effect of nonlinear permeability, without the contribution from the nonlinear elasticity of the solid phase, can be numerically unstable (Suh et al., 1990).

Unconfined Compression

In unconfined compression, a cylindrical cartilage sample is placed between a fixed platen (lower surface) and a moving platen (upper surface). A compressive displacement is applied through the moving platen, leading to a stress relaxation problem. We will use this problem to demonstrate the accuracy of the mixed-penalty and hybrid elements for the linear biphasic equations, modeling the unconfined compression problem in a state of *plane strain*. Recall that a 6-node element is used for both formulations. We assume for the present example that the platens are impermeable and that the interfaces between the specimen and platen surfaces are perfectly adhesive. Figure 4 is a schematic of unconfined compression, with boundary conditions as indicated. Note that the response with an adhesive interface is a function of both x and y position, and that for simplicity of modeling we assume that a displacement boundary condition is also set for the lower platen so that the problem is symmetric about the midheight. As a result, we need only model the upper right quadrant of this symmetric problem. For the present study we use a specimen with height, h = 1.78 mm, and width, 2w = 6.35 mm. The results presented here were obtained using a regular mesh of 144 elements, each element pair comprising a rectangle and the 72 rectangles obtained by dividing the modeled quadrant dimensions w and h/2 into 12 and 6 equal segments, respectively. The stress relaxation test uses a 5% specimen strain that is applied at the upper surface of the sample during a ramp time, t_o = 500 secs. Figure 2 shows the time history of the platen displacements, and the platen velocities can be seen to be constant up to t_o and zero thereafter. The material properties have been selected to correspond to normal, human articular cartilage (Mow, et al., 1980): $\lambda_s = 0.1$ MPa, $\mu_s = 0.3$ MPa, $\phi^s = 0.17$, $\kappa = 7.6 \times 10^{-15}$ m^4/Ns. The penalty number $\beta = 10^{14}$ is used with the mixed penalty method, and the time step is $\Delta t = 5$ secs.

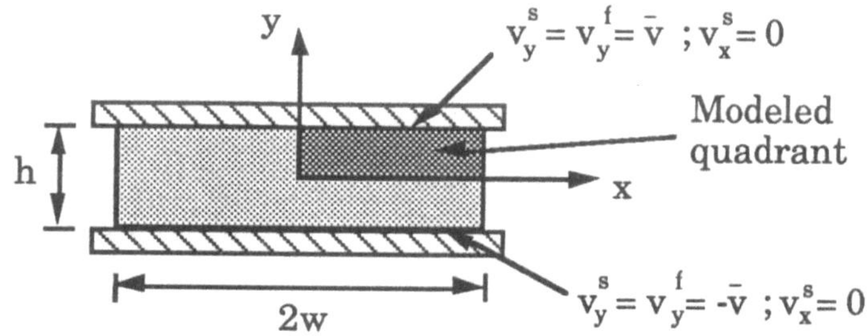

Figure 4. Specimen and modeled quadrant geometry and boundary conditions for the adhesive unconfined compression problem

Results obtained for the mixed-penalty and hybrid methods are presented in Figures 5 and 6. Since no analytical solution exists for this fully two dimensional problem, converged finite element solutions will be presented. These results also agree with those obtained using the 4-node penalty element. Figure 5 shows pressure and stress σ_y along a line located 5.5% from the midheight of the modeled quadrant and extending across its width, at a time of 100 secs from the start of the ramp. Note that the abscissa of this figure represents only half of the specimen width. Figure 6 shows the x component of the solid and fluid phase velocities from time 0 to 1000 secs at the midheight and outer surface of the specimen, or the lower right corner of the modeled quadrant. As can be seen, both methods are able to accurately represent kinematic and kinetic variables for both the solid and fluid phases.

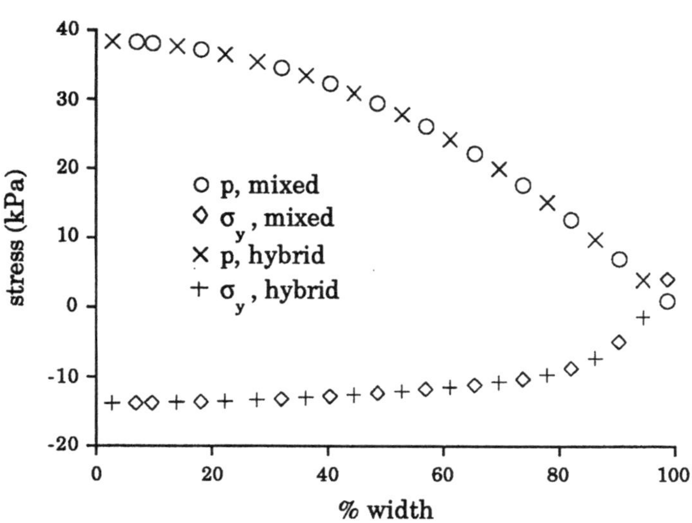

Figure 5. Pressure and stress, σ_y, vs. width for the modeled quadrant at 5.5% height and 100 secs.

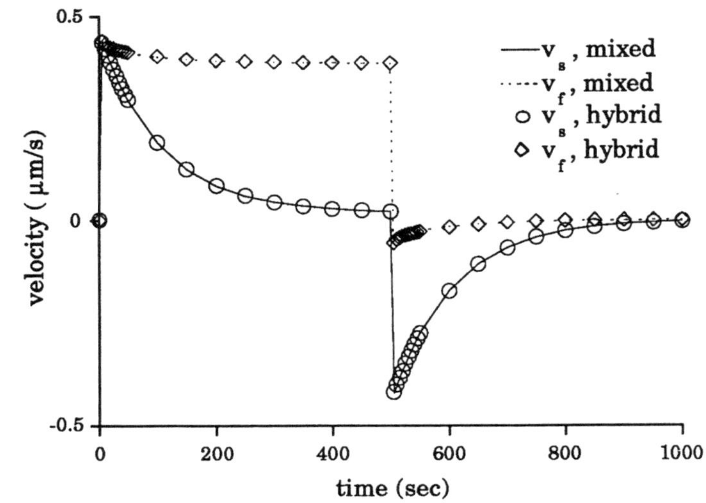

Figure 6. Solid and fluid phase velocities vs. time at the midheight and outer surface of the specimen.

Concluding Remarks

Three alternate finite element formulations have been presented for the biphasic mixture equations which govern the behavior of soft hydrated tissues: a mixed-penalty method in which the penalty form of the continuity equation is included in the weighted residual statement and pressure, solid displacement, and fluid velocity are interpolated; a penalty method in which the pressure is eliminated from the governing equations using the penalty form of the continuity equation, and solid displacement and fluid velocity are interpolated; and a hybrid method in which the momentum equation for the mixture is satisfied exactly, and solid displacement, fluid velocity, and equilibrated stress/pressure are interpolated. The formulations for the penalty and mixed-penalty methods include finite deformation and nonlinear material response. The extension of the hybrid model to finite deformation will require the definition of a complementary free energy density, and will be pursued in future research.

The essential first step in any computational method is the validation of the accuracy of the method for a representative set of example problems, and the demonstration, to the extent possible, that convergence is guaranteed for a general problem. Each of the methods can produce accurate solutions for biphasic problems, as has been demonstrated in the brief results of this manuscript and in Suh, et al. (1990), Spilker, et al. (1990), Spilker and Maxian (1990) and

Vermilyea and Spilker (1990), and can be extended to the development of alternate elements, such as 3-D elements. The penalty method produces an efficient and effective 4-node axisymmetric element, but we have found that the penalty form of the 6-node 2-D triangular element either under-constrains or over-constrains the solution. However, the mixed-penalty 6-node 2-D triangular element is extremely accurate, and should be preferred over its penalty counterpart. While no nonlinear results have been presented with the mixed-penalty method, it should be expected that these advantages will carry over to the nonlinear analysis. Finally, the hybrid element produces results for the 6-node 2-D triangle which are comparable to the mixed-penalty method. The hybrid method has the advantage that no penalty parameter is required. The results of a number of researchers in nonlinear computational mechanics suggest that hybrid methods are more robust than penalty or mixed elements for highly nonlinear problems, and we anticipate that this advantage will ultimately make the hybrid model the method of choice in the analysis of biphasic materials.

The utility of the computational method is measured in the ability to solve problems of clinical importance. There are challenging problems remaining which can be addressed by 2-D analyses, and many demanding problems which will require full 3-D analysis. In either case, as the geometry and boundary conditions become more complicated, automatically defined and adaptively revised meshes will be required in order to obtain accurate solutions with an optimal number of elements. We are pursuing automatic mesh adaptation using finite quadtree and octree mesh generation schemes (Shephard, et al., 1988, 1990) where the mesh will be refined or coarsened as needed during the timewise solution. Triangular elements in 2-D and tetrahedral elements in 3-D are preferred in this analysis since no auxiliary element shapes are required and meshes with acceptable element aspect ratios can be readily formed. Furthermore, second order elements typically provide better approximations and allow for element-level calculation of error estimates and are therefore preferred. Thus, the emphasis in our more recent studies of biphasic finite elements has been on second order 6-node triangular elements in 2-D as a precursor to second order 10-node tetrahedral elements in 3-D. These tools should eventually provide us with accurate analyses of important problems in joint mechanics with relatively little user interaction.

Acknowledgements

The support of the National Science Foundation (EET 87-20314), the National Institute of Arthritis, Musculoskeletal and Skin Diseases (AR 38728), and the Surdna Foundation are gratefully acknowledged. Helpful discussions of biphasic continuum theories with Drs. M. H. Holmes, W. M. Lai, and V. C. Mow are gratefully acknowledged.

References

ABAQUS, ABAQUS theory and user's manual, Version 4.6, Hibbitt, Karlsson and Sorensen Inc., 1987.

Armstrong CG, Lai WM and Mow VC: An analysis of the unconfined compression of articular cartilage, J Biomech Eng 1984;106:pp165-173.

Atluri SN, Murakawa H, and Bratianu C: Use of stress functions and asymptotic solutions in FEM analysis of continua, In New Concepts in Finite Element Analysis, Hughes TJR, Gartling D, and Spilker RL (eds), ASME AMD 1981;44:pp11-28.

Bathe KJ, Finite element procedures in engineering analysis, Prentice-Hall, Englewood Cliffs, NJ, 1982.

Bercovier M and Engelman M: A finite element for the numerical solution of viscous incompressible flows, J Comp Phys 1979;30:pp181-201.

Bercovier M, Hasbani Y, Gilon Y and Bathe K: On a finite element procedure for nonlinear incompressible elasticity, Symp Hybrid and Mixed Finite Elements, Georgia Institute of Technology, 1981.

Biot MA: Mechanics of deformation and acoustic propagation in porous media, J Appl Phys 1962;33(4):pp1482-1498.

Bratianu, C and Atluri SN: A hybrid finite element method for Stokes flow: Part I - formulation and numerical studies, Comp Meth in Appl Mech and Engng 1983;36:pp23-37.

Engelman MS, Sani RL, Gresho PM and Bercovier M: Consistent vs. reduced integration penalty methods for incompressible media using several old and new elements, Int J for Num Meth Fluids 1982;2:pp25-42.

Ghaboussi J and Wilson EL: Seismic analysis of earth dam-reservoir systems, J Soil Mech and Found Div ASCE 1973;(SM10):pp849-862.

Ghaboussi J and Dikman SU: Liquefaction analysis of horizontally layered sands, J Geotech Div ASCE 1978;(GT3):pp341-356.

Holmes MH: Finite deformation of soft tissue: Analysis of a mixture model in uni-axial compression, J Biomech Eng 1986;108:pp372-381.

Holmes MH, Lai WM and Mow VC: Singular perturbation analysis of the nonlinear, flow-dependent compressive stress relaxation behavior of articular cartilage, J Biomech Eng 1985;107:pp206-218.

Holmes MH and Mow VC: The nonlinear characteristics of soft polyelectrolyte gels and hydrated connective tissues in ultrafiltration, J Biomech Eng :To appear.

Hou JS, Holmes MH, Lai WM and Mow VC: Boundary conditions at the cartilage-synovial fluid interface for joint lubrication and theoretical verifications, J Biomech Eng 1989;111(1):pp78-87.

Hughes TJR, Liu WK and Brooks A: Finite element analysis of incompressible viscous flows by the penalty function formulation, J Comp Phys 1979;30.

Hughes TJR: The finite element method; Linear static and dynamic finite element analysis, Prentice-Hall, Englewood Cliffs, NJ, 1987.

Kenyon DE: A mathematical model of water flux through aortic tissue, Bull Math Biol 1979;41:pp79-90.

Kwan MK: A finite deformation theory for nonlinearly permeable cartilage and other soft hydrated connective tissues and rheological study of cartilage PG, Ph.D. Dissertation, RPI, 1985.

Lai WM and Mow VC: Drag-induced compression of articular cartilage during a permeation experiment, Biorheology 1980;17:111-123.

Lai WM, Mow VC and Roth V: Effects of nonlinear strain dependent permeability and rate of compression on the stress behavior of articular cartilage, J Biomech Eng 1981;103:pp61-66.

Lai WM, Hou JS and Mow VC: A triphasic theory for articular cartilage swelling and Donnan osmotic pressure., Torzilli PA and Friedman MH (eds), Biomechanics Symposium, Univ. of Cal., San Diego, ASME 1989;AMD-98.

Lee, SW and Pian THH: Notes on finite elements for nearly incompressible materials, AIAA J 1976;14:pp824-826.

Mak AF, Lai WM and Mow VC: Biphasic indentation of articular cartilage: Part 1 theoretical analysis, J Biomech 1987;20(7):pp703-714.

Malkus DS and Hughes TJR: Mixed finite element methods - Reduced and selective integration techniques: A unification of concepts, Comp Meth in App Mech and Eng 1978;15:pp63-81.

Mau ST, Tong P, and Pian THH: Finite element solutions for laminated anisotropic composite plates, J Comp Mats 1972;6:pp304-311.

Mow VC, Kuei SC, Lai WM and Armstrong CG: Biphasic creep and stress relaxation of articular cartilage in compression: theory and experiments, J Biomech Eng 1980;102:pp73-83.

Mow VC, Holmes MH and Lai WM: Fluid transport and mechanical properties of articular cartilage: A review, J Biomech 1984;17:pp377-394.

Mow VC, Kwan MK, Lai WM and Holmes MH: A finite deformation theory for nonlinearity permeable soft hydrated biological tissues, in Frontiers in Biomechanics, Woo, Schmidt-Schonbein and Zweifach ed. Springer-Verlag, 1985.

Nagtegaal JC, Parks DM and Rice JR: On numerically accurate finite element solutions in the fully plastic range, Comp. Meth. in App. Mech. and Eng. 1974;4:pp153-177.

Nishioka T and Atluri SN: Assumed stress finite element analysis of through - cracks in angle-ply laminates, AIAA J. 1980;18:pp1125-1132.

Oden JT: Finite element of nonlinear continua, McGraw-Hill, NY, 1972.

Oden JT, Kikuchi N and Song YJ: Penalty-finite element methods for the analysis of Stokesian flows, Comp. Meth. in Appl. Mech. and Eng. 1982;31:pp297-329.

Oomens CWJ, Van Campen DH and Grootenboer HJ: A mixture approach to the mechanics of skin, J. Biomech. 1987;20(9):pp877-885.

Prevost JH: Nonlinear transient phenomena in saturated porous media, Comp. Meth. in Appl. Mech. and Eng. 1982;20:pp3-18.

Prevost JH: Non-linear transient phenomena in soil media, in Desai CS and Gallagher RH (eds): Mechanics of Engineering Materials. John Wiley & Sons Ltd., 1984.

Prevost JH: Wave propagation in fluid-saturated porous media: An effective finite element procedure, Soil Dyn. and Earthquake Eng. 1985;4(4):pp183-202.

Shephard MS, Baehmann PL, and Grice KR: The versatility of automatic mesh generators based on tree structures and advanced geometric constructs, Comp. Meth. Appl. Num. Meth. 1988;4:pp379-392.

Shephard MS, Baehmann PL, and Grice KR: Automatic three-dimensional mesh generation by the finite octree technique, Int. J. Num. Meth. in Engng. 1990;To appear.

Simon BR, Wu JSS, Carlton MW, France EP, Evans JH and Kazarian LE: Structural models for human spinal motion segments based on a poroelastic view of the intervertebral disk, J. Biomech. Eng. 1985;107:pp327-335.

Simon BR, Wu JSS and Zienkiewicz OC: Evaluation of higher order, mixed, and hermitian finite element procedures for the dynamic analysis of saturated porous media using one-dimensional models, Int. J. Num. Anal. Meth. Geomech. 1986;10:pp483-499.

Simon BR, Wu JSS, Zienkiewicz OC and Paul DK: Evaluation of U-W and U-P finite element methods for the dynamic response of saturated porous media using one-dimensional models, Int. J. Num. Anal. Meth. Geomech. 1986;10:pp461-482.

Simon BR and Gaballa M: Finite strain poroelastic finite element models for large arterial cross sections, in Spilker RL and Simon BR (eds): Computational Methods in Bioengineering, ASME, 1988.

Spilker RL: Improved hybrid-stress axisymmetric elements including behavior for nearly incompressible materials, Int. J. Num. Meth. Eng. 1981;17:pp483-502.

Spilker RL: Invariant 8-node hybrid-stress elements for thin and moderately thick plates, Int. J. Num. Meth. Eng. 1982;18:pp1153-1178.

Spilker RL, Suh J-K and Mow VC: A finite element formulation of the nonlinear biphasic model for articular cartilage and hydrated soft tissues including strain-dependent permeability, in Spilker RL and Simon BR (eds): Computational Methods in Bioengineering, ASME, 1988;BED-9.

Spilker RL and Suh J-K: Formulation and evaluation of a finite element model for the biphasic model of hydrated soft tissue, Comp. Struc. 1990;To appear.

Spilker RL, Suh J-K and Mow VC: Effects of friction on the unconfined compressive response of articular cartilage: A finite element analysis, J. Biomech. Eng. 1990;To appear.

Spilker RL and Maxian TA: A mixed -penalty finite element formulation of the linear biphasic theory for soft tissues, Int. J. Num. Meth. Eng. 1990;In press.

Suh J-K: A finite element formulation for nonlinear behavior of biphasic hydrated soft tissue under finite deformation, Ph.D. thesis, Rensselaer Polytechnic Institute, 1989.

Suh J-K, Spilker RL, and Holmes MH: A penalty finite element analysis for nonlinear mechanics of biphasic hydrated soft tissue under large deformation, Int J Num Meth Eng. 1990;In press.

Truesdell C and Toupin RA: The classical field theories, in Handbuch der Physik, Flügge S (ed), Springer-Verlag, 3/1, 1960.

Truesdell C and Noll W: The non-linear field theories of mechanics, in Handbuch der Physik, Flügge S (ed), Springer-Verlag, 3/3, 1965.

Vermilyea ME and Spilker RL: A hybrid finite element formulation of the linear biphasic equations for hydrated soft tissue, Int J Num Meth Eng. 1990; In press.

Zienkiewicz OC and Bettess P: Soils and other saturated media under transient, dynamic conditions; General formulation and the validity of various simplifying assumptions, in Soil Mechanics-Transient and Cyclic Loads, Pande and Zienkiewicz (eds), John Wiley & Sons, 1982.

Zienkiewicz OC and Shiomi T: Dynamic behavior of saturated porous media - the generalized Biot formulation and its numerical solution, Int J Num Anal Meth Geom 1984;8:pp71-96.

Chapter 16

Characteristics of Joint Loading as it Applies to Osteoarthrosis

E.L. Radin, D.B. Burr, D. Fyhrie, T.D. Brown, R.D. Boyd

We subscribe to the view that osteoarthrosis is a functional organ failure of the joint caused by mechanical factors (Freeman 1972). Inflammation can play an important role in the osteoarthrotic process, but in this chapter attention will be directed only to those circumstances in which inflammation is not primary.

The pathophysiology of joint failure can be understood only if one appreciates the effect changes in one of the organ's tissues has on the other tissues that make up the organ. For example, the role of subchondral bone contributes to the health of its overlying articular cartilage (Radin and Paul 1971, Radin and Rose 1986; Wu et al in press). The interrelationship among changes of articular cartilage, subchondral bone, and synovium in joints is critical if one is truly to understand the final result that is osteoarthrosis.

Cartilage Damage

The appreciation that cartilage damage need not necessarily be progressive has clarified much of the seemingly contradictory observations about osteoarthrosis in the literature (Byers et al 1970; Radin 1988; Meachim and Emery 1974). We define osteoarthrosis as loss of articular cartilage with eburnation of the underlying bone associated with a proliferative response. Only a few experimental animal models have been shown to reliably create true osteoarthrosis: repetitive impulsive loading (Radin and Paul 1971), proximal tibial osteotomy (varus/valgus angulation) (Wu et al 1990), and cutting the medial collateral and anterior cruciate ligaments with medial meniscectomy, the

Hulth model (Hulth et al 1971).*

Other animal models fail to reliably create full thickness cartilage loss, bony eburnation and osteophytes, or have not been followed long enough to establish these changes (Akeson et al 1969: Pond and Nuki 1973; Altman et al 1984). Studying the repetitive impulsive loading model we find vascular ingrowth of calcified cartilage leading to thickening of the subchondral layer (calcified cartilage and subchondral plate) before cartilage deterioration at the light microscopic level (Table 1). Tidemark advancement in osteoarthrosis, with

TABLE 1
Relation of Vascular Ingrowth and Other Changes in the Repetitive Impulsive Loading Model in the Tibia

3 wks	Decreased vessel density and perimeter, indicative of the filling in of the remodeling space May see collagen crimping in deep cartilage layers, no cloning, or other cellular changes, no biochemical changes in proteoglycans.
6 wks	Increased vessel density and perimeter indicative of new vascular ingrowth Increased small diameter vessels, but decreased size and number of larger vascular or intertrabecular spaces Same cartilage changes histologically as at 3 wks
9 wks	Severe cartilage changes histologically, consisting of gross fibrillation with surface disruption Not all animals show severe changes, but many so, generally no cloning although there may be an increased lacunar volume
9 wks + cage rest for up to 24 wks	Changes as at 9 wks, but with complete loss of cartilage on the weightbearing surface, osteophyte formation, cell cloning in regions with "repair" cartilage, fibroblasts, lots of non-cartilagenous connective tissue

* A recent personal communication (1990) from Kenneth Brandt, M.D., Indiana University, indicates that he and his colleagues have also observed true osteoarthrosis, by our definition, in the canine cruciate section model after 3 3/4 years. The progressive cartilage changes in this model apparently do not begin until thickening of the subchondral plate becomes evident. Similar findings have not yet been reported in rabbits.

thickening of the calcified bed, was suggested by the work of Johnson (1962). Vascular ingrowth of calcified cartilage early in osteoarthrosis has been described in human material by Bullough and Jagannath (1983).

Repetitive Impulsive Loading Model

Comprehensive study of this model (Radin and Paul 1971, Radin et al 1973; Simon et al 1972), which involves the repetitive impulsive loading of splinted rabbit legs in such a manner that the animals cannot actively alternate the physiologically reasonable impulsive repetitive loads, invokes true osteoarthrosis after six to nine weeks of 40 minute loading (at 60 Hz) and a subsequent six months of normal activity. The sequence of events is: subchondral osteophyte remodeling and densification, vascular ingrowth of the subchondral plate, thickening of the subchondral plate, and cartilage deterioration and eventual articular ulceration (Farkas et al 1987). The cartilage changes are initially deep with vertical fibrillations in the transitional and radial zones, but no surface fibrillations (Wu et al in press). Increased water content of the cartilage is not an early finding. This model has no early synovial inflammation, but synovial hyperplasia without inflammation is present by six weeks.

Joint Instability Models

We used the Hulth joint instability model (Hulth et al 1971) to determine the interactive roles of synovial hyperplasia and mechanical alterations on joint destruction. Electron microscopic, light-microscopic and histomorphometric data demonstrated consistent chondrocytic alterations and cartilage destruction. These data show that knee arthrotomy alone is followed by synovial inflammation and cartilage matrix changes. In the sham-operated animals, synovial inflammation followed arthrotomy, and cartilage matrix changes were confined to nonprogressive surface fibrillations. In the Hulth model, the cartilage changes do not progress in the presence of inflammatory changes unless mechanical instability is also present, i.e. mechanical instability is required for progression to osteoarthrosis in this model. Comparison of the histological data of the Hulth model to that of our impulsive loading model (Simon et al 1972) suggests that different inductive mechanisms may be involved in joint destruction in each, but in both models inflammatory changes play a secondary role to mechanical factors in the progression to osteoarthrosis (Radin and Paul 1971; Simon et al 1972; Hulth et al 1971).

Tibial Angulation Model

We have refined a model for osteoarthrosis that relies on changing mechanical forces to a joint by experimentally creating varus or valgus tibial angulations (Wu et al 1990). Thirty-four weeks following osteotomy, changes were accompanied by increased subchondral bone thickening. We found a direct correlation between bone and cartilage changes. Severe cartilage observed severe cartilage changes: osteophytes, cartilage fibrillation, derangement of cell columns and cloning of the overloaded condyle. These deterioration was limited to areas overlying the thickened portion of the subchondral calcified bed.

The pattern and progression of cartilage deterioration following osteotomy and in the Hulth model were different from those in the repetitive impulsive loading model; in the osteotomy models, cartilage changes begin with a loss of superficial and transitional zones, and involve early cellular changes. In the repetitive impulsive loading model, cartilage change usually begins in the intermediate and deep zones; cellular changes are observed only secondarily (Figure 1 A & B). Although increased thickening of the calcified subchondral layer is a common pathogenetic characteristic of mechanically-induced osteoarthrosis, morphological changes in articular cartilage can differ. There appear to be multiple patterns observed in mechanically-induced arthrosis.

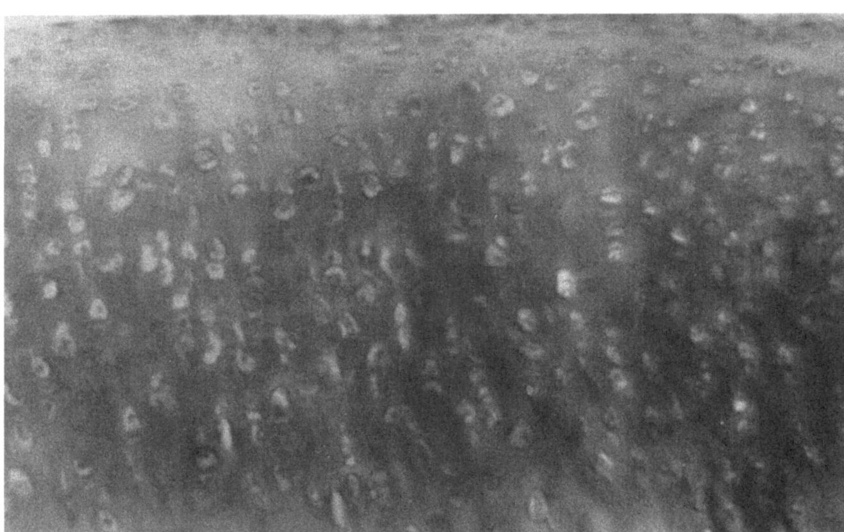

Figure 1A

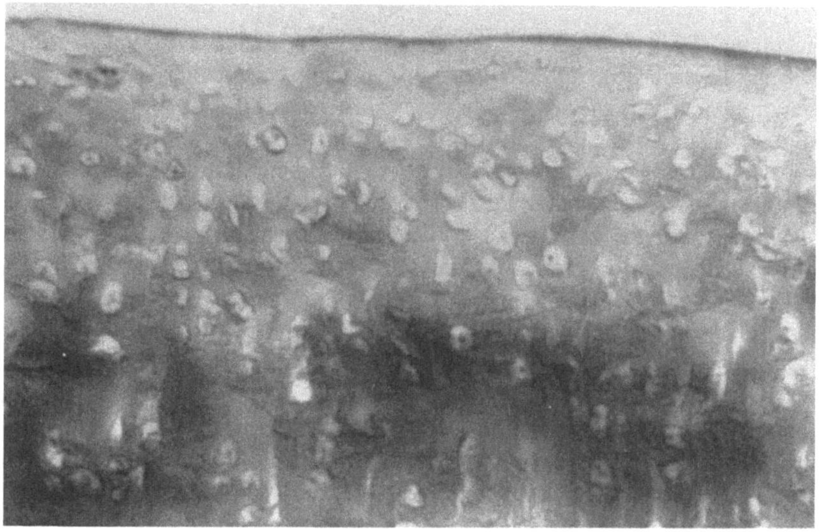

Figure 1B

Figure 1A & B In the repetitive impulsive loading model, cartilage changes begin in the intermediate and deep matrix without disruption of the surface cartilage. Orginal mag 62.5x. (1A Control, 1B Following impact)

Current Hypothesis

Osteoarthrosis is the loss of articular cartilage in the predominately load-bearing areas of the joint associated with eburnation of the underlying subchondral bone and a proliferative response characterized by osteophytosis. Loss of cartilage requires shear stress to be created within its substance. In viscoelastic materials such as articular cartilage, shear stresses are required to damage the cartilage. Stresses are not from rubbing, but from loading.

Substructural disorganization of the collagen matrix probably is the earliest change in the osteoarthrotic articular cartilage, followed by swelling, proteoglycan loss and cellular response (Pelletier et al 1983). These changes are reversible (Radin and Burr 1984). Progression of joint deterioration, which leads to true osteoarthrosis may well be initiated by tidemark and/or osteochondral advancement associated with a vascular invasion of the calcified cartilage. Impulsive loading is required to create the substructural disorganization that reactivates subchondral ossification at the articular cartilage base.

In zones of progressive cartilage damage the cartilage is thinned by tidemark advancement. This increases shear strains deep in the articular cartilage (Armstrong et al 1986), initiating and propagating horizontal splits, which in combination with vertical splits (Meachim and Bentley 1978) allow chunks of articular cartilage to break off, leading to cartilage loss and eburnated bone. Thus osteoarthrosis requires impulsive loading, and animal models of osteoarthrosis must create such loads. We presume that joint instability creates an impulsive force on the joint because joint subluxation under load is an instantaneous phenomenon. In the face of subluxation, we theorize that joint load is increased because muscles spanning the unstable joint rapidly contract to prevent further joint displacement and attempt to restabilize the joint.

The cause of osteoarthrosis following angular deformity at the knee has been related to shifting and diminution of contact surfaces (Pauwels 1980). But the variable penetrance of osteoarthrosis in patients with genu varum and genu valgum (Zayer 1985) suggests other factors may be significant. We hypothesize that osteotomy creates an inclined joint surface which, when compressively loaded, causes the joint to impulsively slip sideways. We believe these three models, although they create differing stress distributions within the joint, will all be shown to have impulsive loading in common. We suggest that impulsive loads create shear stresses, and substructural cartilage damage, and provoke tidemark advancement. Tidemark advancement may be a critical step in the pathophysiology of osteoarthrosis and precede loss of articular cartilage. More rigorous and timely observation of appropriate osteoarthrosis models will confirm or deny this hypothesis.

Shear Stress in Cartilage

It is not yet possible to directly measure the stress within articular cartilage. Stress analysis in articular cartilage can be performed using finite element models. In a one-phase model of cartilage, a local tissue stress tensor can be summarized in terms of shear and hydrostatic (dilatational) stress components (Carter et al 1987). The hydrostatic stress can be compressive or tensile. Shear and tensile hydrostatic stress can produce tensile principal strain in some direction. Due to the weakness of cartilage matrix in monotonic and fatigue tensile extension (Woo et al 1980; Weightman 1976) cartilage shear stresses may introduce microdamage to cartilage (Carter et al 1987). Some models of articular cartilage, in particular that of Mak (1986), include the viscoelasticity of the cartilage matrix in addition to the nonlinear effects due to fluid flow. The widely recognized linear bi-phasic KLM model (Mow et al 1984) includes fluid flow, but treats the matrix as a linear material. Mak (1986) noted that the KLM theory was similar to Biot's (1941) consolidation theory.

Even the most advanced models of cartilage, as part of a joint, fail to model cartilage's inherent and large material nonlinearity. In particular, they ignore the role that fluid pressures have in creating self-equilibrating internal tensile stresses in the cartilage matrix. Because it is not possible to determine these self-equilibrating stresses using standard, single phase, finite element methods, neglect of the fluid component may obscure the mechanisms of the initiation of cartilage damage. The study of whole joint stresses has, nevertheless, given several indications of mechanisms whereby mechanical stresses could cause osteoarthrosis. Simkin et al (1980) observed that the concave and convex sides of a joint are similar to Roman arches. On the convex side of the joint the arch is loaded in such a way that the subchondral bone is compressed (like an arch should be) and on the concave side the arch is loaded "backwards"--the subchondral bone is in tension. Carter et al (1987) verified Simkin's prediction using finite element analysis, and showed that the patterns of principal tensile strains in the subchondral bone of the femoral head and acetabulum were similar to the patterns of cartilage deterioration in osteoarthrosis. A theory of cartilage deterioration has been proposed in which cyclic shear stress tends to increase the chance of osteoarthrosis (Carter et al 1987).

We have demonstrated, using a two-dimensional dynamic contact finite element approach, that regions of deep cartilage peripheral to the main loading area tend to have higher shear stresses than elsewhere in the joint (Anderson et al in press). A potentially significant result of this work (Anderson et al in press) was that the strain rate in the cartilage varied widely with different rates of load application. These analytical studies of joints have provided indications that mechanical stress patterns do correlate with the sites of osteoarthrotic change. Possible mechanisms of causation, however, remain unclear because of the degree of approximation inherent in treating cartilage as a homogenous, linear, single-phase material.

In multi-phasic materials, such as cartilage and bone, deformation under load immediately leads to inter-phasic stresses. For instance, in cartilage, the tendency of fluid to flow under compression is opposed by the resistance of the matrix. The result is that the fluid pressure (a compressive stress) is partially balanced by a tensile stress in the cartilage matrix. Since these stresses are in balance, their net effect on stress in the cartilage is negligible. This is why it is often said that for rapid loading rates cartilage can be modeled as a linear material. However, the internal effect of these stresses on the cartilage matrix is maximum at the very moment that the net effect is minimized. When cartilage is loaded rapidly, the fluid does not have time to flow, and the internal stresses generated can be very large, perhaps leading to fracture of the collagen matrix (Askew and Mow 1978; Dekel and Weissman 1978). It is inherently impossible to calculate these potentially crucial internal stresses using a linear single phase material model for cartilage. To determine the fluid pressure-induced stresses in the cartilage matrix it is essential that both phases, fluid and matrix, be included.

We have investigated, using a biphasic model, the effect of fluid flow on the stiffness of a small disc of cancellous bone (David Fyhrie, personal communication, 1985). An ABAQUS poroelastic model gave results similar to the analytical confined compression solution for cartilage (Mow et al 1984). Because the permeability of cartilage (approximately 10^{-15} m^4 /N-sec) (Mow et al 1984) is 7500 times smaller than the permeability used in this study, the effect of fluid on cartilage matrix tensile stresses will be significant.

Figure 2 illustrates the shear concentration at the cartilage-bone interface using a two-dimensional plane strain model. There is a marked concentration of shear stress at the interface due to a uniform pressure loading, consistent with previous studies (Brown 1984; Carter 1987). At the edge of the contact area the shear stresses are high. Away from the edges, the stresses fall quickly to near zero. This peripheral interface shear was also predicted by Hayes (1972) in his solution for indentation of an elastic layer on a rigid half space (Figure 3).

Impulsive Loading and Subchondral Thickening

The finite element models suggest that strain rate will be an important determinant of the stresses promoted in articular cartilage. Because cartilage and bone are viscoelastic, we expect that tissue damage to them should be load rate dependent. We tested the hypothesis in rabbits that a high rate of loading would cause joints to deteriorate more rapidly than even higher loads applied at lower rates. Severe changes occurred in joints of the high load rate animals

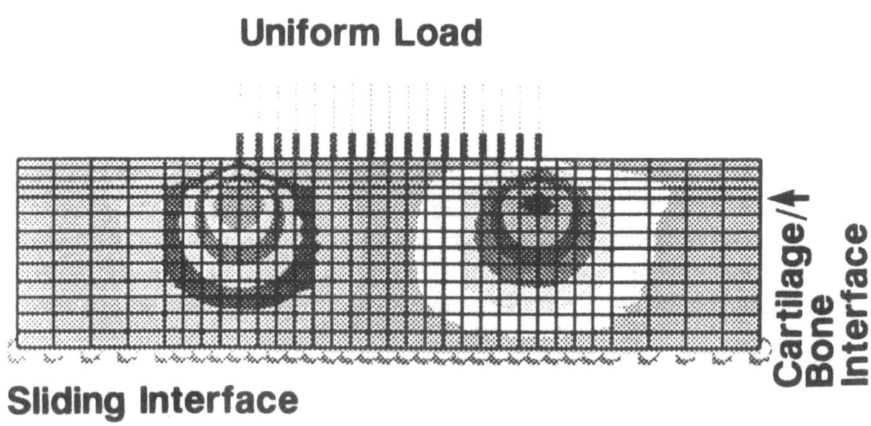

Figure 2 X-Y Shear stresses: Plane strain and analysis with E=5MPa, PR=0.47 in cartilage and E=1000MPa, PR=0.2 in bone

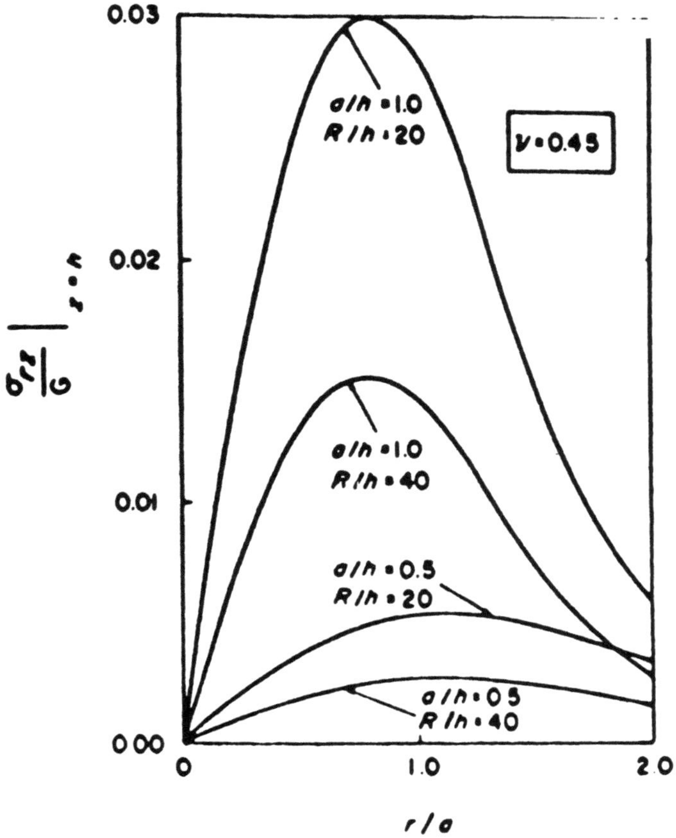

Figure 3 Nondimensional shear stress at the interface, z=h, for the spherical indenter

significantly more often ($p < 0.001$) than in joints of the low load rate animals, even though the load magnitudes in the latter group were greater (Yang et al 1989).

We hypothesize that progressive cartilage deterioration from mechanical means, i.e. osteoarthrosis, requires impulsive loading of the joint. Joint immobilization causes atrophy, but osteoarthrosis only occurs in loaded moving joints. The impulsive load can be a single episode, such as an acute dislocation of the patella creating osteochondral damage, or it can be from small repetitive impulsive loads, over long periods of time. For years we have pioneered experiments in which we repetitively impulsively load the lower extremities of rabbits and are able to provoke osteoarthrosis on a reproducible basis (Radin and Paul 1971, Radin et al 1973, 1984; Simon et al 1972). It takes a long time to occur, nine weeks of daily impulsive loading followed by six months of normal activity, but early cartilage damage is histologically evident after nine weeks (Table 1). This is consistent with the observation that impact loading initiates changes that progress to total cartilage loss even though the insult is followed by a period of reduced loading (Dekel and Weissman 1978; Yang et al 1989).

We have established that a subset of the normal human population impulsively load their legs at heelstrike (Radin et al in press). We refer to this subgroup as "microklutzes." When normals are compared to age-matched subjects with knee pain, whom we diagnose as "pre-arthrotic," (no history of trauma, no signs of inflammation, pain aggravated by exercise and relieved by rest), the "pre-arthrotic" group has a significantly higher loading rate at heelstrike ($p < .01$) than do the normals.

We have shown, *in vivo* and *in vitro*, that to damage joints, the load must be delivered in the impulsive mode (Radin and Paul 1971, Radin et al 1985; Simon et al 1972). What this implies is that under high loading rates, bone and cartilage sustain microscopic or submicroscopic damage that accumulates, finally, to cause a functional failure of the tissues and loss of articular cartilage in habitually loaded areas. Over many years our data have established that repetitive impulsive loading causes stiffening of subchondral bone (Radin et al 1978; 1984, 1985, Radin and Rose 1986). We have shown that such subchondral stiffening increases the shear stresses deep in the overlying articular cartilage (Brown et al 1984).

The stiffening of the subchondral calcified bed (calcified cartilage and subchondral plate) is due both to its increased thickness and to the reduced size and number of normally large vascular and intratrabecular spaces. As this calcified layer grows it invades the articular cartilage base and thins it (Johnson 1962). Using our existing dynamic finite element contact model, we have simulated a case of tidemark advancement leading to articular cartilage thinning. The broad features of the contact event were found to be similar to those for normal cartilage thickness. Load uptake in the tissue occurred more abruptly (63 vs 69 msec) for the thinned-cartilage case. Shear stresses were significantly elevated in the deep-most articular cartilage layer, particularly at the periphery of the contact area.

Why does this seem to require impulsive loading? Articular cartilage and subchondral bone are viscoelastic and under high rates of load become stiffer and less deformable (Ficat 1976; Kwan et al 1984; Radin and Paul 1971, Radin et al 1978; Repo and Finlay 1977). Rapid loading prevents the stress relaxation that occurs in cartilage when water is allowed to flow away from high pressure areas. Reduced deformation minimizes the contact area, further increasing the cartilage stresses (Askew and Mow 1978). The more rapid the impact, the larger the tensile and shear stresses and the greater the probability that substructural matrix damage which leads to fibrillation will be initiated (Armstrong et al 1985; Radin et al 1985).

That shear strains can occur in articular cartilage is not initially obvious. Articular cartilage lubrication with synovial fluid, or even saline, is almost frictionless with coefficients of friction below 0.0050 (Linn and Radin 1968). But shear strains can be generated internally by the deformation of cartilage. Under physiological load, articular cartilage deforms as much as 40% (Linn and Radin 1968). Articular cartilage is rigidly fixed to its calcified bed. The cartilage, deformed by compression, tends to spread laterally, restrained by its calcified bed. When mathematically modeled, this lateral spreading creates shear stresses, particularly deep in the cartilage and at the edges of the compressed zone (Armstrong et al 1985; Askew and Mow 1978; Burnstein 1968; Hayes et al 1972). We hypothesize that this causes deep horizontal splits in cartilage and that these splits are more common in cartilage subjected to high loading rates, particularly when the articular cartilage has been thinned. This is a recognized problem in layered ball bearings, particularly when the outer layer is more compliant than the inner one (Collacott 1981). This is known as "spalling" and is associated with impulsive loading in laminated materials (Johnson 1972).

High shear stresses cause splitting between the layers of bone and cartilage (Imai et al 1989), creating local stress concentrations that can lead to degeneration at the cartilage base even without disruption of the tangential layer at the articular surface (Armstrong et al 1986). Basal degeneration removes some of the constraints on cartilage deformation in the radial direction (Finlay and Repo 1978, 1979), and damages the collagen fibrillar network. We have seen deep horizontal splits, first described by Meachim and Bentley (1978) in our repetitively impulsively loaded rabbits (Radin et al 1984).

It has been presumed that the deteriorating cartilage, osteoarthrosis, swells due to proteoglycan loss and collagen matrix disruption. This unweaving of the collagenous fibers would expose more of their hydrophilic sites. Chunks of cartilage have also been observed in osteoarthrotic synovial fluid (Minns 1976; Tew and Hackett 1981). Those chunks of cartilage cannot be accounted for by abrasive wear. However, if vertical fibrillations were connected at their base by horizontal splits, then large pieces of cartilage would break off, consistent with these observations.

We hypothesize that substructural disorganization of the matrix precedes chondrocytic enzymatic production, and may be the initiating factor that permits entry of catabolic enzymes into the cartilage matrix. We further propose that impulsive loading is an essential factor in the progressive cartilage destruction that characterizes osteoarthrosis. We also hypothesize that tidemark advancement and horizontal cartilage splitting are the primary mechanisms in progressive cartilage loss. We have summarized our hypothesis in Figure 4. We suggest that further study focus on these phenomena.

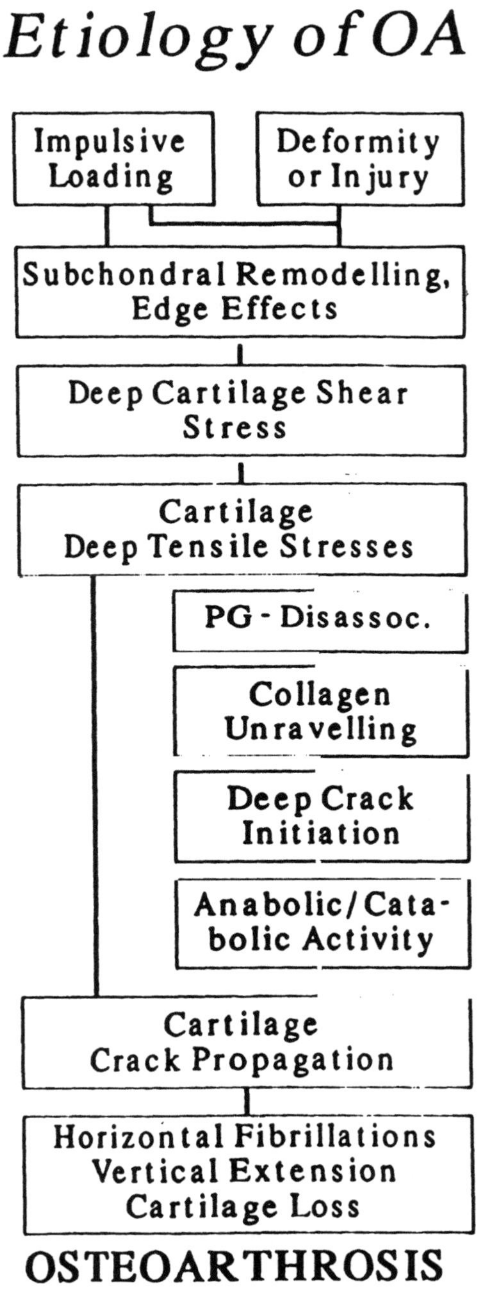
Etiology of OA
Impulsive Loading
Deformity or Injury
Subchondral Remodelling, Edge Effects
Deep Cartilage Shear Stress
Cartilage Deep Tensile Stresses
PG - Disassoc.
Collagen Unravelling
Deep Crack Initiation
Anabolic/Catabolic Activity
Cartilage Crack Propagation
Horizontal Fibrillations
Vertical Extension
Cartilage Loss
OSTEOARTHROSIS

Figure 4

References

Akeson WH, Miyashita C, Taylor TKF, LaViolette D, Amiel D: Experimental arthroplasty of the canine hip: Extracellular matrix composition in cup arthroplasty. J Bone Joint Surg 1968;50A:825.

Altman RD, Tenenbaum J, Latta L, Riskin W, Blanco LN, Howell DS: Biomechanical and biochemical properties of dog cartilage in experimentally induced osteoarthritis. Ann Rheum Dis 1984;43:83-90.

Anderson DD, Brown TD, Yang KH, Radin EL: A dynamic finite element analysis of impulsive loading of the extension splinted rabbit knee. In press

Armstrong CG, Mow VC, Wirth CR: Biomechanics of impact-induced microdamage to articular cartilage -- a possible genesis for chondromalacia patella, in Finnerman G (ed): AAOS Symposium on Sports Medicine. St. Louis, W.B. Saunders, 1985.

Askew MJ, Mow VC: The biomechanical function of the collagen fibril ultrastructure of articular cartilage. J Biomech Eng 1978;100:105-115.

Biot MA: General theory of three-dimensional consolidation. J Appl Physics 1941;12:155.

Brown TD, Radin EL, Martin RB, Burr DB: Finite element studies of juxtarticular stress changes due to localized subchondral stiffening. J Biomech 1984;17:11-24.

Bullough PG, Jagannath A: The morphology of the calcification front in articular cartilage. J Bone Joint Surg 1983;65B:72-78.

Burnstein AH: Elastic Analysis of Condylar Structures. dissertation, New York University, 1968.

Byers PD, Contepomi CA, Farkas TA: A post-mortem study of the hip joint. Ann Rheum Dis 1970;29:15-31.

Carter DR, Rapperport DJ, Fyhrie D, Schurman DJ: Relation of coxarthrosis to stresses and morphogenesis: A finite study. Acta Orthop Scand 1987;58:611-619.

Collacott RA: Mechanical Fault Diagnosis and Condition Monitoring. London, Chapman and Hall, 1981.

Dekel S, Weissman SL: Joint changes after overuse and peak overloading of rabbit knees in vivo. Acta Orthop Scand 1978;49:519-528.

Farkas, T, Boyd RD, Schaffler M, Radin EL, Burr DB: Early vascular changes in rabbit subchondral bone after repetitive impulsive loading. Clin Orthop 1987;219:259-267.

Ficat C: Les contusion du cartilage articulaire. Etude esperimentale. Rev Chir Orthop 1976;62:493-500.

Finlay JB, Repo RU: Energy absorbing ability of articular cartilage during impact. Med Biol Eng Comput 1979;17:397-403.

Finlay JB, Repo RU: Cartilage impact in vitro: Effect of bone and cement. J Biomech 1978;11:379-388.

Freeman MAR: Pathogenesis of osteoarthrosis: A hypothesis, in Apley AG (ed): Modern Trends in Orthopedics. London, Butterworths, 1972.

Hayes WC, Keer LM, Herrmann G, Mockros LF: A mathematical analysis for indentation tests of articular cartilage. J Biomech 1972;5:541-551.

Hulth A, Lindberry L, Telhag H: Experimental osteoarthritis in rabbits. Acta Orthop Scand 1970;41:522-530.

Imai N, Tomatsu T, Okamoto H, Nakamura Y: Clinical and roentgenological studies on malalignment disorders of the patello-femoral joint. III. Lesions of the patellar cartilage and subchondral bone associated with patello-femoral malalignment. J Jpn Orthop Assoc 1989;63:1-17.

Johnson LC: Joint remodelling as a basis for osteoarthritis. J Am Vet Med Assoc 1962;141:1237-41.

Johnson W: Impact Strength of Materials. New York, Crane Research, 1972.

Kwan MK, Lai WM, Mow VC: Fundamentals of fluid transport through cartilage in compression. Ann Biomed Eng 1984;12:537-538.

Linn FC, Radin EL: Lubrication of animal joints. III. The effect of certain chemical alterations of the cartilage and lubricant. Arthr Rheum 1968;11:674-682.

Mak AF: The apparent viscoelastic behavior of articular cartilage - The contributions from the intrinsic matrix (viscoelasticity) and interstitial fluid flows. J Biomed 1986;108:123- 130.

Meachim G, Emery TH: Quantitative aspects of patello-femoral cartilage fibrillation in Liverpool necropsies. Ann Rheum Dis 1974;3 3:39-47.

Meachim G, Bentley G: Horizontal splitting in patella articular cartilage. Arthr Rheum 1978;21:669-674.

Minns RJ: Cartilage ulceration and shear fatigue failure. Lancet 1976; April 24:907-908.

Mow VC, Holmes MH, Lai WM: Fluid transport and mechanical properties of articular cartilage: A review. J Biomech 1984;17:377-394.

Pauwels F: Biomechanics of the Locomotor Apparatus. Berlin, Springer-Verlag, 1980.

Pelletier JP, Martel-Palletier J, Altman RD, Ghandur/Mnaymneh L, Hower DS, Woessner JF, Jr: Collagenolytic activity and collagen matric breakdown of the articular cartilage in the Pond-Nuki dog model of osteoarthritis. Arthr Rheum 1983;26:866-874.

Pond MJ, Nuki G: Experimentally-induced osteoarthritis in the dog. Ann Rheum Dis 1973;32:387-388.

Radin EL, Paul IL: Reponse of joints to impact loading - I. In vitro wear. Arthr Rheum 1971;14:356-362.

Radin EL, Parker HG, Pugh JW, Steinberg RS, Paul IL, Rose RM: Response of joints to impact loading. III. Relationship between trabecular microfractures and cartilage degeneration. J Biomech 1973;6:51-57.

Radin EL, Ehrlich MG, Chernack R, Abernethy P, Paul IL, Rose RM: Effect of repetitive impulsive loading on the knee joint of rabbits. Clin Orthop 1978;131:288-293.

Radin EL, Martin BM, Burr, DB, Caterson B, Boyd RD, Goodwin C: Effects of mechanical loading of the tissues of the rabbit knee. J Orthop Res 1984a;2;221-234.

Radin EL, Burr DB: Hypothesis: Joints can heal. Sem Arthr Rheum 1984b;12:293-302.

Radin EL, Rose RM: Role of subchondral bone in the initiation and progression of cartilage damage. Clin Orthop 1986;213:241-248.

Radin EL, Martin RB, Burr DB, Caterson B, Boyd RD, Goodwin C: Mechanical factors influencing articular cartilage damage, in Peyron JG (ed): Osteoarthritis. Current clinical and fundamental problems. Paris, Ciba-Geigy, 1985.

Radin EL, Yang KH, Riegger C, Kish VL, O'Connor JJ: Relationship between lower limb dynamics and knee joint pain. J Orthop Res, in press.

Repo RU, Finlay JB: Survival of articular cartilage after controlled impact. J Bone Joint Surg 1977;59A:1068-1076

Simkin PA, Gramey DO, Fiechtner JJ: Roman arches, human joints, and disease: Differences between convex and concave sides of joints. Arthr Rheum 1980;23:1308-11

Simon SR, Radin EL, Paul IL, Rose RM: The response of joints to impact loading - II. In vivo behavior of subchondral bone. J Biomech 1972;5:267-272

Tew WP, Hackett RP: Identification of cartilage wear fragments in synovial fluid from equine joints. Arthr Rheum 1981;24:1419-1424

Weightman B: Tensile fatigue of human articular cartilage. J Biomech 1976;9:193-200

Woo SL-Y, Simon BR, Kuei SC, Akeson WH: Quasi-linear viscoelastic properties of normal articular cartilage. J Biomed Eng 198 9;102:85-90

Wu DD, Burr DB, Boyd RD, Radin EL: Bone and cartilage changes following experimental varus and valgus tibial angulation. J Orthop Res, in press

Yang KH, Boyd, RD, Kish VL, Burr DB, Caterson B, Radin EL: Differential effect of load magnitude and rate on the initiation and progression of osteoarthrosis. Trans Orthop Res Soc 1989;14:148

Zayer M: Osteoarthrosis following Blount's disease. Int Orthop 1980;4:63-66.